Clinical Skills for
Paramedic Practice

Clinical Skills for Paramedic Practice

Edited by

Dianne Inglis BN, AdvDip MICA, AssDip HlthSci (Paramedic), CertIV TAE

Jeff Kenneally ASM, BBus, GradCert MICA, AssDip HlthSci (Paramedic), CertIV TAE

ELSEVIER

ELSEVIER

Elsevier Australia. ACN 001 002 357
(a division of Reed International Books Australia Pty Ltd)
Tower 1, 475 Victoria Avenue, Chatswood, NSW 2067

ISBN: 978-0-7295-4263-0

National Library of Australia Cataloguing-in-Publication Data

 A catalogue record for this book is available from the National Library of Australia

Content Strategist: Rachel Ford
Content Project Manager: Fariha Nadeem
Copy edited by Julie Ganner
Proofread by Annabel Adair
Cover by Georgette Hall
Internal Design by Lisa Petroff
Index by Innodata Indexing
Typeset by New Best-set Typesetters Ltd
Printed in Australia

Last digit is the print number: 9 8 7 6 5 4 3 2 1

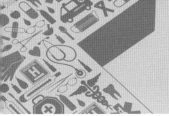

Contents

Contents

About the Editors

Dianne Inglis started her career as a Division 2 nurse in aged care, before completing a nursing degree at La Trobe University. Working in a busy emergency department, she liked the look of life on the other side of the doors – the paramedic side. Crossing over saw the start of her paramedic career. She became a Mobile Intensive Care Ambulance (MICA) paramedic, and worked as a clinical instructor, single responder and clinical support officer. Dianne then became manager of the Ambulance Victoria professional education department, responsible for all ongoing paramedic professional education, and remained in this role for a number of years until the pull of frontline care drew her back. She spent her last few years at Ambulance Victoria as Clinical Manager, overseeing day-to-day clinical operations as part of a regional management team.

Jeff Kenneally ASM wanted to be a paramedic from a young age. Slowed by a minimum age requirement, he worked for the Department of Health as a food analyst. As soon as he could he was successful in obtaining a role of student ambulance officer, became a clinical instructor, completed a Bachelor of Business and then become MICA paramedic. In this role, he worked as a clinical instructor, clinical support officer and team manager of MICA and Advanced Life Support (ALS) teams. Jeff worked for a number of years as Ambulance Victoria's Clinical Effectiveness Manager, responsible for ensuring quality practice and developing clinical guidelines.

A secondment as a lecturer to Victoria University gave Jeff the opportunity to influence students early in their paramedic careers, a role he found particularly rewarding.

Education and clinical excellence have always been priorities for Jeff. He has written his own paramedic practice textbook series, contributed to a number of paramedic and nursing texts and journals and been involved with research throughout his career.

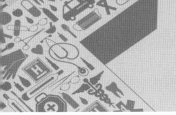

Contributors

Nigel Barr PhD
Senior Fellow HEA, Discipline Leader – Paramedicine, School of Nursing, Midwifery and Paramedicine, Maroochydore DC, Queensland

Paul Burke MEH
Paramedic, Victoria

Chris Cotton ASM
Intensive Care Paramedic
Clinical Support Officer, SA Ambulance Service, South Australia

John Cowell RN, Cert MICA (Paramedic), BBus (Accounting), GradDip Ed, MPhil (Medicine)
Lecturer, College of Health & Biomedicine, Victoria

Breanna Kate Dixon GradCert CEd, BHlthSci (Paramedic)
Lecturer in Paramedicine, School of Nursing, Midwifery, Paramedicine, Australian Catholic University, Melbourne, Victoria

Elizabeth Goble RN, BSc (Hons), MMedSc, PhD
Casual Academic, College of Nursing & Health Sciences, Flinders University, Adelaide, South Australia

Joelene Gott MHlthSCi (Research), BParaSci, GradDip ParaSci (Critical Care)
Lecturer, Paramedic Science & Paramedic, School of Health, Medical & Applied Science, CQ University, Townsville, Queensland

Nick Holden BParaSci, GradDip ParaSci (Critical Care)
Registered Paramedic
Course Coordinator, School of Health, Medical and Applied Sciences, CQ University, Melbourne, Victoria

Amanda Hlushak MHSc, MParamedic Practitioner, EMT-P
Lecturer, Faculty of Nursing Midwifery and Paramedicine, Australian Catholic University, Brisbane, Queensland

Dianne Inglis BN, AdvDip MICA, AssDip HlthSci (Paramedic), CertIV TAE
Intensive Care Paramedic
Clinical Education Manager (ret.), Victoria

Matt Johnson BAppSc, MEmergHlth, GradCert HlthProfEd
Paramedic, Victoria

Joe Karlek FdSc
Paramedic
Lecturer, School of Medicine, University of Tasmania, Sydney, New South Wales

Jeff Kenneally ASM, BBus, GradCert MICA, AssDip HlthSci (Paramedic), CertIV TAE
Intensive Care Paramedic
MICA team manager (ret.)
Lecturer, College of Health and Biomedicine, Victoria University, Victoria

Debra Joy Kiegaldie RN, PhD, MEd, BEdSt
Professor, Faculty of Health Science Youth & Community Studies, Holmesglen Institute & Healthscope Hospitals, Melbourne, Victoria

Liam Langford BHlthSci (Paramedic), MPH
Lecturer of Paramedicine, Faculty of Nursing, Midwifery and Paramedicine, Australian Catholic University, Canberra, Australian Capital Territory
Intensive Care Paramedic, Australian Capital Territory Ambulance Service, Canberra, Australian Capital Territory

Anna Pearce MD, MClinSci, BHlthSci, Dip ParaSci
Medical Officer, Emergency Department, Princess Alexander Hospital, Brisbane, Queensland
Associate Lecturer, Faculty of Medicine, University of Queensland, Brisbane, Queensland

James Pearce BHSc (Paramedic), BN, GradCert InfPrevCtrl, MAdvPrac, GradCert HEd, FACPara
Lecturer in Paramedic Science, College of Medicine and Public Health, Flinders University, Bedford Park, South Australia

Christine Quinn RN, RM, MHPE
Graduate Midwifery Program Lead, Mercy Health, Melbourne, Victoria

Fiona Randall RN, MEd, GradDip InfCtrlN, BN
Sessional Academic, School of Nursing, Midwifery and Paramedicine, University of the Sunshine Coast, Queensland

Mark Rewi BPhysio (Hons), BSc, GradDip EM (Mobile Intensive Care Ambulance), GradCert EMDH, Dip AmbParaSt
Clinical Support Officer, Ambulance Victoria, Melbourne, Victoria

Matt Rose BHlthSci (Paramedic), GradCert HEd
Lecturer, School of Nursing, Midwifery and Paramedicine, Australian Catholic University, Melbourne, Victoria
Paramedic, Ambulance Victoria, Melbourne, Victoria

Gavin Smith PhD, FACP
Registered MICA Paramedic
Adjunct Senior Research Fellow, Monash University, Victoria
Councillor, Royal Society of Victoria, Victoria

John Robert Suringa BHlthSci (Emergency Health Services)
Queensland Chapter, Paramedics Australasia, Townsville, Queensland

Alex Vella BHlthSci (Paramedic), GradDip EH (Intensive Care Paramedic), DIPLM
Intensive Care Paramedic
Paramedic, Victoria

Shaun Wilkinson BSc (Paramedical Science), GradCert TEd, Dip OHS
Advanced Life Support Paramedic
Paramedic, Victoria

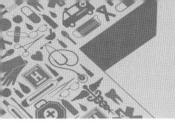

Reviewers

Georgia Clarkson, BA, GradDip Ed, Dip Para, GCTE, MEd, PhD, SFHEA
Senior Lecturer, Learning and Teaching Centre, Australian Catholic University, Melbourne, Victoria, Australia

Richard Galeano, ASM, PhD, MACP
Lecturer, School of Nursing, Midwifery and Paramedicine, Australian Catholic University, Brisbane, Queensland, Australia

Simon Sawyer BParamed, PhD
Lecturer, School of Nursing, Midwifery & Paramedicine (Victoria), Australian Catholic University, Melbourne, Victoria, Australia

Howard Wills BHSc (Paramedic), PGCert HSc (Resuscitation) MProfPrac (Education)
Lecturer in Paramedicine, School of Health and Social Services, Whitireia New Zealand, Porirua, New Zealand

Acknowledgements

The development of this first edition of *Clinical Skills for Paramedic Practice* has been a long and overdue journey. Paramedic practice has evolved considerably in recent years, with a pace that shows no signs of slowing. Paramedic clinical knowledge and the ability to implement complex practice guidelines and pharmacology carry high expectations. Concurrently, clinical skills have also been expected to progress, but with comparatively fewer resources to support that outcome.

A talented and enthusiastic group of prehospital practitioners have contributed to the development of this detailed clinical assessment and skills book, which is specifically intended for paramedic students and practitioners. Our gratitude goes to the many who advised in producing this text and, importantly, to each of those who provided chapter contributions.

Dianne Inglis and **Jeff Kenneally**

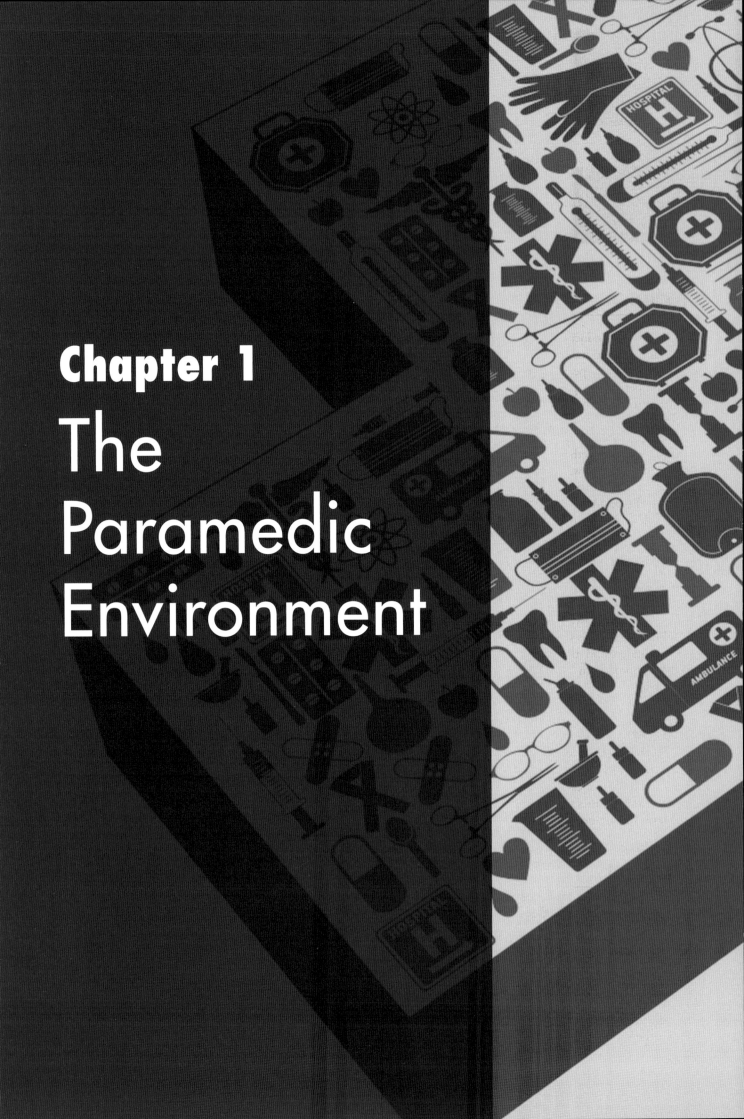

Chapter 1
The Paramedic Environment

1.1 | Clinical skills assessment for paramedics
Debra Kiegaldie

Introduction

Competency-based education focuses on the ability of students and practitioners to use skills, attributes and knowledge to perform specific tasks or roles (Brownie et al., 2011). Competency in paramedic practice is defined as skills, attributes and other characteristics (including values and beliefs) attained by an individual through knowledge (gained through vocational study) and experience (gained 'on road'), which together are considered adequate to enable the individual to work as a paramedic. Competence is defined as the consistent application of knowledge and skill to the standard of performance required in the workplace. It embodies the ability to transfer and apply skills and knowledge to new situations and environments (ASQA, 2019).

Clinical skills are only one aspect of the overall competency of an individual paramedic. In the context of this book, clinical skills represent the performance of health assessment and psychomotor skills to the competent level. While this book is focused on skill performance, it should be understood that using multiple assessments is the best approach in forming a comprehensive view of an individual's level of clinical competence. It is also important to recognise that achieving clinical competence is a career-long learning routine not a one-off event (Epstein, 2007).

This chapter presents an overview of the purpose and principles of clinical skills assessment. It introduces the methods and tools that can be used to assess clinical skills competence and outlines a framework for implementation of these tools in paramedic clinical settings.

Purpose of clinical skills assessment

Assessment of competence in the health professions, working in clinical practice, has been identified as critical in maintaining professional standards (Brownie et al., 2011; Evans, 2008). Professional standards in clinical practice rely on supporting developing practitioners and students in meeting learning objectives (Paramedics Australasia, 2011) including the provision of constructive feedback and assessment (Nursing & Midwifery Board of Australia, 2015). Furthermore, assessment of training is now a well-recognised component of the Australian Commission on Safety and Quality in Health Care Standards (ACSQHC, 2015).

Competence is a complex area and there is widespread debate about the best methods and approaches to use. The purpose of assessment should be to ensure that a minimum level of competence for graduation is achieved. A major challenge in assessing competency is ensuring objectivity. It is generally accepted that assessment of competence should use more than one tool and that assessment of initial competence may require a different approach to assessment of continuing competence (Crossley et al., 2002). The approaches suggested in this book support this view and regardless of the methods used it is essential that paramedic education providers spend time preparing those individuals being assessed and their assessors.

Principles of clinical skills assessment

A model of competence

A traditional model to define a clear and reproducible focus for assessment is Miller's pyramid, which divides up the domains of cognition ('knows'/'knows how') and behaviour ('shows how'/'does') (Miller, 1990) (Fig. 1.1.1).

Miller's pyramid guides the selection of an appropriate assessment method. Demonstration of clinical skills competence falls into the 'shows how' category but this does not always predict day-to-day performance in real life ('does'). The ultimate goal demonstrated in Miller's pyramid is to perform tasks regularly in a competent fashion (ACSQH, 2015). Direct observation of work-based practices is therefore necessary to show how performance is integrated into practice.

Reliability

Reliability is the degree to which a result reflects all possible measurements of the same construct (Crossley et al., 2002). In other words, is the assessment consistent? Reliability in assessment is often under threat and it is one of the most difficult things to control.

There are a number of important strategies that help address issues of reliability, including (Crossley et al., 2002):

- training teachers, supervisors or observers to give consistent scores when measuring performance to reduce subjectivity (this is called inter-rater reliability)
- using a variety of observers to avoid bias
- defining clear performance criteria
- increasing the number of assessments.

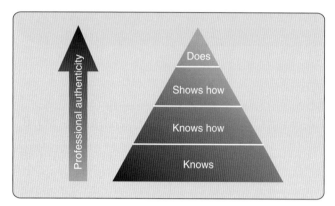

Figure 1.1.1 A simple model of competence
Source: Adapted from Miller, G.E., 1990, The assessment of clinical skills/competence/performance, Academic Medicine, 65(9), S63–67.

Validity

Validity is the degree to which the assessment is measuring what it is supposed to measure. There are three aspects to validity. The assessment must resemble the situation in the real world (face validity); it must include the relevant performance criteria and samples of behaviour (content validity); and it should be able to differentiate between a good and poor performer (construct validity) (Crossley et al., 2002; London Deanery, 2012; Ahmed et al., 2011).

Feasibility and acceptability

All assessments must balance rigour (reliability and validity) against practicality (feasibility, cost and acceptability). Large numbers of skills that are timely to reproduce may increase the chances of validity and reliability but are costly to implement and therefore not feasible (Crossley et al., 2002). Similarly, the subjects involved in the assessment must accept the assessment (Ahmed et al., 2011).

Formative assessment

In the context of clinical skills assessment, formative assessment is critical in the teaching and learning process as it enables learners to receive timely, corrective feedback about their learning with the aim of improving performance. It allows for individual practice until a level of competence is achieved. It also enables teachers or supervisors to determine next steps in the student's learning progression. In the formative assessment process, paramedic students need to be active participants through self-assessment and reflection.

Self-assessment

A key element of good assessment practice is to ensure that there is opportunity for the paramedic learner to self-assess. Self-assessment is a common form of competency

assessment and is a useful starting point (Evans, 2008). It provides paramedic students with an opportunity to identify personal strengths and areas for improvement and allows them to take control over their practice. Ultimately, clinical skills expertise is an outcome of self-assessment and reflection, so repeated opportunities for students to assess their progress towards the achievement of learning outcomes are critical.

Summative assessment

Summative assessment is given at a particular point in time to measure what students actually 'know' and 'can do'. It is used to gauge student learning relative to content standards and requires a judgment of performance against measurement criteria. Most importantly, it takes formative assessment to accomplish summative assessment (Garrison and Ehringhaus, 2007).

Clinical skill work instructions

Clinical skill work instructions are provided for every skill in this book. They are practical lists that detail the specific activities, critical actions and associated rationale relevant for each skill. Each clinical skill work instruction includes the equipment needed to undertake the skill and lists the prerequisite clinical skills.

Performance Improvement Plan (PIP)

A performance improvement action plan is a collaborative tool designed for students and supervisors to document areas requiring improvement in the students' performance of a skill. It can be used to support the learning process by identifying what problems are encountered, the level of support required, and what actions are needed to remedy these problems.

Assessment of competence

While there has been no shortage of published literature identifying tools for assessment of competence, no valid, single effective measure has ever been established (Evans, 2008; Gormley, 2011). This book focuses on health assessment and psychomotor skills, and offers three assessment tools relevant to this area.

Formative Clinical Skill Assessment Tool (F-CSAT)

The F-CSAT relies on the clinical skill work instruction format but includes a rating scale indicating the level of performance to be achieved by the student for each critical action. The use of a scale not only assists in the identification of the degree of competency achieved but also provides an opportunity to identify problem areas for self-assessment, feedback and remediation. The performance improvement is an integral component of the F-CSAT. The key features of the F-CSAT can be seen in Box 1.1.1.

The rating scale used in this book is an adaptation from original work published by Kathleen Bondy in 1983, which has been widely adopted in the nursing context. The literature supports the use of a rubric (rating scale) to ensure a standard assessment and evaluation of performance for each action (Suskie, 2018).

There are four scales, which enable ratings of the:
- required standard of performance of the procedure
- quality of the performance

BOX 1.1.1 KEY FEATURES OF THE F-CSAT

- The F-CSAT:
  - represents the 'shows how' level of Miller's pyramid
  - is formative and used purely as a learning tool for corrective feedback
  - allows for self-assessment and reflection through completion of a performance improvement action plan
  - is conducted in a simulated learning environment (e.g. using part-task trainers).
- A student cannot move to a summative clinical skill assessment until all critical actions are rated as 3 or 4.
- The scale rates each action and should not be summed as part of a cumulative grade.

- intended outcome of the performance
- level of assistance required.

The rating for each action of the skill should stand alone and be an indication of student progress and achievement. It should not be used as a part of a cumulative score. If the student achieves a rating of 3 or more for each action, they can be deemed sufficiently competent in that skill to move on to the next stage of summative assessment.

The example format for the rating scale is found in Table 1.1.1. Skill-specific F-CSATs can be found in each skills chapter.

Summative Clinical Skill Assessment Tool (S-CSAT)

The S-CSAT is a summative assessment that indicates a learner's readiness to undertake the skill in real clinical practice. A student must have passed the F-CSAT before undertaking the S-CSAT. The S-CSAT replicates the activities and critical actions of the clinical skill work instruction but now includes the ability to make a summative judgment on competent performance. Students are deemed to have either achieved or not achieved each critical action with a simple yes/no response from the supervisor. Yes to all actions indicates the student is competent and can proceed to the next stage of assessment. No to **any** critical action requires a PIP and a repeat of the F-CSAT.

Table 1.1.1 Modified Bondy rating scale for skills assessment in the F-CSAT

Skill level	Standard of procedure	Quality of performance	Outcome	Level of assistance required
4 Safe for unsupervised practice	Safe Accurate Behaviour is appropriate to context	Confident Accurate Expedient	Achieved intended outcome	No supporting cues*required
3 Requires supervision	Safe Accurate Behaviour is appropriate to context	Confident Accurate Takes longer than required	Achieved intended outcome	Requires occasional supportive cues*
2 Requires assistance	Safe Accurate Behaviour generally appropriate to context	Lacks certainty	Would not have achieved outcome without support	Requires frequent verbal and occasional physical directives in addition to supportive cues*
1 Requires direction	Safe only with guidance Not completely accurate	Unskilled Inefficient	Would not have achieved outcome without support	Requires continuous verbal and frequent physical directive cues*
0 Unsafe	Unsafe Unable to demonstrate behaviour Lacks insight into behaviour appropriate to context	Unskilled	Would not have achieved outcome	Requires continuous verbal and continuous physical directive cues*

*Refers to physical directives or verbal supportive cues
Source: Adapted from Bondy, 1983; EdCaN, 2009.

The key features of the S-CSAT can be seen in Box 1.1.2. Skill-specific S-CSATs can be found in each skills chapter.

Direct Observation of Procedural Skills (DOPS)

The ultimate goal is for paramedics to perform clinical skills in a competent fashion in everyday clinical practice. The direct observation of skills performed on 'real patients' has therefore become a recognised and necessary approach in health professional education. The final tool included in this book is the DOPS. The DOPS is an assessment of a procedure (clinical skill) involving real patients completed opportunistically during everyday work. For paramedics, this can be implemented 'on the road' when supervising and assessing performance in the paramedic clinical setting (see Appendix 1: The importance of ongoing assessment of clinical skills).

The DOPS assessment tool was first developed by the Royal College of Physicians in the UK (Norcini and McKinley, 2007). It was designed to provide feedback

on skills essential to the provision of good clinical care (McLeod et al., 2007). It is now a widely accepted tool in medicine and has recently become adopted in some international nursing undergraduate and postgraduate nursing contexts (Hengameh et al., 2015; Imanipour and Jalili, 2015; Sadeghigooghari et al., 2013). It involves an assessor observing a learner's performance within the workplace. There is a generic structured checklist that provides guidance for assessors, which avoids the requirement of individualised checklists (work instruction). In the paramedic context, the assessment can include skills such as obtaining informed consent, situational awareness, technical ability, communication skills and overall ability to perform a procedure. For DOPS assessments, assessors need to be familiar with the clinical practice setting of the assessment. Implicit in the DOPS assessment is that the supervisor knows the required standard of performance for each skill and has achieved personal mastery. As an additional component to assessment of competence beyond the work instruction, the DOPS format is included in this book as a valuable tool to be used 'on the road' in paramedic training and continuous professional development.

Table 1.1.2 gives a summary of the benefits and disadvantages of the three assessment tools. Fig. 1.1.3 provides a sample of the generic DOPS form which can be applied to every skill in this book. The four key features of the DOPS can be seen in Box 1.1.3.

Using the assessment tools

Paramedic students

The clinical skills work instructions in this book detail the activities that the paramedic student is expected to demonstrate for each individual skill, along with the required performance criteria. This can help guide the student in the specific actions of the skill to be performed.

BOX 1.1.2 KEY FEATURES OF THE S-CSAT

- The S-CSAT:
  - represents the 'shows how' level of Miller's pyramid
  - is summative and determines a student's readiness for supervised practice on a real patient
  - is conducted in a simulated learning environment (e.g. using part-task trainers).
- The student cannot move to the next stage of assessment until deemed competent (i.e. has achieved all actions without direction).

Table 1.1.2 Benefits and disadvantages of competency checklists, OSCEs and DOPS

Method	Benefits	Disadvantages
Clinical Skills Assessment Tools (F-CSAT and S-CSAT)	• Ease of administration • Conducted in a safe learning environment • Enhances skill acquisition • Allows self-assessment and reflection • Provides opportunities for teaching as well as assessment • Improves learner/clinician confidence • Assesses individual competency in particular situations	• Focuses on elements of a skill, not on holistic performance • Low face validity • Time-consuming to create
DOPS	• High quality instrument that tests 'does' of Miller's pyramid • Assesses technical ability but also interaction with patients • High face validity • Good reliability can be achieved with small numbers of cases and assessors • Easy to implement as it uses a generic template	• Needs multiple assessments from multiple assessors to strengthen reliability • Requires assessor training to ensure inter-rater reliability

Source: Adapted from Bindal et al., 2013; Evans, 2008; McLeod et al., 2012; Naeem, 2013.

BOX 1.1.3 KEY FEATURES OF THE DOPS

- The DOPS:
  - represents the 'does' level of Miller's pyramid
  - is summative and determines a student or clinician's competence for independent practice
  - indicates whether further supervision or training is required
  - is conducted 'on the road'.

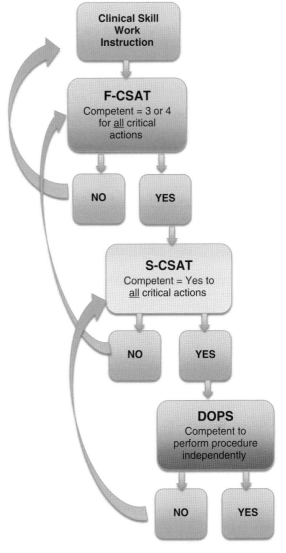

Figure 1.1.2 The progression to clinical skills competence

Source: *Adapted from Bindal, N., Goodyear, H., Bindal T. and Wall, D., 2013, DOPS assessment: a study to evaluate the experience and opinions of trainees and assessors, Medical Teacher, 35, 6, e1230– 1234; Evans, A., 2008, Competency assessment in nursing: A summary of literature published since 2000, Australian Cancer Nursing Education Project (EdCaN), http://edcan.org.au/assets/edcan/files/docs/ EdCancompetenciesliteraturereviewFINAL_0.pdf 2/9/2019; McLeod, R., Mires, G. and Ker, J., 2012, Direct observed procedural skills assessment in the undergraduate setting, Clinical Teacher, 9, 228–232; Naeem, N., 2013, Validity, reliability, feasibility, acceptability and educational impact of direct observation of procedural skills, Journal of the College of Physicians and Surgeons Pakistan, 23(1), 77–82.*

Content experts in paramedicine have developed each skill checklist and a peer review process has been applied during editorial development. Where there is research evidence for the way in which the skill should be performed, this has been included. Students can be confident that the process of performing a skill is based on expert opinion and an underpinning evidence base.

Paramedic undergraduate education providers

The clinical skills work instructions found in this book can be used by undergraduate education providers during skill laboratories when teaching clinical skills to paramedic students, to ensure that there is a standardised and evidence-based approach to the teaching of psychomotor skills.

The F-CSAT can be used for formative assessment of student progress. It provides the opportunity:
- for immediate remediation and feedback
- to provide a safe way to learn without putting patients at risk
- to increase learner confidence.

The S-CSAT can be used as the summative assessment to deem the overall competence of any given skill. It gives education providers confidence that the student is ready and fit to practise as a new graduate.

Ambulance services

The assessment of clinical skills is usually targeted at novice clinicians, to determine their readiness for supervised practice. Ambulance services can incorporate all three assessments into an assessment regime for new graduates. This is to ensure that correct training on each skill is reinforced after graduation and that graduates are deemed competent in each skill before applying it to a real patient situation. The DOPS format provides an additional assessment approach that paramedic supervisors can use 'on the road' to determine how well students have applied the skills in real life.

To ensure the skill continues to be delivered safely, there may also be a need to assess experienced clinicians. The DOPS is also useful for continuing professional development to maintain ongoing competency of the paramedic workforce. Appendix 1 provides more information on the importance of ongoing assessment for experienced clinicians.

The assessment model

The assessment model presented in this book is based on a holistic, cost-effective and evidence-based approach that combines training, assessment, evaluation and feedback. A diagrammatic representation of the model can be seen in Fig. 1.1.2, which shows a student's progression through to clinical skills competence.

Procedure assessed:				
	Aim: To ensure safe, efficient and effective care during this procedure			
	Significant input required from assessor	**Some guidance provided from assessor**	**Able to manage independently**	**Not assessed**
Clinical knowledge	Demonstrates relevant knowledge and understanding of the procedure including indications, contraindications, anatomy, technique, side effects and complications			
	1 2 3	4 5 6	7 8 9	N/A
Preparation	Prepares appropriately for the procedure. Ensures assisting staff are present; checks equipment and prepares drugs, ensures clinically indicated monitoring; arranges workspace ergonomically			
	1 2 3	4 5 6	7 8 9	N/A
Consent	Explains procedure to patient and obtains valid and adequate informed consent			
	1 2 3	4 5 6	7 8 9	N/A
Situational awareness	Demonstrates situational awareness through constant clinical and electronic monitoring. Maintains focus on the patient and avoids distraction			
	1 2 3	4 5 6	7 8 9	N/A
Infection control	Demonstrates aseptic/clean technique and standard (universal) precautions			
	1 2 3	4 5 6	7 8 9	N/A
Technical ability	Demonstrates manual dexterity and confidence; demonstrates correct procedural sequence with minimal hesitation and unnecessary actions			
	1 2 3	4 5 6	7 8 9	N/A
Communication skills	Introduces self, communicates effectively, provides reassurance and checks for any discomfort or concerns from the patient			
	1 2 3	4 5 6	7 8 9	N/A
Insight	Knows when to seek assistance, abandon procedure or arrange alternative care to prevent harm to patient			
	1 2 3	4 5 6	7 8 9	N/A
Documentation/Post-procedure management	Documents the episode including any problems and complications; arranges and documents plans for post-procedural care			
	1 2 3	4 5 6	7 8 9	N/A
Team interactions	Provides clear and concise instructions to assisting staff and hands over relevant information concerning the patient and plans to team members			
	1 2 3	4 5 6	7 8 9	N/A
Overall ability to perform procedure	Needs additional practice under supervision	May need supervision if complications arise	Competent to perform procedure independently	
Strengths:		**Areas to improve:**		
Staff member being assessed:		**Assessor name:** **Signed:**		

Figure 1.1.3 Sample DOPS form

Source: *Adapted from Norcini, J. and McKinley, D., 2007, Assessment methods in medical education,* Teacher and Teaching Education, *23, 239–250.*

Summary

This book contains the major clinical skills taught to paramedics within Australia and New Zealand in either a pre-graduation or post-graduation context. It offers an assessment model, detailed descriptions of each skill and a range of assessment tools. Each clinical skill comes with a set of criteria, indicators and a rating scale that can be used to make judgments on achievement of performance outcomes. This information is relevant for students and providers of paramedic education and ambulance services. The skills included in this book can be adopted in either simulated learning and assessment environments or directly integrated into clinical practice.

Appendix 1: The importance of ongoing assessment of clinical skills

The assessment of clinical skills is usually targeted at novice clinicians, to determine their readiness to commence supervised practice. However, to ensure the skill continues to be delivered safely, it may also be necessary to assess experienced clinicians.

In many centres, the assessment of skill performance is triggered only when a patient suffers a near miss or harm. While the idea of regularly assessing skills that are not linked to harm is unusual, it recognises that there is

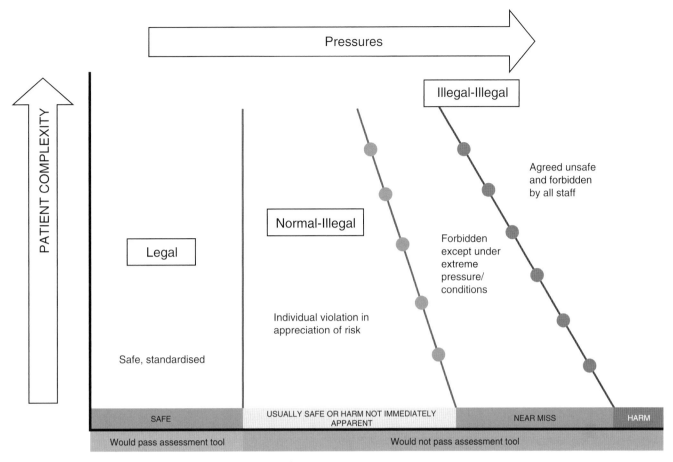

Figure 1.1.4 The migration of practice in the clinical environment

The pressures and variations associated with the clinical environment promote migration from the safe and standardised behaviours required to complete the summative skill assessment tool. Over time, these 'variations' become the normalised (Normal-Illegal) as individual clinicians attempt to reconcile time and resource constraints with best possible practice. In this area, the care is usually safe – although the margin for error is reduced with complex patients – and any harm caused may not be immediately apparent. The DOPS tool is one method of assessing for safe practice from experienced clinicians working in the clinical environment, but assessors must be careful to view the performance of the skill through the lens of the summative assessment tool and not what is 'normally accepted'.

Source: Adapted from Amalberti, R., Vincent, C. Auroy, Y. and de Saint Maurice, G., 2016, Violations and migrations in health care: a framework for understanding and management, Quality & Safety in Health Care, 15 (Suppl I).

a considerable margin between safe practice and actual harm. It may take clinicians some time to migrate from the safe practice demonstrated in a novice assessment to the boundary where injury is caused.

Some authors consider that the 'drift' from the safe practice (as defined by the novice assessment) occurs gradually and sets in over time (Vaughan, 1996). This drift is allowed as the operator is able to gradually deviate from safe practice as long as no harm is observed. From this perspective, increased exposure to a skill may increase the rate of drift and is counterintuitive to the notion that a clinician who regularly performs a skill is inherently safer.

The challenge faced by all clinicians, however, is the almost inevitable variations of practice that are needed to cope with the conflicting demands of complex work situations (Amalberti et al., 2006). From this viewpoint, these variations are often viewed as a strength – the ability to problem solve and increase productivity – associated with experienced clinicians. However, they can increase in both frequency and severity until the skill delivery

migrates to the 'edge' of patient safety and actual harm occurs. This triggers the clinician to either reassess their practice or dismiss the harm as an aberration.

Fig. 1.1.4 illustrates the migration of practice in the clinical environment. The skill assessment provides a structured and standardised approach to patient care but the realities of practice (staff shortages, time pressures, etc) can migrate away from the safe boundary. Practices that would not pass the assessment tool can become routine and are now virtually invisible to both the clinicians and those who work with them.

In most clinical settings, these 'variations' become common but, because few lead to harm, they are tolerated and become the 'Normal-Illegal'. The margin for error is reduced by patient complexity and is represented on the vertical axis.

The tendency for experienced clinicians to drift from safe practice reinforces the need to reassess clinical skills regularly. The skill, the setting and the clinician will determine which assessment tool is the most appropriate to do so.

References

ACSQHC (Australian Commission on Safety and Quality in Health Care), 2015. Assessment of training requirements for credentialed medical and other clinical practitioners and visiting medical officers. Retrieved from http://www.safetyandquality.gov.au/wp-content/uploads/2015/09/Advisory-A13_05-Assessment-of-training-requirements-for-credentialed-medical-and-8-September-2015.pdf

Ahmed, K., Miskovic, D., Darzi, A., Athanasiou, T. and Hanna, G.B., 2011. Observational tools for assessment of procedural skills: a systematic review. *American Journal of Surgery*, 202(4), 469–480.

Amalberti, R., Vincent, C. Auroy, Y. and de Saint Maurice, G., 2006. Violations and migrations in health care: a framework for understanding and management. *Quality & Safety in Health Care*, 15 (Suppl I), i66–i71, doi: 10.1136/qshc.2005.015982.

ASQA (Australian Skills Quality Authority), n.d. Definitions. Retrieved from: https://www.asqa.gov.au/standards-vac/definitions

Bindal, N., Goodyear, H., Bindal T. and Wall, D., 2013. DOPS assessment: a study to evaluate the experience and opinions of trainees and assessors. *Medical Teacher*, 35, 6, e1230–1234.

Bondy, K.,1983. Criterion-referenced definitions for rating scales in clinical evaluation. *Journal of Nursing Education*, 22(9), 376–382.

Brownie, S., Bahnisch, M. and Thomas, J., 2011. Competency-based education and competency-based career frameworks: informing Australia health workforce development. Retrieved from: https://www.hwa.gov.au/sites/uploads/national-competency-report-final-20120410.pdf

Crossley, J., Humphris, G. and Jolly, B., 2002. Assessing health professionals. *Medical Education*, 36, 800–804.

EdCaN (Australian National Cancer Nursing Education Project), 2009. Assessment fact sheet: performance assessment using competency assessment tools. Retrieved from: http://edcan.org.au/assets/edcan/files/docs/EdCan-FactSheet-CATs.pdf 2/9/2019

Epstein, R.M., 2007. Assessment in medical education. *New England Journal of Medicine*, 356(4), 387–396.

Evans, A., 2008. Competency assessment in nursing: a summary of literature published since 2000. Australian Cancer Nursing Education Project (EdCaN). Retrieved from: http://edcan.org.au/assets/edcan/files/docs/EdCancompetenciesliteraturereviewFINAL_0.pdf 2/9/2019

Garrison, C. and Ehringhaus, M., 2007. Formative and summative assessments in the classroom. Retrieved from: http://www.amle.org/Publications/WebExclusive/Assessment/tabid/1120/Default.aspx

Gormley, G., 2011. Summative OSCEs in undergraduate medical education. *Ulster Medical Journal*, 80(3), 127–132.

Hengameh, H., Afsaneh, R., Morteza, K., Hosein, M., Marjan, S.M. and Ebadi, A., 2015. The effect of applying direct observation of procedural skills (DOPS) on nursing students' clinical skills: a randomized clinical trial. *Global Journal of Health Science*, 7(7), 17.

Imanipour, M. and Jalili, M. 2015. Evaluation of nursing students' skills by DOPS. *Journal of Medical Education*, 14(1), 38–44.

London Deanery, 2012. Workplace-based assessment. Retrieved from: http://www.faculty.londondeanery.ac.uk/e-learning/workplace-based-assessment/what-is-workplace-based-assessment

McLeod, R., Mires, G. and Ker, J., 2012. Direct observed procedural skills assessment in the undergraduate setting. *Clinical Teacher*, 9, 228–232.

Miller, G.E., 1990. The assessment of clinical skills/competence/performance. *Academic Medicine*, 65(9), S63–67.

Naeem, N., 2013. Validity, reliability, feasibility, acceptability and educational impact of direct observation of procedural skills. *Journal of the College of Physicians and Surgeons Pakistan*, 23(1), 77–82.

Norcini, J. and McKinley, D., 2007. Assessment methods in medical education. *Teacher and Teaching Education*, 23, 239–250.

Nursing and Midwifery Board of Australia, 2015. Framework for assessing standards for practice for registered nurses, enrolled nurses and midwives. Retrieved from: http://www.nursingmidwiferyboard.gov.au/Codes-Guidelines-Statements/Frameworks/Framework-for-assessing-national-competency-standards.aspx

Paramedics Australasia, 2011. Australasian competency standards for paramedics. Retrieved from: https://paramedics.org/wp-content/uploads/2016/09/PA_Australasian-Competency-Standards-for-paramedics_July-20111.pdf 2/9/2019

Sadeghigooghari, N., Kheiri, M. and Jahantigh, M., 2013. Assessment of acceptability of direct observation of procedural skills (DOPS) among nursing students and faculty members in Zahedane University of Medical Sciences, Iran. *Proceedings from 2nd World Conference on Educational Technology Researchers*, 83, 1023–1026.

Suskie, L., 2018. *Assessing student learning: a common sense guide*. New Jersey: Wiley, p. 190.

Vaughan, D., 1996. *The Challenger launch decision: risky technology, culture, and deviance at NASA*. Chicago: Chicago University Press.

1.2 | The paramedic patient
Jeff Kenneally and Dianne Inglis

The paramedic patient can be any person, with any illness or complaint and present at any time or in any place. Medical or traumatic emergencies can befall anyone, necessitating the paramedic to regularly move through a variety of socioeconomic and cultural circumstances, workplaces, rural and remote settings and roadways. Preparedness and ability to adapt to the presenting situation is a required paramedic attribute. A significant part of the paramedic's role is to provide a professional, caring and reassuring approach to all patients, regardless of circumstance (Halpin et al., 2015; Togher et al., 2015).

Perceptions in emergencies

Commonly, whatever is happening that has prompted the callout will be unexpected and unwanted by patients. Some people might be fearful, distressed and anxious, others comparatively calm and cooperative. For many, these events can be a life-changing event. A normal 'day in the office' for a paramedic may be the worst day of the patient's life, and this consideration should be foremost in each case.

Patients' definitions of an emergency can differ greatly from those of paramedics (Booker et al., 2015; Morgans and Burgess, 2011; Toloo et al., 2013) – so much so that there can seem little correlation between the two groups. Public education campaigns can influence people to call ambulances for defined problems (Bray et al., 2015; Lowthian et al., 2011; Nehme et al., 2017), potentially increasing the workload. Conversely, people with genuine need may not call for assistance until their emergency is advanced, as they don't want to place burden on a busy system. Third parties may call for paramedics on behalf of a patient whom they perceive requires assistance without the patient being aware of this.

Patient presentations within emergencies will also vary considerably. Some will be minimally injured or have injuries that are concealed or less obvious. Others will have major injuries that are gross and confronting. Some will have more than one injury. On other occasions there will be more than one patient, or a scene that is large and complex, involving multiple crews and other emergency services.

Good assessment, the use of prioritising and triage tools and effective procedural ability in differing circumstances will be essential. During student training and afterwards,

when practising, consider utilising more challenging scenarios to prepare for difficult injuries and situations.

Non-acute patients

Not all callouts are for acute emergencies. Some situations will be expected and understood by the patient and their family. Chronic illness is now more prevalent in society, due to aging or poor lifestyle and diet. Patients with chronic illness may experience complications such as chronic respiratory and cardiac diseases, or acquired brain or spinal injuries. These may be encountered in support care centres or in homes substantially modified to provide dependent care (Chan et al., 2013; Hayes et al., 2017; Lee et al., 2014; Savic et al., 2017), including small, government-run homes and larger residential, hospital-like centres. Recurrent problems, or acute exacerbations, including seizures, infection and pressure area/wound care, will require varying degrees of paramedic intervention.

With all chronic illness, guidance from patients and carers, often already following prepared care plans, will be sought and integrated with paramedic care (Berns, 2016; Howcroft et al., 2016).

Palliative care

Increasingly, paramedics are assisting with palliative and end-of-life care. This can include presentations which may have to be managed quite differently from comparable emergency presentations (Rogers et al., 2015). Despite or perhaps because of this, paramedics can find themselves less prepared for the circumstances and how to respond to them (Barnette Donnelly et al., 2017). Withholding assessment and procedures when otherwise indicated can go against normal practice and expectations.

Though the end-of-life circumstance is expected, family members commonly find themselves unprepared for the events that occur near the very end. The patient's and family's expectations can be surprisingly vague or even unrealistic. However, end-of-life documents that can provide a clear guide to patient assessment and procedures are becoming increasing prevalent (Waldrop et al., 2015).

Paramedics can be called to make resuscitation decisions with unclear information and, occasionally, conflicting family messages (Sharp and Thompson, 2016; Waldrop et al., 2015). Decisions to transport patients may have to be negotiated between the patient's best interests and the family's desires (Murphy-Jones and Timmons, 2016). There is greater involvement of families in providing medical care, including the administration of medications to ease patient suffering (Wiese et al., 2011).

In reality, there is often little for paramedics to do other than make patients comfortable and reassure those present that things are as they should be (Pettifer and Bronnert, 2013; Waldrop et al., 2015; Wiese et al., 2011). Some ambulance services are moving to better accommodate these end-of-life situations, including clinical guideline modifications to match patient needs more closely.

Age

Both Australia and New Zealand have aging populations, of which 15% are 65 years of age or older (up from 9% in 1960). These rates are established and will continue to rise, though possibly even faster in New Zealand than in Australia (Kowal et al., 2014). A large proportion of ambulance calls are for patients over the age of 60 and frequently older than 70, with this number rising as the population ages (Cantwell et al., 2016; Lowthian et al., 2011; Pittet et al., 2014; Ross et al., 2017). The age disparity between patients and paramedics may present issues because, as people get older, they can begin to feel stigmatised and relate less well with those who are younger (Chopik et al., 2018).

Age bias can also work in reverse, however: paramedics have demonstrated a range of preconceived notions in regard to the elderly (Ross et al., 2014). Paramedic attitudes towards older patients who have fallen have been shown to be adversely affected by the perception of low acuity of the callout (Simpson et al., 2017). Medical students have been shown to have increased empathy with older patients following interactions with them, rather than relying on education alone (Samra et al., 2013). Bias by either party can impact listening, understanding, interpreting, informing and perceptions formed during clinician–patient interactions (FitzGerald and Hurst, 2017). Generational variations can appear through differences in mannerisms, use of language, dress and appearance, with biases being formed early during any paramedic contact.

Older patients frequently seek assistance later than younger patients (Nguyen et al., 2010). Outside help may seem to them to represent a loss of independent living if they are found to be struggling. Many ambulance calls are for people who live alone (Lowthian et al., 2011), isolated by age or disability, without social or physical support, as a result of the natural segregation of urban lifestyles. This can reduce happiness and the ability to interact with society outside of the patient's home and, importantly, result in a disconnection from family in emergencies (Lowthian et al., 2016; Wong, 2015).

At the same time, social isolation is one reason why ambulances are called for non-emergency primary care situations rather than the more usual or appropriate avenues (Booker et al., 2015; Lowthian et al., 2016; Ross et al., 2017). Paramedics will frequently be called for their social skills, at times being the only communication the patient has had that day or for even longer periods. Paramedics can also often be the only people to view inside a patient's home, as they really live, providing a critical conduit to outside services that can offer greater home help (Ross et al., 2017). In turn, ambulance services are turning to alternative methods of responding to such calls, including the use of non-emergency services and referrals to alternative healthcare providers (Eastwood et al., 2016).

Older patients can have different physiological findings, related to age, to consider during assessment. Comorbidities will commonly be encountered, necessitating comparison to the patient's past history and appreciation for already-known patient assessment variances. Increasing age can also bring a range of adverse variations during assessment and procedures, including reduced patient flexibility and cooperation, decreased muscle mass, differing skin quality and increased ease of injury. Older people are more likely to become sick or injured, and to have serious injuries, and it is more difficult for them to heal and recover.

A smaller number of callouts will be for children. Children differ from adults in many ways, including anatomically, physiologically, behaviourally, emotionally and in the way they communicate. Assessment findings that are considered normal in a young child might be considered widely abnormal in an adult. Clinical guidelines and procedures frequently look similar for adults and children, yet the interpretation and implementation required can vary considerably. The increasing rates of survival at birth and during childhood from diseases that were previously fatal is exposing paramedics to complex congenital diseases they often do not sufficiently understand.

Some procedures are best not performed by paramedics, and are instead left to those with greater expertise. Poor performance can lead to increased errors and patient distress. In turn, this limitation of practice, combined with the lower likelihood of attending paediatric patients, ensures that the necessary expertise will not be gained (Harve et al., 2016; Seppelt, 2015).

Parents and carers can be an excellent source of information for what to anticipate and how to assist with the child patient. Some of these people have become quasi-expert in managing chronic illnesses and can provide excellent insights and guidance. Parents also have intimate knowledge of their child and can identify even subtle differences in appearance and behaviour.

It should not be forgotten, however, that parents are not necessarily medical experts. A sick child can produce great emotion in parents, who themselves will need reassurance to avoid them transmitting their distress back to the child. They will also need to be sufficiently informed as to what is wrong with the child to enable decision making (see Chapter 1.6, Consent).

Gaining compliance in the child patient can be challenging. Parents are again critical in facilitating patient assessment and procedure performance in an otherwise apprehensive and uncooperative patient. In particular, it is important not to separate the child from their parent. Allowing the parent to nurse the child, remove clothing or hold oxygen/nebuliser masks can all be of practical value.

Bariatric patients

The bariatric patient has progressed from an uncommon presentation to regular occurrence in prehospital care. Obesity rates in Australia and New Zealand are among the highest in the world. In New Zealand, the obesity rate for those over 60 years of age is about 26.5% and this is rising. The obesity rate in Australia is slightly lower, at 24.6%, though this is decreasing. As many as one-third of New Zealand children can be considered obese (Shackleton et al., 2018) and as many as 40% of adolescents are considered overweight to obese, with increased prevalence among Pacific Islander and Māori groups (Utter et al., 2015). In Australia, as many as 20% of young children can also be considered overweight to obese. This is strongly associated with increased disease rates, medication use and hospital attendances (Hayes et al., 2016). Comparable rates have been noted among Aboriginal Australian children, though this is far less so in remote communities (Dyer et al., 2017).

Obesity causes a huge range of problems, including the predisposition of patients to disease and increased difficulty for paramedics in performing clinical procedures and moving and transporting patients. Airway procedures, assisted ventilation and cardiopulmonary resuscitation are among the many skills that are more difficult when applied to the bariatric patient (Cushman, 2014). Injections are more likely to find adipose rather than muscle tissue, and intravenous cannulation can be more difficult. On occasion, different equipment may be required, such as obese sphygmomanometer cuffs. Other equipment, such as purpose pelvic splints, may not be large enough to accommodate the patient.

Successful practice may entail effective teamwork. The development of specialist ambulances is a current trend, enabling critical equipment such as stair chairs and lifting devices to be made available, along with appropriately trained personnel. Paramedic skill training in managing, moving and transporting these complex patients improves patient outcomes and reduces the incidence of paramedic injury (Gable et al., 2014).

Patient cooperation

Gaining patient cooperation is essential for performing assessments and procedures. It is frequently challenging to gain cooperation, for a variety of reasons. A patient may not always want others to know what is happening in their life, even if they do request assistance. Occasionally, a patient or family member may not want your assistance at all, whether due to a previous bad experience, distrust or even being tired of their illness and contact with the health system.

Dementia, head trauma, hypoglycaemia, illicit drugs, stimulants, criminal intent and mental health challenges can all create problems such as abuse, threats and violence against paramedics (Cleary et al., 2017; Ross et al., 2017; Pourshaikhian et al., 2016; Usher et al., 2017). All of these difficulties need to be actively overcome to allow safe clinical practice. In some cases, assessments and procedures will be abbreviated, compromised or even absent because of the patient's presentation. However, these compromises must not affect paramedic health or safety, and they must be clearly documented to provide for continuity of care.

Socioeconomic status

A large percentage of people calling for or requiring ambulance assistance are health-system dependent, such as people living with disabilities, or pensioners. Living alone, with a reduced income to pay for services, the reduced availability of and access to alternative sources of health assistance and a lack of personal transport, increases the likelihood of calling for an ambulance (Achat et al., 2010; Kawakami et al., 2007; Toloo et al., 2013).

In turn, this increases the likelihood that ambulance calls to this group will be less acute and will be made for assistance with a broader range of issues that are normally dealt with by alternative primary care means (Booker et al., 2015). Paramedics must be prepared to involve themselves in assessment, assistance and reporting roles that evolve to help meet the varying needs of this patient group.

Race, religion and culture

Clearly, race, religion and culture are three different elements. Conceptually, though, all three are interlinked and can present considerations for paramedics during patient interactions. Differences in race, religion and culture bring differing social and behavioural norms, beliefs and customs that extend beyond biological differences.

Of the three elements, race can arguably be the most visible and obvious. This can lead to bias and stereotyped notions influencing interactions (Stone and Moskowitz, 2011). Cultural differences may not be readily appreciated where any distinguishing ethnic features go unrecognised.

Both Australia and New Zealand are both very ethnically diverse. Despite a background of the now defunct White Australia policy and British law, democracy and heritage, Australia is now comprised of over 200 different ethnic groups. A series of immigration waves saw the arrival of European migrants after the Second World War, followed by Vietnamese migrants after the Vietnam War and, more recently, Middle Eastern and African migrants. Each has brought significant diversity in physical appearance, language and culture (Walters and Zeller, 2018).

In addition, Aboriginal and Torres Strait Islander groups comprise approximately 2.8% of the total Australian population. These peoples are divided further into the usually regional groups they have traditionally identified with, each with its own diversity of culture and language (Taylor and Guerin, 2019). Despite Australia's wealth, this group collectively carries the poorest life expectancy – almost 10 years lower than that of the general population – and substantially higher rates of disease, including diabetes and cardiovascular disease (Azzopardi et al., 2018; Brown and Kritharides, 2017; Davy et al., 2016; Durey and Thompson, 2012). Rates of infant mortality and low birth weight are also higher, as are those of cancer, respiratory disease, ear and eye disease, and this group experiences seven times the national rate of kidney failure. There are also significant concerns with smoking, alcohol and illicit drug use in some communities (Burns et al., 2019).

In many ways, the picture in New Zealand is remarkably similar, underpinned by its British origins and heritage. The Indigenous peoples of New Zealand are the Māori, who comprise 16% of the total population. A similar proportion are Pacific Islander and Asian, the latter group being predominantly Indian and Chinese. Two-thirds of the population are primarily of European descent (Zhao et al., 2018). Just as with Australian Indigenous peoples, the Māori people have higher rates of diabetes, cardiovascular disease, cancer, kidney and lung disease and life expectancy that is nine years lower than that of other New Zealanders. Obesity is a significant problem within Māori communities (Oetzel et al., 2018). As in Australia, some of these health inequities are traceable back to inequities in income, employment, education and healthcare access (Oetzel et al., 2017; Te Karu et al., 2018).

Given the recurring theme of disadvantage and disconnection from health systems, there is always scope for paramedics to assist with education, redirection and reconnection. Cultural awareness and sensitivity is essential in all interactions to help mitigate and erode the already existing disadvantages (Artuso et al., 2013).

For paramedics, gaining an understanding of race, religion and cultural identities within the community of operation can help prepare them for interactions. Added to this will be the need to listen and observe during interactions, maintaining a willingness to accept and respect differences in patient/family responses and requests. This can be challenging when it is inconsistent with the paramedic's own societal norms or interferes with what is perceived to be necessary prehospital care. Patient/family requests can include the removal of footwear on entering the premises, restrictions on skin contact or clothing removal, or the requirement for a chaperone or religious representative to be present. Paramedics' behaviour can be outwardly favourable to patients, including supportive comments and clinical assistance, while remaining implicitly biased through such things as eye contact and mannerisms (Stone and Moskowitz, 2011).

References

Achat, H.M., Thomas, P., Close, G.R., Moerkerken, L.R. and Harris, M.F., 2010. General health care service utilisation: where, when and by whom in a socioeconomically disadvantaged population. *Australian Journal of Primary Health*, 16(2), 132–140.

Artuso, S., Cargo, M., Brown, A. and Daniel, M., 2013. Factors influencing health care utilisation among Aboriginal cardiac patients in central Australia: a qualitative study. *BMC Health Services Research*, 13(1), 83.

Azzopardi, P.S., Sawyer, S.M., Carlin, J.B., Degenhardt, L., Brown, N., Brown, A.D. and Patton, G.C., 2018. Health and wellbeing of Indigenous adolescents in Australia: a systematic synthesis of population data. *Lancet*, 391(10122), 766–782.

Barnette Donnelly C., Armstrong K.A., Perkins M.M., Moulia D., Quest T.E. and Yancey A.H., 2017. Emergency medical services provider experiences of hospice care. *Prehospital Emergency Care*, 9, 1–7.

Berns, N., 2016. Empowering patients through self-management plans. *Prescriber*, 27(4), 41–43.

Booker, M.J., Shaw, A.R. and Purdy, S., 2015. Why do patients with 'primary care sensitive' problems access ambulance services? A systematic mapping review of the literature. *BMJ Open*, 5(5), e007726.

Bray, J.E., Straney, L., Barger, B. and Finn, J., 2015. Effect of public awareness campaigns on calls to ambulance across Australia. *Stroke*, 46(5), 1377–1380.

Brown, A. and Kritharides, L., 2017. Overcoming cardiovascular disease in Indigenous Australians. *Medical Journal of Australia*, 206(1), 10–12.

Burns, J., Drew, N., Elwell, M., Harford-Mills, M., Hoareau, J., Macrae, A., Potter, C., Poynton, M., Ride, K. and Trzesinski, A., 2019. Overview of Aboriginal and Torres Strait Islander health status 2018. Retrieved from: https://healthinfonet.ecu.edu.au

Cantwell, K., Burgess, S., Morgans, A., Smith, K., Livingston, M. and Dietze, P., 2016. Temporal trends in falls cases seen by EMS in Melbourne: the effect of residence on time of day and day of week patterns. *Injury*, 47(1), 266–271.

Chan, V., Zagorski, B., Parsons, D. and Colantonio, A., 2013. Older adults with acquired brain injury: a population based study. *BMC Geriatrics*, 13(1), 97.

Chopik, W.J., Bremner, R.H., Johnson, D.J. and Giasson, H.L., 2018. Age differences in age perceptions and developmental transitions. *Frontiers in Psychology*, 9, 67.

Cleary, M., Jackson, D., Woods, C., Kornhaber, R., Sayers, J. and Usher, K., 2017. Experiences of health professionals caring for people presenting to the emergency department after taking crystal methamphetamine ('ICE'). *Issues in Mental Health Nursing*, 38(1), 33–41.

Cushman, J.T., 2014. Bariatric patient challenges. In *Emergency medical services: clinical practice and systems oversight* (Volume 2). New Jersey: Wiley, p. 407.

Davy, C., Harfield, S., McArthur, A., Munn, Z. and Brown, A. 2016. Access to primary health care services for Indigenous peoples: a framework synthesis. *International Journal for Equity in Health*, 15(1), 163.

Durey, A. and Thompson, S.C., 2012. Reducing the health disparities of Indigenous Australians: time to change focus. *BMC Health Services Approach*, 12(1), 151.

Dyer, S.M., Gomersall, J.S., Smithers, L.G., Davy, C., Coleman, D.T. and Street, J.M., 2017. Prevalence and characteristics of overweight and obesity in Indigenous Australian children: a systematic review. *Critical Reviews in Food Science and Nutrition*, 57(7), 1365–1376.

Eastwood, K., Morgans, A., Smith, K., Hodgkinson, A., Becker, G. and Stoelwinder, J., 2016. A novel approach for managing the growing demand for ambulance services by low-acuity patients. *Australian Health Review*, 40(4), 378–384.

FitzGerald, C. and Hurst, S., 2017. Implicit bias in healthcare professionals: a systematic review. *BMC Medical Ethics*, 18(1), 19.

Gable, B.D., Gardner, A.K., Celik, D.H., Bhalla, M.C. and Ahmed, R.A., 2014. Improving bariatric patient transport and care with simulation. *Western Journal of Emergency Medicine*, 15(2), 199.

Halpin, D., Hyland, M., Blake, S., Seamark, C., Pinnuck, M., Ward, D., Whalley, B., Greaves, C., Hawkins, A. and Seamark, D., 2015. Understanding fear and anxiety in patients at the time of an exacerbation of chronic obstructive pulmonary disease: a qualitative study. *JRSM Open*, 6(12), 2054270415614543.

Harve, H., Salmi, H., Rahiala, E., Pohjalainen, P. and Kuisma, M., 2016. Out-of-hospital paediatric emergencies: a prospective, population-based study. *Acta Anaesthesiologica Scandinavica*, 60(3), 360–369.

Hayes, A., Chevalier, A., D'Souza, M., Baur, L., Wen, L.M. and Simpson, J., 2016. Early childhood obesity: association with healthcare expenditure in Australia. *Obesity*, 24(8), 1752–1758.

Hayes, L., Shaw, S., Pearce, M.S. and Forsyth, R.J., 2017. Requirements for and current provision of rehabilitation services for children after severe acquired brain injury in the UK: a population-based study. *Archives of Disease in Childhood*, 102(9), 813–820.

Howcroft, M., Walters, E.H., Wood-Baker, R. and Walters, J.A., 2016. *Action plans with brief patient education for exacerbations in chronic obstructive pulmonary disease*. Online: The Cochrane Library.

Kawakami, C., Ohshige, K., Kubota, K. and Tochikubo, O., 2007. Influence of socioeconomic factors on medically unnecessary ambulance calls. *BMC Health Services Research*, 7(1).

Kowal, P., Towers, A. and Byles, J., 2014. Ageing across the Tasman Sea: the demographics and health of older adults in Australia and New Zealand. *Australian and New Zealand Journal of Public Health*, 38(4), 377–383.

Lee, B.B., Cripps, R.A., Fitzharris, M. and Wing, P.C., 2014. The global map for traumatic spinal cord injury epidemiology: update 2011, global incidence rate. *Spinal Cord*, 52(2), 110.

Lowthian, J.A., Cameron, P.A., Stoelwinder, J.U., Curtis, A., Currell, A., Cooke, M.W. and McNeil, J.J., 2011. Increasing utilisation of emergency ambulances. *Australian Health Review*, 35(1), 63–69.

Lowthian, J.A., Lennox, A., Curtis, A., Dale, J., Browning, C., Wilson, G., O'Brien, D., Rosewarne, C., Boyd, L., Garner, C. and Cameron, P., 2016. HOspitals and patients WoRking in Unity (HOW RU?): protocol for a prospective feasibility study of telephone peer support to improve older patients' quality of life after emergency department discharge. *BMJ Open*, 6(12), e013179.

Morgans, A. and Burgess, S.J., 2011. What is a health emergency? The difference in definition and understanding between patients and health professionals. *Australian Health Review*, 35(3), 284–289.

Murphy-Jones, G. and Timmons, S., 2016. Paramedics' experiences of end-of-life care decision making with regard to nursing home residents: an exploration of influential issues and factors. *Emergency Medicine Journal*, 33(10), 722–726.

Nehme, Z., Cameron, P.A., Akram, M., Patsamanis, H., Bray, J.E., Meredith, I.T. and Smith, K., 2017. Effect of a mass media campaign on ambulance use for chest pain. *Medical Journal of Australia*, 206(1), 30–35.

Nguyen, H.L., Saczynski, J.S., Gore, J.M. and Goldberg, R.J., 2010. Age and sex differences in duration of prehospital delay in patients with acute myocardial infarction: a systematic review. *Circulation: Cardiovascular Quality and Outcomes*, 3(1), 82–92.

Oetzel, J., Scott, N., Hudson, M., Masters-Awatere, B., Rarere, M., Foote, J., Beaton, A. and Ehau, T., 2017. Implementation framework for chronic disease intervention effectiveness in Māori and other indigenous communities. *Globalization and Health*, 13(1), 69.

Oetzel, J., Wihapi, R., Manuel, C. and Rarere, M., 2018. An integrated approach to prevent chronic lifestyle diseases in Māori men. *International Journal of Integrated Care*, 18(Suppl 2).

Pettifer, A. and Bronnert, R., 2013. End of life care in the community: the role of ambulance clinicians. *Journal of Paramedic Practice*, 5(7), 394–399.

Pittet, V., Burnand, B., Yersin, B. and Carron, P.N., 2014. Trends of pre-hospital emergency medical services activity over 10 years: a population-based registry analysis. *BMC Health Services Research*, 14(1), 380.

Pourshaikhian, M., Gorji, H.A., Aryankhesal, A., Khorasani-Zavareh, D. and Barati, A., 2016. A systematic literature review: workplace violence against emergency medical services personnel. *Archives of Trauma Research*, 5(1).

Rogers, I.R., Shearer, F.M., Rogers, J.R., Ross-Adjie, G., Monterosso, L. and Finn, J.C., 2015. Paramedics' perceptions and educational needs with respect to palliative care. *Australasian Journal of Paramedicine*, 12(5).

Ross, L., Adams, T. and Beovich, B., 2017. Methamphetamine use and emergency services in Australia: a scoping review. *Journal of Paramedic Practice*, 9(6), 244–257.

Ross, L., Duigan, T., Boyle, M.J. and Williams, B., 2014. Student paramedic attitudes towards the elderly: a cross-sectional study. *Australasian Journal of Paramedicine*, 11(3).

Ross, L., Jennings, P.A., Smith, K. and Williams, B., 2017. Paramedic attendance to older patients in Australia, and the prevalence and implications of psychosocial issues. *Prehospital Emergency Care*, 21(1), 32–38.

Ross, L., Jennings, P. and Williams, B., 2017. Psychosocial support issues affecting older patients: a cross-sectional paramedic perspective. *INQUIRY: Journal of Health Care Organization, Provision, and Financing*, 54, 0046958017731963.

Samra, R., Griffiths, A., Cox, T., Conroy, S. and Knight, A. 2013. Changes in medical student and doctor attitudes toward older adults after an intervention: a systematic review. *Journal of the American Geriatrics Society*, 61(7), 1188–1196.

Savic, G., DeVivo, M.J., Frankel, H.L., Jamous, M.A., Soni, B.M. and Charlifue, S., 2017. Long-term survival after traumatic spinal cord injury: a 70-year British study. *Spinal Cord*, 55(7), 651.

Seppelt, I.M., 2015. Who should perform critical procedures on children prehospital, and how often? *Pediatric Critical Care Medicine*, 16(8), 785–786.

Shackleton, N., Milne, B.J., Audas, R., Derraik, J.G., Zhu, T., Taylor, R.W., Morton, S.M.B., Glover, M., Cutfield, W.S. and Taylor, B., 2018. Improving rates of overweight, obesity and extreme obesity in New Zealand 4-year-old children in 2010–2016. *Pediatric Obesity*, 13(12), 766–777.

Sharp, R. and Thompson, S., 2016. Understanding the place of advance directives in paramedic pre-hospital care. *Whitireia Nursing & Health Journal*, 23, 13.

Simpson, P., Thomas, R., Bendall, J., Lord, B., Lord, S. and Close, J., 2017. 'Popping nana back into bed': a qualitative exploration of paramedic decision making when caring for older people who have fallen. *BMC Health Services Research*, 17(1), 299.

Stone, J. and Moskowitz, G.B., 2011. Non-conscious bias in medical decision making: what can be done to reduce it? *Medical Education*, 45(8), 768–776.

Taylor, K. and Guerin, P., 2019. *Health care and Indigenous Australians: cultural safety in practice*. Melbourne: Macmillan International Higher Education.

Te Karu, L., Bryant, L., Harwood, M. and Arroll, B., 2018. Achieving health equity in Aotearoa New Zealand: the contribution of medicines optimisation. *Journal of Primary Health Care*, 10(1), 11–15.

Togher, F.J., O'Cathain, A., Phung, V.H., Turner, J. and Siriwardena, A.N., 2015. Reassurance as a key outcome valued by emergency ambulance service users: a qualitative interview study. *Health Expectations*, 18(6), 2951–2961.

Toloo, G., FitzGerald, G.J., Aitken, P.J., Ting, J.Y., McKenzie, K., Rego, J. and Enraght-Moony, E., 2013. Ambulance use is associated with higher self-rated illness seriousness: user attitudes and perceptions. *Academic Emergency Medicine*, 20(6), 576–583.

Usher, K., Jackson, D., Woods, C., Sayers, J., Kornhaber, R. and Cleary, M., 2017. Safety, risk, and aggression: health professionals' experiences of caring for people affected by methamphetamine when presenting for emergency care. *International Journal of Mental Health Nursing*, 26(5), 437–444.

Utter, J., Denny, S., Teevale, T., Peiris-John, R. and Dyson, B., 2015. Prevalence and recent trends in overweight, obesity, and severe obesity among New Zealand adolescents. *Childhood Obesity*, 11(5), 585–589.

Wiese, C.H., Vagts, D.A., Kampa, U., Pfeiffer, G., Grom, I.U., Gerth, M.A., Graf, B.M. and Zausig, Y.A., 2011. Palliative care and end-of-life patients in emergency situations. Recommendations on optimization of out-patient care. *Der Anaesthesist*, 60(2), 161–171.

Waldrop, D.P., Clemency, B., Lindstrom, H.A. and Cordes, C.C., 2015. 'We are strangers walking into their life-changing event': how prehospital providers manage emergency calls at the end of life. *Journal of Pain and Symptom Management*, 50(3), 328–334.

Walters, R. and Zeller, B., 2018. Citizenship and national identity has strengthened social cohesion in multicultural Australia. Retrieved from: https://papers.ssrn.com/sol3/papers.cfm?abstract_id=3185137

Wong, P.T., 2015. A meaning-centered approach to overcoming loneliness during hospitalization, old age, and dying. *Addressing Loneliness: Coping, Prevention and Clinical Interventions*, 1, 171.

Zhao, J., Gibb, S., Jackson, R., Mehta, S. and Exeter, D.J., 2018. Constructing whole of population cohorts for health and social research using the New Zealand Integrated Data Infrastructure. *Australian and New Zealand Journal of Public Health*, 42(4), 382–388.

1.3 | Infection control
Jeff Kenneally and Dianne Inglis

The paramedic working environment is diverse. The locations attended are dictated by circumstances and events outside the paramedic's control, and the available information about patients is often minimal, sometimes non-existent. Patients may have a medical, traumatic or social complaint, and some will carry infection or transmittable disease, either underlying or as their major problem.

The scope of paramedic clinical practice has greatly increased in the past two decades, including intravenous therapy, airway skills and suturing. This in turn increases the exposure of a much larger number of paramedics to procedures that carry a greater risk of infection (Barr et al., 2017a). Exposure at scenes to sources of infection, including blood, other body fluid, air, surfaces or clothing, occurs frequently, with an increased vulnerability to highly infectious agents such as methicillin-resistant staphylococcus aureus (MRSA), influenza and severe acute respiratory syndrome (SARS) (Thomas et al., 2017).

Exposure can come from proximity to a patient coughing, sneezing or even spitting. It can be from direct skin contact with body fluid through the hands or while kneeling in or having the agent spray or splash or from percutaneous/needlestick injury (Boal et al., 2010). Potential infective agents can remain on uniforms, and are not easy to remove during emergency conditions.

Paramedic preparedness

Paramedic preparedness should include standard vaccinations, with boosters as required, as well as vaccinations against infections carried by high-risk patient groups, including hepatitis. Annual vaccinations, such as influenza, are a critical part of bilaterally protecting both paramedics and at-risk patients, such as those in aged care and the immunocompromised.

Careful attention to dispatch detail may alert the paramedic to the level of personal protection equipment (PPE) required prior to exposure.

Patient protection

The complications of infection are not just for attending paramedics. Managing infection transmission is critical to patients as well. Many patients are immunocompromised or at least vulnerable to infection secondary to other medical problems. Morbidity and mortality in hospitals and intensive care units are greatly increased from nosocomial infection, including that encountered prehospital (Haque et al., 2018) as well as within the hospital system.

During patient contact and procedure performance, paramedics must be mindful of protecting the patient and themselves equally. Cleanliness and even aseptic methods should never be ignored or undermined where they are appropriately required, even in emergencies. The routine approach of maintaining a clean work surface, aseptic needle and drug preparation and injection site preparation should continue regardless of the severity of the patient's illness. Cross-contamination from patient to patient should not occur as a result of paramedic assessment or procedures. Change gloves and dispose of and not reuse items prepared for any other patient.

Paramedics can spread a transmittable illness to patients and other community members just as anyone else would. Presenteeism is the term used for people who attend work when ill, and it incurs a cost, just as absenteeism does. There are a variety of reasons why presenteeism can occur, including workplace culture, the threat of disciplinary action, a lack of alternative cover, demands of the job or personal reasons, including financial concerns (Webster et al., 2019). While workplace strategies are important to reducing this problem, individual responsibility for presenteeism cannot be avoided.

Protection of community

Paramedics will be asked on occasion to provide care for those with known or suspected infection. This can include more serious, contagious and notifiable diseases ranging from active tuberculosis, measles, pertussis or influenza through to pandemic outbreaks such as COVID-19, SARS and swine flu.

Ambulance services frequently provide updates on the identification and required management of diseases. This may include the isolation of patient and caregivers, with care being provided in the home. Where patient transport occurs, it will necessitate warning the hospital in advance to allow enough time for suitable preparation before the patient arrives. Hospital instructions in such cases should be understood prior to arrival. PPE, including overalls, must be disposed of before anyone else is subsequently exposed to the infection. Ambulance vehicles and equipment may have to be decontaminated before further use.

Universal precautions

The management of infectious diseases should not be based on whether or not the paramedic is aware a patient is infective. This information may not be available in an emergency or may be withheld intentionally for personal or confidential reasons. Instead, paramedic practice must be based on presuming every patient is a source of potential infection.

From this ethos has arisen the concept of universal precautions. These were originally devised to provide a level of protection against the transmission of disease from blood or other body fluid (Broussard and Kahwaji, 2018). The use of PPE is considered routine to provide protection against the patient's blood and body fluid (other than sweat) and where the paramedic has any cuts or wounds and their skin integrity is broken. The protection typically included for this purpose includes handwashing and medical nitrile or latex protective gloves.

Protection of mucous membranes includes the mouth and eyes. Protective eyewear/goggles should be worn or, where appropriate, such as when there is splash risk, a face shield. Gowns or disposable coveralls can be worn to protect uniforms and to allow for the disposal of contaminated clothing.

Personal protection choices should be matched to the signs and symptoms that are present and the possible risk and type of exposure. While these choices must be appropriate and offer effective protection, they should also remain balanced against the reality that most people will not offer high infective risk, and so most of the assessments and procedures performed are correspondingly of low risk. Therefore, although the use of gloves and handwashing is standard, the need for the remaining items is less common and usually associated with the potential for being sprayed or splashed (Broussard and Kahwaji, 2018).

The availability of PPE alone, however, will not guarantee that infection transmission can be avoided. Paramedics have been shown to have a reduced understanding of infectious diseases and asepsis/antisepsis (Barr et al., 2017a; Shaban et al., 2012; Szarpak, 2013) and less than optimal compliance with hand cleaning and glove requirements (Barr, Dunn et al., 2017b; Harris and Nicolai, 2010). Although gloves are commonly worn in practice, they are most commonly removed only when the callout has been completed (Barr et al., 2017a).

Handwashing

Paying attention to hand hygiene is in no way negated by the use of gloves. The hands perform assessments and procedures, making them major sources of infection transmission to and from the patient. Effective hand hygiene is the single most effective method of reducing healthcare-associated infections (White et al., 2015). Performed before and after patient contact, it can significantly decrease infection transmission (Jefferson et al., 2011; Tran et al., 2012).

The ability to cleanse hands prior to and following a procedure is limited by lack of normal handwashing facilities in paramedic practice. There is greater reliance on using handwash gels and antimicrobial agents (Barr et al., 2017a), though soap and water wash will suffice if available provided sufficient hand rubbing occurs (Freeman et al., 2014; Smith et al., 2015). Alcohol-based liquids and gels can provide high bacterial reduction (Kawagoe et al., 2011; White et al., 2015).

Guiding infection control are the 2009 World Health Organization guidelines for five critical moments in hand hygiene (White et al., 2015). These are:
1. Before touching any patient
2. Before performing any procedure
3. After performing any procedure
4. After touching any patient
5. After touching any patient's surroundings.

The aseptic non-touch technique (ANTT®; see Chapter 2.20) is an essential part of infection transmission management. It involves six principles, including use of sterile or non-sterile gloves and maintaining an aseptic field when required.

Asepsis is not always required for many procedures; more often cleanliness is sufficient. To assist with cleanliness, consider first spreading out a clean surface on which to lay out equipment for use. This could be a clean linen item, such as a towel or pillowcase, or a product specific for this purpose. Such a surface looks professional and provides an orderly single place for the location of equipment. Any item that requires sterility can be maintained in its original packaging when laid out on the surface.

Before any procedure, clean the hands and then don disposable gloves. These gloves are protective to paramedics; they can become contaminated as easily as bare skin. Following patient contact, change or discard the gloves to avoid contamination of other equipment, surfaces and the ambulance vehicle.

Where there is more than one patient, either wear multiple gloves and remove the outer one between each patient or replace them with new gloves between patients. Importantly, avoid touching the face, mouth, eyes and nose (Smith et al., 2015).

Airborne infection protection

Respiratory illness allows exposure to aerosol/droplets from coughing- and sneezing-generated airborne agents and minute microorganisms/infective agents that distribute and settle on surfaces for subsequent contact (Bischoff et al., 2013; Jones and Brosseau, 2015; Ather and Edemekong, 2018). Smaller particle agents, such as many viruses, can remain airborne for longer periods, heightening their prospect for transmission. While some risk sources will be comparatively obvious, others are less so; for example, vomiting into a toilet and then flushing is a less obvious means of producing airborne agents (Fernstrom and Goldblatt, 2013). Respiratory infection is the third leading cause of death worldwide (Richard and Fouchier, 2015).

When attending respiratory infective patients, consider wearing respiratory P-rated protective masks or, alternatively, having the patient wear one. Purpose respiratory masks are a key method of reducing respiratory transmission (Broussard and Kahwaji, 2018; Jefferson et al., 2011). There are different levels designed to filter out fine viral particles: while P2 is typically sufficient, superior options are also available, including P3 and N-95 masks, although most circumstances do not generally warrant the extra expense. Surgical masks are usually not sufficient, particularly if working in close proximity to the patient (Bischoff et al., 2013; Smith et al., 2015).

Despite the potential for infection transmission and adverse outcomes, respiratory mask protection remains inadequately used. This is partly from ignorance but also because masks can be uncomfortable or cause fogging of eyewear. Compliance requires multiple inputs including regulation/supervision, effective equipment and training (Verbeek et al., 2015). Where appropriate, respiratory masks, including P2 and surgical masks, can be provided to patients who are coughing or sneezing to minimise their transmission potential (Patel et al., 2016).

Airway procedures

Airway procedures are high risk for infectious transmission. This risk can extend two metres from a patient and increases considerably when in proximity to the face (Bischoff et al., 2013). Invasive procedures, including endotracheal intubation, airway suctioning, assisted ventilation and non-invasive ventilation methods, are all high risk for creating aerosol/droplets (Chan et al., 2018; Flores and Cohen, 2014; Hui et al., 2014; Scala and Soroksky, 2014; Tran et al., 2012). Where airway procedures are being performed, respiratory protection should be worn (Bischoff et al., 2013), accompanied by protective eyewear or face shields.

A common therapy considered for patients with respiratory illness is nebulised medication administration. Unfortunately, the nebulisation process helps distribute any infective agent into the air, making it risky for paramedics (Ather and Edemekong, 2018; Hui et al., 2014; O'Neil et al., 2017). Where possible, use nebulisers in well-ventilated areas and ensure that all others present wear respiratory masks. Alternatively, use metered dose inhalers or administer drug therapy via a different route.

Full body protection

For some diseases, standard PPE will not provide sufficient protection. Where the prospect of an adverse or fatal outcome is higher, increased respiratory protection and full body protection are necessary.

This chapter does not intend to discuss this higher level of specialty response. However, use of full body protection will occasionally be required where clothing contact and the transmission of disease are likely (Jefferson et al., 2011; Verbeek et al., 2015); for example, when attending a known highly infectious agent during pandemics such as COVID-19, SARS and H1N1, or an aged care centre where a gastrointestinal disease outbreak has occurred. In these cases, the prevalence of disease and likelihood of contamination warrants donning disposable gowns or protective-rated disposable overalls before entering. On leaving, these are carefully removed and disposed of in clinical waste bags. Protective clothing removal, or doffing, must follow a careful process, avoiding contact with uncontaminated clothing, skin or surfaces, as there is significant risk of disease transmission through doing this (Verbeek et al., 2015).

Sharps use and disposal

Invasive procedures involving needles (sharps waste) necessitate particular vigilance. These include all forms of injection, needle decompression and blood sugar assessment. Appropriate containers for sharps/needle disposal should be procured and placed in a convenient location before commencing the procedure. These must be stored with all intravenous therapy equipment and placed strategically during any such procedure to allow immediate disposal of contaminated sharps. They should not be out of reach or in an awkward position that would prompt stretching or reaching across the body or towards any other person.

The containers should be of a size suitable to receive the contaminated waste item. Used sharps should never be recapped. Where sharps containers are partly filled from previous use, consider replacing them with new ones before problems can occur when subsequent items are inserted. Dispose of the sharps container itself appropriately once it is finished with. Never attempt to open a sharps container to inspect or retrieve any item within it.

When using sharp devices, inform others within the vicinity of operation, including colleagues and the patient. Patient compliance is essential; incorporate assistance if you are concerned about the prospect of unwanted patient movement. Ensure no other person, aside from the patient, is within the immediate area of the sharp so as to avoid accidental needlestick injury. Assistants should position themselves safely away from area of needle likely movement. Remove and discard the sharp safely before requesting any assistant to move into that immediate area again.

Where possible, have available and make use of sharp items that have inbuilt safety features such as self-sheathing.

Contaminated material

Contaminated materials are handled carefully and disposed of in specific-purpose infectious waste bags.

Removal of used PPE should involve 'reversal' of items. That is, remove face shields from the rear and pull gloves from the uppermost, peeling them towards the fingers so that the inner layer finishes on the outside with the first glove left inside the second. Gowns should be untied and pulled from the neck, turning them inside out (Broussard and Kahwaji, 2018). Overalls are similarly unzipped and turned inside out as they are removed.

Dispose of contaminated materials immediately. Paramedic uniforms contaminated during patient contact should not be worn to attend further patients. Ideally, they should be changed as soon as practicable and laundered following ambulance service guidelines for such circumstances.

Equipment and ambulance vehicle surfaces are regularly exposed to infectious agents. Blood and body fluids can leak onto floors and trolleys. Contaminated hand contact spreads agents to the walls, cupboard doors, drawers and even consumables inside them (Barr et al., 2017a). Inside a hospital, a purpose cleaner might take responsibility for floor and bed cleaning, while hospital staff try to limit the equipment used to trolleys with disposable coverings atop. In ambulances, however, many surfaces are within reach during emergency care and it is not possible to cover them in advance. Post-incident cleaning is therefore necessary, although time-consuming and difficult to achieve with certainty. This can be compounded by pressure from ambulance services to have paramedics clear as quickly as possible to attend subsequent callouts.

Ambulance equipment will typically be divisible into disposable and non-disposable items. The increasing trend is towards disposable items wherever possible to reduce need for and risk of inadequate cleaning. This includes many items that were previously not disposable such as laryngoscope blades, ventilator hoses and masks, and even tourniquets for intravenous therapy. On all occasions, disposable items should be placed immediately and carefully into a waste bag. PPE should be replaced and worn during the cleaning process to avoid droplet splashing.

The urgency of a patient's condition can distract the paramedic from unseen pathogens. Ambulances can notoriously become sites of untidiness, with waste material strewn about during the haste of emergency care. This should be considered unnecessary in many instances, however, as it only takes a few moments to place discarded items into clinical waste bags at time of use.

Ambulance services all have detailed work instructions for infection control, personal protection and equipment/vehicle cleaning. Understanding of and adherence to these is an essential part of paramedic practice. Non-disposable equipment can be challenging, however, particularly if the item is small or awkward to clean, with difficult-to-see components such as pulse oximetry probes and electrocardiograph leads.

Contamination can be subtle and have no visible evidence. Contaminated items can be easily overlooked or inadequately attended to, and some contaminants can remain active for prolonged periods, risking disease transmission. Airway and respiratory care items are particularly high risk for disease transmission if not disposed of or appropriately cleaned, including physical wiping, scrubbing and chemical disinfectant. Poor disinfectant compliance among hospital and paramedic staff is common and is associated with nosocomial infection (Boyce, 2016; McDonell, 2015).

Paramedic follow-up

Despite best endeavours, paramedic exposure to infection can still occur. Accidental needlestick injury and blood or body fluid splash are a concern as they occur at significant rates (Auta et al., 2018; Gray and Collie, 2016; Murphy, 2018). The paramedic can be exposed before realising a patient is a potential transmitter of a disease. Exposure to a high-risk disease, such as meningococcal infection, may occur even where all PPE is employed.

In all cases, paramedics should seek advice and instruction on how to proceed. This can include receiving first aid, medical assessment, responsive medical therapies and subsequent follow-up and review.

Human factors

Finally, it should be remembered that all precautions against infection must still be balanced against human considerations. Providing patient contact for reassurance can be important on occasions, and personal protection items can impede this. Explaining the items' use and using effective interpersonal skills can assist in combating this problem, along with wearing only those items that are needed for the particular level of risk involved.

References

Ather, B. and Edemekong, P.F., 2018. Precautions, airborne. Retrieved from: https://www.statpearls.com

Auta, A., Adewuyi, E.O., Tor-Anyiin, A., Edor, J.P., Kureh, G.T., Khanal, V., Oga, E. and Adeloye, D., 2018. Global prevalence of percutaneous injuries among healthcare workers: a systematic review and meta-analysis. *International Journal of Epidemiology*, 47(6), 1972–1980.

Barr, N., Holmes, M., Roiko, A. and Lord, W., 2017a. A qualitative exploration of infection prevention and control guidance for Australian paramedics. *Australasian Journal of Paramedicine*, 14(3).

Barr, N., Holmes, M., Roiko, A., Dunn, P. and Lord, B., 2017b. Self-reported behaviors and perceptions of Australian paramedics in relation to hand hygiene and gloving practices in paramedic-led health care. *American Journal of Infection Control*, 45(7), 771–778.

Bischoff, W.E., Swett, K., Leng, I. and Peters, T.R., 2013. Exposure to influenza virus aerosols during routine patient care. *Journal of Infectious Diseases*, 207(7), 1037–1046.

Boal, W.L., Leiss, J.K., Ratcliffe, J.M., Sousa, S., Lyden, J.T., Li, J. and Jagger, J., 2010. The national study to prevent blood exposure in paramedics: rates of exposure to blood. *International Archives of Occupational and Environmental Health*, 83(2), 191–199.

Boyce, J.M., 2016. Modern technologies for improving cleaning and disinfection of environmental surfaces in hospitals. *Antimicrobial Resistance & Infection Control*, 5(1), 10.

Broussard, I.M. and Kahwaji, C.C., 2018. Precautions universal. Retrieved from: https://www.statpearls.com

Chan, M.T., Chow, B.K., Lo, T., Ko, F.W., Ng, S.S., Gin, T. and Hui, D.S., 2018. Exhaled air dispersion during bag-mask ventilation and sputum suctioning: implications for infection control. *Scientific Reports*, 8(1), 198.

Fernstrom, A. and Goldblatt, M., 2013. Aerobiology and its role in the transmission of infectious diseases. *Journal of Pathogens*, doi: 10.1155/2013/493960.

Flores, M.V. and Cohen, M., 2014. Preventing airborne disease transmission: implications for patients during mechanical ventilation. In *Noninvasive ventilation in high-risk infections and mass casualty events*. Vienna: Springer, pp. 305–313.

Freeman, M.C., Stocks, M.E., Cumming, O., Jeandron, A., Higgins, J., Wolf, J., Prüss-Ustün, A., Bonjour, S., Hunter, P.R., Fewtrell, L. and Curtis, V., 2014. Systematic review: hygiene and health: systematic review of handwashing practices worldwide and update of health effects. *Tropical Medicine & International Health*, 19(8), 906–916.

Gray, S. and Collie, A., 2016. *Workers' compensation claims among nurses and ambulance officers in Australia, 2008/09 to 2013/14*. Melbourne: Monash University.

Haque, M., Sartelli, M., McKimm, J. and Bakar, M.A., 2018. Health care-associated infections – an overview. *Infection and Drug Resistance*, 11, 2321.

Harris, S.A. and Nicolai, L.A., 2010. Occupational exposures in emergency medical service providers and knowledge of and compliance with universal precautions. *American Journal of Infection Control*, 38(2), 86–94.

Hui, D.S., Chan, M.T. and Chow, B., 2014. Aerosol dispersion during various respiratory therapies: a risk assessment model of nosocomial infection to health care workers. *Hong Kong Medical Journal*, 20(Suppl 4), S9–S13.

Jefferson, T., Del Mar, C.B., Dooley, L., Ferroni, E., Al-Ansary, L.A., Bawazeer, G.A., van Driel, M.L., Nair, S., Jones, M.A., Thorning, S. and Conly, J.M., 2011. *Physical interventions to interrupt or reduce the spread of respiratory viruses*. Online: The Cochrane Library.

Jones, R.M. and Brosseau, L.M., 2015. Aerosol transmission of infectious disease. *Journal of Occupational and Environmental Medicine*, 57(5), 501–508.

Kawagoe, J.Y., Graziano, K.U., Martino, M.D.V., Siqueira, I. and Correa, L., 2011. Bacterial reduction of alcohol-based liquid and gel products on hands soiled with blood. *American Journal of Infection Control*, 39(9), 785–787.

McDonell, A., 2015. Issues of infection control in prehospital settings. *Australasian Journal of Paramedicine*, 6(4).

Murphy, C., 2018. How many more Australian healthcare workers have to sustain a needlestick injury before safety engineered devices become routine. *Australian Nursing and Midwifery Journal*, 25(9), 16.

O'Neil, C.A., Li, J., Leavey, A., Wang, Y., Hink, M., Wallace, M., Biswas, P., Burnham, C.A.D. and Babcock, H.M., 2017. Characterization of aerosols generated during patient care activities. *Clinical Infectious Diseases*, 65(8), 1335–1341.

Patel, R.B., Skaria, S.D., Mansour, M.M. and Smaldone, G.C., 2016. Respiratory source control using a surgical mask: An in vitro study. *Journal of Occupational and Environmental Hygiene*, 13(7), 569–576.

Richard, M. and Fouchier, R.A., 2015. Influenza A virus transmission via respiratory aerosols or droplets as it relates to pandemic potential. *FEMS Microbiology Reviews*, 40(1), 68–85.

Scala, R. and Soroksky, A., 2014. Noninvasive ventilation interfaces for high-risk infections: implications for health care workers. In *Noninvasive ventilation in high-risk infections and mass casualty events*. Vienna: Springer, pp. 29–34.

Shaban, R., Creedy, P. and Clark, P., 2012. Paramedic knowledge of infectious disease aetiology and transmission in an Australian emergency medical system. *Australasian Journal of Paramedicine*, 1(3), 10.

Smith, E., Coghlan, B. and Leder, K., 2015. Avian influenza: Clinical and epidemiological information for paramedics and emergency healthcare workers. *Australasian Journal of Paramedicine*, 4(1).

Szarpak, Ł., 2013. Knowledge of aseptics and antisepsis and following their rules as elements of infection prevention in the work of paramedics. *Medycyna Pracy*, 64(2), 239–243.

Thomas, B., O'Meara, P. and Spelten, E., 2017. Everyday dangers – the impact infectious disease has on the health of paramedics: a scoping review. *Prehospital and Disaster Medicine*, 32(2), 217–223.

Tran, K., Cimon, K., Severn, M., Pessoa-Silva, C.L. and Conly, J., 2012. Aerosol generating procedures and risk of transmission of acute respiratory infections to healthcare workers: a systematic review. *PLOS ONE*, 7(4), e35797.

Verbeek, J.H., Ijaz, S., Mischke, C., Ruotsalainen, J.H., Makela, E. and Neuvonen, K., 2015. *Personal protective equipment for preventing highly infectious diseases due to contact with contaminated body fluids in health care staff*. Online: The Cochrane Library.

Webster, R.K., Liu, R., Karimullina, K., Hall, I., Amiot, R. and Rubin, G.J., 2019. A systematic review of infectious illness presenteeism: prevalence, reasons and risk factors. *BMC Public Health*, 19(1), 799.

White, K.M., Jimmieson, N.L., Obst, P.L., Graves, N., Barnett, A., Cockshaw, W., Gee, P., Haneman, L., Page, K., Campbell, M. and Martin, E., 2015. Using a theory of planned behaviour framework to explore hand hygiene beliefs at the '5 critical moments' among Australian hospital-based nurses. *BMC Health Services Research*, 15(1), 59.

1.4 | Situational awareness

Jeff Kenneally and Dianne Inglis

The paramedic situation can be in a crowded public place or a deserted laneway, a typical family home or a farm paddock, a public roadway or a factory workplace, night or day, summer or winter. The paramedic's emergency resuscitation cubicle might be a back bedroom, a public toilet block, the floor of a train, the front seat of a twisted, wrecked car or the confines of the patient compartment of an ambulance.

Just as the paramedic patient can potentially be anyone, the paramedic situation can similarly be anywhere – endlessly varied and difficult to control.

Danger, hazard and risk

The prehospital environment, given its uncontrolled and unpredictable nature, carries a wide variety of hazards. These include less obvious hazards such as exposure to infectious disease and post-traumatic stress or physical injuries from manual handling and other accidents. On a broader scale, hazards can be found with major incidents such as road trauma and chemical, biological and radiological events. The list includes exposure on roads or railways, leaking fuels, fire, atmospheric contamination, slippery surfaces and confined spaces. These major incidents will certainly require specialist management from a combating authority such as police, fire or state emergency services.

The consistent paramedic maxim must be personal safety first *then* patient safety. Dangerous situations may require a patient to be moved prior to thorough assessment or any procedures. Alternatively, presenting hazards may mean it is unsafe for the paramedic to approach at all, even though there is a patient in obvious need of care. Such hazards can include live powerlines, an unstable vehicle during trauma, an active shooter or an explosive or radiological situation. There may be delays while and until the hazard is negated. Patient assessment and procedures will follow only after a specific assessment of the situation risk has been made and it has been determined that it is safe to continue.

More recently, occupational violence towards paramedics has increased; this is partly attributable to illicit drug use. Improved situational awareness through training and experience, avoiding working alone when concerned and utilising support resources such as police

are all useful strategies to mitigate this hazard (Maguire et al., 2018).

Not all hazards will be present at the scene outset. Anxious or aggressive friends or family can arrive after the paramedics. And paramedics themselves can introduce hazards through unsafe practices such as inadequate sharps safety, inappropriate manual handling or inattention to personal protection.

Familiarity with particular events and hazards can influence the paramedic's perception of the risk involved (Smith et al., 2011). Injuries to paramedics occur at a rate seven times the national average in Australia, double the rate of police officers (Maguire et al., 2014). In particular, accidents associated with ambulance vehicles, both responding and within the patient compartment, are overrepresented and problematic for ambulance services (Maguire, 2011).

Environment

The environment can influence and even dictate paramedic actions. Decisions will frequently have to be made to modify or delay assessment and procedures to safely accommodate adverse environmental factors. Extremes in temperature can adversely impact both the patient and the paramedic responder in terms of physiological responses and the ability to operate. Rain, wind and fog also have a similar impact.

Coats, gloves and other cold/wet weather protection limit what can be performed. It may be necessary to first transfer the patient to a protected environment, such as within the ambulance itself. Conversely, it can be equally difficult to perform more demanding physical tasks such as cardiopulmonary resuscitation and manual handling in hot environments. Improvised shading can sometimes be organised by co-responding rescue agencies or even by bystanders.

Some procedures might be considered necessary for patient care, such as splinting for musculoskeletal trauma. The benefits of such care may need to be weighed against pressing environmental factors. Burning hot road surfaces may cause worse injury than the patient already has, while cold and rain may exacerbate hypothermia, increasing morbidity and mortality. The prolonged exposure of a patient to an austere environment can worsen their presentation and is associated with poorer outcomes with extremes of temperature (Balvers et al., 2016; Forristal et al., 2019; Gupta et al., 2016; Ireland et al., 2011; Keqne, 2016).

Finally, time of day is a factor. Night operations vary considerably from those during the day. Fatigue is common at night (and is discussed later in this chapter). Fewer people will be available at night where information or assistance from bystanders is required. Hazards will be more difficult to see, necessitating alternative lighting options including torches, temporary lighting or even the use of vehicle headlights and external lighting. Reduced light can make it far more challenging to assess patients thoroughly and to perform some procedures. Conversely, bright sunshine can bring its own difficulties, including making equipment screens difficult to read or impeding visualisation during laryngoscopy.

Limited time

Paramedics are often the first in attendance to initiate care. They are required to estimate the urgency of clinical presentations and refer the patient, usually by expeditious ambulance transport, to an appropriate receiving hospital. This all takes time – and the more the paramedic does, the more time it will likely take.

Prehospital times are typically measured by both ambulance services and governments. These can impact on ambulance availability, operational costs and, most importantly, adverse patient outcomes. Many health systems include measures of time to hospital treatment, including stroke, cardiac and trauma systems (Brown et al., 2016; Farshid et al., 2015; Harmsen et al., 2015; Pulvers and Watson, 2017).

Decreases in prehospital time are not best brought about simply by rushing and urgency. This can lead to errors and accidents. Instead, efficient patient assessment and examination methods, competent procedural performance, sometimes delayed until within the confines of the ambulance, and correct patient movement methods are the tools to minimise time and delays.

Even with severe limitations on patient contact time, there is scope for the management of priority signs or symptoms, including lifesaving defibrillation or tension pneumothorax decompression. Even dressing minor wounds or administering analgesia can still be performed during patient transport to hospital. The extent of prehospital practice will vary with the severity of the patient's illness and the proximity to more definitive medical support.

Limited information

The prehospital world lacks many advanced diagnostic methods, including x-ray, blood analysis and diagnostic scans. Similarly, paramedics do not usually have access to detailed or accurate medical records and patient histories, nor rely on precise diagnosis or the availability of specialist expertise. Paramedic assessment tools are designed to identify critical signs, symptoms and compromise in one or more body systems that prompt likely interventions.

Paramedics have clinical practice guidelines to follow, and rely on recognising the emergency then applying the appropriate guideline effectively. These guidelines form the visible edge of the balance between following directions and the clinical judgment required to address the varied clinical problems. Clinical judgment is most effective when supported by evaluation and decision-making tools (Fullerton et al., 2012; Kleber et al., 2014; Wallgren et al., 2014). The application of many practical procedures can be guided by algorithms to improve patient outcomes.

Uncertainty is a constant companion for the paramedic – a feeling that must be overcome to allow effective practice (Harenčárová, 2017). In hospital, the treating practitioner will frequently devise differential diagnoses and follow a path, including pathology and radiological investigations, before forming a conclusion. This will not usually be the case for paramedics.

Rather, overcoming uncertainty is attempted using such principles as 'do no harm', 'treat for the most likely worst case' and 'avoid excluding serious options too quickly', along with making use of checklists, algorithms, communication with colleagues and occasional external consultation. However, this can lead to an overestimation of the problem's severity (Miles et al., 2018). Even where these algorithmic tools exist, paramedics have still been shown to be strongly influenced by experience, cognition and 'gut feeling'. This can be at the expense of gathering the critical information that is available, including vital signs and other physical assessment (Newgard et al., 2011). Situational experience should not be thought of as something disadvantageous, however, as it is strongly associated with broader problem consideration and an increased accuracy and speed of decision making (Smith et al., 2013).

The very nature of emergency situations creates conditions that are likely to lead to errors and cognition overload (Croskerry, 2014). Inexperience reduces cognitive ability and the ability to recognise important cues and explore a range of assessments and options (Smith et al., 2013). Errors do not always have a simple human cause. They often follow a series of events or system inadequacies that combine with 'time pressure, diagnostic uncertainty and cognitive overload, limited information and hazardous conditions' (Lammers et al., 2012).

Real-life training involving simulations blended with classroom learning can improve paramedics' ability to identify the conditions that produce errors (Lammers et al., 2012) and to use paramedic skills (Cowling and Birt, 2018; Herbstreit et al., 2017; Teteris et al., 2012; Van Dillen et al., 2016). Regular training with repeated feedback on progress can improve performance (Bosse et al., 2015) and help maintain readiness for and proficiency in rarely performed skills (Andreatta et al., 2016; Campbell et al., 2015).

When training in skills, vary the mode, including mannequins, mock-ups, cadaver labs and clinical placements, to avoid developing a false sense of success (Austlid et al., 2017). And wherever possible, make use of simulated patients, accurately acting in roles, to enhance clinical performance (Herbstreit et al., 2017).

Limited resources

Paramedics have relatively few invasive skills and medications available to them. Everything for prehospital use must be compact and lightweight, much of it squeezed into portable bags. Heavier or otherwise preferred hospital options might not be logistically viable for prehospital responders. This frequently compromises the selection of equipment and encourages multiple or hybridised use (Bigham and Welsford, 2015).

Some situations may require more personnel than are immediately or even ultimately available. Complex cases such as cardiac arrest or multi-trauma scenes are such examples. This may require prioritising, delaying or omitting some elements, and these cases should never be allowed to introduce risk for the paramedic.

Incidents where patient numbers overwhelm the available paramedic resources, including mass casualty events, may dictate the extent of the patient assessment or procedures that are possible. To provide care for the highest number of patients, the individual care given, if any, may vary with the scale of the incident.

Crowds and audience

Interviewing and assessing a patient in prominent view or outside of the home can be daunting for all. Paramedic practice in front of a crowd, particularly where the likelihood of being filmed or recorded is omnipresent, is challenging and confronting. The paramedic situation can include considerable public scrutiny at sporting, roadway and other major incidents. Being able to continue to perform the paramedic role under this scrutiny can clearly be distracting. Use can be made of police or security in some cases to move people back. In other cases, it may be possible to create an artificial screen for privacy or to move the patient to the privacy of the ambulance.

Even in the relatively safe confines of patients' homes or the ambulance vehicle itself, family members and friends can provide a variety of challenges. These people may require explanation of assessment or procedures or they may require reassurance and emotional support. People at a scene can sometimes be problematic, behaving in an obstructive or confrontational manner. In some cases it can be more beneficial to keep these people within the immediate vicinity of the patient, particularly where children are involved or there are cultural issues that necessitate this. In others, scene management may require having people being moved away for privacy or restrained by police.

Patients who must be managed in public view may still wish to maintain their privacy and dignity. The removal of clothing and exposure of intimate parts of their body will be undesirable for many people, even those with serious illness or injury. The need to provide emergency assessment and care should not automatically be allowed to override these important patient considerations. Look for methods to maintain privacy as far as is practicable, ideally by removing either onlookers or the patient to provide seclusion.

Teamwork and leadership

Patient assessment and procedures may not always be effectively performed in isolation. Integrating specific patient treatment into a holistic package of care requires tasks being prioritised and shared between those present. Some procedures will require cooperation to complete, including patient restraint or physical support. More active involvement may occasionally be necessary to provide direct assistance during the procedure.

As with any team effort, roles must be delineated and a leader decided on. The functioning of a team involves the potential for errors in communication, interpretation of problems, vigilance during performance and the management provided to the patient (Sarcevic et al., 2012). Clarifying the team leadership and roles can help avoid these problems.

Paramedic operations are not performed in isolation in health or emergency systems. Major incidents, including vehicle collisions, entrapments, industrial accidents and building fires, all require integrated teamwork. Paramedic managers are frequently embedded within the emergency management team structure to coordinate inter-agency cooperation. Paramedics themselves are integral members of urban search and rescue, road rescue and industrial rescue teams.

Patient care must also be integrated into the overall health system, ideally providing a seamless transition from one to the next. Paramedic practice should be consistent with emergency department expectations and the subsequent hospital and healthcare chain. It is pointless operating independently if that does not improve the collective effort. Input and endorsement is sought from peak bodies, including those for emergency, trauma, obstetrics and paediatrics, before any practice enters normal prehospital operations.

Rather than de-skilling and encroachment, a more sensible outcome is observed where the most appropriate person provides care at the most appropriate time. A good example of this is the shift to paramedic prehospital 12-lead electrocardiograph and thrombolysis delivery. The available evidence indicated the most logical point of delivery was prehospital, pushing the paramedic scope to increase rather than decrease (Davis et al., 2017; Doan et al., 2019; Khan et al., 2016; Mannsverk et al., 2019). Subsequent evidence is continually gathered in detail to define its effectiveness. Activities that were once only within the scope of traditional senior medical practitioners are progressively making their way into prehospital practice.

Single responder operations

Paramedics have been operating in Australia and New Zealand in solo emergency roles for many years. Though these typically do not involve patient transport, they do include assessing patients and performing procedures. This adds an extra dimension to clinical practice, due to the reduced ability to double check or to have assistance at hand when needed.

A new role of paramedic practitioner has appeared, with increased scope for less urgent in-home care, particularly in rural and more isolated areas (Hoyle et al., 2012). Paramedics are often called to manage patients who have complex chronic health problems and great social difficulties that lie outside the traditional definition of an emergency (Goldstein et al., 2015; Paul et al., 2017; Ross et al., 2017; Simpson et al., 2013; Tiedemann et al., 2013). This occupational transition can further relieve the overwhelmed hospital and nursing services who would otherwise be turned to for these situations. Evidence will continue to be gathered as to patient outcomes with this new approach (Bigham et al., 2013; Tohira et al., 2014; Woollard, 2015).

Paramedics must always recognise and operate within their scope of practice. If a procedure cannot be safely or effectively completed alone, call for and await support. On occasion, use can be made of bystanders and others at a callout. Medical consultation, which effectively, even if not physically, brings the expert to the scene, helps support that line (Gonzalez et al., 2011).

Stressors

Patient presentation can occasionally be stressful for paramedics, leading to such unwanted outcomes as post-traumatic stress disorder and medical errors, particularly when the patient is a child (Hegg-Deloye et al., 2014; Fowler et al., 2018; Guise et al., 2017; Regehr and LeBlanc, 2017; Streb et al., 2014). Stress associated with critically ill patients and complex procedures contributes to cognitive overload, impairing decision making and situational awareness and leading to the paramedic 'becoming task focused' (Frerk et al., 2015).

Difficult exposures can include people who are deceased or have disadvantaged lifestyles, graphic injuries or incredible misfortune. Every type of case will have to be attended for the first time, increasing the novice's vulnerability (Fjeldheim et al., 2014). Post case debriefing and the use of psychological support mechanisms should be normal paramedic practice. Operational requirements may dictate this immediately after a callout or, alternatively, at a more suitable time later.

Fatigue

Fatigue is frequently associated with paramedic practice, particularly given the association with long and night shift requirements. Rest breaks can be unpredictable, interrupted and even delayed or absent. Shift work, particularly the rotating style of work paramedics frequently perform, can have an adverse impact on sleep (Anderson, 2019; Kirby et al., 2016). This can, in turn, impact adversely on injuries, mental health and the ability to drive to, from and at work (Donnelly et al., 2019; Pyper and Paterson, 2016; Ramey et al., 2019; Rawat et al., 2015).

Increased errors and adverse patient events are associated with fatigue (Donnelly et al., 2019; Pyper and Paterson, 2016; Ramey et al., 2019). Many paramedic assessments and procedures require careful focus, a complex assembly of the available information or fine motor skills. There is considerable scope for error to occur, and fatigue is a very unwanted accompaniment.

Compromised sleep patterns are associated with reduced empathy for patients (Guadagni et al., 2018). Empathy is a key part of a positive interaction between patient and paramedic. This is important not only for achieving best patient care outcomes, but equally so for maintaining resilience and a positive attitude among paramedics (Rawat et al., 2015; Williams et al., 2017).

Fatigue can also occur as a result of work practice. Long periods of relative inactivity at prolonged standby scenes or, conversely, intense physical activities such as cardiopulmonary resuscitation or heavy manual handling can be equally fatiguing and compromise the paramedic's continuing performance.

Some procedures can be fatiguing on different parts of the body. This is particularly so where cramping hand positions or awkward postures must be maintained for extended periods of time.

The ambulance vehicle

Regardless of the situational nature of any call, the final part of the paramedic's scope of operation is within the ambulance vehicle itself. Frequently, this will be the place to retreat to when external factors are too challenging or troublesome. Most calls – and certainly when any patient is transported – will involve some patient care being provided within the ambulance itself.

The design and layout of ambulance vehicles is an increasingly complex and purposeful science. Extensive consultation is typically involved before they finally enter production. A standard configuration for an ambulance includes a bed for the patient and at least one seat (with restraining belts) for the paramedic(s). External opening lockers allow quick access to portable equipment when attending calls, while there are multiple cupboards, drawers and shelves inside the vehicle for storage, working and equipment restraint.

Space is the always present challenge in ambulance design. The smaller the vehicle, the smaller the amount of space in which to work. Even larger ambulances entail some challenges moving around, accessing cupboards with the patient/stretcher in place and providing patient care. Two elements are always in conflict:

1. Providing effective patient care when accessing multiple items, cupboards and patient vantage points, which is exacerbated when there is more than one crew member in the patient cabin.
2. Ensuring safety, restraint and good posture while in an unpredictably moving ambulance.

Ironically, ambulance vehicles are not always the best places to provide patient care. The cramped space forces poor postures, reduced patient access options and limited ability for assistants during procedures. Moving ambulances increase the challenges and reduce safety considerably.

Give thought to what equipment may be needed before moving away, to reduce the challenges of accessing it afterwards. Restrain all equipment in the position in which it will be most effective, and position people in the ambulance where they can best perform their allocated tasks. Stop the ambulance whenever difficult or delicate skills are being performed to reduce noise and movement. This includes performing injections and assessments such as blood pressure, chest auscultation and electrocardiography.

The ambulance should not be considered the ideal place to work, nor ignored during student training. Perform training exercises and scenarios with some time spent routinely in the ambulance compartment to ensure the idiosyncrasies of this part of the paramedic role are truly understood.

References

Anderson, L., 2019. The impact of paramedic shift work on the family system: a literature review. *Journal of Paramedic Practice*, 11(8), 335–341.

Andreatta, P.B., Dooley-Hash, S.L., Klotz, J.J., Hauptman, J.G., Biddinger, B. and House, J.B., 2016. Retention curves for pediatric and neonatal intubation skills after simulation-based training. *Pediatric Emergency Care*, 32(2), 71–76.

Austlid, I., Arkestaal, K.L. and Kibsgaard, H.P., 2017. Skill learning and retention. *Journal of Trauma and Acute Care Surgery*, 82(6S), S103–S106.

Balvers, K., Van der Horst, M., Graumans, M., Boer, C., Binnekade, J.M., Goslings, J.C. and Juffermans, N.P., 2016. Hypothermia as a predictor for mortality in trauma patients at admittance to the Intensive Care Unit. *Journal of Emergencies, Trauma, and Shock*, 9(3), 97.

Bigham, B.L., Kennedy, S.M., Drennan, I. and Morrison, L.J., 2013. Expanding paramedic scope of practice in the community: a systematic review of the literature. *Prehospital Emergency Care*, 17(3), 361–372.

Bigham, B. and Welsford, M., 2015. Applying hospital evidence to paramedicine: issues of indirectness, validity and knowledge translation. *Canadian Journal of Emergency Medicine*, 17(3), 281–285.

Bosse, H.M., Mohr, J., Buss, B., Krautter, M., Weyrich, P., Herzog, W., Jünger, J. and Nikendei, C., 2015. The benefit of repetitive skills training and frequency of expert feedback in the early acquisition of procedural skills. *BMC Medical Education*, 15(1), 22.

Brown, J.B., Rosengart, M.R., Forsythe, R.M., Reynolds, B.R., Gestring, M.L., Hallinan, W.M., Peitzman, A.B., Billiar, T.R. and Sperry, J.L., 2016. Not all prehospital time is equal: influence of scene time on mortality. *Journal of Trauma and Acute Care Surgery*, 81(1), 93.

Campbell, D., Shepherd, I., McGrail, M., Kassell, L., Connolly, M., Williams, B. and Nestel, D., 2015. Procedural skills practice and training needs of doctors, nurses, midwives and paramedics in rural Victoria. *Advances in Medical Education and Practice*, 6, 183.

Cowling, M. and Birt, J., 2018. Pedagogy before technology: a design-based research approach to enhancing skills development in paramedic science using mixed reality. *Information*, 9(2), 29.

Croskerry, P., 2014. ED cognition: any decision by anyone at any time. *Canadian Journal of Emergency Medicine*, 16(1), 13–19.

Davis, P., Howie, G. and Dicker, B., 2017. New Zealand paramedics are ready for an autonomous pre-hospital thrombolysis protocol. *Australasian Journal of Paramedicine*, 14(3).

Doan, T.N., Schultz, B.V., Rashford, S., Rogers, B., Prior, M., Vollbon, W. and Bosley, E., 2019. Prehospital ST-segment elevation myocardial infarction (STEMI) in Queensland, Australia: findings from 11 years of the statewide prehospital reperfusion strategy. *Prehospital Emergency Care*, 1–9.

Donnelly, E.A., Bradford, P., Davis, M., Hedges, C., Socha, D. and Morassutti, P., 2019. Fatigue and safety in paramedicine. *Canadian Journal of Emergency Medicine*, 1–4.

Farshid, A., Allada, C., Chandrasekhar, J., Marley, P., McGill, D., O'Connor, S., Rahman, M., Tan, R. and Shadbolt, B., 2015. Shorter ischaemic time and improved survival with pre-hospital STEMI diagnosis and direct transfer for primary PCI. *Heart, Lung and Circulation*, 24(3), 234–240.

Fjeldheim, C.B., Nöthling, J., Pretorius, K., Basson, M., Ganasen, K., Heneke, R., Cloete, K.J. and Seedat, S., 2014. Trauma exposure, posttraumatic stress disorder and the effect of explanatory variables in paramedic trainees. *BMC Emergency Medicine*, 14(1), 11.

Forristal, C., Van Aarsen, K., Columbus, M., Wei, J., Vogt, K. and Mal, S., 2019. Predictors of hypothermia upon trauma center arrival in severe trauma patients transported to hospital via EMS. *Prehospital Emergency Care*, 1–8.

Fowler, J., Beovich, B. and Williams, B., 2018. Improving paramedic confidence with paediatric patients: A scoping review. *Australasian Journal of Paramedicine*, 15(1).

Frerk, C., Mitchell, V.S., McNarry, A.F., Mendonca, C., Bhagrath, R., Patel, A., O'Sullivan, E.P., Woodall, N.M., Ahmad, I., 2015. Difficult Airway Society intubation guidelines working group: Difficult Airway Society 2015 guidelines for management of unanticipated difficult intubation in adults. *British Journal of Anaesthesia*, 115(6), 827–848.

Fullerton, J.N., Price, C.L., Silvey, N.E., Brace, S.J. and Perkins, G.D., 2012. Is the Modified Early Warning Score (MEWS) superior to clinician judgement in detecting critical illness in the pre-hospital environment? *Resuscitation*, 83(5), 557–562.

Goldstein, J., Jensen, J.L., Carter, A.J., Travers, A.H. and Rockwood, K., 2015. The epidemiology of prehospital emergency responses for older adults in a provincial EMS system. *Canadian Journal of Emergency Medicine*, 17(5), 491–496.

Gonzalez, M.A., Hanna, N., Rodrigo, M.E., Satler, L.F. and Waksman, R., 2011. Reliability of prehospital real-time cellular video phone in assessing the simplified National Institutes of Health Stroke Scale in patients with acute stroke: a novel telemedicine technology. *Stroke*, 42(6), 1522–1527.

Guadagni, V., Cook, E., Hart, C., Burles, F. and Iaria, G., 2018. Poor sleep quality affects empathic responses in experienced paramedics. *Sleep and Biological Rhythms*, 16(3), 365–368.

Guise, J.M., Hansen, M., O'Brien, K., Dickinson, C., Meckler, G., Engle, P., Lambert, W. and Jui, J., 2017. Emergency medical services responders' perceptions of the effect of stress and anxiety on patient safety in the out-of-hospital emergency care of children: a qualitative study. *BMJ Open*, 7(2), e014057.

Gupta, B., Gautam, P.L., Katyal, S. and Gautam, N., 2016. Hot climate and perioperative outcome in trauma patients. *Journal of Clinical and Diagnostic Research*, 10(4), UC01.

Harenčárová, H., 2017. Managing uncertainty in paramedics' decision making. *Journal of Cognitive Engineering and Decision Making*, 11(1), 42–62.

Harmsen, A.M.K., Giannakopoulos, G.F., Moerbeek, P.R., Jansma, E.P., Bonjer, H.J. and Bloemers, F.W., 2015. The influence of prehospital time on trauma patients' outcome: a systematic review. *Injury*, 46(4), 602–609.

Hegg-Deloye, S., Brassard, P., Jauvin, N., Prairie, J., Larouche, D., Poirier, P., Tremblay, A. and Corbeil, P., 2014. Current state of knowledge of post-traumatic stress, sleeping problems, obesity and cardiovascular disease in paramedics. *Emergency Medicine Journal*, 31(3), 242–247.

Herbstreit, F., Merse, S., Schnell, R., Noack, M., Dirkmann, D., Besuch, A. and Peters, J., 2017. Impact of standardized patients on the training of medical students to manage emergencies. *Medicine*, 96(5).

Hoyle, S., Swain, A.H., Fake, P. and Larsen, P.D., 2012. Introduction of an extended care paramedic model in New Zealand. *Emergency Medicine Australasia*, 24(6), 652–656.

Ireland, S., Endacott, R., Cameron, P., Fitzgerald, M. and Paul, E., 2011. The incidence and significance of accidental hypothermia in major trauma – a prospective observational study. *Resuscitation*, 82(3), 300–306.

Keane, M., 2016. Triad of death: the importance of temperature monitoring in trauma patients. *Emergency Nurse*, 24(5).

Khan, A.A., Williams, T., Savage, L., Stewart, P., Ashraf, A., Davies, A.J., Faddy, S., Attia, J., Oldmeadow, C., Bhagwandeen, R. and Fletcher, P.J., 2016. Pre-hospital thrombolysis in ST-segment elevation myocardial infarction: a regional Australian experience. *Medical Journal of Australia*, 205(3), 121–125.

Kirby, K., Moreland, S. and Pollard, J., 2016. The impact of working shifts: exploring the views of UK paramedics. *Journal of Paramedic Practice*, 8(5), 252–257.

Kleber, C., Giesecke, M.T., Lindner, T., Haas, N.P. and Buschmann, C.T., 2014. Requirement for a structured algorithm in cardiac arrest following major trauma: epidemiology, management errors, and preventability of traumatic deaths in Berlin. *Resuscitation*, 85(3), 405–410.

Lammers, R., Byrwa, M. and Fales, W., 2012. Root causes of errors in a simulated prehospital pediatric emergency. *Academic Emergency Medicine*, 19(1), 37–47.

Maguire, B.J., 2011. Transportation-related injuries and fatalities among emergency medical technicans and paramedics. *Prehospital and Disaster Medicine*, 26(5), 346–352.

Maguire, B.J., O'Meara, P.F., Brightwell, R.F., O'Neill, B.J. and Fitzgerald, G.J., 2014. Occupational injury risk among Australian paramedics: an analysis of national data. *Medical Journal of Australia*, 200(8), 477–480.

Maguire, B.J., O'Neill, B.J., O'Meara, P., Browne, M. and Dealy, M.T., 2018. Preventing EMS workplace violence: a mixed-methods analysis of insights from assaulted medics. *Injury*, 49(7), 1258–1265.

Mannsverk, J., Steigen, T., Wang, H., Tande, P.M., Dahle, B.M., Nedrejord, M.L., Hokland, I.O. and Gilbert, M., 2019. Trends in clinical outcomes and survival following prehospital thrombolytic therapy given by ambulance clinicians for ST-elevation myocardial infarction in rural sub-arctic Norway. *European Heart Journal: Acute Cardiovascular Care*, 8(1), 8–14.

Miles, J., Coster, J. and Jacques, R., 2018. Thinking on scene: using vignettes to assess the accuracy and rationale of paramedic decision making. *BMJ Open*, doi: 10.1136/bmjopen-2018-EMS.62.

Newgard, C.D., Nelson, M.J., Kampp, M., Saha, S., Zive, D., Schmidt, T., Daya, M., Jui, J., Wittwer, L., Warden, C. and Sahni, R., 2011. Out-of-hospital decision-making and factors influencing the regional distribution of injured patients in a trauma system. *Journal of Trauma*, 70(6), 1345.

Paul, S.S., Harvey, L., Carroll, T., Li, Q., Boufous, S., Priddis, A., Tiedemann, A., Clemson, L., Lord, S.R., Muecke, S. and Close, J.C., 2017. Trends in fall-related ambulance use and hospitalisation among older adults in NSW, 2006–2013: a retrospective, population-based study. *Public Health Research and Practice*, 27(4), e27341701–e27341701.

Pulvers, J.N. and Watson, J.D., 2017. If time is brain where is the improvement in prehospital time after stroke? *Frontiers in Neurology*, 8, 617.

Pyper, Z. and Paterson, J.L., 2016. Fatigue and mental health in Australian rural and regional ambulance personnel. *Emergency Medicine Australasia*, 28(1), 62–66.

Ramey, S., MacQuarrie, A., Cochrane, A., McCann, I., Johnston, C.W. and Batt, A.M., 2019. Drowsy and dangerous? Fatigue in paramedics: an overview. *Faculty & Staff Publications – Public Safety*, 27. Retrieved from: https://first.fanshawec.ca/fhcsps_publicsafety_facultystaffpublications/27

Rawat, V., Dawson, D., Schilders, M.R. and Kennedy, G.A., 2015. *Sleep disturbances among Victorian paramedics and the impact of demographic and biopsychosocial factors. The time of your life*. Melbourne: Australasian Chronobiology Society, pp. 12–17.

Regehr, C. and LeBlanc, V.R., 2017. PTSD, acute stress, performance and decision-making in emergency service workers. *Journal of the American Academy of Psychiatry and the Law*, 45(2), 184–192.

Ross, L., Jennings, P.A., Smith, K. and Williams, B., 2017. Paramedic attendance to older patients in Australia, and the prevalence and implications of psychosocial issues. *Prehospital Emergency Care*, 21(1), 32–38.

Sarcevic, A., Marsic, I. and Burd, R.S., 2012. Teamwork errors in trauma resuscitation. *ACM Transactions on Computer-Human Interaction (TOCHI)*, 19(2), 13.

Simpson, P.M., Bendall, J.C., Patterson, J., Tiedemann, A., Middleton, P.M. and Close, J.C., 2013. Epidemiology of ambulance responses to older people who have fallen in New South Wales, Australia. *Australasian Journal on Ageing*, 32(3), 171–176.

Smith, M.W., Bentley, M.A., Fernandez, A.R., Gibson, G., Schweikhart, S.B. and Woods, D.D., 2013. Performance of experienced versus less experienced paramedics in managing challenging scenarios: a cognitive task analysis study. *Annals of Emergency Medicine*, 62(4), 367–379.

Smith, E.C., Burkle, F.M. and Archer, F.L., 2011. Fear, familiarity, and the perception of risk: a quantitative analysis of disaster-specific concerns of paramedics. *Disaster Medicine and Public Health Preparedness*, 5(1), 46–53.

Streb, M., Häller, P. and Michael, T., 2014. PTSD in paramedics: resilience and sense of coherence. *Behavioural and Cognitive Psychotherapy*, 42(4), 452–463.

Teteris, E., Fraser, K., Wright, B. and McLaughlin, K., 2012. Does training learners on simulators benefit real patients? *Advances in Health Sciences Education*, 17(1), 137–144.

Tiedemann, A., Mikolaizak, A.S., Sherrington, C., Segin, K., Lord, S.R. and Close, J.C., 2013. Older fallers attended to by an ambulance but not transported to hospital: a vulnerable population at high risk of future falls. *Australian and New Zealand Journal of Public Health*, 37(2), 179–185.

Tohira, H., Williams, T.A., Jacobs, I., Bremner, A. and Finn, J., 2014. The impact of new prehospital practitioners on ambulance transportation to the emergency department: a systematic review and meta-analysis. *Emergency Medicine Journal*, 31(e1), e88–e94.

Van Dillen, C.M., Tice, M.R., Patel, A.D., Meurer, D.A., Tyndall, J.A., Elie, M.C. and Shuster, J.J., 2016. Trauma simulation training increases confidence levels in prehospital personnel performing life-saving interventions in trauma patients. *Emergency Medicine International*, doi: 10.1155/2016/5437490.

Wallgren, U.M., Castrén, M., Svensson, A.E. and Kurland, L., 2014. Identification of adult septic patients in the prehospital setting: a comparison of two screening tools and clinical judgment. *European Journal of Emergency Medicine*, 21(4), 260–265.

Williams, B., Lau, R., Thornton, E. and Olney, L.S., 2017. The relationship between empathy and burnout – lessons for paramedics: a scoping review. *Psychology Research and Behavior Management*, 10, 329.

Woollard, M., 2015. The role of the paramedic practitioner in the UK. *Australasian Journal of Paramedicine*, 4(1).

1.5 | Communication
Jeff Kenneally and Dianne Inglis

There are two great challenges for paramedics that are integral to every callout: logistics and communication. 'Logistics' refers to the practice of safely and effectively moving things about, including ambulances, equipment and patients.

Communication is continuous in one form or other from the very moment the call is received. Information is gathered by the call taker about location, safety and what is wrong with the patient. Advice is provided to bystanders, family and the patient. Pertinent information is then relayed to the paramedic crew dispatched to the scene.

Communication continues with the patient interview, family/carer/bystander questioning, reassurance, explanation, informed consent and decision making. Expert consultation can occur, as well as early hospital notification, followed by the handover from paramedic to triage nurse and then medical care. Medical documentation is produced as a record of what has occurred to ensure continuity of care.

Non-verbal communication

Assessing a patient and performing procedures requires cooperation and trust, and first impressions can be particularly important. Well groomed, hygienic, uniformed presentation is the ideal starting point. A genuine, welcoming facial expression, the introduction of all paramedics in attendance and enquiry as to the patient's name follows. And don't forget the family members.

If possible, adopt a relaxed position at the patient's eye level and avoid standing over the patient if they are in bed or on the floor (Kollhoff et al., 2017). It is also preferable to ask permission first before sitting on the patient's bed (Gupta et al., 2015).

Non-verbal cues through body language help convey or dissuade interest, compassion and empathy. Negative facial expressions, arms crossed or hands on hips and leaning against a wall are all examples of body language that conveys a lack of interest and empathy. When spoken words and body language do not match, the tendency will be to disbelieve the words or consider them insincere.

Equally, watch the patient and family for their body language. This can betray apprehension, fear, distrust or a failure to understand. Potentially aggressive or threatening people at any scene can be identified through their mannerisms, posture or other non-verbal cues. Conversely, their body language can also convey that they feel trusting and cooperative and are confident in your approach.

Non-verbal options including the use of appropriate touch, distraction, pets or clowning behaviour can be effective in reducing child anxiety (Abdelmoniem et al., 2016; Çelebioğlu et al., 2015; Kuo et al., 2016; Moore et al., 2015; Tener et al., 2016; Vagnoli et al., 2015). Some of these options might be suitable for adults too, particularly humour. However, this can be risky if the mood is not picked correctly, leading to puzzlement at least or disapproval and anger at worst (Togher et al., 2015).

Verbal patient communication

Verbal communication is paramount for paramedics, including radio communications, reassuring the family and patient, taking a history and providing patient information, education and medical handover. The paramedic must become adept at gathering specific information quickly, knowing the right sources. They must be able to throw out a net that is broad enough to be thorough and not miss anything key, yet not so broad as to cause a lengthy delay or be ineffective. Paramedic assessment typically has to be brief, gathering key information quickly but without jumping to incorrect conclusions.

Patient communication involves more than taking a logical history and gathering clinical information. It must include a significant emphasis on reassurance and explanation. There should also be provision for non-clinical conversation, where time permits. At all times the paramedic is expected to provide a professional demeanour. This can be hard to define and very individualised but typically includes courtesy, patience, kindness and generous listening skills. Patients and family do not necessarily understand what is wrong with them or what paramedics are doing to assist. Explain findings and procedures so that the patient and family all understand and are complicit in consent.

Those on scene look to the paramedic for guidance and an indication of the seriousness of the situation. Remain calm, interested and with a competent demeanour (Halpin et al., 2015; Togher et al., 2015). Alternatively, poor communication can lead to misunderstanding and complaints against paramedics (Anderson, 2019).

Communication must be empathetic. While this might be just another day in the office for a paramedic, it could be the worst day in memory for the patient and their family. Acknowledge patient complaints, even if they seem distracting, irrelevant or unimportant: they are important to the patient. If necessary, the patient interview can be brought back to the paramedic assessment again soon after the complaints have been addressed (Kollhoff et al., 2017). Offering dignity and compassion, listening and making a difference with the small things might make a huge difference in events. These are the things people will remember later and appreciate. Their worst day ever can be made even worse with poor communication or even no communication (Togher et al., 2015).

Students' communication skills can deteriorate with the greater focus on the medical components of their education. Role play or simulated training with actor-patients can help develop and maintain these skills (Kaplonyi et al., 2017; Keifenheim et al., 2015). When in the actual paramedic role, observe the communication skills and interactions of colleagues. Identify what works, what doesn't and why. Learn from these experiences, while always being mindful to be true to your own personality. You cannot simply act like someone else and still be genuine.

Patient language

There is no one language style that is applicable to all patients. For most occasions, language should be kept plain and free from technical words and jargon. These mean little if the patient does not understand them. However, some patients and family members may be more adept in this regard if they have a medical background themselves or where there is chronic illness.

The aim must be for the patient to feel comfort and ease from the outset. While relaxed language using the patient's own words can help reassure, form trust and elicit greater understanding, it can also be perceived as condescending and demeaning if used incorrectly. Confirm the patient's understanding through summation and having them repeat back key points. Acknowledge any key words the patient uses, such as 'turn', 'wonky' or 'gammy', and ensure you understand precisely what they mean. It is acceptable to then use those terms during the assessment, provided both parties are clear on what is being conveyed by them.

A relaxed style of communication that is effective with patients and family will not necessarily translate to other medical professionals, and may sound unprofessional and diminished. The language style must therefore be transformed into professional medical communication for the triage nurse, emergency physician or consultant/specialist. For example, what the patient describes as 'having a turn' might become 'a syncopal episode' in handover.

Language barriers

A major barrier to communication occurs where the patient does not share a common language with the paramedic.

Where there is sufficient time, and a telephone, use can be made of an interpreter service. However, this can be cumbersome, necessitating three-way conversations. Determining what language the patient speaks can be more difficult than it sounds, with the added complication of dialects and pronunciation. Family members, bystanders and non-verbal body language cues, which are more immediately at hand, can all assist, though there will always be uncertainty about what may be lost or added in the translation (Tate et al., 2016). Provide straightforward questions or information to make interpreting easier. Clarify each answer or response before continuing, and direct conversation at the patient rather than the interpreter to avoid any unwanted feelings of exclusion.

Language barriers can lead to varied or compromised patient care if not resolved (Tate, 2015). Hand gestures and pointing to body regions may have limited use. Nonetheless, paramedics become quite adept at dealing with these circumstances, often without any compromise in patient care or prehospital delays (Weiss et al., 2015). Demonstrating the desired procedure or miming your intentions may help you explain what it is you wish to do for the patient.

Hearing difficulty is another barrier to communication that can adversely impact on medical assessment (Cohen et al., 2017) and patient understanding, and increase the risk of misdiagnosis (Mormer et al., 2017). Communication with patients with poor hearing may be improved using simple strategies. Ensure the patient has their hearing aid in use. Where possible, reduce background noise and interference. Face the person and make eye contact while speaking; many people can follow lips during speech. Speak clearly and steadily. Beware of speaking too slowly or speaking unnecessarily loudly. These don't help and can appear condescending – the patient has a hearing problem, not an intellectual one. Repeat and clarify the main points. Particularly in the case of deafness, is there an interpreter who can sign? Can reading and writing be used to communicate?

Communication can be challenging where patients have cognitive difficulties. Dementia, stroke, acquired brain trauma or even confusion post trauma can form an effective barrier to communication, including dysphasia and issues with understanding (Jones, 2018). These challenges increase again where the patient cannot speak at all.

Honesty

Be honest with patients. This can be challenging for some if the news is bad. The patient or their family will often sense there is something wrong. Get the bad news out of the way as succinctly as you can, then replace it with whatever good news you can. The latter may be minimal and as simple as an offer of analgesia or other medical assistance.

Breaking bad news is one of the most challenging communication roles a paramedic can take on. Many feel unprepared and reluctant to do so (Anderson et al., 2019).

The process can be broken into key steps. Ideally, find an appropriate place for this to happen – although in emergencies there may be few options in this regard. Religious and cultural sensitivity is necessary. Provide the information necessary for patient/family understanding and answer any questions or fill in any information shortfalls that exist. Clarify any misunderstanding, ensuring the news is understood (Monden et al., 2016). There can be a considerable gap in understanding between the patient and paramedic prior to bad news being discussed (Maunder and Maguire, 2017).

If performing a procedure will cause the patient pain or discomfort, don't try to deceive them otherwise. This is particularly so for children, in whom distrust can be lasting. Parental touch and words, including an explanation of the procedure, can be valuable in settling vital signs and reducing anxiety in both patient and parent (Brown et al., 2018; Carmichael et al., 2015; Corniero et al., 2011; Jacobsen et al., 1990; Johnston et al., 2012; McAlvin and Carew-Lyons, 2014). Parental anxiety can enhance any child patient's anxiety, as can the inadequate performance of any procedure (Racine et al., 2015).

Patient inclusion

Communication allows patients to feel included in decision making and informed by having their many questions answered and anxieties eased, even if only slightly. Patients feel the need to be listened to (Togher et al., 2015). They will know when you simply have no more to offer. Listening is a critical part of the patient interview process. Take in the patient's actual words, reluctances and hesitation; remove distractions; encourage answers to be provided; and reflect back to the patient what they have said, for accuracy (Kollhoff et al., 2017).

Decision making can vary with urgency and capacity. There are two methods of patient inclusion in decision making: shared, where information is provided and an agreed decision is made, or motivational interviewing, where some aspect of patient behaviour needs to be overcome. The latter, involving leading to a conclusion and placating objections, is particularly useful where major or urgent decisions are required in the face of reluctance (Elwyn et al., 2014).

Disagreement is not common but it can occur. Questions of consent, end-of-life discussions or simply what a paramedic might consider to be bad decisions can arise. An understanding of consent is necessary to work through what can appear to be an emotional quagmire, and it is essential to use de-escalation strategies. There is no point allowing a situation to escalate to the point where communication and trust completely break down. It is also important to remember that, in most instances, anger is not personally directed towards the paramedic; rather, it is a response to the situation that is evolving. Responding to anger with anger will only cause the situation to deteriorate.

Patient cooperation, beyond the essential consent, is often required for the performance of procedures. Patients may have to follow a line of questioning or instructions, make particular movements, change positions or remain compliant during brief pain or discomfort. This will require explanation and trust.

It has been shown that even unresponsive patients can actually have varying levels of unrecognised consciousness, allowing for limited memory recall and experience of sensation, including pain (Rohaut et al., 2019). Where possible, verbal communications regarding assessment and procedures should include the usual patient explanations and reassurances, notwithstanding variations in consent with this cohort (see Chapter 1.6, Consent).

With paramedics trained and accustomed to working as a team, it can be easy to forget about the patient and their family. Technical discussions regarding clinical decisions, drug doses/calculations or electrocardiograph analysis have the potential to draw paramedics away from direct patient contact. These discussions can imply there is something for the patient to be concerned about while being not included. Minimise such discussions and, when they do occur, explain to the patient afterwards what was said.

Social media

Social media can create as many difficulties for paramedics and ambulance services as advantages. There has been a growing trend by paramedics to communicate, using social media platforms, details of what they are doing in their work. This can lead to complications of patient privacy, professional expectations from employers and the broader community (Baron and Townsend, 2017).

Similarly, other people can report on events as they occur, with almost every mobile phone being a video recorder and creating images that are immediately available to upload. Interpretations of events can be made that are out of context, such as while trying to de-escalate an agitated patient. Not all paramedic social media exposure will be intentional or even desired. This third-party recording can be intentionally directed at paramedics, producing uncomfortable circumstances to operate within.

Not specifically social media, mobile telephones can be used to take photographs to provide to receiving hospitals to assist with accident scenes and mechanism of injuries. These should be deleted afterwards and not used for any other purpose. Discretion should also be employed when taking any such photographs to avoid public misconception of their purpose.

Patient care documentation and handover

Patient documentation/records and immediate medical handover are a critical part of patient care and the communication process. A considerable amount of information can be gathered by paramedics, including much that would be difficult to gain otherwise. Details of medications found at a patient's home, descriptions by witnesses to events, mechanisms of injury that are appreciable only by seeing the aftermath, the manner in which a patient lives in their own home and the levels of social support might all be available only to treating paramedics. Medical professionals who are subsequent in the health chain might fail to receive or appreciate some of this information, or their awareness of it may be delayed.

Verbal handover typically precedes documentation to allow the immediate continuation of patient care. What is provided in the handover can vary with the urgency of the patient's condition. More urgent situations might require a briefer initial description followed by greater detail afterwards, allowing for assessment and intervention to begin without delay, while less urgent situations can allow for greater detail in the first instance.

Handover should include (Shah et al., 2016):
1. Introducing the patient
2. A brief description of what has happened or the major complaint
3. A list of the major injuries or associated information of the complaint
4. Vital signs; emphasis can be placed on abnormalities and those details that are particularly relevant to the complaint
5. A list of any therapies provided, including their effectiveness.

These elements are the primary elements necessary. To this can then be added supportive patient information:
6. Allergies and sensitivities
7. Past medical history
8. Medications taken by the patient
9. Any other factors of relevance, including social circumstances.

Handover effectiveness is adversely impacted by surrounding noise, urgency and haste to initiate patient management (Wood et al., 2015). Providing information in a standardised order may help avoid the omission of important information and improve listening and the retention of information by the receiver (Shah et al., 2016).

As with other forms of communication, non-verbal cues are important during handover to avoid patient errors and miscommunication. A paramedic's demeanour can emphasise or undermine verbal handover (Mattsson, 2017).

Verbal handovers will likely have gaps and be less comprehensive than the subsequent patient care record documentation. Further, the written record will still be present with the patient long after the paramedic crew has departed (Shelton and Sinclair, 2016).

The documentation must include, along with standard patient details including address and birthdate, a more detailed description of the way a patient presented and what therapies were provided, including specific times, complications/difficulties, any responses to therapies and changes in condition during care. Incomplete or incorrect documentation is a source of avoidable error (Drach-Zahavy and Hadid, 2015).

In some emergency situations, patients and sometimes even family members will not be in a position to offer consent to procedures. Such situations include unconsciousness, drug-affected patients and mental health emergencies. In some cases, the only record of events prior to any procedure will be the patient care record. These documents will not only maintain the continuity of care for in-hospital practice, but they can also form the basis of evidence in a coroner's and other legal courts. Such documentation should always include not only the procedural details, but justification and explanation for any patient exposure, contact or invasive therapy that is reliant on implicit consent. Documentation must provide accurate details and records of events, and be completed as soon as practicable following the events.

References

Abdelmoniem, S.A. and Mahmoud, S.A., 2016. Comparative evaluation of passive, active, and passive-active distraction techniques on pain perception during local anesthesia administration in children. *Journal of Advanced Research*, 7(3), 551–556.

Anderson, B., 2019. Reflecting on the communication process in health care. Part 1: clinical practice – breaking bad news. *British Journal of Nursing*, 28(13), 858–863.

Anderson, N., Slark, J. and Gott, M., 2019. How are ambulance personnel prepared and supported to withhold or terminate resuscitation and manage patient death in the field? A scoping review. *Australasian Journal of Paramedicine*, 16.

Baron, A. and Townsend, R., 2017. Live tweeting by ambulance services: a growing concern. *Journal of Paramedic Practice*, 9(7), 282–286.

Brown, E.A., De Young, A., Kimble, R. and Kenardy, J., 2018. Review of a parent's influence on pediatric procedural distress and recovery. *Clinical Child and Family Psychology Review*, 1–22.

Carmichael, N., Tsipis, J., Windmueller, G., Mandel, L. and Estrella, E., 2015. 'Is it going to hurt?': the impact of the diagnostic odyssey on children and their families. *Journal of Genetic Counseling*, 24(2), 325–335.

Çelebioğlu, A., Gürol, A., Yildirim, Z.K. and Büyükavci, M., 2015. Effects of massage therapy on pain and anxiety arising from intrathecal therapy or bone marrow aspiration in children with cancer. *International Journal of Nursing Practice*, 21(6), 797–804.

Cohen, J.M., Blustein, J., Weinstein, B.E., Dischinger, H., Sherman, S., Grudzen, C. and Chodosh, J., 2017. Studies of physician-patient communication with older patients: How often is hearing loss considered? A systematic literature review. *Journal of the American Geriatrics Society*, 65(8), 1642–1649.

Corniero, P., Gamell, A., Cotanda, C.P., Trenchs, V. and Cubells, C.L., 2011. Family presence during invasive procedures at the emergency department: what is the opinion of Spanish medical staff? *Pediatric Emergency Care*, 27(2), 86–91.

Drach-Zahavy, A. and Hadid, N., 2015. Nursing handovers as resilient points of care: linking handover strategies to treatment errors in the patient care in the following shift. *Journal of Advanced Nursing*, 71(5), 1135–1145.

Elwyn, G., Dehlendorf, C., Epstein, R.M., Marrin, K., White, J. and Frosch, D.L., 2014. Shared decision making and motivational interviewing: achieving patient-centered care across the spectrum of health care problems. *Annals of Family Medicine*, 12(3), 270–275.

Gupta, A., Harris, S. and Naina, H., 2015. To sit or stand during the medical interview: a poll of Caucasian patients. *Journal of Medical Practice Management: MPM*, 31(2), 110–112.

Halpin, D., Hyland, M., Blake, S., Seamark, C., Pinnuck, M., Ward, D., Whalley, B., Greaves, C., Hawkins, A. and Seamark, D., 2015. Understanding fear and anxiety in patients at the time of an exacerbation of chronic obstructive pulmonary disease: a qualitative study. *JRSM Open*, 6(12), 2054270415614543.

Jacobsen, P.B., Manne, S.L., Gorfinkle, K., Schorr, O., Rapkin, B. and Redd, W.H., 1990. Analysis of child and parent behavior during painful medical procedures. *Health Psychology*, 9(5), 559.

Johnston, C.C., Rennick, J.E., Filion, F., Campbell-Yeo, M., Goulet, C., Bell, L., Tucci, M. and Ranger, M., 2012. Maternal touch and talk for invasive procedures in infants and toddlers in the pediatric intensive care unit. *Journal of Pediatric Nursing: Nursing Care of Children and Families*, 27(2), 144–153.

Jones, V., 2018. Experiences of paramedics when dealing with patients with communication difficulties (Doctoral dissertation). Cardiff Metropolitan University. Retrieved from: http://hdl.handle.net/10369/9910

Kaplonyi, J., Bowles, K.A., Nestel, D., Kiegaldie, D., Maloney, S., Haines, T. and Williams, C., 2017. Understanding the impact of simulated patients on health care learners' communication skills: a systematic review. *Medical Education*, 51(12), 1209–1219.

Keifenheim, K.E., Teufel, M., Ip, J., Speiser, N., Leehr, E.J., Zipfel, S. and Herrmann-Werner, A., 2015. Teaching history taking to medical students: a systematic review. *BMC Medical Education*, 15(1), 159.

Kollhoff, M., Owings, C.S. and Cathcart-Rake, W., 2017. Preparing medical students for the medical interview. *Kansas Journal of Medicine*, 10(1), 22.

Kuo, H.C., Pan, H.H., Creedy, D.K. and Tsao, Y., 2016. Distraction-based interventions for children undergoing venipuncture procedures: a randomized controlled study. *Clinical Nursing Research*, 1054773816686262.

Mattsson, J., 2017. The non-verbal communication in handover situations are the spice between the lines, to understand the severity of the patient's condition. *Journal of Nursing Education and Practice*, 7(5).

Maunder, E.Z. and Maguire, D., 2017. Breaking bad news: the need for a coping mechanism in paramedicine. *International Paramedic Practice*, 7(1), 3–7.

McAlvin, S.S. and Carew-Lyons, A., 2014. Family presence during resuscitation and invasive procedures in pediatric critical care: a systematic review. *American Journal of Critical Care*, 23(6), 477–485.

Monden, K.R., Gentry, L. and Cox, T.R., 2016, January. Delivering bad news to patients. In *Baylor University Medical Center Proceedings*, 29 (1). Dallas: Taylor & Francis, pp. 101–102.

Moore, E.R., Bennett, K.L., Dietrich, M.S. and Wells, N., 2015. The effect of directed medical play on young children's pain and distress during burn wound care. *Journal of Pediatric Health Care*, 29(3), 265–273.

Mormer, E., Cipkala-Gaffin, J., Bubb, K. and Neal, K., 2017, May. Hearing and health outcomes: recognizing and addressing hearing loss in hospitalized older adults. In *Seminars in Hearing*, 38(2). New York: Thieme Medical Publishers, pp. 153–159.

Racine, N.M., Pillai Riddell, R.R., Khan, M., Calic, M., Taddio, A. and Tablon, P., 2015. Systematic review: predisposing, precipitating, perpetuating, and present factors predicting anticipatory distress to painful medical procedures in children. *Journal of Pediatric Psychology*, 41(2), 159–181.

Rohaut, B., Eliseyev, A. and Claassen, J., 2019. Uncovering consciousness in unresponsive icu patients: technical, medical and ethical considerations. *Critical Care*, 23(1), 78.

Shah, Y., Alinier, G. and Pillay, Y., 2016. Clinical handover between paramedics and emergency department staff: SBAR and IMIST-AMBO acronyms. *International Paramedic Practice*, 6(2), 37–44.

Shelton, D. and Sinclair, P., 2016. Availability of ambulance patient care reports in the emergency department. *BMJ Open Quality*, 5(1), u209478–w3889.

Tate, R.C., 2015. The need for more prehospital research on language barriers: a narrative review. *Western Journal of Emergency Medicine*, 16(7), 1094.

Tate, R.C., Hodkinson, P.W., Meehan-Coussee, K. and Cooperstein, N., 2016. Strategies used by prehospital providers to overcome language barriers. *Prehospital Emergency Care*, 20(3), 404–414.

Tener, D., Ofir, S., Lev-Wiesel, R., Franco, N.L. and On, A., 2016. Seriously clowning: medical clowning interaction with children undergoing invasive examinations in hospitals. *Social Work in Health Care*, 55(4), 296–313.

Togher, F.J., O'Cathain, A., Phung, V.H., Turner, J. and Siriwardena, A.N., 2015. Reassurance as a key outcome valued by emergency ambulance service users: a qualitative interview study. *Health Expectations*, 18(6), 2951–2961.

Vagnoli, L., Caprilli, S., Vernucci, C., Zagni, S., Mugnai, F. and Messeri, A., 2015. Can presence of a dog reduce pain and distress in children during venipuncture? *Pain Management Nursing*, 16(2), 89–95.

Weiss, N.R., Weiss, S.J., Tate, R., Oglesbee, S. and Ernst, A.A., 2015. Language disparities in patients transported by emergency medical services. *American Journal of Emergency Medicine*, 33(12), 1737–1741.

Wood, K., Crouch, R., Rowland, E. and Pope, C., 2015. Clinical handovers between prehospital and hospital staff: literature review. *Emergency Medicine Journal*, 32(7), 577–581.

1.6 | Consent

Jeff Kenneally and Dianne Inglis

Paramedicine in New Zealand and Australia has increasingly been considered 'professional' in recent decades. The term 'professional' is difficult to define, but it can be considered in one respect to mean holding particular knowledge that others do not have, creating a dependent state that requires trust (Townsend and Luck, 2019). Progressive and continually evolving efforts continue to break this down into constituent elements, including competency and standards of expected behaviour and conduct.

The governance of paramedic practice has been overseen traditionally by regional, state or territory ambulance services. These are structured variously via government-run or charitable organisations, predominantly St John Ambulance or Wellington Free Ambulance. In 2018, Australia extended this into a system of national registration for paramedics, in line with that for nurses, medical practitioners and other health professionals. Legislation and regulations, administered by an oversight peak body, now sit alongside employer policies, established common-law principles and other associated health legislation.

Few would doubt that paramedics attending sick and injured patients typically bring best intentions to every callout. The clinical framework for this is built on tertiary education, ongoing training, professional development and the implementation of evidence-based clinical guidelines. Despite this, paramedics cannot simply assume they have autonomy to do whatever they want on every occasion because it is 'clinically correct'. Every patient must receive assessment and procedures that are performed with empathy, understanding, explanation and reassurance; they do not need you to simply do things to them (Wong, 2015). There also needs to be a mechanism of understanding that any assessment or procedure is agreed to by the patient. This is referred to as 'consent'.

Informed consent

To assess a patient, perform any procedure or administer any medication, patient approval or permission is first required (Hein et al., 2015). The need to obtain permission acknowledges that the autonomy actually resides with the patient and not the paramedic (or any other medical professional). Consent is required for any patient contact, regardless of whether it is considered major or minor.

There are various ways for a patient to provide consent. The simplest, of course, is for the paramedic to simply ask the patient for permission and for them to verbally agree. However, this approach alone is not sufficient for consent to be valid.

Consent requires three elements for it to be considered validly provided (Lamont et al., 2016):

1. The consent must be freely and voluntarily given by the patient. The patient cannot be threatened or intimidated into any approval. There can be a fine line here if cajoling occurs because a therapy is considered imperative and a patient is being unreasonably obstructive (Kinnersley et al., 2013). The risk of ignoring a patient's true wishes is very high. In particular, a patient's family members may be employed to cajole the patient even though these same people may also be integral in providing the essential support that enables the patient to make decisions. In emergencies, consent might be sought when the patient is under duress and far from able to think clearly (Spatz et al., 2016). Notwithstanding this, the patient always has the right to disapprove of a decision.

2. The patient must be competent to provide their consent. Not everybody is able to make reasonable decisions for themselves. Competence requires a patient to have the capacity to understand what is wrong with them and why an assessment or procedure is necessary, and then act reasonably (Khoury and Khoury, 2015; Neilson and Chaimowitz, 2015). They need to be able to truly understand they are ill, be able to identify the risks versus benefits of refusal or consent, and then be able to communicate (in some unequivocal form) that decision (Kinnersley et al., 2013; Khoury and Khoury, 2015).

3. The consent provided must be informed. That is, the medical professional in the room is the paramedic and not usually the patient. The paramedic is the one who holds the knowledge the patient requires to make an informed decision. Once the patient is deemed competent, they need to be provided with sufficient information to be able to weigh up the decision (Neilson and Chaimowitz, 2015).

Of these three elements, informed consent is the most likely to demand paramedic input. There will often be some urgency during the interaction. Most likely there will seem – to the paramedic at least – to be a clear need to assess or provide some treatment. However, that need must be equally clear to the patient, so it is essential that the paramedic provides sufficient explanation or justification to achieve this.

While statements such as 'if it were me' or 'if it were my child' can be compelling, they are emotive and lack sufficient detail for making any informed decision. The person making the decision in this instance is not the person making the statement. Further, simply asking a patient what they wish to do without having discussed options and their particular merits is equally lacking in informative content.

Acceptable decision making in this context requires four key elements (Grootens-Wiegers et al., 2017):

1. The expression of the choice
2. An understanding of what has been stated, including the ability to focus on the information available and process it beyond the short term
3. A reasoning to support that understanding
4. An appreciation of the benefits and ramifications that accompany the decision.

Informed consent can be described as a discussion between paramedic (in this case) and patient (or legal representative, such as power of attorney), following which there will be an understanding of the expectations, risks, benefits and reasonable alternatives to any assessment or procedure and consequences of not having it (Khoury and Khoury, 2015; Kinnersley et al., 2013; Neilson and Chaimowitz, 2015). The scale of consent will likely be consistent with the scale of the event. For instance, the consent conversation to assess a patient's blood sugar would be significantly different from a conversation about administering thrombolysis medication during an acute coronary event.

A consent conversation may develop in steps throughout a single patient encounter. There may be a request to complete a thorough clinical assessment, supported by a further conversation about a specific element of the assessment, such as exposure of the chest to perform an electrocardiograph. Following this, a further conversation may occur where findings are discussed and a plan of management ensues, including the procedures to be performed and medications administered. In this case, informed consent would be difficult to achieve in a single conversation, as each action depends on the findings of the previous one. Consent is usually specific to the intended action and cannot necessarily be extended to any range of alternative or subsequent options unless they are also included in the original discussion (Neilson and Chaimowitz, 2015).

Consent is required even if the patient will clearly benefit from a procedure, as there is frequently a disadvantage to be considered too. Even if the patient does not ask sufficient questions to explore the consequences of the proposed action, this information should be volunteered by the paramedic anyway. However, how much information is considered necessary can be subjective. There is no easy and precise answer to this issue, though the test is 'what would the reasonable patient be likely to find significant?' (Kinnersley et al., 2013). The test for what is important is based not on what 'reasonable' paramedics would think, but on what 'reasonable' patients would think (Spatz et al., 2016). This will in all likelihood vary not only between procedures but also between patients.

The process of gaining informed consent satisfies a number of purposes. It helps protect patient rights, allows for patient-centred decision making, provides an effective record of the process and allows trust to be built for present and future interventions (Hall et al., 2012).

There are many reasons that informed consent can fail or be inadequate. Prehospital practice is typically fraught with time pressures; time is a significant factor in providing sufficiently informed consent (Fink et al., 2010; Steer, 2015). The need to give a detailed explanation of procedures, risks and benefits may be at odds with the perceived time available. Ideally, a patient should be allowed sufficient time to consider their decision (Neilson and Chaimowitz, 2015). However, it may be envisaged that providing further detail to the patient might only add to their distress during an emergency, or the information provided might be comprised of difficult medical terms and jargon. There may be conflict or extreme emotion at a scene that prohibits detailed informed discussion, and paramedics themselves may be insufficiently trained in what constitutes informed consent (Steer, 2015). The interpretation of consent can vary between what a reasonable patient/family would want to know and what a reasonable paramedic would usually discuss (Hall et al., 2012; Kinnersley et al., 2013; Neilson and Chaimowitz, 2015; Schenker et al. 2011; Spatz et al., 2016).

Though competent at law, there can be language and comprehension barriers between paramedic and patient/family that can form an impediment (Fink et al., 2010; Schenker et al., 2011). Comprehension is easily overestimated and influenced by age, education and anxiety (Hall et al., 2012).

There are four ethical principles around consent (Selinger, 2009):

1. Justice – the fairness and equality of any patient contact and treatment
2. Non-maleficence – the obligation not to inflict harm
3. Autonomy – the main principle defining informed consent
4. Beneficence – to have the clear intention that any patient interaction should be for their good; justice needs to be applied when deciding on treatments.

These principles should underpin all healthcare activities and should certainly be applied to any patient assessment or procedure. Honesty and truthfulness are vital elements of ensuring patient dignity.

Patient competency (capacity)

Patient competency can be difficult to determine, frequently relying on the ability of the assessor, compounded by the subjectivity of their observations and the complexity of any associated ethical issues (Grisso and Appelbaum, 1998). Judgments and determinations of capacity are not usually within the domain of paramedics, more frequently being determined at law (Lee and Goldstein, 2017). Questions of competency arise over children, the aged (particularly where there are dementia concerns), those with cognitive impairment and patients who are severely ill (Hiriscau and Reiter-Theil, 2017).

Impairment of cognitive reasoning can adversely affect the patient's capacity to provide consent. Some clinical conditions, including psychosis, severe mood disorder, drug or alcohol intoxication, or confusion following head injury, can remove the capacity for consent (Neilson and Chaimowitz, 2015). However, the existence of a mental health disorder does not automatically exclude capacity. Many people will still have capacity to make valid decisions for themselves. Patients with mild dementia and cognitive impairment can have decreased decision-making ability yet still retain sufficient capacity (Appelbaum, 2010; Lee and Goldstein, 2017). Consideration must also be given to multiple capacities in one person. A person may have sufficient capacity to understand and make decisions on lesser interventions but not meet the standard for more complex decisions.

At the other extreme, informed consent may be suspended entirely when a mental health condition is such that a patient is made an involuntary patient. The governance over these circumstances is substantial but not without potential for human rights violations (McSherry and Waddington, 2017). Prescribed practitioners are required to provide interventions. In some instances this includes paramedics. Mental health legislation typically includes provision for emergency patient management in an acute crisis where involuntary status has not been invoked. Risk of harm to self or others is a typical precipitating factor.

A patient must have sufficient cognitive capacity to consent before it is accepted as valid. Like all others, a patient must be able to understand the consequences of treatment and future repercussions (Fields and Calvert, 2015). Where choices are provided by a person who has competence, these should continue to be supported if it is then later lost (Neilson and Chaimowitz, 2015). Incapacity should not be viewed by the clinician simply as an opportunity to intervene.

The common law doctrine of necessity is an English law that has passed down into New Zealand and Australian law. This doctrine allows an incapacitated person to be provided assessment or treatment that is deemed necessary. The risk of this is the removal of normal consent safeguards (Douglass, 2018). It does not override circumstances where a person has already defined their wishes previously (Lamont et al., 2016).

This doctrine has been enshrined into legislation such as the *Health and Disability Commissioner Act 1994* (NZ). It also enshrines the notion that even those with diminished capacity must be included in decision making as far as reasonably possible. Acting in someone else's best interests does not negate the need to involve the incapacitated person as much as possible and considering their 'wishes

and feelings'. Medical (clinical) paternalism is an inherent challenge to this (Douglass, 2018). Similar legislation exists throughout Australian state jurisdictions (Lamont et al., 2016).

In addition, New Zealand's Treaty of Waitangi outlines the relationship obligations between government (the Crown) and the Māori people. In particular, the Treaty underscores Māori beliefs, values, diversity and cultural differences, adding a level of protection where the doctrine of necessity is in question (Douglass, 2018).

Children and consent

By legal definition, every person under the age of 18 years is considered a child under the United Nations Convention on the Rights of the Child (Casby and Lyons, 2018). This same convention confers rights to consultation and consideration of the child's wishes. The huge variation in physical and mental aspects through age, experience, culture, illness and family all blur the line on just how different the right to self-determination of any individual child should be from that of a corresponding adult.

Where a child does not have capacity for consent, this will usually rest with the parents or, less commonly, with adopted parents or legal guardians and in court orders.

Capacity can be difficult to apply to children, though many will be considered to have necessary capacity (Neilson and Chaimowitz, 2015). The specific age at which it does exist is unclear and can depend on the individual and their life experience (Fives, 2016; Hein et al., 2015). With children, capacity is not assumed but established, first with some form of assessment, which varies with the significance of what is proposed. Age is a variable factor for capacity in children, with capacity for consent developing between 9 and 12 years of age. Children as young as 7 years old can begin to develop logical reasoning and decision making (Committee on Bioethics, 2016). Sufficient cognitive capacity is frequently achieved once the child is over 12 years, and usually developed by mid-adolescence (Committee on Bioethics, 2016).

The upper age limit for capacity questions is 17–18 years (Hein et al., 2015), with the presumption that most medical decisions can be reasonably handled by 16–18-year-olds (Casby and Lyons, 2018). As age decreases, so does maturity, making it increasingly relevant in informed decision making (Hein et al., 2015; Katz et al., 2016). For children younger than 16 years of age, the Gillick principle is generally applied; this assesses for *sufficient understanding and intelligence to enable full understanding of what is proposed* (Casby and Lyons, 2018; Kang and Kim, 2019; Moran-Ellis and Tisdall, 2019). Unfortunately, there is little in the way of sound guidance for determining this.

Child capacity can be unwittingly and incorrectly reduced simply because a child may not be compliant and agreeable with adults – a problem that does not happen as often to adult patients (Moran-Ellis and Tisdall, 2019). In the first instance, the child should be encouraged to involve the parents in decision making.

Paramedics and health professionals should deliver information to children in an age-appropriate manner (Katz et al., 2016) that acknowledges the true cognitive abilities of the child (Committee on Bioethics, 2016). The usual requirements of freedom of decision making, capacity and being informed continue to apply.

Parents have unique understanding of their child's needs, and typically focus on the child and the family rather than expressing their own personal choice (Hein et al., 2015). Where the child is too young to have capacity, parents have automatic consent provided they themselves have capacity (Fives, 2016; Hein et al., 2015). Despite this, parents have been shown to be unable to understand or recall the details on which they based their consent, which calls into question whether the consent was truly informed (Nadeau et al., 2010).

The automatic rights of parents are also not absolute. Parents do not have the right to allow harm to come to a child, and they have a duty to act in the child's best interests (Steer, 2015). If a child's life is threatened, essential therapy should not be withheld while trying to gain consent from an adult who is not present (Casby and Lyons, 2018; Committee on Bioethics, 2016; Sirbaugh and Diekema, 2011).

Dissent and refusal in an adolescent can be even more challenging than when it occurs in adults. Where proposed interventions are not considered essential, it is reasonable to accept this. Similarly, where there is a chronic condition or a particularly poor prognosis anyway, an adolescent's right to refuse should be strongly considered (Committee on Bioethics, 2016). Where a child's consent is in question, the situation can vary in a similar way to that of others with doubtful capacity. The lesser the risk and complexity of the assessment or procedure, the more control the child can be allowed (Casby and Lyons, 2018).

A particular difficulty with adolescent children is confidentiality. Where consent is considered appropriate, difficulty can then arise where the parents wish to know information that the child has provided in confidence (Dreisinger and Zapolsky, 2018; Murphy and Goldstein, 2017). Situations where confidentiality is particularly favoured include sexual health (including pregnancy), mental health and substance abuse (Committee on Bioethics, 2016; Murphy and Goldstein, 2017). Though uncommonly encountered, this can be particularly challenging for paramedics. Attempt to convince (not coerce) the child to agree to parental involvement, but also try to understand their objections. If the child is considered to have capacity, their right to confidentiality must be respected (Kang and Kim, 2019). It is important to keep appropriate documentation of the attempts to convince the child otherwise and the reasons for respecting their capacity.

Implied consent

Consent can be implied. Patients who collapse in the street without anyone knowing anything about them are typically assumed to want resuscitation. Indeed, some treatments will likely restore the capacity of a patient to subsequently provide consent (Lee and Goldstein, 2017). It would be impractical if not impossible to seek permission when only minutes were available in any emergency. In this situation, the implication is paramedics will exercise their best judgment to provide the expected standard of care a reasonable patient would normally expect in this circumstance (Kinnersley et al., 2013). In other words, act in the best interests of the patient (Lamont et al., 2016; Townsend et al., 2019).

Consent is so well implied that it is the reason orders for the refusal of treatment are created for terminally ill or aged care residents who specifically do not want these efforts.

Implied consent does not always refer to unconscious or gravely ill patients. If a patient recognises an item of equipment, such as a stethoscope or sphygmomanometer, and positions themselves or begins adjusting clothing to allow for its use, the implication is the patient is approving of the assessment/procedure. This sort of implied consent more commonly applies to lower level assessment and procedures (Townsend et al., 2019).

The inference of consent can also be in part drawn from where a patient has made calls for assistance, such as the act of calling an ambulance, though this should not be considered carte blanche for subsequent actions (Neilson and Chaimowitz, 2015).

Advance care directives

People who envisage losing capacity in the foreseeable future, particularly the aged or those with a degenerative illness, can elect to provide written (or sometimes verbal) instruction to their wishes in regard to healthcare issues. This instruction may be made in an official document such as an advance care directive, making it clear how a person wishes to be cared for if they become incapacitated. Advance care planning allows individuals to plan their goals and preferences, while competent, for future medical treatment and care in conjunction with family and medical practitioners (Rietjens et al., 2017; Stuart et al., 2017). The advance care directive is intended to be interactive between these parties and can allow for a proxy to take over when necessary (Mignani et al., 2017). It may predetermine power of attorney, giving a third party(s) authority to make medical decisions in the event of incapacitation. In such cases, consent passes to the third party.

These instructions more commonly spell out what treatments people do not want, and it may be the proxy who is the person paramedics must speak with for consent and instruction. These documents frequently focus on whether lifesaving interventions may be used or not (Lamont et al., 2016). In the absence of an advance care directive, family or carers are compelled to make emergency health decisions on behalf of the patient despite confronting their own often strong emotions and not always knowing the person's wishes (Pearse et al., 2019).

Despite the value of advance care directives and patients' willingness to participate in them, the conversations to initiate such directives can be difficult and are often avoided. Further, directives are not always immediately at hand when needed. This can leave a void for wishes and instructions that paramedics must overcome in the short term (Detering et al., 2017; Hemsley et al., 2019). In settings where an advance care directive is likely to exist, such as for aged care or terminal illness, paramedics should ask immediately if any such instructions are available. Where doubt exists, assessment and procedures can be commenced and then stopped again if further information comes to light. This may be in the form of verbal reiteration without actually sighting the formal document.

The documentation expressing the patient's wishes may be far less complex and detailed than a directive. These include emergency bracelets, chains and wallet documents that identify specific illnesses the patient may have and how they prefer to be treated. Diabetics, epileptics and anaphylactic patients fall into this group. Paramedics should inspect the patient for these when assessing someone who is unresponsive or incapacitated.

Refusal of treatment

Provided all of the requirements are met for informed consent, every person has the right to refuse treatment of any part of it, even to their own detriment (Hall et al., 2012; Kinnersley et al., 2013; Lamont et al., 2016). They are not compelled to agree with paramedic or any other medical requests, even if their decision is likely to be to their own detriment. This can include refusing transport by ambulance.

The paramedic may have difficulty with this. Attempts can be made to convey the gravity of any situation and the ramifications of persisting with refusal, include utilising family members to provide their point of view. However, these attempts must stop short of threat or undue influence in order to avoid the risk of the patient losing their freedom to make decisions.

The definition of urgency and emergency may not be shared between patient and paramedic. Conditions where an ambulance is called for assistance do not automatically mean there is not a requirement to seek consent. A good

example of this is during normal childbirth. As this is considered a normal life event rather than any emergency, maternal capacity is not lost and informed consent remains essential (Nour and Griffiths, 2016; Stohl, 2018).

Refusal of treatment may not be comprehensive. The patient may accept some assessment or therapy but not everything. Any refusal should be clarified with the patient and then documented in the patient care record.

Failure to receive consent

Performing an assessment or procedure without receiving consent can be considered variously as assault – an intentional act that creates a fearful mindset – or battery, where there is actual contact and touch that creates harm or offence (Lamont et al., 2016). Even minor touch or the belief that touch will occur can meet the definition of assault if it is unwanted (Khoury and Khoury, 2015). Patient compliance alone may not be sufficient to overcome this issue if other aspects of consent cannot be shown (Lane, 2016). This can be so even when the patient appears to cooperate or allow events to proceed. Patients can withdraw consent after commencement, at which point whatever is occurring should stop (Neilson and Chaimowitz, 2015).

For treating paramedics, unwanted assessment and particularly procedures/treatments given without valid consent can be considered assault. Further, consent might be invalidated if the information provided was insufficient or misrepresented. Where adverse outcome eventuates, duty of care failure and negligence might be the eventual remedy (Lamont et al., 2016).

In-hospital processes often involve written consent documentation and formal checklists for staff to work through with patients. They usually require signing to reflect the patient's agreement. Consent forms are not commonly associated with paramedic practice, aside from where the treatment and transport offered is refused. However, this is changing with the advent of invasive and comparatively elective procedures such as thrombolysis administration, where an extensive pre-checklist must be first completed. A patient's signing of consent forms does not necessarily demonstrate that the provisions of consent have been fully met (Jukic et al., 2011; Spatz et al., 2016).

References

Appelbaum, P.S., 2010. Consent in impaired populations. *Current Neurology and Neuroscience Reports*, 10(5), 367–373.

Casby, C. and Lyons, B., 2018. Consent and children. *Anaesthesia & Intensive Care Medicine*, doi: https://doi.org/10.1016/j.mpaic.2018.11.007.

Committee on Bioethics, 2016. Informed consent in decision-making in pediatric practice. *Pediatrics*, 138(2), e20161484.

Detering, K.M., Carter, R.Z., Sellars, M.W., Lewis, V. and Sutton, E.A., 2017. Prospective comparative effectiveness cohort study

comparing two models of advance care planning provision for Australian community aged care clients. *BMJ Supportive & Palliative Care*, bmjspcare-2017.

Douglass, A., 2018. Rethinking necessity and best interests in New Zealand mental capacity law. *Medical Law International*, 18(1), 3–34.

Dreisinger, N. and Zapolsky, N., 2018. Complexities of consent: ethics in the pediatric emergency department. *Pediatric Emergency Care*, 34(4), 288–290.

Fields, L.M. and Calvert, J.D., 2015. Informed consent procedures with cognitively impaired patients: a review of ethics and best practices. *Psychiatry and Clinical Neurosciences*, 69(8), 462–471.

Fink, A.S., Prochazka, A.V., Henderson, W.G., Bartenfeld, D., Nyirenda, C., Webb, A., Berger, D.H., Itani, K., Whitehill, T., Edwards, J. and Wilson, M., 2010. Predictors of comprehension during surgical informed consent. *Journal of the American College of Surgeons*, 210(6), 919–926.

Fives, A., 2016. Who gets to decide? Children's competence, parental authority, and informed consent. In *Justice, education and the politics of childhood*. Cham: Springer, pp. 35–47.

Grisso, T. and Appelbaum, P.S., 1998. *Assessing competence to consent to treatment: a guide for physicians and other health professionals*. New York: Oxford University Press.

Grootens-Wiegers, P., Hein, I.M., van den Broek, J.M. and de Vries, M.C., 2017. Medical decision-making in children and adolescents: developmental and neuroscientific aspects. *BMC Pediatrics*, 17(1), 120.

Hall, D.E., Prochazka, A.V. and Fink, A.S., 2012. Informed consent for clinical treatment. *Canadian Medical Association Journal*, 184(5), 533–540.

Hein, I.M., De Vries, M.C., Troost, P.W., Meynen, G., Van Goudoever, J.B. and Lindauer, R.J., 2015. Informed consent instead of assent is appropriate in children from the age of twelve: Policy implications of new findings on children's competence to consent to clinical research. *BMC Medical Ethics*, 16(1), 76.

Hemsley, B., Meredith, J., Bryant, L., Wilson, N.J., Higgins, I., Georgiou, A., Hill, S., Balandin, S. and McCarthy, S., 2019. An integrative review of stakeholder views on Advance Care Directives (ACD): barriers and facilitators to initiation, documentation, storage, and implementation. *Patient Education and Counseling*, January.

Hiriscau, E.I. and Reiter-Theil, S., 2017. Competence. *Encyclopedia of Global Bioethics*, 1–11.

Jukic, M., Kozina, S., Kardum, G., Hogg, R. and Kvolik, S., 2011. Physicians overestimate patients' knowledge of the process of informed consent: a cross-sectional study. *Medicinski Glasnik*, 8, 39–45.

Kang, M. and Kim, K., 2019. Prescribing for adolescents. *Australian Prescriber*, 42(1), 20.

Katz, A.L., Webb, S.A. and Committee on Bioethics, 2016. Informed consent in decision-making in pediatric practice. *Pediatrics*, e20161485.

Kinnersley, P., Phillips, K., Savage, K., Kelly, M.J., Farrell, E., Morgan, B., Whistance, R., Lewis, V., Mann, M.K., Stephens, B.L. and Blazeby, J., 2013. Interventions to promote informed consent for patients undergoing surgical and other invasive healthcare procedures. *Cochrane Database of Systematic Reviews*, 7.

Khoury, B.S. and Khoury, J.N., 2015. Consent: a practical guide. *Australian Dental Journal*, 60(2), 138–142.

Lamont, S., Stewart, C. and Chiarella, M., 2016. Decision-making capacity and its relationship to a legally valid consent: ethical, legal and professional context. *Journal of Law and Medicine*, 24, 371–386.

Lane, A.N., 2016. Medical imaging and consent: when is an X-ray assault? *Journal of Medical Radiation Sciences*, 63(2), 133–137.

Lee, L.M.M. and Goldstein, S., 2017. *EMS, capacity and competence*. Retrieved from: https://www.ncbi.nlm.nih.gov/books/NBK470178/

McSherry, B. and Waddington, L., 2017. Treat with care: the right to informed consent for medical treatment of persons with mental impairments in Australia. *Australian Journal of Human Rights*, 23(1), 109–129.

Mignani, V., Ingravallo, F., Mariani, E. and Chattat, R., 2017. Perspectives of older people living in long-term care facilities and of their family members toward advance care planning discussions: a systematic review and thematic synthesis. *Clinical Interventions in Aging*, 12, 475.

Moran-Ellis, J. and Tisdall, E.K.M., 2019. The relevance of 'competence' for enhancing or limiting children's participation: unpicking conceptual confusion. *Global Studies of Childhood*, 9 (3), 212–223.

Murphy, M. and Goldstein, M.A., 2017. The adolescent patient interview: adolescent confidentiality and consent. In *The MassGeneral Hospital for Children adolescent medicine handbook*. Cham: Springer, pp. 11–17.

Nadeau, D.P., Rich, J.N. and Brietzke, S.E., 2010. Informed consent in pediatric surgery: do parents understand the risks? *Archives of Otolaryngology – Head & Neck Surgery*, 136(3), 265–269.

Neilson, G. and Chaimowitz, G., 2015. Informed consent to treatment in psychiatry. *Canadian Journal of Psychiatry (Revue Canadienne de Psychiatrie)*, 60(4), 1.

Nour, S. and Griffiths, S., 2016. Obtaining consent for obstetric procedures. *Anaesthesia & Intensive Care Medicine*, 17(8), 408–410.

Pearse, W., Oprescu, F., Endacott, J., Goodman, S., Hyde, M. and O'Neill, M., 2019. Advance care planning in the context of clinical deterioration: a systematic review of the literature. *Palliative Care: Research and Treatment*, 12, 1178224218823509.

Rietjens, J.A., Sudore, R.L., Connolly, M., van Delden, J.J., Drickamer, M.A., Droger, M., van der Heide, A., Heyland, D.K., Houttekier, D., Janssen, D.J. and Orsi, L., 2017. Definition and recommendations for advance care planning: an international consensus supported by the European Association for Palliative Care. *Lancet Oncology*, 18(9), e543–e551.

Schenker, Y., Fernandez, A., Sudore, R. and Schillinger, D., 2011. Interventions to improve patient comprehension in informed consent for medical and surgical procedures: a systematic review. *Medical Decision Making*, 31(1), 151–173.

Selinger, C.P., 2009. The right to consent: Is it absolute? *British Journal of Medical Practitioners*, 2(2).

Sirbaugh, P.E. and Diekema, D.S., 2011. Consent for emergency medical services for children and adolescents. *Pediatrics*, 128(2), 427–433.

Spatz, E.S., Krumholz, H.M. and Moulton, B.W., 2016. The new era of informed consent: getting to a reasonable-patient standard through shared decision making. *JAMA*, 315(19), 2063–2064.

Steer, B., 2015. Paramedics, consent and refusal – are we competent? *Australasian Journal of Paramedicine*, 5(1).

Stohl, H., 2018. Childbirth is not a medical emergency: maternal right to informed consent throughout labor and delivery. *Journal of Legal Medicine*, 38(3–4), 329–353.

Stuart, B., Volandes, A. and Moulton, B.W., 2017. Advance care planning: ensuring patients' preferences govern the care they receive. *Generations*, 41(1), 31–36.

Townsend, R. and Luck, M., 2019. Paramedic professionalism. *Applied paramedic law, ethics and professionalism: Australia and New Zealand*. Sydney: Elsevier, p. 1.

Townsend, R., Willis, S. and Mehmet, N., 2019. *Legal and ethical aspects of paramedic practice. Fundamentals of paramedic practice: a systems approach*. New Jersey: Wiley-Blackwell.

Wong, P.T., 2015. A meaning-centered approach to overcoming loneliness during hospitalization, old age, and dying. *Addressing Loneliness: Coping, Prevention and Clinical Interventions*, 1, 171.

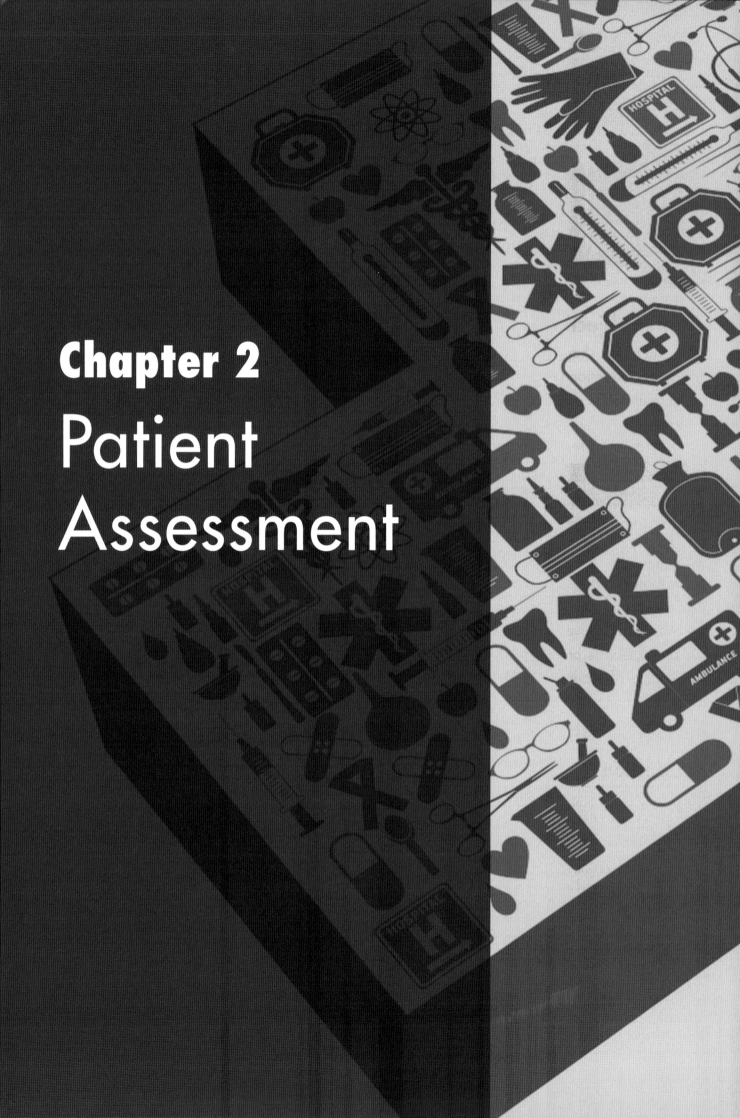

Chapter 2
Patient Assessment

Assessment using the modified Glasgow Coma Scale

Matt Johnson and Jeff Kenneally

Chapter objectives

At the end of this chapter the reader will be able to:

1. Describe the rationale for assessment using the modified Glasgow Coma Scale (GCS)
2. Demonstrate the assessment process using the modified GCS
3. Interpret and report on common pathologies identified by the modified GCS

Resources required for this assessment

- Standardised patient to provide sensory and motor responses or mannequin with instructor to provide responses
- Hand decontamination agent
- Disposable gloves
- Clinical waste bag
- Method of documenting results

Skill matrix

This assessment requires:

- Infection control (CS 1.3)
- Communication (CS 1.5)
- Consent (CS 1.6)

This assessment is a component of:

- Patient assessment (Chapter 2)

Introduction

The Glasgow Coma Scale (GCS) was devised in 1974 to provide a standardised means of assessing changes in consciousness in traumatic brain injured (TBI) patients in a neurosurgical unit (Teasdale and Jennett, 1974). Despite this tightly defined origin, it has since found much broader use as an almost universal measure of acute conscious state assessment (Green, 2011). The original GCS comprised 14 points, with a score out of five for motor response, and was later modified to include 'abnormal flexion', making the highest score 15.

The GCS is the most widely used tool to assess initial, and subsequent, level of consciousness (Gonzalez and Moore, 2012). It is a standard component of prehospital vital sign assessment and can be used for all patients, particularly where alteration or deterioration of consciousness may

be suspected. It must be well understood for it to be performed correctly.

Anatomy and physiology

The brain and spinal cord comprise the central nervous system. Most of the brain, including cerebrum and diencephalon, are within the protective confine of the skull. The brain is largely made up of fluids, the volumes of which can vary. This includes cerebrospinal fluid (CSF) within and around the brain, intracellular fluid and blood flowing through the brain.

Brain content is limited in its ability to escape the confines of the skull. If a significant increase in volume occurs within the skull, increased pressure is placed on the brain. Causes of such an increase include haemorrhage, tumour, oedema and CSF outflow obstruction.

Rising intracranial pressure adversely impacts normal brain functions. This can produce assessable changes, including to conscious thought, speech ability and motor function.

Normal brain can be adversely affected by a wider variety of factors, including medications, environment, endocrine emergencies and blood gas or perfusion derangement.

Key brain structures for consciousness include the reticulating activating system (RAS), thalamus and cortex. The RAS controls wakefulness and sleep. It receives a wide array of stimuli from all over the body and, when functioning, can cause arousal. Pain is a particularly good stimulus. The thalamus helps direct attention of stimuli to the appropriate part of the cortex and produces wakefulness. Where the RAS or thalamus are adversely affected, the ability to achieve arousal, wakefulness or direct appropriate cortex responses can all be impacted as responses become subcortical.

Clinical rationale

Consciousness can be assessed for arousal and wakefulness. There are two essential GCS elements: score and scale. The score ranges from 3 (unresponsive) to 15 (fully conscious). A total GCS score can be compiled by adding three individual assessment scores: eye opening, scoring 1 to 4; verbal response, scoring 1 to 5; and motor response, scoring 1 to 6 (Gonzalez and Moore, 2012).

However, the GCS score is not intended for use as a sum (Teasdale and Jennett, 1974), with each individual component more useful than any total (Teasdale et al., 2014; Green, 2011). The scale reports responses as 'E', 'V' and 'M' with numerical value beside each letter.

For reliability and consistency, GCS assessment must be performed the same way by each subsequent person. This is done by using standard stimuli during testing and reporting on response findings in the same manner (Gonzalez and Moore, 2012).

Standard stimuli

The standard stimuli for the scale are as follows.

Eye opening (E, indicating arousal)

4. Spontaneous and purposeful.
3. After verbally being asked 'Can you open your eyes?' (if not *spontaneously* open).
2. Following painful stimuli to sternum or nailbed. Supraorbital and jaw angle pain can cause eye squinting.
1. None.

Verbal responses (V, indicating awareness)

5. Oriented answers to 'Can you tell me your name?', 'Do you know where you are?', 'Do you know the time/day/date?'.
4. Confused, being unclear on any of the person/time/place questions even if some answers are correct.
3. Inappropriate, where the answers have no correlation with the question. Swearing is common.
2. Incomprehensible, where noise from the mouth occurs (moaning/groaning) that is intentional and not inadvertent respiratory noise such as snoring.
1. None.

Motor (arm) responses (M)

6. Spontaneously obeys the command, 'Can you reach out and squeeze my hands with yours?'.
5. Localises to painful central stimulus such as sternum pressure, supraorbital notch or trapezius pinch.
4. Withdraws from painful nailbed pressure.
3. Abnormally flexes from nailbed pressure.
2. Abnormally extends from nailbed pressure.
1. None.

It is important that, when asked, the patient reaches out and grasps the assessor's hands. Do not place your own hands into the patient's hands as a prompt, as this can cause misleading reflex grasping.

Painful stimuli come in two levels: centrally brain stimulating (including sternum) and peripheral nailbed that may be adversely affected by spinal cord injury (Braine and Cook, 2017). Pain is applied only when there is no response to verbal stimuli.

Sternum painful stimulus is created by continuous downward pressure, typically using the knuckle, against the middle of the sternum for up to 10 seconds. Rubbing is not necessary. It should be firm enough to cause pain but not injury, which can be considered assault (Fig. 2.1.1). This is the first level of painful stimulus for motor response, assessing the ability to feel pain, locate it, then reach up with an arm to push it away. Both arms should be able to achieve this. If necessary, restrain a responding arm to assess the second. If one or both limbs fail, move to the nailbed stimulus. Motor responses are where most errors are made (Bledsoe et al., 2015).

Nailbed painful stimulus can use a firm object such as a pen pressed firmly against the fingernail for up to 10 seconds to cause pain but not injury (Fig. 2.1.2). This stimulus is necessary to identify withdrawal, abnormal flexion and extension responses. Assess both limbs; if

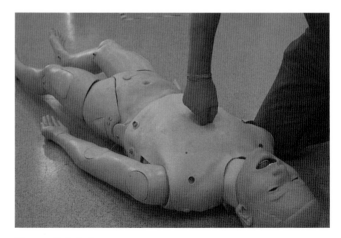

Figure 2.1.1 Sternum pressure

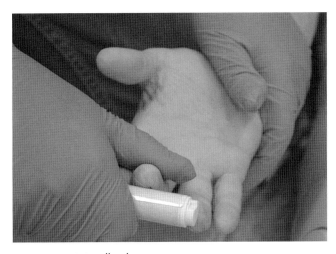

Figure 2.1.2 Nailbed pressure

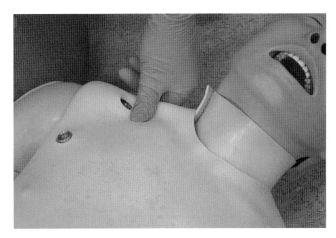

Figure 2.1.4 Trapezius squeeze

Paediatric variations

Paediatric conscious state (CS) assessment can be challenging. In particular, verbal response in the younger child may be impossible to determine. Where the child is too young to speak or provide reliable answers, consider estimating appropriate facial expressions or appropriate baby noises for the child as oriented and score 5. If the verbal sounds are not appropriate but are spontaneous, score 4. If they are only produced following verbal stimuli, score 3. If only produced following painful stimuli, score 2. No verbal response scores 1.

Despite limb assessment being the most prone to error, motor response is most the reliable indicator in small children if done correctly (Acker et al., 2014; Fortune and Shann, 2010). Use of the AVPU score (see Chapter 2.2) is frequently preferred for the younger child.

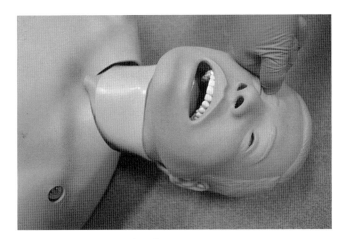

Figure 2.1.3 Supraorbital pressure

they are different, score the highest but document both responses.

Alternative stimuli

Supraorbital notch pressure (Fig. 2.1.3) aimed at the supraorbital nerve and the trapezius muscle pinch (Fig. 2.1.4) aimed at the cranial nerve XI are alternative central painful stimuli (Braine and Cook, 2017; Waterhouse, 2017; Reith et al., 2016). They can be used to assess for localising, to elicit the eye opening response or to assist with differentiation between flexion and localising responses in limbs to nailbed pressure.

Clinical skill assessment process

The following section outlines the clinical skill assessment tools that should be used to determine a student's ability to demonstrate safe and accurate application of the modified GCS.

1. Clinical Skill Work Instruction
2. Formative Clinical Skill Assessment (F-CSAT)
3. Performance Improvement Plan (PIP)
4. Summative Clinical Skill Assessment (S-CSAT)
(5. Direct Observation of Procedural Skills (DOPS) – see Chapter 1.1)

Clinical Skill Work Instruction

Equipment and resources: Standardised patient to provide sensory and motor responses or mannequin with instructor to provide responses; hand decontamination agent; disposable gloves; clinical waste bag; method of documenting results

Associated Clinical Skills: Infection control; Communication; Consent

Assessing the modified GCS

Activity	Critical Action	Rationale
Position patient	Patient positioned to ensure airway patency, comfort and safety.	Primary survey takes precedence over GCS.
Check readiness	Check for factors that will interfere with communication or ability to respond.	Speech, hearing, language difficulty, pain, injuries, distractions, can lead to an inaccurate result.
Assess eye response	Observe for spontaneous purposeful eye opening. If open, score 4. If eyes are not open, ask the patient loudly and clearly to open them. If the eyes open, score 3. If no response to verbal request, elicit pain response by applying sternal pressure. If the eyes open, score 2. If the eyes do not open, score 1.	Eye opening requires higher brain function but can require stimulus to provoke. Inadequate response suggests brain function decline.
Assess verbal response	Assess orientation to person, time and place by asking, 'What is your name?', 'What time/day is it today'? and 'Do you know where you are now?'. Oriented responses score 5. If the patient answers these questions but provides incorrect answer(s), they are confused and score 4. Random or muddled speech unrelated to questioning is inappropriate and scores 3. Intentional orally formed sounds that are not clear as words or are incomprehensible score 2. No reaction scores 1.	Verbal response requires higher brain function. Inadequate response suggests brain function decline.
Assess motor response	Ask patient to reach up with both hands to grasp paramedic's corresponding hands. Obeying scores 6. If the patient does not obey with both arms, apply central pressure stimulus and observe for ability to localise to pain with purposeful attempts to remove/push away the stimulus. Localising scores 5. If one or both hands do not localise, apply painful nailbed stimulus to the unresponsive limb(s). If the patient purposefully withdraws away from the stimulus, score 4. If the patient's arm moves towards the chest, with fingers and wrists flexed, elbow bent (decorticate posturing), this is abnormal flexing and scores 3. If the patient's arms and legs extend, wrists rotate away from their body (decerebrate posturing), this is abnormal extension and scores 2. No motor response scores 1. Assess both sides for best result of each.	Controlled motor response requires higher brain function. Inadequate response suggests brain function decline. Left and right sides must both be assessed to allow for both brain hemispheres. Central pressure must be applied with local nailbed only if response is inadequate.
Interpret and report findings	Accurately interpret, document and report on each subset.	Accurate record kept and continuity of patient care.

Source: *Adapted from Teasdale et al., 2014.*

Formative Clinical Skill Assessment (F-CSAT)

Equipment and resources: Standardised patient to provide sensory and motor responses or mannequin with instructor to provide responses; hand decontamination agent; disposable gloves; clinical waste bag; method of documenting results

Associated Clinical Skills: Infection control; Communication; Consent

Staff/Student being assessed: _____

Assessing the modified GCS

Activity	Critical Action	Performance				
Positions patient	Patient positioned to ensure airway patency, comfort and safety.	0	1	2	3	4
Checks readiness	Checks for factors that will interfere with communication or ability to respond.	0	1	2	3	4
Assesses eye response	Observes patient's eyes for purposeful spontaneous eye opening and scores 4. If necessary, asks the patient loudly and clearly to open their eyes. If they respond by opening their eyes they score 3. If necessary, elicits a pain response by applying painful sternal stimuli. If the eyes open, they score 2. If there is no response to pain, the patient scores 1.	0	1	2	3	4
Assesses verbal response	Determines orientation to person/time/place by asking questions 'What is your name?', 'What time/day is it today?', 'Do you know where you are at the moment?'. Scores 5 for oriented answers. Scores 4 for confused answers. Scores 3 for inappropriate answers. Scores 2 for incomprehensible answers. Scores 1 for no response.	0	1	2	3	4
Assesses motor response	Asks patient to reach up and squeeze paramedic's hands with both limbs. Scores 6 if commands obeyed. If the patient doesn't obey with both arms, provides sternum pressure. Scores 5 if able to localise. If the patient does not localise, provides nailbed painful stimulus. If withdraw/pulls away from stimulus, scores 4. Scores 3 for abnormal flexion. Scores 2 for abnormal extension. No reaction to stimuli scores 1. Examines both sides for best result.	0	1	2	3	4
Interprets and reports findings	Accurately interprets, documents and reports on each subset.	0	1	2	3	4

Source: *Adapted from Teasdale et al., 2014.*

Standard Achieved: (please circle one)

Competent (C)   Not Yet Competent* (NYC)

Staff/Student Name: _____

Assessor (please print name)**:** _____

Signed (Assessor)**:** _____

Date of Assessment: _____

Comments:

*If Not Yet Competent (NYC) a PIP needs to be completed and a repeat of the F-CSAT

Formative Clinical Skill Assessment (F-CSAT) Key

Skill level	Standard of procedure	Quality of performance	Outcome	Level of assistance required
4 Safe for unsupervised practice	Safe Accurate Behaviour is appropriate to context	Confident Accurate Expedient	Achieved intended outcome	No supporting cues* required
3 Requires supervision	Safe Accurate Behaviour is appropriate to context	Confident Accurate Takes longer than required	Achieved intended outcome	Requires occasional supportive cues*
2 Requires assistance	Safe Accurate Behaviour generally appropriate to context	Lacks certainty	Would not have achieved outcome without support	Requires frequent verbal and occasional physical directives in addition to supportive cues*
1 Requires direction	Safe only with guidance Not completely accurate	Unskilled Inefficient	Would not have achieved outcome without support	Requires continuous verbal and frequent physical directive cues*
0 Unsafe	Unsafe Unable to demonstrate behaviour Lack of insight into behaviour appropriate to context	Unskilled	Would not have achieved outcome	Requires continuous verbal and continuous physical directive cues*

*Refers to physical directives or verbal supportive cues

Performance Improvement Plan (PIP)

Please document the agreed education plan and completion timelines for areas assessed as less than 4.

This plan should be presented to assessor prior to commencement of summative assessment.

Where was supervisor support required?	Student summary of deficit. (Why was there a problem?)	Improvement Plan	Completed (Y/N)

Staff/Student Name: _____

Staff/Student Signature: _____

Educator Name: _____

Educator Signature: _____

Summative Clinical Skill Assessment (S-CSAT)

Equipment and resources: Standardised patient to provide sensory and motor responses or mannequin with instructor to provide responses; hand decontamination agent; disposable gloves; clinical waste bag; method of documenting results

Associated Clinical Skills: Infection control; Communication; Consent

Staff/Student being assessed: _____

- Completed Formative Clinical Skill Assessment (F-CSAT):   **YES   NO**

- Completed Performance Improvement Plan (PIP):   **YES   NO   N/A**

Assessing the modified GCS

Activity	Critical Action	Achieved	Without Direction
Positions patient	Patient positioned to ensure airway patency, comfort and safety.	NO	YES
Checks readiness	Checks for factors that will interfere with communication or ability to respond.	NO	YES
Assesses eye response	Observes patient's eyes for purposeful spontaneous eye opening and scores 4. If necessary, asks the patient loudly and clearly to open their eyes. If they respond by opening their eyes they score 3. If necessary, elicits a pain response by applying painful sternal stimuli. If the eyes open they score 2. If there is no response to pain the patient scores 1.	NO	YES

Assessing the modified GCS continued

Activity	Critical Action	Achieved Without Direction	
Assesses verbal response	Asks patient what their name is, what day/date/year it is and where they are. Scores 5 for oriented answers. Scores 4 for confused answers. Scores 3 for inappropriate answers. Scores 2 for incomprehensible answers. Scores 1 for no response.	NO	YES
Assesses motor response	Asks patient to reach up and squeeze paramedic's hands with both limbs. Scores 6 if commands obeyed. If the patient does not obey, provides sternum pressure. Scores 5 if able to localise. If the patient does not localise, provides nailbed painful stimulus to failing limb(s). If withdraw/pulls away from stimulus, scores 4. Scores 3 for abnormal flexion. Scores 2 for abnormal extension. No reaction to stimuli scores 1. Examines both sides for best result.	NO	YES
Interprets and reports findings	Accurately interprets, documents and reports on each subset.	NO	YES

Source: *Adapted from Teasdale et al., 2014.*

Standard Achieved: (please circle one)

Competent (C)   Not Yet Competent* (NYC)

Staff/Student Name: _____

Assessor (please print name)**:** _____

Signed (Assessor)**:** _____

Date of Assessment: _____

Comments:

*If Not Yet Competent (NYC) a PIP needs to be completed and a repeat of the F-CSAT

Clinical findings

Interpreting the GCS

GCS scores range between 3 and 15, with the three levels allowing 120 different combinations (Healey et al., 2003). Though not recommended, GCS scores are used by paramedics to differentiate between acceptable and low conscious states to provide a trigger for airway protection interventions, including intubation. Low is commonly defined as a score of <10.

Since the GCS was derived as a tool for tracking progression and recovery from TBI, the score itself is not a good predictor for cause of unconsciousness or response to treatment. For example, common emergencies such as opioid overdose or hypoglycaemia can produce low GCS scores that respond readily to standard therapies.

Suitability for GCS assessment

There are several confounding provisos when assessing any patient using the GCS. These should be checked before assessment.

- *Eyes:* Eye opening must be purposeful to be representative of higher brain function. If the eyes are found open despite the patient being otherwise unresponsive, gently close them and ask to open them again.
- *Speech:* The patient must be able to hear, speak and understand the language used. If they are deaf, aphasic or not understanding the questions asked, verbal responses will be unreliable. If the patient is intubated,

mark this criteria as 'T' without scoring a value (Teasdale et al., 2014).

- *Injuries:* Patient injuries can interfere with responses. Swollen eyes can prevent eye opening, facial trauma can prevent speech and limb or spinal injuries can prevent normal responses to stimuli. Instead, describe what is observed, noting any impediment. If injury prevents eye opening, mark this criteria as 'C' (closed) without scoring a value. If limb injuries prevent the patient from responding, ask them to perform a task

they can achieve, such as poking out their tongue. Document the stimulus used (Teasdale et al., 2014).

- *Chronic changes:* Dementia, past stroke and other past problems can leave permanent changes in GCS findings. Score as presenting, noting any chronic abnormality and any new change observed.
- *Non-cooperation:* Occasionally, patients refuse to comply with GCS assessment for a variety of reasons, including drugs and mental health. Score as they present, noting suspected purposeful non-compliance.

PRACTICE TIP!

When applying painful stimulus, be aware of patient striking out in response. A self-protective position should always be adopted.

PRACTICE TIP!

Painful stimulus can cause physical harm. It must be applied respectfully and not exceed the level that would normally be expected to elicit a result. Excessive force is unnecessary and inappropriate.

PRACTICE TIP!

To localise to painful stimuli, the patient must raise up their arm and attempt to remove the central stimulus. Limb movement without successful localising requires nailbed stimulus to clarify the next best result. Where only one limb localises, restrain it and assess the best performance of the other arm.

PRACTICE TIP!

A GCS score <8–10 can trigger escalating care to an extended care or intensive care paramedic. Ensure appropriate interim therapies are provided while waiting for these to arrive. Ensure a recent GCS assessment is performed prior to handover.

PRACTICE TIP!

Eyes must open purposefully. If they are open but the patient is otherwise unresponsive, gently close their eyes and have them reopen them if they can.

PRACTICE TIP!

The GCS score is notoriously unreliable to calculate (Green, 2011). To reduce inaccuracy, communicate each finding to your partner, who can then calculate using a scale.

TEST YOUR KNOWLEDGE QUESTIONS

1. **What are the three categories of physical assessment in GCS?**
    Eye opening; verbal response; motor function.

2. **What is the difference between score and scale in GCS?**
    Score is the numerical value from the three sections; scale is the descriptor criteria for each category.

3. **How is GCS made reliable and consistent?**
    Assessment is performed the same way by each subsequent person, using standard stimuli and reporting on response findings in the same manner.

4. **How many person/time/place questions does a patient need to get incorrect to be confused?**
    Any one or more.

5. **How are snoring sounds scored during GCS?**
    They score 1 if there are no other speech sounds, since this is not purposeful.

6. **What are the two levels of standard painful stimuli?**
    Central (sternum pressure, trapezius pinch, supraorbital pressure); localised nailbed.

7. **Why is GCS in small children considered differently?**
    Children provide different verbal responses, sometimes requiring different interpretation.

8. **How are chronic changes scored during GCS?**
    As they are found but with notation of new versus old findings.

9. **What should you do if the eyes are found not purposefully open?**
    If the eyes are open despite being otherwise unresponsive, gently close them and ask the patient to open them again.

10. **What is the next action if only one arm is able to obey or to localise to pain?**
    Nailbed painful stimulus is provided to the other limb to assess its best response. The GCS score uses the best result, with the other being noted.

References

Acker, S.N., Ross, J.T., Partrick, D.A., Nadlonek, N.A., Bronsert, M. and Bensard, D.D., 2014. Glasgow motor scale alone is equivalent to Glasgow Coma Scale at identifying children at risk for serious traumatic brain injury. *Journal of Trauma and Acute Care Surgery*, 77(2), 304–309.

Bledsoe, B.E., Casey, M.J., Feldman, J., Johnson, L., Diel, S., Forred, W. and Gorman, C., 2015. Glasgow Coma Scale scoring is often inaccurate. *Prehospital and Disaster Medicine*, 30(1), 46–53.

Braine, M.E. and Cook, N., 2017. The Glasgow Coma Scale and evidence-informed practice: a critical review of where we are and where we need to be. *Journal of Clinical Nursing*, 26, 280–293.

Fortune, P.M. and Shann, F., 2010. The motor response to stimulation predicts outcome as well as the full Glasgow Coma Scale in children with severe head injury. *Pediatric Critical Care Medicine*, 11(3), 339–342.

Green S., 2011. Cheerio, laddie! Bidding farewell to the Glasgow Coma Scale. *Annals of Emergency Medicine*, 58(5), 426–429.

Gonzalez, E. and Moore, E.E., 2012. Glasgow Coma Scale. In *Encyclopedia of intensive care medicine*. Berlin/Heidelberg: Springer, pp. 982–984.

Healey, C., Osler, T.M., Rogers, F.B., Healey, M.A., Glance, L.G., Kilgo, P.D., Shackford, S.R. and Meredith, J.W., 2003. Improving the Glasgow Coma Scale score: motor score alone is a better predictor. *Journal of Trauma and Acute Care Surgery*, 54(4), 671–680.

Reith, F.C., Brennan, P.M., Maas, A.I. and Teasdale, G.M., 2016. Lack of standardization in the use of the Glasgow Coma Scale: results of international surveys. *Journal of Neurotrauma*, 33(1), 89–94.

Teasdale, G., Maas, A., Lecky, F., Manley, G., Stocchetti, N. and Murray, G., 2014. The Glasgow Coma Scale at 40 years: standing the test of time. *Lancet Neurology*, 13(8), 844–854.

Teasdale, G. and Jennett, B., 1974. Assessment of coma and impaired consciousness. *Lancet*, 2, 81–84.

Waterhouse, C., 2017. Practical aspects of performing Glasgow Coma Scale observations. *Nursing Standard*, 31(35), 40–46.

Assessing the Alert, Voice, Pain, Unresponsiveness (AVPU) score

Matt Johnson and Jeff Kenneally

Chapter objectives

At the end of this chapter the reader will be able to:

1. Describe the rationale for AVPU assessment
2. Demonstrate the AVPU assessment

Resources required for this assessment

- Standardised patient to provide sensory and motor responses or mannequin with instructor to provide sensory and motor responses
- Hand decontamination agent
- Disposable gloves
- Clinical waste bag
- Method of documenting results

Skill matrix

This assessment requires:

- Infection control (CS 1.3)
- Situational awareness (CS 1.4)
- Communication (CS 1.5)
- Consent (CS 1.6)

This assessment is a component of:

- Patient assessment (Chapter 2)

Introduction

The 15-point Glasgow Coma Scale (GCS; see Chapter 2.1) has repeatedly been shown to lack inter-rater reliability. Despite appearance of accuracy, several of its categories remain highly subjective (Bassi et al., 1999; Bledsoe et al., 2015; Fischer et al., 2010; Gill et al., 2004; Green, 2011; Holdgate et al., 2006; Juarez and Lyons, 1995; Lindsay et al., 1983; Rowley et al., 1991; Teasdale et al., 1978; Tesseris et al., 1991; Zuercher et al., 2009).

Of the three subsets that comprise the GCS (eyes, verbal and motor), the motor subset is the most sensitive, with some evidence it could be used in isolation (Acker et al., 2014; Al-Salamah et al., 2004; Fortune and Shann, 2010; Green, 2011; Ross et al., 1998; Van de Voorde et al., 2008).

Other researchers have sought even simpler tools to provide adequate information for safe decisions in the emergency setting. The AVPU (Alert, Voice, Pain, Unresponsive) scale is one such abbreviated assessment

that is easier to calculate yet remains sufficiently accurate (Hoffmann et al., 2016; Kelly et al., 2004). It is intended as a rapid initial consciousness assessment tool in emergencies, while GCS allows for the assessment of more subtle changes over time. The AVPU scale is discussed in this chapter.

Anatomy and physiology

The brain contains several structures that are together responsible for consciousness and awareness. The thalamus sits slightly superior to the brainstem. Within the brainstem itself is a dispersed series of nuclei known as the reticulating activating system (RAS), which is largely responsible for the secretion of neurotransmitters, including acetylcholine, noradrenaline, serotonin and dopamine.

The RAS is substantially connected to the motor cortex. Sensory signals are received by the RAS from all over the body. The ability for these to cause response, including awakening or motor response, is called arousal.

Pain, frequently requiring the brain to respond, is a good stimulus for the RAS.

Consciousness can be described as the level of arousal and/or awareness of the internal and external environment. Any injury or adverse impact to these structures can lead to decreased arousal, wakefulness and even coma. This can be caused by rising intracranial pressure from an increase in volume due to haemorrhage, tumour, oedema or CSF outflow obstruction. Other causes include the effects of medication, environment, endocrine emergencies and blood gas or perfusion derangement.

Clinical rationale

Like the GCS, the AVPU tool considers eye opening, verbal responses and motor function as criteria for the assessment of arousal, wakefulness and cortical control. Although not intended for long-term observations of recovery, the AVPU tool is much easier to calculate than the GCS, with only the following four responses to consider.

Alert: Responds spontaneously to external environment

The eyes are open purposefully with the patient able to communicate and move limbs spontaneously. If a patient opens their eyes to command then remains as just described, they are also described as 'A' on the AVPU, which allows for patients who are simply disturbed from rest. The alert patient can variously be calm, restless, agitated or even drowsy (Rajabi Kheirabadi et al., 2015).

Voice: Responds to verbal instructions

The broad way to score 'V' is when verbal commands are required to produce any eye, voice or motor response. As with the GCS, verbal response should ideally include standard stimuli, including a request to open the eyes, reach up and move limbs and answer questions about person, time and place. 'V' will include confused or inappropriate responses and may include eyes closed. 'V' is arguably the most difficult level to assess (Brunker and Harris, 2015).

Pain: Responds to painful stimuli

Pain can be applied as central or nailbed pressure, as for the GCS (see Chapter 2.1). Nailbed or continuous blunt pressure to the sternum (without rubbing) is preferred. Some advocate supraorbital pressure or pinching the trapezius muscle, but be mindful that this can be construed as patient assault if poorly applied. Any response including eyes, voice or motor function will score as 'P'.

Table 2.2.1 The AVPU scale

AVPU	Criteria
Alert	Fully awake although not necessarily oriented. This patient will have spontaneously open eyes, respond to voice (although may be confused) and have bodily motor function.
Voice	The patient makes some response to verbal stimulus: the response could be from any of the three component measures of eyes, voice or motor (e.g. patient's eyes open on being addressed, grunting, moaning, or movement of a limb when requested).
Pain	The patient makes some response to painful stimuli. The response could be any of the three component measures of eyes, voice or motor (e.g. patient's eyes open, grunting, moaning, or movement of a limb to painful stimulus).
Unresponsive	The patient does not give any eye, voice or motor response to voice or pain.

Unresponsive: Does not respond

'U' is without response from eyes, verbal or motor to any stimuli including painful sternum pressure (see Table 2.2.1).

Paediatric variations

The GCS is difficult to use to assess small children, particularly when assessing their verbal responses. In contrast, since AVPU is less reliant on specific responses, it is widely considered suitable for paediatric patients as an alternative (Fortune and Shann, 2010; Hoffmann et al., 2016; Nuttall et al., 2016; Sam et al., 2016).

Clinical skill assessment process

The following section outlines the clinical skill assessment tools that should be used to determine a student's ability to demonstrate safe and accurate AVPU assessment.
1. Clinical Skill Work Instruction
2. Formative Clinical Skill Assessment (F-CSAT)
3. Performance Improvement Plan (PIP)
4. Summative Clinical Skill Assessment (S-CSAT)
(5. Direct Observation of Procedural Skills (DOPS) – see Chapter 1.1)

Clinical Skill Work Instruction

Equipment and resources: Standardised patient to provide sensory and motor responses or mannequin with instructor to provide sensory and motor responses; hand decontamination agent; disposable gloves; clinical waste bag; method of documenting results

Associated Clinical Skills: Infection control; Situational awareness; Communication; Consent

Assessing the AVPU score

Activity	Critical Action	Rationale
Prepare patient	Patient positioned for airway patency, comfort and safety.	Primary survey takes precedence over GCS.
	Assess factors that can interfere with communication or ability to respond.	Speech, hearing, language difficulty, pain, injuries, distractions, can lead to an inaccurate result.
Alert	Assess for spontaneous eye opening. Observe for spontaneously open eyes, or verbally responding (even confused) or demonstrating bodily motor function.	Eliminates need to assess remaining components of AVPU, as patient can be considered alert.
Voice	If no spontaneous response, assess for response to voice. Assess for response to verbal stimulus: the response could be one or more from eyes, voice or motor.	Compromised brain function can produce responses include eyes opening, speaking, grunting, moaning or limb movement.
Pain	If no response to voice, assess for response to pain. Assess for response to painful stimulus. The response could be one or more of eyes, voice or motor including abnormal posturing.	Severely compromised brain function responses can be any from eyes, verbal or movement.
Unresponsive	The patient does not provide any eye, voice or motor response to any stimulus.	Patient is unconscious and requires appropriate care for the unconscious patient.
Report	Document/hand over findings.	Accurate record kept and continuity of patient care.

Source: *Adapted from Hoffmann et al., 2016; Kelly et al., 2004.*

Formative Clinical Skill Assessment (F-CSAT)

Equipment and resources: Standardised patient to provide sensory and motor responses or mannequin with instructor to provide sensory and motor responses; hand decontamination agent; disposable gloves; clinical waste bag; method of documenting results

Associated Clinical Skills: Infection control; Situational awareness; Communication; Consent

Staff/Student being assessed: _____

Assessing the AVPU score

Activity	Critical Action	Participant Performance				
Prepares patient	Positions patient for airway patency, comfort and safety.	0	1	2	3	4
	Assesses factors that can interfere with communication or ability to respond.	0	1	2	3	4
Alert	Assesses for spontaneous eye opening. Observes for spontaneously open eyes, or verbally responding (even confused) or demonstrating bodily motor function.	0	1	2	3	4
Voice	If no spontaneous response, assesses for response to voice. Assesses for response to verbal stimulus, including from eyes, voice or motor.	0	1	2	3	4
Pain	If no response to voice, assesses for response to pain. Assesses for response to painful stimulus including from eyes, voice or motor including abnormal posturing.	0	1	2	3	4
Unresponsive	The patient does not give any eye, voice or motor response to voice or pain.	0	1	2	3	4
Reports	Documents/hands over findings.	0	1	2	3	4

Source: *Adapted from Hoffmann et al., 2016; Kelly et al., 2004.*

Standard Achieved: (please circle one)

Competent (C)   Not Yet Competent* (NYC)

Staff/Student Name: _____

Assessor (please print name)**:** _____

Signed (Assessor)**:** _____

Date of Assessment: _____

Comments:

*If Not Yet Competent (NYC) a PIP needs to be completed and a repeat of the F-CSAT

Formative Clinical Skill Assessment (F-CSAT) Key

Skill level	Standard of procedure	Quality of performance	Outcome	Level of assistance required
4 Safe for unsupervised practice	Safe Accurate Behaviour is appropriate to context	Confident Accurate Expedient	Achieved intended outcome	No supporting cues* required
3 Requires supervision	Safe Accurate Behaviour is appropriate to context	Confident Accurate Takes longer than required	Achieved intended outcome	Requires occasional supportive cues*
2 Requires assistance	Safe Accurate Behaviour generally appropriate to context	Lacks certainty	Would not have achieved outcome without support	Requires frequent verbal and occasional physical directives in addition to supportive cues*
1 Requires direction	Safe only with guidance Not completely accurate	Unskilled Inefficient	Would not have achieved outcome without support	Requires continuous verbal and frequent physical directive cues*
0 Unsafe	Unsafe Unable to demonstrate behaviour Lack of insight into behaviour appropriate to context	Unskilled	Would not have achieved outcome	Requires continuous verbal and continuous physical directive cues*

*Refers to physical directives or verbal supportive cues

Performance Improvement Plan (PIP)

Please document the agreed education plan and completion timelines for areas assessed as less than 4.

This plan should be presented to assessor prior to commencement of summative assessment.

Where was supervisor support required?	Student summary of deficit. (Why was there a problem?)	Improvement Plan	Completed (Y/N)

Staff/Student Name: _____

Staff/Student Signature: _____

Educator Name: _____

Educator Signature: _____

Summative Clinical Skill Assessment (S-CSAT)

Equipment and resources: Standardised patient to provide sensory and motor responses or mannequin with instructor to provide sensory and motor responses; hand decontamination agent; disposable gloves; clinical waste bag; method of documenting results

Associated Clinical Skills: Infection control; Situational awareness; Communication; Consent

Staff/Student being assessed: _____

- Completed Formative Clinical Skill Assessment (F-CSAT): **YES NO**
- Completed Performance Improvement Plan (PIP): **YES NO N/A**

Assessing the AVPU score			
Activity	**Critical Action**	**Achieved Without Direction**	
Prepares patient	Positions patient for airway patency, comfort and safety.	NO	YES
	Assesses factors that can interfere with communication or ability to respond.	NO	YES
Alert	Assesses for spontaneous eye opening. Observes for spontaneously open eyes, or verbally responding (even confused) or demonstrating bodily motor function.	NO	YES
Voice	If no spontaneous response, assesses for response to voice. Assesses for response to verbal stimulus, including from eyes, voice or motor.	NO	YES
Pain	If no response to voice, assesses for response to pain. Assesses for response to painful stimulus, including from eyes, voice or motor including abnormal posturing.	NO	YES
Unresponsive	The patient does not give any eye, voice or motor response to voice or pain.	NO	YES
Reports	Documents/hands over findings.	NO	YES

Source: *Adapted from Hoffmann et al., 2016; Kelly et al., 2004.*

Standard Achieved: (please circle one)

Competent (C)   Not Yet Competent* (NYC)

Staff/Student Name: _____

Assessor (please print name): _____

Signed (Assessor): _____

Date of Assessment: _____

Comments:

*If Not Yet Competent (NYC) a PIP needs to be completed and a repeat of the F-CSAT

Clinical findings

Interpreting AVPU

AVPU scores in the prehospital setting are usually used to differentiate between 'high' and 'low' conscious states, with 'low' acting as a trigger for interventions such as airway protection, including intubation. 'Low' is usually defined as response to pain (P) or unresponsive (U). The AVPU score can quickly exclude patients who do not require airway intervention (alert/A or voice/V).

The AVPU scale is useful as a quick assessment tool of a patient's consciousness at any moment. It acts as a quick 'triage' of conscious state with those failing to meet the alert or voice criteria being subject to a more exacting GCS assessment. Any score lower than V should prompt the paramedic to consider and manage any reversible cause of an altered conscious state.

Like the GCS score, a single AVPU score is not a good predictor for the cause of unconsciousness (Brunker and Harris, 2015), nor is it a good predictor of response to treatment. Patients presenting with narcotic overdose or hypoglycaemia, for example, can often present with an initial AVPU score of U but can respond rapidly to treatment and return to a score of A within minutes.

AVPU and GCS

The AVPU scale has been shown to have rough equivalency with the ranges in the GCS. Though it cannot be interpreted precisely in this way, the comparison provides a general context of any AVPU finding (see Table 2.2.2). All unresponsive 'U' patients according to AVPU correspond to a GCS score <8 (Hoffmann et al., 2016; Weeks et al., 2016), including in children.

Minor head trauma remains an uncertain area in acute medicine, with mild to severe concussion (e.g. following sporting accidents) presenting with little or no variance in GCS or AVPU scores. A more detailed neurological examination should be used to assess this group.

Table 2.2.2 AVPU equivalence with the Glasgow Coma Scale

AVPU	GCS
A	15–12
V	14–10
P	10–5
U	5–3

Source: *Kelly et al., 2004; MacKay et al., 2000; McNarry and Goldhill, 2004; Raman, 2011; Sam et al., 2016.*

Traumatic brain injuries are a relatively uncommon cause of altered consciousness, with diseases (stroke, dementia, delirium, infection), drugs (alcohol, antidepressants, opioids, illicit) and metabolic causes (hypoglycaemia, electrolyte imbalances) all more likely to be the cause. The AVPU score can provide a level of accuracy similar to the GCS in these cases (MacKay et al., 2000; Nuttall et al., 2016; Rajabi Kheirabadi et al., 2015; Raman, 2011).

Suitability for AVPU assessment

There are several confounding provisos when assessing any patient with AVPU. These should be checked before assessment.

- *Eyes:* Eye opening must be purposeful to be representative of higher brain function. If the eyes are found open despite the patient being otherwise unresponsive, gently close them to observe if the patient opens them again or use other response criteria.
- *Speech:* The patient must have the ability to hear, speak and understand the language used. If they are deaf, aphasic or not able to understand the questions asked, the responses to verbal stimuli will be unreliable.

- *Injuries:* Patient injuries can interfere with responses. Swollen eyes can prevent eye opening, facial trauma can prevent speech and limb or spinal injuries can prevent normal responses to stimuli. Where this is so, observe for other responses.

- *Non-cooperation:* Occasionally patients will refuse to comply with an AVPU assessment for a variety of reasons, including drugs and mental health issues. Make note of suspected purposeful non-compliance and instead observe for any other response to stimuli.

PRACTICE TIP!

Mastoid pressure, supraorbital pressure and sternal pressure are all forms of 'painful stimuli' and carry greater risk of physical harm to the patient than does nailbed pressure. Any pain stimulus can be used in AVPU assessment provided it elicits responses from the brain.

PRACTICE TIP!

A primary function of the AVPU score in prehospital care is to determine the need for airway support. Generally, patients with no response to the pain stimulus require some form of airway support and ventilation monitoring. This can trigger the need for escalating care to an extended care or intensive care paramedic.

PRACTICE TIP!

Extending the arm laterally before applying nailbed pressure allows the paramedic to be essentially 'out of reach' if the patient unexpectedly lashes out in response to the stimulus.

PRACTICE TIP!

Speaking to patients who have altered consciousness as if they are conscious and explaining your actions to them and others can reduce the chance of anyone reacting poorly to painful stimuli.

TEST YOUR KNOWLEDGE QUESTIONS

1. **What are the three patient response criteria assessed for when using AVPU?**
   Eye opening; verbal response; motor response.

2. **Which of the following is not a response component of the AVPU scale?**
   a. Airway
   b. Response to verbal stimulation
   c. Response to painful stimulation
   d. Unresponsive
   Airway.

3. **The AVPU scale can be used to aid the paramedic in assessment of neurologic status and disability much like the Glasgow Coma Scale. What does the P stand for in AVPU?**
   a. Pupils are reactive and equal
   b. Responds only to pain
   c. Private medical history such as alcoholic withdrawal seizures
   d. Pain
   Responds only to pain.

4. **A patient who opens their eyes only after painful stimulus would receive an AVPU rating of:**
   a. A
   b. V
   c. P
   d. U
   P.

5. **A patient who opens their eyes only after a verbal stimulus would receive an AVPU rating of:**
   a. A
   b. V
   c. P
   d. U
   V.

6. **A patient has their eyes closed due to injury in trauma. How do you respond to this interference with the AVPU assessment?**
   Look for other responses including verbal or motor to the stimulus provided.

7. **Is the AVPU considered a useful tool in the paediatric patient?**
   Yes, it is a very useful alternative to GCS.

8. **What AVPU result may prompt airway intervention?**
   Low (P or U) responses.

9. **Can AVPU results be equated to GCS findings in any way?**
   Yes, AVPU results fit roughly into broad GCS ranges for comparison.

10. **If a patient makes incomprehensible verbal responses to painful stimulus, how are they described in AVPU?**
    P – responds to pain.

References

Acker, S.N., Ross, J.T., Partrick, D.A., Nadlonek, N.A., Bronsert, M. and Bensard, D.D., 2014. Glasgow Motor Scale alone is equivalent to Glasgow Coma Scale at identifying children at risk for serious traumatic brain injury. *Journal of Trauma and Acute Care Surgery*, 77(2), 304–309.

Al-Salamah, M.A., McDowell, I., Stiell, I.G., Wells, G.A., Perry, J., Al-Sultan, M. and Nesbitt, L., 2004. Initial emergency department trauma scores from the OPALS study: the case for the motor score in blunt trauma. *Academic Emergency Medicine*, 11(8), 834–842.

Bassi, S., Buxton, N., Punt, J.A. and O'Reilly, G., 1999. Glasgow Coma Scale: a help or hindrance? *British Journal of Neurosurgery*, 13(5), 526–539.

Bledsoe, B.E., Casey, M.J., Feldman, J., Johnson, L., Diel, S., Forred, W. and Gorman, C., 2015. Glasgow Coma Scale scoring is often inaccurate. *Prehospital and Disaster Medicine*, 30(1), 46–53.

Brunker, C. and Harris, R., 2015. How accurate is the AVPU scale in detecting neurological impairment when used by general ward nurses? An evaluation study using simulation and a questionnaire. *Intensive and Critical Care Nursing*, 31(2), 69–75.

Fischer, M., Rüegg, S., Czaplinski, A., Strohmeier, M., Lehmann, A., Tschan, F., Hunziker, P.R. and Marsch, S.C., 2010. Inter-rater reliability of the Full Outline of UnResponsiveness score and the Glasgow Coma Scale in critically ill patients: a prospective observational study. *Critical Care*, 14(2), R64.

Fortune, P.M. and Shann, F., 2010. The motor response to stimulation predicts outcome as well as the full Glasgow Coma Scale in children with severe head injury. *Pediatric Critical Care Medicine*, 11, 339–342.

Gill, M., Reiley, D.G. and Green, S.M., 2004. Interrater reliability of Glasgow Coma Scale scores in the emergency department. *Annals of Emergency Medicine*, 43, 215–223.

Green, S.M., 2011. Cheerio, laddie! Bidding farewell to the Glasgow Coma Scale. *Annals of Emergency Medicine*, 58(5), 427–430.

Hoffmann, F., Schmalhofer, M., Lehner, M., Zimatschek, S., Grote, V. and Reiter, K., 2016. Comparison of the AVPU scale and the Pediatric GCS in prehospital setting. *Prehospital Emergency Care*, 20(4), 493–498.

Holdgate, A., Ching, N. and Angonese, L., 2006. Variability in agreement between physicians and nurses when measuring the Glasgow Coma Scale in the emergency department limits its clinical usefulness. *Emergency Medicine Australia*, 18, 379–384.

Juarez, V.J. and Lyons, M., 1995. Interrater reliability of the Glasgow Coma Scale. *Journal of Neuroscience Nursing*, 27, 283–286.

Kelly, C.A., Upex, A. and Bateman, D.N., 2004. Comparison of consciousness level assessment in the poisoned patient using the alert/verbal/painful/unresponsive scale and the Glasgow Coma Scale. *Annals of Emergency Medicine*, 44(2), 108–113.

Lindsay, K.W., Teasdale, G.M. and Knill-Jones, R.P., 1983. Observer variability in assessing the clinical features of subarachnoid hemorrhage. *Journal of Neurosurgery*, 58, 57–62.

MacKay, C.A., Burke, D.P., Burke, J.A., Porter, K.M., Bowden, D. and Gormen, D., 2000. Association between the assessment of conscious level using AVPU system and GCS. *Prehospital Immediate Care*, 4, 17–19.

McNarry, A.F. and Goldhill, D.R., 2004. Simple bedside assessment of level of consciousness: comparison of two simple assessment scales with the Glasgow Coma Scale. *Anaesthesia*, 59(1), 34–37.

Nuttall, A., Patton, K. and Kemp, A.M., 2016. G224 (P) Glasgow Coma Scale or AVPU: what do clinicians use in head injury? Does it matter? *Archives of Disease in Childhood*, 101, A123–A124.

Rajabi Kheirabadi, A., Tabeshpour, J. and Afshari, R., 2015. Comparison of three consciousness assessment scales in poisoned patients and recommendation of a new scale: AVPU Plus. *Asia Pacific Journal of Medical Toxicology*, 4(2), 58–63.

Raman, S., 2011. Comparison of Alert-Verbal-Painful-Unresponsiveness Scale and the Glasgow Coma Score. *Indian Pediatrics*, 48, 330–332.

Ross, S.E., Leipold, C., Terregino, C. and O'Malley, K.F., 1998. Efficacy of the motor component of the Glasgow Coma Scale in trauma triage. *Journal of Trauma and Acute Care Surgery*, 45(1), 42–44.

Rowley, G. and Fielding, K., 1991. Reliability and accuracy of the Glasgow Coma Scale with experienced and inexperienced users. *Lancet*, 337, 535–538.

Sam, N.T.H., Toan, P.N. and Hong, T.T.M., 2016. Comparison of AVPU scale and the Glasgow Coma Scale score in assessing encephalitis in children. *Pediatric Infectious Diseases: Open Access*, 1(4).

Teasdale, G., Knill-Jones, R. and Vander Sande, J., 1978. Observer variability in assessing impaired consciousness and coma. *Journal of Neurology, Neurosurgery, and Psychiatry*, 41, 603–610.

Tesseris, J., Pantazidis, N., Routsi, C. and Fragoulakis, D., 1991. A comparative study of the Reaction Level Scale (RLS 85) with Glasgow Coma Scale (GCS) and Edinburgh-2 Coma Scale (modified) (E 2 CS (M)). *Acta Neurochirurgica*, 110(1), 65–76.

Van de Voorde, P., Sabbe, M., Rizopoulos, D., Tsonaka, R., De Jaeger, A., Lesaffre, E., Peters, M. and PENTA Study Group, 2008. Assessing the level of consciousness in children: a plea for the Glasgow coma motor subscore. *Resuscitation*, 76(2), 175–179.

Weeks, S.R., Stevens, K.A., Haider, A.H., Efron, D.T., Haut, E.R., MacKenzie, E.J. and Schneider, E.B., 2016. A modified Kampala Trauma Score (KTS) effectively predicts mortality in trauma patients. *Injury*, 47(1), 125–129.

Zuercher, M., Ummenhofer, W., Baltussen, A. and Walder, B., 2009. The use of Glasgow Coma Scale in injury assessment: a critical review. *Brain Injury*, 23(5), 371–384.

Chapter objectives

At the end of this chapter the reader will be able to:

1. Describe the rationale for palpating a pulse
2. Demonstrate the palpation of the radial and brachial pulse
3. Accurately report on the findings of the assessment
4. Identify pathologies associated with abnormal pulses

Resources required for this assessment

- Simulated patient with skin exposed to mid upper arm or mannequin capable of producing radial and brachial pulses
- Hand decontamination agent such as an alcohol-based hand gel
- Disposable gloves
- Clinical waste bag
- Method of documenting results

Skill matrix

This assessment requires:

- Infection control (CS 1.3)
- Communication (CS 1.5)
- Consent (CS 1.6)

This assessment is a component of:

- Patient assessment (Chapter 2)
- Cardiac arrest (Chapter 6)

Introduction

The ability of the heart to perfuse the tissues is an essential component of homeostasis. Pulse abnormalities can be indicative of compromised perfusion. The skill of assessing a pulse is quick and easy to perform, requires no equipment and can act as a simple start to the physical examination. Conducted effectively, the pulse check discussed in this chapter provides the paramedic with clear clinical information and builds trust and engagement with the patient and carers.

Anatomy and physiology

The pulse is the palpable expansion and contraction of an artery when a pressure-generated wave is produced by left ventricular systolic contraction and diastolic relaxation. Normal adult left ventricular ejection is approximately 95 mL (+/−14 mL) of blood into the arterial system with each contraction (Waugh and Grant, 2014). This surge of blood travels down and stretches the muscular wall of the artery. A finger placed against the artery can best feel this expansion where an artery runs near to the body surface. The most common sites used are the radial, brachial, carotid and femoral. In between pulses, the muscular artery walls force it to return to its resting diameter.

The pulse is one element of the cardiovascular system. It varies with input from the autonomic nervous system to respond to normal variations to maintain homeostasis and in response to disease. The sympathetic nervous system is involved in increasing heart and pulse rate, and the parasympathetic nervous system for slowing them.

Arguably, the most common site for pulse detection is the radial pulse, which is felt by palpating 2 cm proximal to the anterior and lateral wrist overlying the radial artery (Fig. 2.3.1). This is the most accessible and least intrusive site.

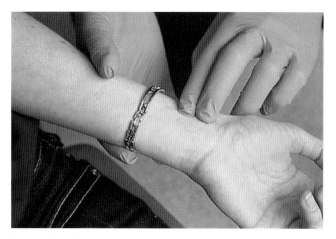

Figure 2.3.1 Radial pulse palpation

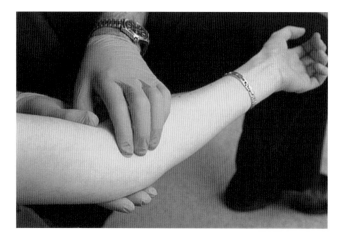

Figure 2.3.2 Brachial pulse palpation

The brachial pulse can be detected in adults on the anterior arm, medial of the biceps tendon in the elbow crease overlying the brachial artery. This site is used for palpating and auscultating blood pressure with a sphygmomanometer (Fig. 2.3.2).

Clinical rationale

The pulse is an extremely sensitive variable, making it useful for patient assessment and trend monitoring. In all patients, the main characteristics of the pulse, rate, rhythm and strength can provide a suggestion of perfusion compromise or indicate the presence of underlying pathology that requires further investigation.

In patients with an altered conscious state, the presence of a normal pulse strongly suggests that the cause of the abnormal conscious state is not inadequate perfusion. The absence of a pulse (or a very slow pulse) in the unconscious patient suggests circulatory failure and is an indication to commence cardiopulmonary resuscitation (CPR).

A gentle inward pressure will need to be applied to feel the pulse. Hold this and time the pulse to detect beats per minute. This can be done using a shorter timeframe such as 15 seconds then multiplying the counts by 4 if the pulse is regular and of normal rate. If it becomes irregular and abnormally slow or fast, count the pulse for a longer period such as 30 seconds and then double the result.

As blood moves further from the left ventricle, the pressure decreases. The brachial pulse may remain palpable when there is insufficient blood pressure to detect a radial pulse.

Clinical skill assessment process

The following section outlines the clinical skill assessment tools that should be used to determine a student's ability to demonstrate safe and accurate palpation and recording of a radial and brachial pulse.
1. Clinical Skill Work Instruction
2. Formative Clinical Skill Assessment (F-CSAT)
3. Performance Improvement Plan (PIP)
4. Summative Clinical Skill Assessment (S-CSAT)
(5. Direct Observation of Procedural Skills (DOPS) – see Chapter 1.1)

Clinical Skill Work Instruction

Equipment and resources: Simulated patient with skin exposed to mid upper arm or mannequin with palpable radial/brachial pulse; hand decontamination agent; disposable gloves; clinical waste bag; a method of documenting results

Associated Clinical Skills: Infection control; Communication; Consent

Assessing the radial and brachial pulse

Activity	Critical Action	Rationale
Position patient	The arm used should be relaxed, preferably resting on a flat surface. The point of palpation should not be higher than the heart.	Contracting forearm muscles increases difficulty palpating the radial artery.

Assessing the radial and brachial pulse continued

Activity	Critical Action	Rationale
Locate radial/ brachial artery	Radial: Place the pads of two fingers over the radial artery on the anterior surface of the wrist 2 cm proximal to the crease, 1–2 cm from the lateral aspect. Brachial: Place the pads of two fingers over the brachial artery on the anterior surface of the arm, medial to the biceps tendon in the elbow crease.	Do not use the thumb to palpate the artery as it may have its own pulse.
Palpate radial/ brachial pulse	Gently push fingers inwards, sensing for artery pulsing.	
Assess	Count pulses for 15 seconds and multiply by 4. Note rate. Note rhythm. Note strength.	Slow and irregular rhythms can increase calculation errors. Counting for longer will improve accuracy (e.g. 30 seconds and multiply by 2, or even 1 whole minute).
Record findings	Accurately document/hand over findings.	Accurate record kept and continuity of patient care.

Formative Clinical Skill Assessment (F-CSAT)

Equipment and resources: Simulated patient with skin exposed to mid upper arm or mannequin with palpable radial/ brachial pulse; hand decontamination agent; disposable gloves; clinical waste bag; a method of documenting results

Associated Clinical Skills: Infection control; Communication; Consent

Staff/Student being assessed: _____

Assessing the radial and brachial pulse

Activity	Critical Action	Performance				
Positions patient	The arm used is relaxed, preferably resting on a flat surface. The point of palpation is not higher than the heart.	0	1	2	3	4
Locates radial/ brachial artery	Radial: Places the pads of two fingers over the radial artery on the anterior surface of the wrist 2 cm proximal to the crease, 1–2 cm from the lateral aspect. Brachial: Places the pads of two fingers over the brachial artery on the anterior surface of the arm, medial to the biceps tendon in the elbow crease.	0	1	2	3	4
Palpates radial/ brachial pulse	Gently pushes inwards until pulsing is detected.	0	1	2	3	4
Assesses	Counts pulses for 15 seconds and multiplies by 4 (or 30 seconds and multiplies by 2 if pulse slow or irregular). Notes rate. Notes rhythm. Notes strength.	0	1	2	3	4
Records findings	Accurately documents/hands over findings.	0	1	2	3	4

Standard Achieved: (please circle one)

Competent (C)   Not Yet Competent* (NYC)

Staff/Student Name: _____

Assessor (please print name)**:** _____

Signed (Assessor)**:** _____

Date of Assessment: _____

Comments:

*If Not Yet Competent (NYC) a PIP needs to be completed and a repeat of the F-CSAT

Formative Clinical Skill Assessment (F-CSAT) Key

Skill level	Standard of procedure	Quality of performance	Outcome	Level of assistance required
4 Safe for unsupervised practice	Safe Accurate Behaviour is appropriate to context	Confident Accurate Expedient	Achieved intended outcome	No supporting cues* required
3 Requires supervision	Safe Accurate Behaviour is appropriate to context	Confident Accurate Takes longer than required	Achieved intended outcome	Requires occasional supportive cues*
2 Requires assistance	Safe Accurate Behaviour generally appropriate to context	Lacks certainty	Would not have achieved outcome without support	Requires frequent verbal and occasional physical directives in addition to supportive cues*
1 Requires direction	Safe only with guidance Not completely accurate	Unskilled Inefficient	Would not have achieved outcome without support	Requires continuous verbal and frequent physical directive cues*
0 Unsafe	Unsafe Unable to demonstrate behaviour Lack of insight into behaviour appropriate to context	Unskilled	Would not have achieved outcome	Requires continuous verbal and continuous physical directive cues*

*Refers to physical directives or verbal supportive cues

Performance Improvement Plan (PIP)

Please document the agreed education plan and completion timelines for areas assessed as less than 4.

This plan should be presented to assessor prior to commencement of summative assessment.

Where was supervisor support required?	Student summary of deficit. (Why was there a problem?)	Improvement Plan	Completed (Y/N)

Staff/Student Name: _____

Staff/Student Signature: _____

Educator Name: _____

Educator Signature: _____

Summative Clinical Skill Assessment (S-CSAT)

Equipment and resources: Simulated patient with skin exposed to mid upper arm or mannequin with palpable radial/brachial pulse; hand decontamination agent; disposable gloves; clinical waste bag; a method of documenting results

Associated Clinical Skills: Infection control; Communication; Consent

Staff/Student being assessed: _____

- Completed Formative Clinical Skill Assessment (F-CSAT): **YES   NO**
- Completed Performance Improvement Plan (PIP): **YES   NO   N/A**

Assessing the radial and brachial pulse

Activity	Critical Action	Achieved Without Direction	
Positions patient	The arm used is relaxed, preferably resting on a flat surface. The point of palpation is not higher than the heart.	NO	YES
Locates radial/brachial artery	Radial: Places the pads of two fingers over the radial artery on the anterior surface of the wrist 2 cm proximal to the crease, 1–2 cm from the lateral aspect. Brachial: Places the pads of two fingers over the brachial artery on the anterior surface of the arm, medial to the biceps tendon in the elbow crease.	NO	YES
Palpates radial/brachial pulse	Gently pushes inwards until pulsing is detected.	NO	YES
Assesses	Counts pulses for 15 seconds and multiplies by 4 (or for 30 seconds and multiplies by 2 if pulse slow or irregular). Notes rate. Notes rhythm. Notes strength.	NO	YES
Records findings	Accurately documents/hands over findings.	NO	YES

Standard Achieved: (please circle one)

Competent (C)   Not Yet Competent* (NYC)

Staff/Student Name: _____

Assessor (please print name)**:** _____

Signed (Assessor)**:** _____

Date of Assessment: _____

Comments:

*If Not Yet Competent (NYC) a PIP needs to be completed and a repeat of the F-CSAT

Clinical findings

The pulse should be assessed for the following characteristics:
- absence/presence
- rate
- rhythm
- strength.

Absence/presence

The absence of a palpable pulse raises two broad concerns. The first is that the clinician is unable to locate it. This may be due to a failure to identify the correct site, significant overlaying adipose tissue covering the site or underlying vascular disease (Claassen et al., 2010; Mohammedi et al., 2016). In such cases, attempt to locate the pulse using a different site. The second, more serious, concern is that the patient may be failing to produce a reasonable pulse, for reasons such as profound hypotension or cardiac arrest.

Rate

The typical resting adult pulse has a rate of between 60 and 80 beats per minute (bpm) (Cox, 2013). Variations outside of these parameters do not necessarily indicate abnormality, however, as exertion, pain and stress can raise the resting heart rate, while some medications and high levels of fitness can produce acceptable rates below 60 bpm.

Pulse rates are:
- normal: 60–100 bpm
- abnormal: <60 or >100 bpm

Any rate over 100 bpm or lower than 60 bpm should be investigated further by electrocardiogram (ECG) and patient assessment. A rate between 60 and 100 bpm does not exclude significant injuries or pathologies, as pain, stress and medications can all interfere with autonomic nervous system heart rate control.

The factors that affect the heart rate include:
- physical activity
- sleep
- fever
- medical conditions affecting the cardiovascular system

- pain
- circulating blood volume loss
- street drugs
- emotional states
- prescribed medications.

Rhythm

Pulse rhythms are described as:
- regular
- irregularly irregular: with no discernible pattern
- regularly irregular: with a discernible pattern.

The time between each pulsatile wave should usually be the same (Waugh and Grant, 2014). A regular heart rate indicates the rhythm is being generated by autorhythmic nodal tissue, most likely the sinoatrial (SA) node. Occasional irregularity caused by ectopic beats or associated with breathing can be normal.

An irregularly irregular rhythm with no predictable pattern is most often caused by atrial fibrillation. This may be normal for some patients but should trigger further assessment, including ECG confirmation.

Very fast tachycardia rhythms may not have sufficient time for ventricular filling between contractions, producing weakness and irregularity of the pulses felt. The pulse rate might be difficult to detect and be markedly different from the monitored ECG heart rate.

The factors that affect pulse regularity include:
- prescribed medications
- cardiovascular diseases
- diseases of the myocardial electrical conduction system.

Strength

The volume and viscosity of blood pushed into the artery with each ventricular contraction are the primary determinants of pulse strength. Arteriosclerosis can reduce the force detected during palpation.

Pulse strength is reported as:
- normal
- weak or thready
- bounding.

Decreased left ventricular function or hypovolemia can produce a 'weak' expansion of the artery and a pulse that is difficult to feel. In comparison, a normal heart pumping blood of increased viscosity (dehydration from heat stress or severe hyperglycaemia) produces a sharp and sudden expansion described as 'bounding'.

The factors that affect the strength of the pulse include any factor affecting:

- myocardial preload (initial monocyte stretching prior to contraction)
- myocardial afterload (resistance to ejection into aorta)
- stroke volume (amount of blood ejected by the ventricles).

PRACTICE TIP!

Do not confuse pulse rate with the electrical heart rate that stimulates ventricular contraction. At rapid rates and/or certain arrhythmias, ventricular filling can be compromised, with not every electrical ventricular depolarisation generating a contraction and subsequent pulse. An ECG is required to determine heart rate and should always be performed any time abnormality of the pulse or perfusion is detected. Pulse and heart rate should be the same but are not always so.

PRACTICE TIP!

Pulses on the left and right sides should be equal in strength; it is uncommon to find significant differences between them. A weak pulse on one arm generally indicates an obstruction to the arteries between the point of palpation and the left ventricle. Unilateral difference in pulse strength can be caused by thoracic aorta dissection blocking blood flow into one arm. Comparing pulse strengths on both sides is worthwhile if this condition is suspected; however, the absence of any difference does not exclude it.

PRACTICE TIP!

The absence of a pulse in the unconscious patient is a trigger to commence CPR. Outside of this circumstance, no decision should be finalised on pulse palpation alone and options should be considered in the context of overall perfusion status assessment.

TEST YOUR KNOWLEDGE QUESTIONS

1. **Define the term 'pulse'.**
    A pulse is the expansion in diameter of an artery following the contraction of the left ventricle and the subsequent movement of blood through the arterial system.

2. **Why is pulse rate not the same as heart rate?**
    Electrical heart rate stimulates ventricular contraction. At rapid rates and/or certain arrhythmias, ventricular filling can be compromised, with not every electrical ventricular depolarisation generating a contraction and subsequent pulse. An ECG is required to determine heart rate, which can then be compared to pulse.

3. **How does the autonomic nervous system control heart rate?**
    The sympathetic division increases the firing rate of the SA node whereby the parasympathetic division inhibits it, causing the rate to slow.

4. **When assessing a pulse, what three characteristics should a paramedic assess for?**
    Rate; rhythm; strength.

5. **List five abnormalities in a pulse.**
    Too fast; too slow; irregular; too strong; weak.

6. **List five causes of a fast pulse.**
    Exercise; sleep; fever; medications; street drugs; pain; blood loss; emotion.

7. **At what points during pulse assessment should a paramedic decontaminate their hands?**
    Before and after the procedure.

8. **What are two reasons for assessing brachial pulse?**
    This site is used for palpating and auscultating blood pressure with a sphygmomanometer; as blood pressure falls, the brachial pulse may remain palpable when a radial pulse may not be able to be detected.

9. **Fill in the missing number: When the pulse is regular, count for .... seconds then multiply the number of beats by 4.**
    15.

10. **Fill in the missing number: When the pulse is irregular, count for .... seconds then multiply the number of beats by 2.**
    30.

References

Cox, C., 2013. *Physical assessment for nurses*. Oxford: Wiley.

Claassen, H., Schmitt, O., Werner, D., Schareck, W., Kröger, J.C. and Wree, A., 2010. Superficial arm arteries revisited: brother and sister with absent radial pulse. *Annals of Anatomy (Anatomischer Anzeiger)*, 192(3), 151–155.

Mohammedi, K., Woodward, M., Zoungas, S., Li, Q., Harrap, S., Patel, A., Marre, M., Chalmers, J. and ADVANCE Collaborative Group, 2016. Absence of peripheral pulses and risk of major vascular outcomes in patients with type 2 diabetes. *Diabetes Care*, dc161594.

Waugh, A. and Grant, A., 2014. *Ross and Wilson anatomy and physiology in health and illness*. 12th edn. Sydney: Elsevier.

Bibliography

Koeppen, B.M. and Stanton, B.A., 2010. *Berne and Levy physiology*. 6th edn. St Louis: Mosby/Elsevier.

Patton, K.T. and Thibodeau, G.A., 2014. *Mosby's handbook of anatomy and physiology*. 2nd edn. St Louis: Mosby.

2.4 | Assessing blood pressure

Matt Johnson

Chapter objectives

At the end of this chapter the reader will be able to:

1. Describe the rationale for measuring blood pressure
2. Demonstrate auscultation and palpation of brachial blood pressure
3. Accurately report on assessment findings

Resources required for this assessment

- Standardised patient with skin exposed to mid upper arm or mannequin capable of producing brachial pulses or Korotkoff sounds
- Sphygmomanometer and stethoscope
- Disposable gloves
- Method of documenting the results

Skill matrix

This assessment requires:

- Infection control (CS 1.3)
- Communication (CS 1.6)
- Consent (CS 1.6)
- Assessing the radial and brachial pulse (CS 2.3)

This assessment is a component of:

- Patient assessment (Chapter 2)

Introduction

Blood pressure (BP) is one of four necessary components of perfusion status assessment, including heart rate, conscious state and skin appearance. Perfusion is assessed considering all factors.

Assessing blood pressure is a baseline observation paramedics assess in almost every patient. It is a relatively simple skill but can be challenging when working in a confined space, with an agitated patient or under time pressure. Mastering this skill, which is discussed in this chapter, is essential for paramedics.

Blood pressure can be assessed by either auscultation or palpation. The auscultation method is more common and useful. Occasions where palpation may be preferred are discussed below.

Anatomy and physiology

With each contraction, the adult left ventricle ejects around 100 millilitres (mL) of blood into the aorta. This in turn forces blood already in the arterial system to move away from the heart towards the capillaries. The pressure generated by the left ventricle with each contraction (systole) and resistance of the blood in the arterial system combine to cause a peak in fluid pressure within the blood vessel walls. This is blood pressure.

Some pressure remains between contractions (diastole), as the elastic contraction of the arterial walls maintains residual pressure in the system. Measuring systolic and diastolic pressures provides a guide to the level of blood flow through the arterial system and subsequent tissue perfusion.

Although there are 'normal' values prescribed to blood pressure, these can vary considerably with body size and health. Small females may have low 'normal' blood pressures while large males with undiagnosed hypertension may display other signs of poor perfusion while maintaining high blood pressure. The actual value is often of less diagnostic use than any trend in subsequent assessments (Sheppard et al., 2016).

Clinical rationale

A single blood pressure measurement is simply a snapshot of condition at that moment. Trends in blood pressure (rising or falling) can indicate injury progression (including lowering blood pressure with ongoing haemorrhage or rising blood pressure with closed head injury and rising intracranial pressure). Trends indicate a response (or lack of one) to treatment, necessitating accurate measurements every time.

The sphygmomanometer comprises a Velcro®-fastened fabric cuff containing a rubber bladder with a pressure gauge attached and a valved pump to inflate it. The cuff is wrapped around the upper arm and inflated to a pressure that temporarily occludes blood flow through the artery (Fig. 2.4.1). When the cuff pressure compressing the artery drops below the pressure of the blood inside the artery, blood flow resumes. This is the systolic blood pressure. This method, performed correctly, should be within 3–4 mmHg of actual intra-arterial pressure (Smulyan and Safar, 2011).

The brachial artery is the standard location for auscultating blood pressure, though the radial pulse is useful for palpation methods (Ogedegbe et al., 2010). Placing the stethoscope bell over the brachial artery before the cuff is inflated reveals no sounds as blood is able to flow through the artery in a silent, smooth, laminar fashion. Inflate the cuff until Korotkoff sounds are heard (McCutcheon et al., 1967).

Continue inflating until the sounds are lost again. Inflate approximately 40 mmHg more to ensure flow is impeded and to allow sufficient time to detect sounds returning as the cuff is deflated. As the cuff is slowly deflated from this pressure there will be silence until the pressure in the cuff is equal (or slightly less) than the pressure generated during systole.

At this point, the turbulent flow of blood through the partially occluded artery registers as 'taps' consistent with each contraction. Note the reading, as this is the systolic blood pressure.

As the cuff is slowly deflated the 'taps' become softer in volume and lower in pitch. When these muffled sounds completely disappear, the pressure exerted by the cuff is no longer distorting the walls of the artery and is equivalent to the diastolic pressure in the artery within 10 mmHg of intra-arterial pressure (Smulyan and Safar, 2011). Note this reading as the diastolic blood pressure.

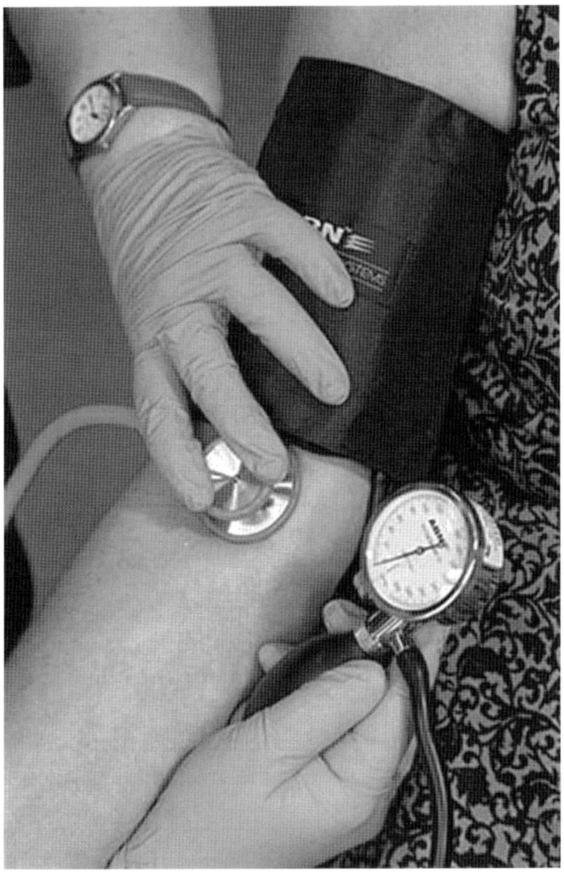

Figure 2.4.1 Auscultating blood pressure

KOROTKOFF SOUNDS

There are five Korotkoff sounds:

Phase I: The first faint but clear tapping sounds – the *systolic* blood pressure.

Phase II: The sounds soften with a swishing quality.

Phase III: The sounds become sharper, regaining, or exceeding, first sound intensity.

Phase IV: A distinct, abrupt muffling.

Phase IV: The sounds disappear – the *diastolic* pressure.

Only the first and final Korotkoff sounds have any clinical significance. In some patients, the sounds may disappear for a short time between phases II and III, which is referred to as 'the auscultatory gap' (McCutcheon et al., 1967).

Documenting blood pressure

Blood pressure is documented as:

systolic reading/diastolic reading mmHg

In controlled clinical settings, blood pressures are normally auscultated with the patient sitting and their arm resting on a table. In the paramedic setting where location, privacy, weather, noise, entrapment or injury don't allow for auscultation, the return of brachial/radial

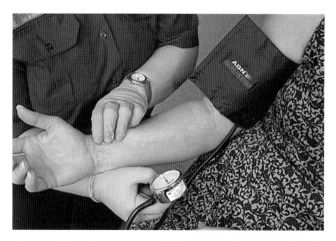

Figure 2.4.2 Assessing (radially) palpated systolic blood pressure

pulse as the cuff is deflated as a measure of systolic blood pressure is often used (Fig. 2.4.2). This palpated value is usually close to an auscultated systolic pressure.

The systolic value is sensitive to changes in blood volume, heart failure and acute changes in the vascular system, and so can be a sufficient first-line measurement of blood pressure.

Blood pressure by palpation is documented as:

systolic reading/palp mmHg

or as:

systolic reading/sys mmHg

denoting the absence of a diastolic value.

Cuffs come in various sizes for paediatric, adult and obese use. Incorrect cuff sizing can generate reading errors. The cuff bladder width should be at least 40% of the circumference of the limb at the point of application, with the length being about 75% to 80% of the circumference.

If the cuff is too small the Velcro® may not hold it during inflation.

For brachial blood pressure, an appropriately sized cuff should leave 2–3 cm between the distal cuff edge to where the stethoscope bell is placed. The hose to the cuff should sit approximately over the brachial artery, running distally.

Ideally, the cuff is applied with the point of measure at an equivalent height to the heart (seated with the arm resting on table for brachial, supine with legs flat for popliteal). Treat variations in consecutive readings with caution if there is any change in body position between measurements.

The cuff should not be placed over an arm receiving intravenous fluid therapy, as it can interfere with flow. Arms with arteriovenous fistula should be avoided due to the risk of injuring the graft.

Blood pressure can be measured by listening over the popliteal artery posterior to the knee with an appropriately sized cuff applied at the mid-thigh. Systolic blood pressures in the legs are usually 10–20% higher than the brachial artery.

Clinical skill assessment process

The following section outlines the clinical skill assessment tools that should be used to determine a student's ability to safely and accurately auscultate, palpate and record a blood pressure.

1. Clinical Skill Work Instruction
2. Formative Clinical Skill Assessment (F-CSAT)
3. Performance Improvement Plan (PIP)
4. Summative Clinical Skill Assessment (S-CSAT)
(5. Direct Observation of Procedural Skills (DOPS) – see Chapter 1.1)

Clinical Skill Work Instruction

Equipment and resources: Standardised patient with skin exposed to mid upper arm or mannequin capable of producing brachial pulses or Korotkoff sounds; sphygmomanometer; stethoscope; disposable gloves; method of documenting the results

Associated Clinical Skills: Infection control; Communication; Consent; Assessing the brachial and radial pulse

Assessing blood pressure

Activity	Critical Action	Rationale
Prepare patient	Seated or reclined with back support, legs uncrossed, feet flat on floor, arm bare and supported.	This position is critical to increase accuracy.
	Inform/explain procedure.	Gain cooperation.
Prepare cuff	Choose the correct size of cuff.	Incorrect size can cause inaccurate reading.
	Ensure the cuff is fully deflated.	Partially inflated cuffs cause inaccurate over-reading.

Assessing blood pressure continued

Activity	Critical Action	Rationale
Auscultate blood pressure	Palpate brachial pulse. Position cuff so the artery marker points along brachial artery. Wrap cuff firmly around the arm, confirming Velcro® adhesion.	Ensures correct position and cuff tightness.
	Place stethoscope bell over the brachial pulse 2–3 cm from distal edge of cuff, with stethoscope in ears.	Optimal for detecting sounds.
	Close valve and inflate cuff, listening for Korotkoff sounds. Continue inflating until sound ceases. Add a further 40 mmHg.	Provides indication of required cuff inflation.
	Open valve and release air slowly at 2–3 mmHg per second.	Slow release of cuff allows for first sound to be heard.
	Detect Korotkoff sounds return. Note gauge reading. Continue slow deflation.	Denotes systolic reading.
	Detect loss of Korotkoff sounds. Note gauge reading. Release remainder of air from cuff. Remove from limb.	Denotes diastolic reading.
Palpate radial blood pressure	For palpable BP assessment, locate and maintain brachial or radial pulse palpation. Watch gauge and compress cuff inflator until cuff inflates and pulse is lost. Continue 40 mmHg further, then slowly release air until pulse returns. Note systolic reading.	To ensure accurate recording of systolic pressure.
Report	Accurately document/hand over findings.	To enable trend identification and to ensure continuity of care.

Formative Clinical Skill Assessment (F-CSAT)

Equipment and resources: Standardised patient with skin exposed to mid upper arm or mannequin capable of producing brachial pulses or Korotkoff sounds; sphygmomanometer; stethoscope; disposable gloves; method of documenting the results

Associated Clinical Skills: Infection control; Communication; Consent; Assessing the brachial and radial pulse

Staff/Student being assessed: _____

Assessing blood pressure

Activity	Critical Action	Participant Performance				
Prepares patient	Seats or reclines with back support, legs uncrossed, feet flat on floor, arm bare and supported.	0	1	2	3	4
	Informs/explains procedure.	0	1	2	3	4
Prepares cuff	Chooses the correct size of cuff.	0	1	2	3	4
	Ensures the cuff is fully deflated.	0	1	2	3	4

Assessing blood pressure continued

Activity	Critical Action	Participant Performance				
Auscultates blood pressure	Palpates brachial pulse. Positions cuff so artery marker points along brachial artery. Wraps cuff firmly around the arm, confirming Velcro® adhesion.	0	1	2	3	4
	Places stethoscope bell over the brachial pulse 2–3 cm from distal edge of cuff, with stethoscope in ears.	0	1	2	3	4
	Closes valve and inflates cuff, listening for Korotkoff sounds. Continues inflating until sound ceases. Adds a further 40 mmHg.	0	1	2	3	4
	Opens valve and releases air slowly at 2–3 mmHg per second.	0	1	2	3	4
	Detects Korotkoff sounds return. Notes gauge reading. Continues slow deflation.	0	1	2	3	4
	Detects loss of Korotkoff sounds. Notes gauge reading. Releases remainder of air from cuff. Removes from limb.	0	1	2	3	4
Palpates radial blood pressure	For palpable BP assessment, locates and maintains brachial or radial pulse palpation. Watches gauge and compresses cuff inflator until cuff inflates and pulse is lost. Continues 40 mmHg further, then slowly releases air until pulse returns. Notes systolic reading.	0	1	2	3	4
Reports	Accurately documents/hands over the findings.	0	1	2	3	4

Standard Achieved: (please circle one)

Competent (C)   Not Yet Competent* (NYC)

Staff/Student Name: _____

Assessor (please print name): _____

Signed (Assessor): _____

Date of Assessment: _____

Comments:

*If Not Yet Competent (NYC) a PIP needs to be completed and a repeat of the F-CSAT

Formative Clinical Skill Assessment (F-CSAT) Key

Skill level	Standard of procedure	Quality of performance	Outcome	Level of assistance required
4 Safe for unsupervised practice	Safe Accurate Behaviour is appropriate to context	Confident Accurate Expedient	Achieved intended outcome	No supporting cues* required
3 Requires supervision	Safe Accurate Behaviour is appropriate to context	Confident Accurate Takes longer than required	Achieved intended outcome	Requires occasional supportive cues*

Skill level	Standard of procedure	Quality of performance	Outcome	Level of assistance required
2 Requires assistance	Safe Accurate Behaviour generally appropriate to context	Lacks certainty	Would not have achieved outcome without support	Requires frequent verbal and occasional physical directives in addition to supportive cues*
1 Requires direction	Safe only with guidance Not completely accurate	Unskilled Inefficient	Would not have achieved outcome without support	Requires continuous verbal and frequent physical directive cues*
0 Unsafe	Unsafe Unable to demonstrate behaviour Lack of insight into behaviour appropriate to context	Unskilled	Would not have achieved outcome	Requires continuous verbal and continuous physical directive cues*

*Refers to physical directives or verbal supportive cues

Performance Improvement Plan (PIP)

Please document the agreed education plan and completion timelines for areas assessed as less than 4.

This plan should be presented to assessor prior to commencement of summative assessment.

Where was supervisor support required?	Student summary of deficit. (Why was there a problem?)	Improvement Plan	Completed (Y/N)

Staff/Student Name: _____

Staff/Student Signature: _____

Educator Name: _____

Educator Signature: _____

Summative Clinical Skill Assessment (S-CSAT)

Equipment and resources: Standardised patient with skin exposed to mid upper arm or mannequin capable of producing brachial pulses or Korotkoff sounds; sphygmomanometer; stethoscope; disposable gloves; method of documenting the results

Associated Clinical Skills: Infection control; Communication; Consent; Assessing the brachial and radial pulse

Staff/Student being assessed: _____

- Completed Formative Clinical Skill Assessment (F-CSAT): **YES** **NO**

- Completed Performance Improvement Plan (PIP): **YES** **NO** **N/A**

Assessing blood pressure

Activity	Critical Action	Achieved Without Direction	
Positions patient	Seats or reclines with back support, legs uncrossed, feet flat on floor, arm bare and supported.	NO	YES
	Informs/explains procedure.	NO	YES
Prepares cuff	Chooses the correct size of cuff.	NO	YES
	Ensures the cuff is fully deflated.	NO	YES
Auscultates blood pressure	Palpates brachial pulse. Positions cuff so artery marker points along brachial artery. Wraps cuff firmly around the arm, confirming Velcro® adhesion.	NO	YES
	Places stethoscope bell over the brachial pulse 2–3 cm from distal edge of cuff, with stethoscope in ears.	NO	YES
	Closes valve and inflates cuff, listening for Korotkoff sounds. Continues inflating until sound ceases. Adds a further 40 mmHg.	NO	YES
	Opens valve and releases air slowly at 2–3 mmHg per second.	NO	YES
	Detects Korotkoff sounds return. Notes gauge reading. Continues slow deflation.	NO	YES
	Detects loss of Korotkoff sounds. Notes gauge reading. Releases remainder of air from cuff. Removes from limb.	NO	YES
Palpates radial blood pressure	For palpable BP assessment, locates and maintains brachial or radial pulse palpation. Watches gauge and compresses cuff inflator until cuff inflates and pulse is lost. Continues 40 mmHg further, then slowly releases air until pulse returns. Notes systolic reading.	NO	YES
Reports	Accurately documents/hands over the findings.	NO	YES

Standard Achieved: (please circle one)

Competent (C)   Not Yet Competent* (NYC)

Staff/Student Name: _____

Assessor (please print name)**:** _____

Signed (Assessor)**:** _____

Date of Assessment: _____

Comments:

*If Not Yet Competent (NYC) a PIP needs to be completed and a repeat of the F-CSAT

Clinical findings

Systolic value

Normal systolic blood pressure in an adult is 100–120 mmHg. Values up to 139 mmHg are considered above normal, with persistent values >140 mmHg diagnostic for hypertension (James et al., 2014; Qaseem et al., 2017).

Blood pressures <100 mmHg are usually considered as hypotension but some guidelines will tolerate a BP of 90 mmHg before recommending intervention.

Diastolic value

Normal diastolic blood pressure is <80 mmHg. Diastolic values >90 mmHg are considered significant for hypertension and cardiovascular risk (James et al., 2014).

For short-term clinical decisions, diastolic value is of limited paramedic use.

Pulse pressure

Pulse pressure is the difference between systolic and diastolic. A narrowing pulse pressure in trauma may indicate significant blood loss. In other situations it may be an indication that stroke volume is low.

Hypotension

Systolic hypotension can be categorised into three causes:
1. *Reduction in blood volume* from haemorrhage or plasma loss (burns, anaphylaxis, dehydration, sepsis)
2. *Increased vascular capacity* from vasodilation (sepsis, anaphylaxis, drug effects)
3. *Decrease in cardiac output* from decreased contraction or inadequate heart rate (ventricular failure, arrhythmia, pulmonary embolus, tension pneumothorax).

Hypertension

Hypertension, which is generally a chronic condition, is rarely an indication for paramedic intervention. Hypertensive emergencies with associated end organ dysfunction are a notable exception, as this represents substantial risk factor for cardiovascular disease (Qaseem et al., 2017; Savoia and Touyz, 2017).

Hypertension can be observed associated with head injury, autonomic dysreflexia, rising intracranial pressure, and eclampsia of pregnancy.

Limb variations

Blood pressures are not routinely taken on both sides, as the values are generally similar. Differences of less than 10 mmHg can be normal. However, differences greater than 20 mmHg left and right can indicate significant cardiovascular disease, including aortic aneurysm (Clark et al., 2012), aortic dissection or peripheral artery disease.

Incorrect readings

Sphygmomanometers that are not properly calibrated can provide incorrect readings, as can poor technique (Sheppard et al., 2016; Ward et al., 2012). Nervousness during assessment can increase reading values (Myers et al., 2010).

Positioning, such as not supporting the patient's back or arm, can raise the systolic finding between 5 and 10 mmHg, crossing the legs can add up to 8 mmHg, and the patient talking during the reading can add up to 15 mmHg. The greatest potential for error is taking measurements over clothing, which can add up to 40 mmHg to the finding (Campbell et al., 2005).

PRACTICE TIP!

Poor weather, entrapment and heavy clothing can all make arm exposure and accurate blood pressure assessment difficult. It is acceptable to temporarily delay assessment in such cases if this is quickly rectifiable in the ambulance. Checking other perfusion indicators can provide some information. Guidelines reliant on accurate blood pressure should not be started unless the measurement is attained.

PRACTICE TIP!

Make sure the patient is relaxed, with their arm supported, to ensure the most accurate reading.

PRACTICE TIP!

Remember that blood pressure is one perfusion component to consider in context with the others: skin appearance, pulse and conscious state.

TEST YOUR KNOWLEDGE QUESTIONS

1. **Blood pressure is the force exerted by the blood against what?**
   The arterial wall.

2. **What is the unit of blood pressure measurement?**
   Millimetres of mercury (mmHg).

3. **What is the pulse site commonly used for auscultating blood pressure?**
   Brachial pulse.

4. **What pulse sites can be commonly used for palpating blood pressure and how does the result differ from auscultation?**
   Radial or brachial pulse; there is no diastolic reading.

5. **Once a cuff is inflated and the sound or pulse is lost, what extra inflation occurs and why?**
   40 mmHg over; to allow careful air release to precisely detect when sound/pulse returns.

6. **What patient position is normally preferred for assessing blood pressure?**
   Sitting or semi-reclined, with back and arm support.

7. **What gap is allowed between brachial pulse and cuff?**
   2–3 cm from distal cuff edge to stethoscope bell placement.

8. **What limb variation in reading is considered significant?**
   20 mmHg.

9. **What are the most common causes of incorrect blood pressure readings?**
   Improperly calibrated sphygmomanometers; patient nervousness; unsupported patient back or arm; crossing legs; patient talking throughout; assessing over clothing.

10. **Which of the five Korotkoff sounds are most important to blood pressure and why?**
    Five; the first is the systolic blood pressure reading, the fifth is the diastolic reading.

References

Campbell, N.R., Culleton, B.W. and McKay, D.W., 2005. Misclassification of blood pressure by usual measurement in ambulatory physician practices. *American Journal of Hypertension*, 18(12), 1522–1527.

Clark, C.E., Taylor, R.S., Shore, A.C. and Campbell, J.L., 2012. The difference in blood pressure readings between arms and survival: primary care cohort study. *British Medical Journal*, 344, e1327.

James, P.A., Oparil, S., Carter, B.L., Cushman, W.C., Dennison-Himmelfarb, C., Handler, J., Lackland, D.T., LeFevre, M.L., MacKenzie, T.D., Ogedegbe, O. and Smith, S.C., 2014. 2014 evidence-based guideline for the management of high blood pressure in adults: report from the panel members appointed to the Eighth Joint National Committee (JNC 8). *JAMA*, 311(5), 507–520.

McCutcheon, E.P., Rushmer, R.F., Jacobson, O. and Sandier, H., 1967. Korotkoff sounds: an experimental critique. *Circulation Research*, 20(2), 149–161.

Myers, M.G., Godwin, M., Dawes, M., Kiss, A., Tobe, S.W. and Kaczorowski, J., 2010. Measurement of blood pressure in the office. *Hypertension*, 55(2), 195–200.

Ogedegbe, G. and Pickering, T., 2010. Principles and techniques of blood pressure measurement. *Cardiology Clinics*, 28(4), 571–586.

Qaseem, A., Wilt, T.J., Rich, R., Humphrey, L.L., Frost, J. and Forciea, M.A., 2017. Pharmacologic treatment of hypertension in adults aged 60 years or older to higher versus lower blood pressure targets: a clinical practice guideline from the American College of Physicians and the American Academy of Family Physicians pharmacologic treatment of hypertension in adults. *Annals of Internal Medicine*, 166(6), 430–437.

Savoia, C. and Touyz, R.M., 2017. Hypertension, diabetes mellitus, and excess cardiovascular risk: importance of baseline systolic blood pressure. *Hypertension*, 70(5), 882–883.

Sheppard, J.P., Martin, U., Gill, P., Stevens, R. and McManus, R.J., 2016. Prospective Register Of patients undergoing repeated OFfice and Ambulatory Blood Pressure Monitoring (PROOF-ABPM): protocol for an observational cohort study. *BMJ Open*, 6(10), e012607.

Smulyan, H. and Safar, M.E., 2011. Blood pressure measurement: retrospective and prospective views. *American Journal of Hypertension*, 24(6), 628–634.

Ward, A.M., Takahashi, O., Stevens, R. and Heneghan, C., 2012. Home measurement of blood pressure and cardiovascular disease: systematic review and meta-analysis of prospective studies. *Journal of Hypertension*, 30(3), 449–456.

Recording the 12-lead electrocardiogram

Jeff Kenneally

Chapter objectives

At the end of this chapter the reader will be able to:

1. Describe the rationale for applying a 12-lead electrocardiogram (ECG)
2. Demonstrate the application of the 12-lead ECG
3. Report on common difficulties encountered when recording the 12-lead ECG

Resources required for this assessment

- Standardised or simulated patient with upper body exposed
- Disposable gloves
- 12-lead ECG device with leads and electrodes
- Method of documenting results

Skill matrix

This assessment requires:

- Infection control (CS 1.3)
- Communication (CS 1.5)
- Consent (CS 1.6)

This assessment is a component of:

- Patient assessment (Chapter 2)

Introduction

Despite being a century old, the electrocardiogram (ECG) remains a widely used medical diagnostic tool. For many occasions, the 3-lead ECG will be sufficient for cardiac rhythm monitoring, while the 12-lead ECG adds to this acute coronary syndrome diagnostics. This chapter focuses on the key ECG, capturing aspects of correct methods of use and lead placement.

Anatomy and physiology

Myocardial muscle depolarisation/repolarisation and conduction from cell to cell through the heart produces detectable electrical energy. Normal impulse initiates in the sinoatrial (SA) node in the anterosuperior right atrial wall. Conduction flows through the atria before passing through the atrioventricular (AV) node in the septal wall. Conduction continues down the septum in the bundle branches before distributing from the apex to the remainder of the ventricles through the Purkinje fibres.

The heart sits behind the sternum, leaning backwards and to the right. Right of the sternum, beneath the third and fourth ribs, is the right atrium, including the SA node. The right ventricle and AV node are behind the sternum and the septum just to its left, beneath the fourth and fifth ribs. These ribs angle inferiorly, with the bulk of the left ventricle and apex found in the lower left chest.

Despite electrical conduction flow distributing globally through the atria and ventricles, the normal overall flow from SA node to AV node to apex follows a predictable right-upper to left-lower chest vector. Strategic ECG electrode placement is necessary as positive or negative terminals form 'leads' to detect electricity flowing towards or away from them. A depolarisation wave towards a positive electrode causes upward deflection of the ECG graph. Depolarisation away from the positive terminal causes downward deflection.

Each ECG lead provides a different electrical perspective or 'view' of the heart. When all leads are combined, they provide a nearly complete view of myocardium electrical activity. Where electrical conduction does not follow normal flow directions, this can be identified by variations in the ECG patterns.

Clinical rationale

Electrodes

Electrodes are the conduit between the human body and the ECG device, detecting and measuring electricity flow. Electrode types vary, but the basic principle is an adhesiveness to human skin that allows ECG monitor wires to be attached. The most common are Ag/AgCl gel electrodes, which are typically able to perform effectively in most settings (Meziane et al., 2013). Paediatric-sized electrodes should be used for children, so that they all fit onto small chests.

Gel-based electrodes lose their conductivity unpredictably as they dry out (Wiese et al., 2005), and should be inspected for expiry date and quality before use. The ECG wires should be able to be attached without easily detaching. Attach them before the electrode is applied to patient, as attaching the wire afterwards requires pushing hard, which is uncomfortable for the patient and displaces gel from the electrode.

Electrodes can have difficulty attaching to wet/clammy skin, necessitating drying before attachment. Excess body hair can also interfere with adherence. If necessary, relocate the electrode to a less hairy but still correct place or clip the body hair with scissors.

Limb leads I, II, III

The first clinical use of ECG was to detect cardiac arrhythmias. For this purpose, the 3-lead ECG remains sufficiently sensitive and specific. This 'views' the heart from a frontal plane perspective, detecting electrical flow moving from the upper right to lower left chest.

Limb leads should be placed as follows (Fig. 2.5.1):
- Lead I view is from left (positive) arm/shoulder to right (negative) arm/shoulder, which is useful in assessing atrial activity and high lateral left ventricular ischemia.
- Lead II, left (positive) leg to right (negative) arm/shoulder, is the best view of normal conduction system. Flow towards the positive lead forms the normal upright QRS.
- Lead III, left (positive) leg to left (negative) arm/shoulder, looks inferiorly at the left ventricle.

None of these look at anterior or low lateral ischemia changes.

Limb leads are 'bipolar', since one electrode acts as a positive terminal while the other as negative. Ideally, limb leads are placed distally on the limbs, despite the vulnerability to interference from the electricity produced by muscle movement.

Electrode locations on the upper chest and lower abdomen are partly acceptable alternatives, and are referred to as Mason-Likar lead positions. These are associated with underdiagnosis and are not preferred placement options except for cardiac monitoring (Farrell et al., 2008;

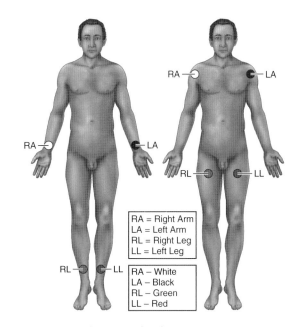

Figure 2.5.1 Limb electrode placement
Limb lead placement for a standard 12-lead ECG.
Source: *Ostendorf, W.R., Potter, P.A. and Griffin Perry, A., 2020, Nursing interventions & clinical skills, 7th edn, Elsevier.*

Jowett et al., 2005; Man et al., 2008; Sejersten et al., 2006) unless the cardiac monitor being used has been calibrated specifically for this purpose. This calibration is increasingly common in portable devices specifically intended for prehospital use.

Another alternative is the Lund positions, placing electrodes on the upper arms and left iliac crest in the mid-axillary line (Pahlm and Wagner, 2008; Trägårdh-Johansson et al., 2011; Welinder et al., 2010).

An additional fourth lead is in some cases placed on the right leg to provide an earth signal for the other leads. It does not add an additional view (see Table 2.5.1).

Augmented limb leads

The 12-lead ECG includes augmented unipolar views using the existing attached leads. The ECG device uses the positive bipolar electrode from one of the three limb leads and draws a line to a calculated midway negative reference point between the remaining two electrodes. They are prefixed 'aV' for augmented voltage. Lead aVL uses the left arm electrode, aVR the right arm lead and aVF (foot) the left leg electrode.

Collectively, the six limb leads create a 360-degree frontal plane view of the heart.

Precordial or chest leads

The precordial leads view the heart in a horizontal plane. A 'theoretical central' negative electrode is created to connect to the placed positive electrode theoretically positioned anywhere circling the chest. The standard six electrodes that form the 'unipolar' or 'chest' leads are placed to look at anterior, septal and lateral left ventricle walls (Fig. 2.5.2).

The 'chest' leads are prefixed by the letter 'V' (V1–V6) (Table 2.5.2). To attach these leads, remove the upper body garments to allow chest access, remembering to do so respectfully and with the patient's consent.

Locate leads V1 and V2 first as identifiable reference points. Locating the fourth intercostal space is critical, with V1 and V2 either side of the sternum at that level. Run the finger from V2 down along the fourth intercostal

space until reaching the mid-clavicular line. Move directly down over the rib into the fifth intercostal space. This is where the V4 electrode is located. V3 can then be located directly between V2 and V4. Continue running along the fifth intercostal space from V4 as it curves slightly upwards until located in the mid-axillary line. V6 is positioned here. V5 can then be located between V4 and V6.

V1 and V2 look inwards at the septum, V3 and V4 at the anterior surface and V5 and V6 from the side at the lower lateral wall. Although these views are not as ideal as limb leads for electricity conduction through the heart, they are good for analysis of the left ventricle wall for injury and ischemia.

If required, chest electrodes can be positioned mirrored on the right side of the chest. This provides a view of the right side of the heart and requires specific labelling if performed.

Recording

On most modern ECG machines, interpretation will not start immediately with the device analysing the heart for minimal interference. This usually occurs within a

Table 2.5.1 Limb electrode placement

Electrode	Location
Left arm	Preferred: Anterior aspect of left wrist Mason-Likar: Left upper chest between deltoid and pectoral muscle Lund: Lateral aspect of mid upper arm between lateral deltoid and bicep
Right arm	Preferred: Anterior aspect of right wrist Mason-Likar: Right upper chest between deltoid and pectoral muscle Lund: Lateral aspect of mid upper arm between lateral deltoid and bicep
Left leg	Preferred: Anterior aspect of left lower leg or anterior aspect of mid upper leg Mason-Likar: Lower abdomen, 7.6 cm below a horizontal line from the umbilicus, 5 cm left of the umbilical vertical line (Khan, 2015) Lund: Left iliac crest, mid-axillary line
Right leg	Preferred: Anterior aspect of right lower leg or anterior aspect of mid upper leg Mason-Likar: Lower abdomen, 7.6 cm below a horizontal line from the umbilicus, 5 cm right of the umbilical vertical line Lund: Right iliac crest, mid-axillary line

Source: Adapted from Khan, 2015; Pahlm and Wagner, 2008; Trägårdh-Johansson et al., 2011; Welinder et al., 2010.

Table 2.5.2 Chest electrode placement

Electrode	Location
V1	Fourth intercostal space, just right of the sternum
V2	Fourth intercostal space, just left of the sternum
V3	Midway between V2 and V4
V4	Fifth intercostal space, mid-clavicular line
V5	Midway between V4 and V6
V6	Fifth intercostal space, mid-axillary line

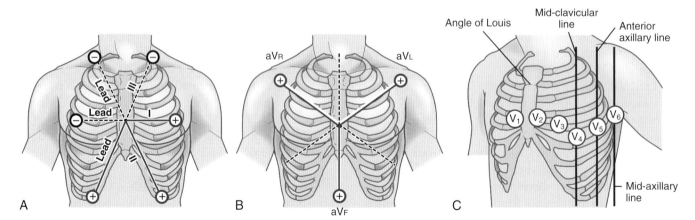

Figure 2.5.2 Chest electrode placement

Placement for the unipolar chest leads: V1, fourth intercostal space at the right sternal border; V2, fourth intercostal space at the left sternal border; V3, halfway between V2 and V4; V4, fifth intercostal space at the left mid-clavicular line; V5, fifth intercostal space at the left anterior axillary line; V6, fifth intercostal space at the left mid-axillary line.

Source: Edwards, H., Seaton, I., McLean Heitkemper, M., Buckley, T., Brown, D., Ruff Dirksen, S., Lewis, S.L. and Bucher, L., 2015, Lewis's medical–surgical nursing: assessment and management of clinical problems, 4th edn (Chapter 32, Figure 32-2), Elsevier.

few seconds, and the patient is instructed to remain as still as possible. Skeletal muscle contraction can generate electrical activity and may distort ECG clarity.

Clinical skill assessment process

The following section outlines the clinical skill assessment tools that should be used to determine a student's ability to demonstrate safe and accurate recording of the 12-lead electrocardiogram.

1. Clinical Skill Work Instruction
2. Formative Clinical Skill Assessment (F-CSAT)
3. Performance Improvement Plan (PIP)
4. Summative Clinical Skill Assessment (S-CSAT)
(5. Direct Observation of Procedural Skills (DOPS) – see Chapter 1.1)

Clinical Skill Work Instruction

Equipment and resources: Standardised or simulated patient with upper body exposed; 12-lead ECG device with leads and electrodes; disposable gloves; method of documenting the results

Associated Clinical Skills: Infection control; Communication; Consent

Recording the 12-lead ECG

Activity	Critical Action	Rationale
Prepare equipment	Check system and confirm paper speed, calibration and transmission ability if available. Inspect wires and electrodes.	Interpretations require paper speed and amplitude set to a standard setting.
	Attach electrodes to ECG lead wires.	Pre-attaching is easier than pressing wires firmly against patient after electrode attachment.
Prepare patient	Patient semi-reclined or supine is preferred; can be seated. Support feet and arms, legs uncrossed.	Skeletal muscle contraction generates electrical artifact.
	Explain procedure. Obtain informed consent.	Legal and ethical requirement for cooperation.
	Expose patient sufficiently for limb and chest electrode application.	Requires undressing or loosening clothing. Ensure privacy.
Place limb lead	Attach white right arm wire and electrode to right anterior wrist or right upper arm or right upper chest.	There are multiple options in that order of preference.
	Attach black left arm wire and electrode to left anterior wrist or right upper arm or right upper chest.	
	Attach red left leg wire and electrode to left anterior lower leg or left anterior upper leg or left lower abdomen.	
	Attach green right leg wire and electrode to right anterior lower leg or right anterior upper leg or right lower abdomen if there is this fourth lead.	
Place chest lead	Locate fourth intercostal space, immediately right of the sternum. Place V1 electrode.	Standard positions to ensure accurate reading.
	Locate fourth intercostal space, immediately left of the sternum. Place V2 electrode.	
	Locate fifth intercostal space, mid-clavicular line. Place V4 electrode.	
	Locates mid-point between V2 and V4. Place V3 electrode.	
	Locate fifth intercostal space, mid-axillary line. Place V6 electrode.	
	Locate mid-point between V4 and V6. Place V5 electrode.	

Recording the 12-lead ECG continued

Activity	Critical Action	Rationale
Acquire ECG	Ensure ambulance or stretcher not moving. Have patient remain as still as possible, breathing normally.	To avoid artifact.
	Press acquisition on ECG device. Correctly enter patient details as prompted.	To identify printout as belonging to patient.
	Inspect ECG recording for sufficient quality.	Repeat if necessary.
Report	Report on ECG rhythm and diagnostic observations.	Accurate record kept and continuity of patient care.

Formative Clinical Skill Assessment (F-CSAT)

Equipment and resources: Standardised or simulated patient with upper body exposed; 12-lead ECG device with leads and electrodes; disposable gloves; method of documenting the results

Associated Clinical Skills: Infection control; Communication; Consent

Staff/Student being assessed: _____

Recording the 12-lead ECG

Activity	Critical Action	Participant Performance				
Prepares equipment	Checks system and confirms paper speed, calibration and transmission ability if available. Inspects wires and electrodes.	0	1	2	3	4
	Attaches electrodes to ECG lead wires.	0	1	2	3	4
Prepares patient	Positions patient as necessary with feet and arms supported, legs uncrossed.	0	1	2	3	4
	Explains procedure. Obtains informed consent.	0	1	2	3	4
	Exposes patient sufficiently for limb and chest electrode application.	0	1	2	3	4
Places limb lead	Attaches white right arm wire and electrode to right anterior wrist or right upper arm or right upper chest.	0	1	2	3	4
	Attaches black left arm wire and electrode to left anterior wrist or right upper arm or right upper chest.	0	1	2	3	4
	Attaches red left leg wire and electrode to left anterior lower leg or left anterior upper leg or left lower abdomen.	0	1	2	3	4
	Attaches green right leg wire and electrode to right anterior lower leg or right anterior upper leg or right lower abdomen if there is this fourth lead.	0	1	2	3	4
Places chest lead	Locates fourth intercostal space, immediately right of the sternum. Places V1 electrode.	0	1	2	3	4
	Locates fourth intercostal space, immediately left of the sternum. Places V2 electrode.	0	1	2	3	4
	Locates fifth intercostal space, mid-clavicular line. Places V4 electrode.	0	1	2	3	4
	Locates mid-point between V2 and V4. Places V3 electrode.	0	1	2	3	4
	Locates fifth intercostal space, mid-axillary line. Places V6 electrode.	0	1	2	3	4
	Locates mid-point between V4 and V6. Places V5 electrode.	0	1	2	3	4

Recording the 12-lead ECG continued

Activity	Critical Action	Participant Performance				
Acquires ECG	Ensures ambulance or stretcher not moving. Has patient remain as still as possible, breathing normally.	0	1	2	3	4
	Presses acquisition on ECG device. Correctly enters patient details as prompted.	0	1	2	3	4
	Inspects ECG recording for sufficient quality.	0	1	2	3	4
Reports	Reports on ECG rhythm and diagnostic observation.	0	1	2	3	4

Standard Achieved: (please circle one)

Competent (C)   Not Yet Competent* (NYC)

Staff/Student Name: _____

Assessor (please print name): _____

Signed (Assessor): _____

Date of Assessment: _____

Comments:

*If Not Yet Competent (NYC) a PIP needs to be completed and a repeat of the F-CSAT

Formative Clinical Skill Assessment (F-CSAT) Key

Skill level	Standard of procedure	Quality of performance	Outcome	Level of assistance required
4 Safe for unsupervised practice	Safe Accurate Behaviour is appropriate to context	Confident Accurate Expedient	Achieved intended outcome	No supporting cues* required
3 Requires supervision	Safe Accurate Behaviour is appropriate to context	Confident Accurate Takes longer than required	Achieved intended outcome	Requires occasional supportive cues*
2 Requires assistance	Safe Accurate Behaviour generally appropriate to context	Lacks certainty	Would not have achieved outcome without support	Requires frequent verbal and occasional physical directives in addition to supportive cues*
1 Requires direction	Safe only with guidance Not completely accurate	Unskilled Inefficient	Would not have achieved outcome without support	Requires continuous verbal and frequent physical directive cues*
0 Unsafe	Unsafe Unable to demonstrate behaviour Lack of insight into behaviour appropriate to context	Unskilled	Would not have achieved outcome	Requires continuous verbal and continuous physical directive cues*

*Refers to physical directives or verbal supportive cues

Performance Improvement Plan (PIP)

Please document the agreed education plan and completion timelines for areas assessed as less than 4.

This plan should be presented to assessor prior to commencement of summative assessment.

Where was supervisor support required?	Student summary of deficit. (Why was there a problem?)	Improvement Plan	Completed (Y/N)

Staff/Student Name: _____

Staff/Student Signature: _____

Educator Name: _____

Educator Signature: _____

Summative Clinical Skill Assessment (S-CSAT)

Equipment and resources: Standardised or simulated patient with upper body exposed; 12-lead ECG device with leads and electrodes; disposable gloves; method of documenting the results

Associated Clinical Skills: Infection control; Communication; Consent

Student/Staff member being assessed: _____

- Completed Formative Clinical Skill Assessment (F-CSAT):   **YES**   **NO**

- Completed Performance Improvement Plan (PIP):   **YES**   **NO**   **N/A**

Recording the 12-lead ECG			
Activity	**Critical Action**	**Achieved**	**Without Direction**
Prepares equipment	Checks system, confirms paper speed, calibration and transmission ability if available. Inspects wires and electrodes.	NO	YES
	Attaches electrodes to ECG lead wires.	NO	YES
Prepares patient	Positions patient as necessary with feet and arms supported, legs uncrossed.	NO	YES
	Explains procedure and obtains informed patient consent.	NO	YES
	Exposes patient sufficiently for limb and chest electrode application.	NO	YES

Recording the 12-lead ECG continued

Activity	Critical Action	Achieved Without Direction	
Places limb lead	Attaches white right arm wire and electrode to right anterior wrist or right upper arm or right upper chest.	NO	YES
	Attaches black left arm wire and electrode to left anterior wrist or right upper arm or right upper chest.	NO	YES
	Attaches red left leg wire and electrode to left anterior lower leg or left anterior upper leg or left lower abdomen.	NO	YES
	Attaches green right leg wire and electrode to right anterior lower leg or right anterior upper leg or right lower abdomen if there is this fourth lead.	NO	YES
Places chest lead	Locates fourth intercostal space, immediately right of the sternum. Places V1 electrode.	NO	YES
	Locates fourth intercostal space, immediately left of the sternum. Places V2 electrode.	NO	YES
	Locates fifth intercostal space, mid-clavicular line. Places V4 electrode.	NO	YES
	Locates mid-point between V2 and V4. Places V3 electrode.	NO	YES
	Locates fifth intercostal space, mid-axillary line. Places V6 electrode.	NO	TES
	Locates mid-point between V4 and V6. Places V5 electrode.	NO	YES
Acquires ECG	Ensures ambulance or stretcher not moving. Has patient remain as still as possible, breathing normally.	NO	YES
	Presses acquisition on ECG device. Correctly enters patient details as prompted.	NO	YES
	Inspects ECG recording for sufficient quality.	NO	YES
Reports	Reports on ECG rhythm and diagnostic observation.	NO	YES

Standard Achieved: (please circle one)

Competent (C)   Not Yet Competent* (NYC)

Staff/Student Name: _____

Assessor (please print name)**:** _____

Signed (Assessor)**:** _____

Date of Assessment: _____

Comments:

*If Not Yet Competent (NYC) a PIP needs to be completed and a repeat of the F-CSAT

Clinical findings

ECG interpretation

The ECG allows assessment of three diagnostic functions:
1. Arrhythmias
2. Conduction defects
3. Ischemic or infarcted myocardium.

Detecting ST segment elevation consistent with myocardial infarction is the primary diagnostic aim of performing a 12-lead ECG. It allows paramedic 12-lead ECG transmission to receiving hospitals for reperfusion interventions. ECG patterns can allow the identification of a variety of other medical conditions.

Breast interference

The placement of anterior chest electrodes may be confounded by female breasts. Larger breasts (occasionally also noted in men) can force placement that is too high, low or incorrectly angled (Colaco et al., 2000). The preferred electrode position is on top of the breast (Kania et al., 2014; Rautaharju et al., 1998). Where the electrode cannot be placed correctly on top, respectfully lift the breast gently upwards with the back of the hand and place the electrodes beneath it. The patient can lift their own breast if preferred.

Electrode misplacement

The incorrect placement of electrodes alters diagnostic ability (Bond et al., 2012; Drew, 2006; Harrigan et al.,

2012) and QRS appearance (Anter et al., 2012; Batchvarov et al., 2007; Drew, 2006; McCann et al., 2007; Rudiger et al., 2007). Misplacement of limb leads has less impact than misplaced chest leads, making placement of the latter more critical (Kania et al., 2014; Sheppard et al., 2011). A common error is placing the chest leads anatomically too high (Kania et al., 2014).

Artifact

Electrical interference creates detectable artifact ('noise'). There are numerous sources, managed by recognition and removal of either the source or the patient. This includes external/nearby electrical devices, electric blankets and mobile telephones.

Motion is a major source of noise caused by electrode movement, including patient movement/trembling or stretcher or ambulance movement. ECG devices have filters built in to reduce this impact. Ask patients to remain still during assessment. Any other motion must be temporarily ceased (Buxi et al., 2012; Harrigan et al., 2012; Panda and Pati, 2012; Suchetha and Kumaravel, 2013; Tong et al., 2002).

Absent limb(s)

In the case of one or more absent limbs, place the leads at the most suitable available sites.

PRACTICE TIP!

Large breasts can pose difficulty when applying the 12-lead ECG. If necessary, use the back of a gloved hand to lift the breast and allow electrode access beneath it. Alternatively, have the patient lift the breast.

PRACTICE TIP!

Electrode placement is important, particularly in diagnostic use. Ensure careful placement and verify for correctness. If the ECG pattern is unusual, reassess the electrode placement and correct wire attachment.

PRACTICE TIP!

As removing or adjusting upper garments and potentially touch contact with skin and breasts is needed, consider changing the ECG operator where gender or cultural circumstances prompt this.

PRACTICE TIP!

The 12-lead ECG is typically only required for diagnostic use. Monitoring cardiac rhythm only requires the standard three (or four) leads, allowing for the removal of chest leads and covering the patient.

PRACTICE TIP!

Balance the need for and performance of the procedure with completing other assessments, including history taking and urgency.

TEST YOUR KNOWLEDGE QUESTIONS

1. **What should electrodes be inspected for before use?**
    Sufficient gel and expiry date.

2. **Why are ECG wires attached to the electrodes before they are applied to the patient?**
    Attaching them afterwards can require pushing hard, causing discomfort and displacing the electrode gel.

3. **List two factors that can cause electrodes to not adhere properly.**
    Clammy skin; excess body hair.

4. **What is the preferred placement of limb electrodes?**
    Anterior aspect of distal limb.

5. **Why are alternative placements of limb electrodes sometimes used?**
    For patient ease and reduced interference during ongoing monitoring.

6. **What are the common causes of ECG artifact?**
    Electrical/nearby power sources; mobile telephones; movement of the patient, stretcher or ambulance.

7. **How is artifact managed?**
    Have the patient remain still; cease all other movement; remove electrical interference; remove the patient from source/s of interference.

8. **What happens if the chest electrodes are not correctly placed?**
    Diagnostic ability is reduced and QRS appearance is altered.

9. **What is the purpose of the green fourth limb lead?**
    To provide an earth signal for the other leads. It does not add an additional view.

10. **What is the most common misplacement of the chest lead electrodes?**
    V1 and V2 are placed too high.

References

Anter, E., Frankel, D.S., Marchlinski, F.E. and Dixit, S., 2012. Effect of electrocardiographic lead placement on localization of outflow tract tachycardias. *Heart Rhythm*, 9(5), 697–703.

Batchvarov, V.N., Malik, M. and Camm, A.J., 2007. Incorrect electrode cable connection during electrocardiographic recording. *Europace*, 9(11), 1081–1090.

Bond, R.R., Finlay, D.D., Nugent, C.D., Breen, C., Guldenring, D. and Daly, M.J., 2012. The effects of electrode misplacement on clinicians' interpretation of the standard 12-lead electrocardiogram. *European Journal of Internal Medicine*, 23(7), 61–615.

Buxi, D., Kim, S., Van Helleputte, N., Altini, M., Wijsman, J., Yazicioglu, R.F., Penders, J. and Van Hoof, C., 2012. Correlation between electrode-tissue impedance and motion artifact in biopotential recordings. *IEEE Sensors Journal*, 12, 3373–3383.

Colaco, R., Reay, P., Beckett, C., Aitchison, T.C. and Macfarlane, P.W., 2000. False positive ECG reports of anterior myocardial infarction in women. *Journal of Electrocardiology*, 33, 239–244.

Drew, B.J., 2006. Pitfalls and artifacts in electrocardiography. *Cardiology Clinics*, 24(3), 309–315.

Farrell, R.M., Syed, A., Syed, A. and Gutterman, D.D., 2008. Effects of limb electrode placement on the 12-and 16-lead electrocardiogram. *Journal of Electrocardiology*, 41(6), 536–545.

Harrigan, R.A., Chan, T.C. and Brady, W.J., 2012. Electrocardiographic electrode misplacement, misconnection, and artifact. *Journal of Emergency Medicine*, 43(6), 1038–1044.

Jowett, N.I., Turner, A.M., Cole, A. and Jones, P.A., 2005. Modified electrode placement must be recorded when performing 12-lead electrocardiograms. *Postgraduate Medical Journal*, 81(952), 122–125.

Kania, M., Rix, H., Fereniec, M., Zavala-Fernandez, H., Janusek, D., Mroczka, T., Stix, G. and Maniewski, R., 2014. The effect of precordial lead displacement on ECG morphology. *Medical & Biological Engineering & Computing*, 52(2), 10–119.

Khan, G.M., 2015. A new electrode placement method for obtaining 12-lead ECGs. *Open Heart*, 2(1).

Man, S.C., Maan, A.C., Kim, E., Draisma, H.H., Schalij, M.J., van der Wall, E.E. and Swenne, C.A., 2008. Reconstruction of standard 12-lead electrocardiograms from 12-lead electrocardiograms recorded with the Mason-Likar electrode configuration. *Journal of Electrocardiology*, 41(3), 211–219.

McCann, K., Holdgate, A., Mahammad, R. and Waddington, A., 2007. Accuracy of ECG electrode placement by emergency department clinicians. *Emergency Medicine Australasia*, 19(5), 44–448.

Meziane, N., Webster, J.G., Attari, M. and Nimunkar, A.J., 2013. Dry electrodes for electrocardiography. *Physiological Measurement*, 34(9), R47.

Pahlm, O. and Wagner, G.S., 2008. Proximal placement of limb electrodes: a potential solution for acquiring standard electrocardiogram waveforms from monitoring electrode positions. *Journal of Electrocardiology*, 41(6), 454–457.

Panda, R. and Pati, U.C., 2012. Removal of artifacts from electrocardiogram using digital filter. In *2012 IEEE Students' Conference on Electrical, Electronics and Computer Science (SCEECS)*. New Jersey: IEEE, pp. 1–4.

Rautaharju, P.M., Park, L., Rautaharju, F.S. and Crow, R., 1998. A standardized procedure for locating and documenting ECG chest electrode positions: consideration of the effect of breast tissue on ECG amplitudes in women. *Journal of Electrocardiology*, 31(1), 17–29.

Rudiger, A., Hellermann, J.P., Mukherjee, R., Follath, F. and Turina, J., 2007. Electrocardiographic artifacts due to electrode misplacement and their frequency in different clinical settings. *American Journal of Emergency Medicine*, 25(2), 17–178.

Sejersten, M., Pahlm, O., Pettersson, J., Zhou, S., Maynard, C., Feldman, C.L. and Wagner, G.S., 2006. Comparison of EASI-derived 12-lead electrocardiograms versus paramedic-acquired 12-lead electrocardiograms using Mason-Likar limb lead configuration in patients with chest pain. *Journal of Electrocardiology*, 39(1), 13–21.

Sheppard, J.P., Barker, T.A., Ranasinghe, A.M., Clutton-Brock, T.H., Frenneaux, M.P. and Parkes, M.J., 2011. Does modifying electrode placement of the 12 lead ECG matter in healthy subjects? *International Journal of Cardiology*, 152(2), 184–191.

Suchetha, M. and Kumaravel, N., 2013. Empirical mode decomposition based filtering techniques for power line interference reduction in electrocardiogram using various adaptive structures and subtraction methods. *Biomedical Signal Processing and Control*, 8(6), 575–585.

Tong, D.A., Bartels, K.A. and Honeyager, K.S., 2002. Adaptive reduction of motion artifact in the electrocardiogram. In *Proceedings of the Second Joint 24th Annual Conference and the Annual Fall Meeting of the Biomedical Engineering Society (Engineering in Medicine and Biology)* (Volume 2). New Jersey: IEEE, pp. 1403–1404.

Trägårdh-Johansson, E., Welinder, A. and Pahlm, O., 2011. Similarity of ST and T waveforms of 12-lead electrocardiogram acquired from different monitoring electrode positions. *Journal of Electrocardiology*, 44(2), 109–114.

Welinder, A., Wagner, G.S., Maynard, C. and Pahlm, O., 2010. Differences in QRS axis measurements, classification of inferior myocardial infarction, and noise tolerance for 12-lead electrocardiograms acquired from monitoring electrode positions compared to standard locations. *American Journal of Cardiology*, 106(4), 58–586.

Wiese, S.R., Anheier, P., Connemara, R.D., Mollner, A.T., Neils, T.F., Kahn, J.A. and Webster, J.G., 2005. Electrocardiographic motion artifact versus electrode impedance. *IEEE Transactions on Biomedical Engineering*, 52(1), 136–139.

2.6 | Assessment of respiratory rate and rhythm

Jeff Kenneally

Chapter objectives

At the end of this chapter the reader will be able to:

1. Describe the rationale for assessing respiratory rate and rhythm
2. Demonstrate the method of assessing respiratory rate and rhythm
3. Accurately report on assessment findings
4. Identify pathologies associated with abnormal respiratory rate and rhythm

Resources required for this assessment

- Standardised patient with observable breathing movements
- Disposable gloves
- Method of documenting the results

Skill matrix

This assessment requires:
- Infection control (CS 1.3)
- Communication (CS 1.5)
- Consent (CS 1.6)

This assessment is a component of:
- Patient assessment (Chapter 2)

Introduction

Evaluating respiratory rate and rhythm is an important part of baseline assessment, to monitor trends in the patient's condition and their response to the treatment provided (Barthel et al., 2013; Philip et al., 2015). It is a key element of patient triage and early warning systems, and variations from normal can indicate significant illness (Arnold et al., 2016). It is equally valid when assessing patients of any age, provided variations in 'expected normal' are allowed for.

This chapter discusses respiratory assessment for rate and rhythm of breathing.

Anatomy and physiology

Breathing is predominantly involuntary, with capacity for transient conscious control to allow for higher functions such as speaking or voluntary breath holding. Inspiration is provided through diaphragm and external intercostal muscle actions. Expiration is mostly passive, relying on chest wall elastic recoil.

Primary respiratory control is in the medulla, with secondary pons input. Oxygen and carbon dioxide equilibrium is maintained through variations in breathing rate and effort. The input for control includes pH receptors in the cerebrospinal fluid (CSF) and chemoreceptors in the carotid and aortic bodies monitoring arterial oxygen and carbon dioxide levels. The carotid and aortic bodies are sensitive to lowering oxygen levels and provide stimulus to breathe with hypoxemia. CSF receptors are more sensitive to stimulus, making carbon dioxide and not oxygen the usual primary stimulus to breathe.

Finally, there are receptors within the lungs and airways themselves. These allow for airway constriction and relaxation to prevent the entry of irritants and for lung volume changes when required. They also limit maximum inspiratory volume by restricting overstretch of the lungs (Cretikos et al., 2008).

Respiration is usually regular, at equally spaced intervals. The inspiration to expiration ratio is part of respiratory rhythm. Active inspiration and predominantly passive expiration means more time is required for emptying the lungs. A normal adult and child ratio is around 1:2 for inspiration–expiration. Problems affecting expiration can prolong the expiratory phase (Arnold et al., 2016).

Changes in rate and rhythm are normally in response to demand and can trend up or down with illness, exercise and recovery (Barthel et al., 2013).

Clinical rationale

At rest, regular breathing patterns maintain necessary blood gas and pH levels. To regularly activate underutilised alveoli, periodic sighing occurs, temporarily increasing inspiratory effort. As metabolic demand increases or blood gases move outside tolerable ranges, respiratory rate and effort increase to compensate (Cretikos et al., 2008).

Minute ventilation is a product of the respiratory rate and volume of each breath (Cretikos et al., 2008). Increasing the respiratory rate increases minute volume but also reduces the time for exhalation to occur.

Normal respiratory rate is typically between 12 and 20 breaths per minute in adults, most commonly around 14–15.

The elderly frequently face respiratory system decline for reasons including disease, muscle weakness and a reduced capacity for carrying blood oxygen. To compensate, respiratory rates slightly increase to 14–25 breaths per minute. This reduces the ability of elderly patients to provide respiratory compensation during illness, making even small variations from normal significant (McFadden et al., 1982).

There is a range of respiratory rates considered normal for children, reflecting significant differences with age (Fleming et al. 2011). The newborn has the fastest normal respiratory rate, which decreases with age (see Table 2.6.1).

Children have a relatively small alveolar surface area, which increases slowly with age. A more vertical and compliant chest does not provide the same chest expansion with intercostal muscle contraction as that of adults, leading to smaller tidal volumes. Because children have greater metabolic rates, with an increased demand for oxygen and a higher production of waste carbon dioxide, they compensate by breathing faster.

Table 2.6.1 Paediatric respiratory rates

Age	Respiratory range (breaths per minute)
Newborn	40–60
Infant	30–40
Pre-school	25–30
Primary school	20–25
Adolescent	15–20

Source: *Sanders et al., 2007.*

When assessing breathing, avoid allowing the patient to know that their respiration is being counted, as they may alter their breathing if they are aware of this. Perform the assessment without warning, ideally under the guise of another assessment being performed, such as pulse counting.

Watch the chest rise and fall with each breath. Commence timing and count the inspiration rate over a 30-second period; then multiply by 2 to get the rate per minute.

Where the patient is in an altered conscious state and breathing is shallow, one hand can be placed over the chest or abdomen to help detect breathing movement.

Compare the duration of inspiration and compare it to the following expiration. A ratio of 1:2 is usual. A ratio of greater than this is unusual and prompts further investigation.

Don't rush by assessing the patient over too short a time, as changes in pattern may not be noted. Inaccurate recording can create an underestimation of the severity of illness (Badawy et al., 2017).

Clinical skill assessment process

The following section outlines the clinical skill assessment tools that should be used to determine a student's ability to demonstrate safe and accurate assessment of respiratory rate and rhythm.
1. Clinical Skill Work Instruction
2. Formative Clinical Skill Assessment (F-CSAT)
3. Performance Improvement Plan (PIP)
4. Summative Clinical Skill Assessment (S-CSAT)
(5. Direct Observation of Procedural Skills (DOPS) – see Chapter 1.1)

Clinical Skill Work Instruction

Equipment and resources: Standardised patient with detectable breathing movements; disposable gloves; method of documenting results

Associated Clinical Skills: Infection control; Communication; Consent

Assessment of respiratory rate and rhythm

Activity	Critical Action	Rationale
Prepare patient	Counting respiration and assessing rhythm can be performed in any position, including upright or lateral.	All that is required is vision or feel of the chest movement.
	If it is impractical to view or feel chest breathing movement, upper body garments may have to be removed to allow access. Minimise exposure.	Allow for environment and dignity.
	Avoid the patient knowing their respiration is being counted. Perform assessment without warning, ideally under the guise that another assessment is being performed, such as counting the pulse.	If the patient is aware breathing is being counted they may modify their rate.
Assess respiratory rate	Watch the chest rise and fall with each breath. When ready, commence timing and count inspiration rate over a 30-second period. Multiply by 2 to obtain the value per minute.	Alternatively, a full minute can be used to count respiration rate.
	Where the patient is in an altered conscious state and breathing is shallow, one hand can be placed over the chest or abdomen to help detect breathing movement.	Detecting breathing via touch can assist where visual assessment is difficult.
Assess respiratory rhythm	Compare duration of inspiration compared to the following expiration. A ratio of 1 : 2 is usual. A ratio of greater than this is unusual. Compare time between breaths during timing interval to assess for regularity.	Expiration takes longer than inspiration since it is passive. Even timing between breaths indicates irregular rhythm.
Report	Accurately document/hand over findings, including any abnormal rate or inspiratory–expiratory ratio detected.	To ensure continuity of care.

Formative Clinical Skill Assessment (F-CSAT)

Equipment and resources: Standardised patient with detectable breathing movements; disposable gloves; method of documenting results

Associated Clinical Skills: Infection control; Communication; Consent

Staff/Student being assessed: _____

Assessment of respiratory rate and rhythm

Activity	Critical Action	Participant Performance				
Prepares patient	Counts respiration and assesses rhythm in position.	0	1	2	3	4
	If it is impractical to view or feel chest breathing movement, removes upper body garments to allow access. Minimises patient exposure.	0	1	2	3	4
	Avoids allowing the patient to know respiration is being counted.	0	1	2	3	4

Assessment of respiratory rate and rhythm continued

Activity	Critical Action	Participant Performance				
Assesses respiratory rate	Watches the chest rise and fall with each breath. Commences timing and counts inspiration rate over a 30-second period. Multiplies by 2 to obtain the value per minute.	0	1	2	3	4
	Where the patient is in an altered conscious state and breathing is shallow, places one hand over the chest or abdomen to help detect breathing movement.	0	1	2	3	4
Assesses respiratory rhythm	Compares inspiration duration and compares it to the following expiration. Notes any abnormality. Compares time between breaths during timing interval to assess for regularity.	0	1	2	3	4
Reports	Accurately documents/hands over findings, including any abnormal rate or inspiratory–expiratory ratio detected.	0	1	2	3	4

Standard Achieved: (please circle one)

Competent (C)   Not Yet Competent* (NYC)

Staff/Student Name: _____

Assessor (please print name): _____

Signed (Assessor): _____

Date of Assessment: _____

Comments:

*If Not Yet Competent (NYC) a PIP needs to be completed and a repeat of the F-CSAT

Formative Clinical Skill Assessment (F-CSAT) Key

Skill level	Standard of procedure	Quality of performance	Outcome	Level of assistance required
4 Safe for unsupervised practice	Safe Accurate Behaviour is appropriate to context	Confident Accurate Expedient	Achieved intended outcome	No supporting cues* required
3 Requires supervision	Safe Accurate Behaviour is appropriate to context	Confident Accurate Takes longer than required	Achieved intended outcome	Requires occasional supportive cues*
2 Requires assistance	Safe Accurate Behaviour generally appropriate to context	Lacks certainty	Would not have achieved outcome without support	Requires frequent verbal and occasional physical directives in addition to supportive cues*

Skill level	Standard of procedure	Quality of performance	Outcome	Level of assistance required
1 Requires direction	Safe only with guidance Not completely accurate	Unskilled Inefficient	Would not have achieved outcome without support	Requires continuous verbal and frequent physical directive cues*
0 Unsafe	Unsafe Unable to demonstrate behaviour Lack of insight into behaviour appropriate to context	Unskilled	Would not have achieved outcome	Requires continuous verbal and continuous physical directive cues*

Refers to physical directives or verbal supportive cues

Performance Improvement Plan (PIP)

Please document the agreed education plan and completion timelines for areas assessed as less than 4.

This plan should be presented to assessor prior to commencement of summative assessment.

Where was supervisor support required?	Student summary of deficit. (Why was there a problem?)	Improvement Plan	Completed (Y/N)

Staff/Student Name: _____

Staff/Student Signature: _____

Educator Name: _____

Educator Signature: _____

Summative Clinical Skill Assessment (S-CSAT)

Equipment and resources: Standardised patient with detectable breathing movements; disposable gloves; method of documenting results

Associated Clinical Skills: Infection control; Communication; Consent

Staff/Student being assessed: _____

- Completed Formative Clinical Skill Assessment (F-CSAT):   **YES   NO**

- Completed Performance Improvement Plan (PIP):   **YES   NO   N/A**

Assessment of respiratory rate and rhythm

Activity	Critical Action	Achieved Without Direction	
Prepares patient	Counts respiration and assesses rhythm in any position.	NO	YES
	If it is impractical to view or feel chest breathing movement, removes upper body garments to allow access. Minimises patient exposure.	NO	YES
	Avoids allowing the patient to know respiration is being counted.	NO	YES
Assesses respiratory rate	Watches the chest rise and fall each breath. Commences timing and counts inspiration rate over 30-second period. Multiplies by 2 to obtain the value per minute.	NO	YES
	Where the patient is in an altered conscious state and breathing is shallow, places one hand over the chest or abdomen to help detect breathing movement.	NO	YES
Assesses respiratory rhythm	Compares inspiration duration and compares it to the following expiration. Notes any abnormality. Compares time between breaths during timing interval to assess for regularity.	NO	YES
Reports	Accurately documents/hands over findings, including any abnormal rate or inspiratory–expiratory ratio detected.	NO	YES

Standard Achieved: (please circle one)

Competent (C)   Not Yet Competent* (NYC)

Staff/Student Name: _____

Assessor (please print name)**:** _____

Signed (Assessor)**:** _____

Date of Assessment: _____

Comments:

*If Not Yet Competent (NYC) a PIP needs to be completed and a repeat of the F-CSAT

Clinical findings

The key variables in respiratory assessment are respiratory rate, depth and inspiration/expiration ratio (rhythm).

Respiratory rates can be faster or slower than normal values. Rhythm, though usually regular, can vary in response to clinical conditions.

Clinical assessment looks for variation in one or more of these.

Rate-related findings

Tachypnoea

Tachypnoea is a respiratory rate above the normal 20 bpm (in adults). Causes can include fear, emotion, pain, anxiety, exercise, febrile illness or pulmonary disease (Cretikos et al., 2008).

Tachypnoea is a natural sympathetic nervous system response to physiological threat, making it a serious finding until proven otherwise (Barthel et al., 2013, McFadden et al., 1982; Philip et al., 2015). Occasionally, an increased breathing rate can cause blood gas derangement (Arnold et al., 2016).

Paediatric normal respiration rates vary considerably, as shown Table 2.6.1. The definition of tachypnoea varies with the usual upper limit of normal for the child's age (Fleming et al., 2011).

Hyperventilation

Hyperventilation is a specific form of tachypnoea in which excessive alveolar ventilation, from increased respiratory depth and/or rate, causes excessive carbon dioxide removal and respiratory alkalosis.

Hyperventilation is a misunderstood term that is often confused with other respiratory terms. There are two broad causes for hyperventilation: benign or sinister.

Benign hyperventilation covers a range of problems, including anxiety and emotion. It can be intentional, such as preceding breath holding. It is commonly encountered and is not usually harmful.

It is essential to not mistake a benign cause for a sinister cause of hyperventilation. The causes of sinister hyperventilation causes vary and include Kussmaul breathing, as seen during diabetic ketoacidosis, and Cheyne-Stokes respiration, which can occur during acute stroke.

Hypoventilation and bradypnoea

Hypoventilation includes decreased respiration depth and/or rate. Precise prehospital assessment of tidal volume is difficult if not impossible. Reduced depth can reduce chest movement to barely noticeable.

Increased depth is a normal response to exercise and many illnesses, to increase ventilation, and typically accompanies increased respiratory rate.

The reasons for decreased depth include pulmonary disease, neuromuscular disease or painful chest injury.

Hypoventilation due to slower than normal respiratory rate is termed 'bradypnoea'. In many ways, it is the opposite of hyperventilation. The usual cause of bradypnoea is brain failure to stimulate a faster rate. The reasons for this include depressive drug effects, such as opioids, or rising intracranial pressure.

Any decrease rate decreases minute volume. The lower limit of respiratory rate is 10–12 bpm (in adults).

Agonal breathing

This is an ominous sign, frequently associated with cardiac arrest, characterised by slow, stertorous, gasping breathing. It is unlikely to produce sufficient chest movement for airflow. Its mechanism is not well understood but likely involves several key factors involved in controlling respiration. Insufficient blood flow to carotid and aortic chemoreceptors or the medulla adversely impacts the ability to dictate normal breathing.

Primitive gasping respiration in response to deranged blood oxygen and carbon dioxide levels can follow early in cardiac arrest before eventually falling away to apnoea. This breathing pattern may also be seen in extremely low perfusion states such as cardiogenic shock, where it may persist longer than in cardiac arrest.

Agonal breathing during early cardiac arrest may help maintain viability and increase resuscitation prospect. It can return during cardiac arrest. However, agonal breathing can present an ethical dilemma if it is associated with an end-of-life situation and withholding resuscitation when success is unlikely.

This form of breathing must be recognised, since it is not effective breathing (Haouzi et al., 2010; Perkin and Resnik, 2002; Zuercher et al., 2010) and requires intervention.

Rhythm-related findings

Kussmaul breathing

Kussmaul breathing is a recognisable respiratory pattern responding to metabolic acidosis, most commonly seen during diabetic ketoacidosis (Johnson et al., 2009).

It involves deep breaths; the rate can be fast or slow. The intent is to increase exhalation and carbon dioxide removal to create compensatory respiratory alkalosis for the metabolic acidosis.

Cheyne-Stokes breathing

Cheyne-Stokes breathing is an irregular cyclical pattern of alternating hyperventilation with bradypnoea/apnoea. Its causes include altered sensitivity to carbon dioxide levels by chemoreceptors, left heart failure, altitude sickness or brainstem respiratory control dysfunction from rising intracranial pressure (Duning et al., 2013; Naughton, 2012, 2014).

Prolonged expiratory phase

The inspiratory–expiratory ratio changes from the usual 1:2 to 1:4 or even more. Any impediment to airflow escape has the potential to increase expiratory time. Causes include asthma and chronic obstructive airways disease. Resting time between breaths decreases (Arnold et al., 2016).

PRACTICE TIP!

There are many reasons for a respiratory rate outside of the normal range. It is essential that respiratory rate be counted for every patient, as it can provide important early clues to clinical problems.

PRACTICE TIP!

Counting respiratory rate is easily corrupted through the patient's ability to consciously modify their own breathing. To avoid this, the patient should not know their respiratory rate is being counted. Count the rate while purporting to perform some other assessment, such as pulse counting.

PRACTICE TIP!

Respiratory rate must be placed into the context of other assessment findings. On its own, respiratory rate could indicate a serious problem or it may represent little more than an expected emotional or anxiety response.

TEST YOUR KNOWLEDGE QUESTIONS

1. **What is the normal adult respiratory rate?**
   12–20 breaths per minute.

2. **Which are three key factors monitored by receptors to control breathing rate?**
   pH; pO_2; pCO_2.

3. **What are two key variables that form minute volume in respiration?**
   Respiratory rate per minute multiplied by tidal volume of each breath.

4. **Why do children typically have faster normal respiratory rates than adults?**
   Children have a relatively small alveolar surface area, which increases slowly with age. A more vertical and compliant chest provides less chest expansion than that of adults, leading to smaller tidal volumes. Children have greater metabolic rates, with an increased oxygen demand and higher production of waste carbon dioxide, and so they compensate by breathing faster.

5. **What is the normal respiratory rhythm?**
   Respiratory rhythm is usually breaths taken at equally spaced intervals, with the ratio between inspiration and expiration being around 1:2.

6. **What is a common cause of gross irregularity of inspiratory rhythm?**
   Cheyne-Stokes breathing is an alternation between apnoea/bradypnoea with hyperventilation, typically caused by brainstem dysfunction or altered sensitivity to carbon dioxide levels by chemoreceptors.

7. **What is a common cause of prolonged expiration?**
   Reductions in expiratory airflow, typically from diseases such as asthma or chronic obstructive pulmonary disease.

8. **Why is it important for the patient to not know their respiration is being counted?**
   Some may attempt to control or change the rate, so distorting the observation.

9. **What is the difference between tachypnoea and hyperventilation?**
   Hyperventilation is a specific form of ventilation that can include increased rate and/or depth to move blood gas parameters outside of normal ranges. Tachypnoea is simply increased respiratory rate.

10. **How is respiratory rate assessed differently where consciousness is altered?**
    One hand can be placed over the chest or abdomen to help detect breathing movement.

References

Arnold, D.H., Penrod, C.H., Sprague, D.J. and Hartert, T.V., 2016. Count on it! Accurately measured respiratory rate is associated with lung function and clinical severity in children with acute asthma exacerbations. *Journal of Pediatrics*, 175, 236–236.

Badawy, J., Nguyen, O.K., Clark, C., Halm, E.A. and Makam, A.N., 2017. Is everyone really breathing 20 times a minute? Assessing epidemiology and variation in recorded respiratory rate in hospitalised adults. *BMJ Quality & Safety*, 26(10), 832–836.

Barthel, P., Wensel, R., Bauer, A., Müller, A., Wolf, P., Ulm, K., Huster, K.M., Francis, D.P., Malik, M. and Schmidt, G., 2013. Respiratory rate predicts outcome after acute myocardial infarction: a prospective cohort study. *European Heart Journal*, 34(22), 1644–1650.

Cretikos, M.A., Bellomo, R., Hillman, K., Chen, J., Finfer, S. and Flabouris, A., 2008. Respiratory rate: the neglected vital sign. *Medical Journal of Australia*, 188(11), 657.

Duning, T., Deppe, M., Brand, E., Stypmann, J., Becht, C., Heidbreder, A. and Young, P., 2013. Brainstem involvement as a cause of central sleep apnea: pattern of microstructural cerebral damage in patients with cerebral microangiopathy. *PLOS ONE*, 8(4), e60304.

Fleming, S., Thompson, M., Stevens, R., Heneghan, C., Plüddemann, A., Maconochie, I., Tarassenko, L. and Mant, D., 2011. Normal ranges of heart rate and respiratory rate in children from birth to 18 years of age: a systematic review of observational studies. *Lancet*, 377(9770), 1011–1018.

Haouzi, P., Ahmadpour, N., Bell, H.J., Artman, S., Banchs, J., Samii, S., Gonzalez, M. and Gleeson, K., 2010. Breathing patterns during cardiac arrest. *Journal of Applied Physiology*, 109(2), 405–411.

Johnson, S.K., Naidu, R.K., Ostopowicz, R.C., Kumar, D.R., Bhupathi, S., Mazza, J.J. and Yale, S.H., 2009. Adolf Kussmaul: distinguished clinician and medical pioneer. *Clinical Medicine & Research*, 7(3), 107–112.

McFadden, J.P., Price, R.C., Eastwood, H.D. and Briggs, R.S., 1982. Raised respiratory rate in elderly patients: a valuable physical sign. *BMJ Clinical Research*, 284(6316), 626–627.

Naughton, M.T., 2012. Cheyne–Stokes respiration: friend or foe? *Thorax*, 67(4), 357–360.

Naughton, M.T., 2014. Cheyne-Stokes respiration. *Sleep Medicine Clinics*, 9(1), 13–25.

Perkin, R. and Resnik, D., 2002. The agony of agonal respiration: is the last gasp necessary? *Journal of Medical Ethics*, 28(3), 164–169.

Philip, K.E., Pack, E., Cambiano, V., Rollmann, H., Weil, S. and O'Beirne, J., 2015. The accuracy of respiratory rate assessment by doctors in a London teaching hospital: a cross-sectional study. *Journal of Clinical Monitoring and Computing*, 29(4), 455–460.

Sanders, M.J., McKenna, K.D., Quick, G. and Lewis, L.M., 2007. *Mosby's paramedic textbook*. 3rd edn. St Louis: Mosby/Elsevier.

Zuercher, M., Ewy, G.A., Hilwig, R.W., Sanders, A.B., Otto, C.W., Berg, R.A. and Kern, K.B., 2010. Continued breathing followed by gasping or apnea in a swine model of ventricular fibrillation cardiac arrest. *BMC Cardiovascular Disorders*, 10(1), 1.

Bibliography

Craft J., Gordon C., Huether, S.E., McCance K.L. and Brashers V.L., 2015. *Understanding pathophysiology (ANZ adaptation)*. Sydney: Elsevier.

McCance K.L. and Huether, S.E., 2015. *Pathophysiology: the biologic basis for disease in adults and children*. Sydney: Elsevier.

Chapter objectives

At the end of this chapter the reader will be able to:

1. Describe the rationale for assessing work of breathing
2. Demonstrate the method of assessing work of breathing
3. Accurately report on the findings of the assessment
4. Identify pathologies associated with abnormal work of breathing

Resources required for this assessment

- Standardised patient with observable breathing movements
- Disposable gloves
- Method of documenting the results

Skills matrix

This assessment requires:

- Infection control (CS 1.3)
- Communication (CS 1.5)
- Consent (CS 1.6)
- Assessment of respiratory rate and rhythm (CS 2.6)

This assessment is a component of:

- Patient assessment (Chapter 2)

Introduction

Evaluating work of breathing, previously referred to as respiratory effort, is an important part of respiratory assessment, for monitoring the trend in a patient's condition and their response to the treatment provided (Barthel et al., 2013; Philip et al., 2015). It provides a guide to the severity of disease and physiological compensation to exercise or illness (Arnold et al., 2011).

This chapter discusses assessment of work of breathing.

Anatomy and physiology

The ability to draw air into the lungs to ventilate alveoli is integral to respiration. Inspiration requires strong muscular action and the diaphragm is the principal muscle of inspiration, supported by external intercostal muscles. When the need for gas exchange increases, so must the rate and depth of ventilation. To increase breathing depth (inspiratory reserve volume), diaphragm and external intercostal muscle action intensifies. During respiratory difficulty, accessory breathing muscles of the sternocleidomastoid, scalene and pectoral muscles (Arnold et al., 2011) pull the sternum upwards and maximise chest and lung expansion.

Expiration is typically passive, relying on inspiratory muscle relaxation and elastic recoil of the lung and chest wall. During respiratory difficulty, the internal intercostal muscles pull the chest inwards and abdominal wall muscles push the diaphragm upwards to increase expiratory effort. This is important when obstructions are encountered.

Clinical rationale

Normal breathing appears relaxed, with minimal chest and diaphragm movement visible. It may be so relaxed that palpation of breathing may be necessary. Place one hand lightly over the diaphragm to feel movement. Similarly, placing one hand against either side of the chest can help you to view chest expansion with each breath. These actions are useful when breathing effort is shallow and difficult to discern.

There is a problem with using the hands to assess breathing effort. Once a patient becomes aware that their breathing is being assessed they can, wittingly or otherwise, make changes to it. Breathing assessment should therefore be performed without the patient being aware of it.

With increasing demand for gas exchange, there must be a corresponding increase in ventilation. This means increased muscle activity. During extreme physical exercise, minute volume can increase from 5–6 L every minute to more than 100 L, partly by increasing both respiratory rate and tidal volume (Burton et al., 2004).

Increasing tidal volume provides strong visible clues from the key contributing muscles. Assess the activity of the diaphragm, intercostal muscles and resulting chest excursion, the abdominal wall contraction during expiration and, importantly, the addition of accessory muscles during inspiration.

Posture becomes important with increasing effort. The patient may have to stand or sit leaning forwards with their arms braced against their knees or a suitable surface. This tripod position (Fig. 2.7.1) allows the arms to work with upper accessory muscles to expand the lungs during inspiration (Arnold et al., 2011). Conversely, a relaxed, natural posture suggests less effort of breathing.

Patients with breathing difficulty will usually not want to be positioned supine. If the patient is found supine, either they are not in great respiratory difficulty or they are in severe respiratory distress and in an altered conscious state.

The child patient differs from patients of other ages when assessing respiration. Children's airway diameters are narrower, with the structures in the mouth, including the tongue and epiglottis, being relatively larger. Any airway narrowing or swelling of those structures can significantly reduce airflow (Sahin-Yilmaz and Naclerio, 2011).

Further, the smaller child's chest is more vertical than that of adults, with less input from intercostal muscles. The diaphragm is relatively more important, making its evaluation critical during assessment. The softer chest wall of the child makes its inward retraction more likely during breathing difficulty, particularly the sternum and the subcostal chest margin.

There are several facial features that indicate increased breathing effort. In children, the most notable is nasal flaring. The opening of the nose is only about one-quarter the diameter of the nasal cavity itself. This is particularly important in children, as any change in their airway diameter is significant. With nasal flaring, muscles

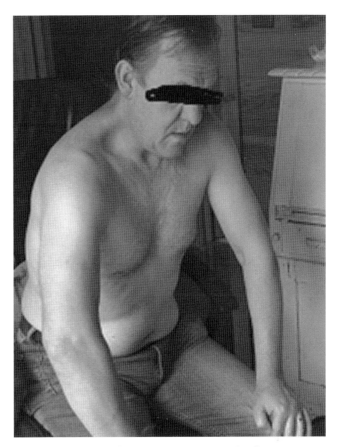

Figure 2.7.1 Tripod position using upper body accessory muscles

inside the nose cause nostrils to flare during inspiration, increasing inward airflow. These muscles relax during expiration, slowing air escape and prolonging the time for gas exchange (Sahin-Yilmaz and Naclerio, 2011).

Other common features of the child with breathing difficulty are grunting and head bobbing. Grunting is forced expiration against partial closure of the glottis, briefly opposing air escape. Pressure in the lower airway increases, keeping the bronchioles and alveoli open longer and so improving overall alveolar air escape and gas exchange. Head bobbing is the evident extension of the neck during inspiration as the chest wall and accessory muscles retract away. This is a sign that the accessory muscles are being used (Yost et al., 2001).

Adults tend to be mouth-breathers rather than nose-breathers. Instead of nasal flaring, pursed lips are commonly observed (Cabral et al., 2014). Some respiratory diseases, particularly those involving gas retention such as asthma, emphysema and chronic bronchitis, involve the lower airway collapsing during expiration. Air on the proximal side of any lower airway obstruction escapes, lowering the pressure in the upper airway. The lower airways, which are commonly inflamed, collapse inwards, trapping alveolar air behind them. This contributes to gas retention and airflow reduction. Pursed lip breathing (Fig. 2.7.2) slows expiration and maintains pressure in the lower airways, keeping them open longer and increasing alveolar gas escape (Cabral et al., 2014; Visser et al., 2010).

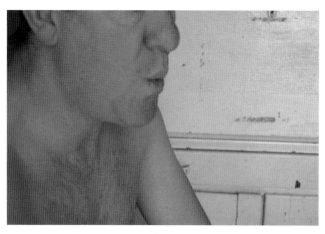

Figure 2.7.2 Pursed lip expiration

Clinical skill assessment process

The following section outlines the clinical skill assessment tools that should be used to determine a student's ability to demonstrate safe and accurate assessment of work of breathing.

1. Clinical Skill Work Instruction
2. Formative Clinical Skill Assessment (F-CSAT)
3. Performance Improvement Plan (PIP)
4. Summative Clinical Skill Assessment (S-CSAT)
(5. Direct Observation of Procedural Skills (DOPS) – see Chapter 2)

Clinical Skill Work Instruction

Equipment and resources: Standardised patient with detectable breathing movements; disposable gloves; method of documenting results

Associated Clinical Skills: Infection control; Communication; Consent; Assessment of respiratory rate and rhythm

Assessment of work of breathing

Activity	Critical Action	Rationale
Prepare patient	Assessing work of breathing can be performed with patient in any position.	In distress the patient will find the most effective position.
	To assess chest and abdominal movement during breathing, remove upper body garments to allow visibility and palpation. Minimise exposure, gaining the patient's consent and protecting their dignity.	Allows visibility of retraction and work of breathing.
Assess work of breathing	Observe patient posture: sitting, standing or lying.	Position will give clues to degree of distress.
	Observe any nasal flaring, grunting, head bobbing or pursed lip breathing.	Signs of increased work of breathing, particularly in children.
	Observe any visible accessory muscle use, including suprasternal, supraclavicular, sternal and subcostal retraction.	Accessory muscle use implies increased work of breathing.
	Observe chest rise and fall with each breath. Evaluate expansion of both sides of the chest. Where there is difficulty assessing chest wall movement, place one hand on either side of the chest to aid assessment. Determine if movement is shallow, normal, increased or maximal.	Determine equal air entry and chest wall movement when respiration is shallow.
	Observe the upper abdomen to assess movement of the diaphragm. One hand can be placed over the upper abdomen to help assess breathing movement.	Detecting breathing via touch can assist where visual assessment is difficult.
Report	Accurately document/hand over findings, including abnormal position, accessory muscle use, chest wall retraction, chest expansion and abdominal movement.	Continuity of care.

Formative Clinical Skill Assessment (F-CSAT)

Equipment and resources: Standardised patient with detectable breathing movements; disposable gloves; method of documenting results

Associated Clinical Skills: Infection control; Communication; Consent; Assessment of respiratory rate and rhythm

Staff/Student being assessed: _____

Assessment of work of breathing

Activity	Critical Action	Participant Performance				
Prepares patient	Assesses patient work of breathing in position presenting.	0	1	2	3	4
	Removes upper body garments to allow visibility and palpation. Minimises patient exposure, gaining the patient's consent and protecting their dignity.	0	1	2	3	4
Assesses work of breathing	Observes patient posture: sitting, standing or lying.	0	1	2	3	4
	Observes any nasal flaring, grunting, head bobbing or pursed lip breathing.	0	1	2	3	4
	Observes any visible accessory muscle use, including suprasternal, supraclavicular, sternal and subcostal retraction.	0	1	2	3	4
	Observes chest rise and fall with each breath. Evaluates expansion of both sides of the chest. Where there is difficulty assessing chest wall movement, places one hand on either side of the chest to aid assessment. Determines if the movement is shallow, normal, increased or maximal.	0	1	2	3	4
	Observes the upper abdomen to assess diaphragm movement. Places one hand over the upper abdomen to help assess breathing movement if necessary.	0	1	2	3	4
Reports	Accurately documents/hands over findings, including any abnormal position, accessory muscle use, chest wall retraction, chest expansion and abdominal movement.	0	1	2	3	4

Standard Achieved: (please circle one)

Competent (C)   Not Yet Competent* (NYC)

Staff/Student Name: _____

Assessor (please print name): _____

Signed (Assessor): _____

Date of Assessment: _____

Comments:

*If Not Yet Competent (NYC) a PIP needs to be completed and a repeat of the F-CSAT

Formative Clinical Skill Assessment (F-CSAT) Key

Skill level	Standard of procedure	Quality of performance	Outcome	Level of assistance required
4 Safe for unsupervised practice	Safe Accurate Behaviour is appropriate to context	Confident Accurate Expedient	Achieved intended outcome	No supporting cues* required
3 Requires supervision	Safe Accurate Behaviour is appropriate to context	Confident Accurate Takes longer than required	Achieved intended outcome	Requires occasional supportive cues*
2 Requires assistance	Safe Accurate Behaviour generally appropriate to context	Lacks certainty	Would not have achieved outcome without support	Requires frequent verbal and occasional physical directives in addition to supportive cues*
1 Requires direction	Safe only with guidance Not completely accurate	Unskilled Inefficient	Would not have achieved outcome without support	Requires continuous verbal and frequent physical directive cues*
0 Unsafe	Unsafe Unable to demonstrate behaviour Lack of insight into behaviour appropriate to context	Unskilled	Would not have achieved outcome	Requires continuous verbal and continuous physical directive cues*

*Refers to physical directives or verbal supportive cues

Performance Improvement Plan (PIP)

Please document the agreed education plan and completion timelines for areas assessed as less than 4.

This plan should be presented to assessor prior to commencement of summative assessment.

Where was supervisor support required?	Student summary of deficit. (Why was there a problem?)	Improvement Plan	Completed (Y/N)

Staff/Student Name: _____

Staff/Student Signature: _____

Educator Name: _____

Educator Signature: _____

Summative Clinical Skill Assessment (S-CSAT)

Equipment and resources: Patient with detectable breathing difficulty signs; gloves; method of documenting results

Associated Clinical Skills: Infection control; Communication; Consent; Assessment of respiratory rate and rhythm

Staff/Student being assessed: _____

- Completed Formative Clinical Skill Assessment (F-CSAT): **YES** **NO**
- Completed Performance Improvement Plan (PIP): **YES** **NO** **N/A**

Assessment of work of breathing

Activity	Critical Action	Achieved Without Direction	
Prepares patient	Assesses patient work of breathing in position found.	NO	YES
	Removes upper body garments to allow visibility and palpation. Minimises patient exposure, gaining the patient's consent and protecting their dignity.	NO	YES
Assesses work of breathing	Observes patient posture: sitting, standing or lying.	NO	YES
	Observes any nasal flaring, grunting, head bobbing or pursed lip breathing.	NO	YES
	Observes any visible accessory muscle use, including suprasternal, supraclavicular, sternal and subcostal retraction.	NO	YES
	Observes chest rise and fall with each breath. Evaluates expansion of both sides of the chest. Where there is difficulty assessing chest wall movement, places one hand on either side of the chest to aid assessment. Determines if the movement is shallow, normal, increased or maximal.	NO	YES
	Observes the upper abdomen to assess diaphragm movement. Places one hand over the upper abdomen to help assess breathing movement if necessary.	NO	YES
Reports	Accurately documents/hands over findings, including any abnormal position, accessory muscle use, chest wall retraction, chest expansion and abdominal movement.	NO	YES

Standard Achieved: (please circle one)

Competent (C)   Not Yet Competent* (NYC)

Staff/Student Name: _____

Assessor (please print name)**:** _____

Signed (Assessor)**:** _____

Date of Assessment: _____

Comments:

*If Not Yet Competent (NYC) a PIP needs to be completed and a repeat of the F-CSAT

Clinical findings

Abnormal findings in illness context

Abnormal breathing changes can be a result of primary respiratory disease and can provide useful clues to the severity of illness and assist in diagnosis.

In other cases, breathing changes can be secondary compensation for another underlying problem. In each case, abnormal findings must be interpreted in the context of the patient's past and current history.

Chronic respiratory disease

Some chronic respiratory illness can produce variations to a patient's normal day-to-day breathing pattern. After establishing abnormal breathing variations, these must be compared to how the patient's 'normal' would usually present. In some cases, what is being observed as variation from standard parameters is not significant for the patient being assessed.

Patient age

Adults' airway and chest anatomy and respiratory physiology vary significantly from those of children, particularly newborn and smaller children. Key signs of breathing difficulty in the child patient may therefore differ from that of the adult patient.

PRACTICE TIP!

Children can be difficult to assess when they are anxious and apprehensive. Use the parent to help build confidence, and allow them to remove child's clothing and gain their compliance. Explain to the parent precisely what you want to observe, so that they can help you access the child's torso.

PRACTICE TIP!

Patients with underlying chronic respiratory illness will also have a reduced ability to compensate for any worsening of their condition. In such cases, it must be remembered during assessment that even relatively small adverse changes may be difficult to tolerate.

PRACTICE TIP!

Work of breathing must be assessed in the context of any underlying condition. Some patients have chronic increased breathing effort; while abnormalities observed as increased work of breathing may appear severe, they may in fact represent only a small worsening of the patient's condition. The patient's 'normal' must be established in such situations.

TEST YOUR KNOWLEDGE QUESTIONS

1. **What is the normal dominant respiratory muscle?**
   The diaphragm.

2. **How is this muscle assessed for effort?**
   It can be felt by placing the hand over it or it can be visually observed.

3. **Why are intercostal muscle use and chest movement less likely to be helpful in the child patient?**
   A child's chest wall is more vertical and less able to swing outwards than it does with adults, so the diaphragm is more important to observe in children.

4. **What two key variables suggest the patient is trying to slow their own expiratory airflow?**
   Pursed lips in adult patients and grunting in smaller children both suggest the patient is resisting expiration.

5. **Which signs of increase of the work of breathing are more likely in the child patient?**
   The small child is more likely to demonstrate nasal flaring, head bobbing and grunting than adults, and to have increased diaphragm movement and soft tissue retraction.

6. **What are the key variables in work of breathing to assess for?**
   Posture; increased work of the diaphragm; increased chest movement; use of accessory muscles; nasal flaring; grunting; head bobbing; or pursed lips during expiration.

7. **What problem can arise if the patient is aware their respiration is being assessed?**
   The patient can instinctively control and change their respiratory rate and effort.

8. **What are the accessory muscles and how are they observed?**
   These are the sternocleidomastoid, pectoral and scalene muscles of the upper chest used to pull the sternum upwards and outwards. They can be observed in use by upper body movement and tripod positioning. They are joined by the abdominal muscles to raise abdominal pressure and push the diaphragm upwards, which is observable by watching for increased movement.

9. **What breathing effort is usually observable with normal breathing?**
   Minimal chest and diaphragm movement is visible and may be so relaxed that palpation of breathing may be necessary.

10. **What is the significance of chronic underlying illness when assessing a patient's normal breathing?**
    The patient's 'normal' can involve signs usually associated with respiratory difficulty, including increased effort, accessory muscle use and facial signs. Assessment must include observation and deviation from the patient's normal features rather than from standard normal findings.

References

Arnold, D.H., Gebretsadik, T., Sheller, J.R., Abramo, T.J. and Hartert, T.V., 2011. The value of observation for accessory muscle use in pediatric patients with acute asthma exacerbations: severity-dependent associations with fev1 and hospitalization decisions. *Annals of Allergy, Asthma & Immunology*, 106(4), 344.

Barthel, P., Wensel, R., Bauer, A., Müller, A., Wolf, P., Ulm, K., Huster, K.M., Francis, D.P., Malik, M. and Schmidt, G., 2013. Respiratory rate predicts outcome after acute myocardial infarction: a prospective cohort study. *European Heart Journal*, 34(22), 1644–1650.

Burton, A.B., Stokes, K., Hall, G.M., 2004. Physiological effects of exercise. *Continuing Education in Anaesthesia, Critical Care & Pain*, 4(6), 185–188.

Cabral, L.F., D'Elia, T.C., Marins, D.S., Zin, W.A. and Guimaraes, F.S., 2014. Pursed lip breathing improves exercise tolerance in COPD: a randomized crossover study. *European Journal of Physical Rehabilitation Medicine*, 51(1), 79–88.

Philip, K.E., Pack, E., Cambiano, V., Rollmann, H., Weil, S. and O'Beirne, J., 2016. The accuracy of respiratory rate assessment by doctors in a London teaching hospital: a cross-sectional study. *Journal of Clinical Monitoring and Computing*, 29(4), 455–460.

Sahin-Yilmaz, A. and Naclerio, R.M., 2011. Anatomy and physiology of the upper airway. *Proceedings of the American Thoracic Society*, March, 8(1), 31–39.

Visser, F.J., Ramlal, S., Dekhuijzen, P.R. and Heijdra, Y.F., 2010. Pursed-lips breathing improves inspiratory capacity in chronic obstructive pulmonary disease. *Respiration*, 81(5), 372–378.

Yost, G.C., Young, P.C. and Buchi, K.F., 2001. Significance of grunting respirations in infants admitted to a well-baby nursery. *Archives of Pediatric Adolescent Medicine*, 155(3), 372–375.

Bibliography

Craft, J., Gordon, C., Huether, S.E., McCance K.L. and Brashers V.L., 2015. *Understanding pathophysiology (ANZ adaptation)*. Sydney: Elsevier.

McCance, K.L. and Huether, S.E., 2015. *Pathophysiology: the biologic basis for disease in adults and children*. Sydney: Elsevier.

Chapter objectives

At the end of this chapter the reader will be able to:

1. Describe the rationale for chest auscultation
2. Demonstrate the method of chest auscultation
3. Accurately report on assessment findings
4. Identify pathologies associated with abnormal respiratory sounds

Resources required for this assessment

- Standardised patient with anterior, lateral and posterior chest exposed to skin
- Stethoscope with diaphragm suited to chest auscultation
- Disposable gloves
- Method of documenting the results

Skill matrix

This assessment requires:
- Infection control (CS 1.3)
- Communication (CS 1.5)
- Consent (CS 1.6)
- Assessment of respiratory rate and rhythm (CS 2.6)
- Assessment of work of breathing (CS 2.7)

This assessment is a component of:
- Patient assessment (Chapter 2)

Introduction

Assessing breathing status is a core vital sign component. Variations from 'normal' can provide important assessment clues.

The act of moving air during breathing creates two broad groups of signs. The first describe work of breathing and are observable. They include muscle activity and respiratory rate (see Chapters 2.6 and 2.7).

Chest auscultation is the second sign. It assesses sounds as air moves through airways to detect and identify abnormalities. This chapter discusses chest auscultation.

Anatomy and physiology

The airway is divided into upper and lower. The upper airway extends from mouth and nose, inwards to the nasopharynx and oropharynx then distally to the larynx and trachea. It continues downwards into right and left bronchi and further bronchial bifurcations. Lower airways complete the respiratory tree with the smallest air-conducting branches of the bronchioles and distal alveoli.

The lung tissue surrounding the distal airways includes interstitial fluid, supportive connective tissue and the vascular network.

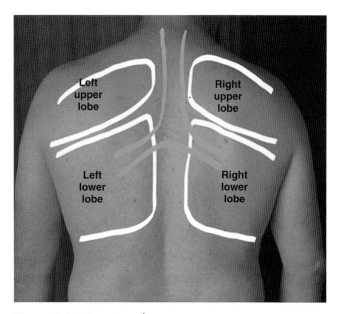

Figure 2.8.1 Posterior chest

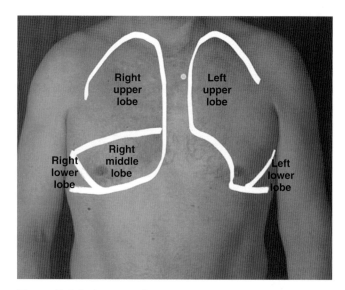

Figure 2.8.2 Anterior chest

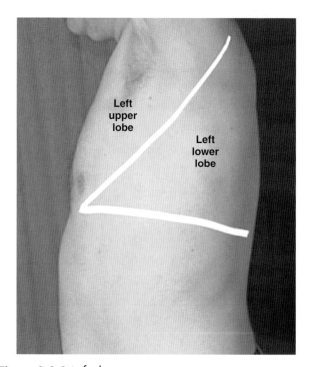

Figure 2.8.3 Left chest

Inspiratory airflow is created mostly through diaphragm contraction supported by the external intercostal muscles. Expiratory airflow is normally passive, with inspiratory muscle relaxation and elastic recoil of the lungs and chest wall.

Supporting the chest is the sternum and rib cage. Two pleural serous membrane layers line the chest wall and lungs.

The two lungs further divide into five distinctive lobes, three on the larger right side and two on the left. The mediastinum containing the heart intrudes into the left lung space.

Posterior chest

The lower three-quarters of the chest covers the left and right lower lobes. The upper quarter covers the left and right upper lobes (Fig. 2.8.1).

Anterior chest

The left side of the chest covers the left upper lobe, with an indent at the medial base where the heart sits. The right side upper two-thirds cover the right upper lobe, and the lower third the right lower lobe (Fig. 2.8.2).

Viewed from the side, the anterior lung base is higher than the posterior base. Chest sounds are audible further down the posterior chest.

Left lateral

A diagonal line can be drawn from the posterior shoulder to the lower anterior base. The upper triangle is the left upper lobe, while the lower triangle is the lower left lobe (Fig. 2.8.3).

Right lateral

A line can be drawn from the posterior shoulder down to the anterior base. The right lower lobe is posterior and the right upper lobe is superior. The right middle lobe – the

third lobe – is smaller and located towards the right base and anterior chest (Fig. 2.8.4).

Clinical rationale

Chest auscultation is listening for sounds heard:
- near the mouth with an unaided ear
- over the chest using a stethoscope.

Classical stethoscopes have two earpieces, one or two 45–65 cm hollow tubes and a single- or double-sided distal chest piece end (Sarkar, 2015).

Earpieces can be soft or hard, for comfort preference. The metal earpiece arms should each face slightly towards the assessor's nose, to align towards the eardrum (Fig. 2.8.5).

Chest pieces sometimes have a smaller, cup-shaped end called the bell, which is designed for lower frequency

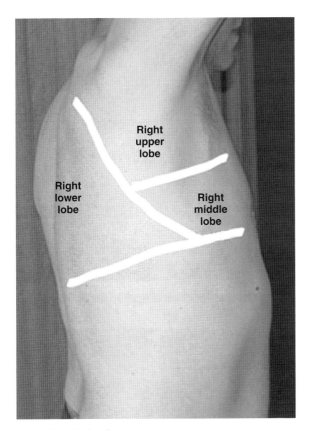

Figure 2.8.4 Right chest

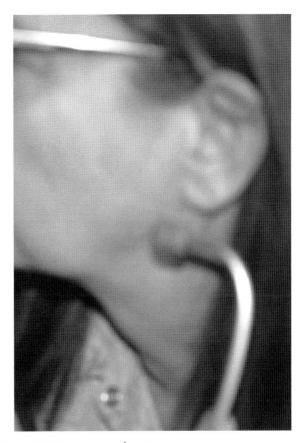

Figure 2.8.5 Earpiece direction

sounds such as heart murmurs and bowel sounds. It is placed lightly over the skin, though pushing down harder can improve higher pitched sounds. The bell is less likely to trap and rub over hairs and produce sound on hairy-chested patients.

The flatter, wider disc is the diaphragm, which is preferred for higher frequency sounds including lung and normal heart sounds. The diaphragm is a membrane that vibrates like the eardrum, transmitting and magnifying noise along the tubes.

The chest piece is held between the first and second fingers to minimise the noise produced by rubbing the assessor's own fingers (Fig. 2.8.6).

The sounds created by the patient vocalising must be distinguished first from those being created within the lungs themselves. Patients should typically be asked to not speak throughout the assessment so as to remove vocal sounds. While vocal sounds can occasionally be useful for assessment, this is not common during paramedic prehospital assessment.

Vocal sounds

Vocal sounds are generated within the larynx as air passes through and vibrates the vocal cords. They vary between high and low frequency and are altered by lung pathology, and are assessable by bronchophony, egophony and whispered pectoriloquy (Bohadana et al., 2014; Boucher et al., 2013; Sarkar et al., 2015).

Normally, vocal sounds become less audible in the lungs. Bronchophony is vocal sounds that are louder than

expected in distal lungs. Air displacement from the lungs by fluid, typically pneumonia, can increase the resonance and loudness of sound. To identify bronchophony, have the patient say 'ninety-nine' repeatedly during auscultation (Bohadana et al., 2014; Boucher et al., 2013; Sarkar et al., 2015).

Whispered pectoriloquy is a variation of bronchophony, and is assessed in the same manner, except by whispering rather than saying 'ninety-nine', to identify the amplification of low-volume sounds (Bohadana et al., 2014; Sarkar et al., 2015).

Egophony is another variation. Rather than saying 'ninety-nine', the patient slowly says the letter 'E' repeatedly. Over consolidation areas, the pronunciation sounds more like the letter 'A' (Bohadana et al., 2014; Sarkar et al., 2015).

Lung sounds

Lung sounds are separable into normal and abnormal (adventitious) sounds (Boucher et al., 2013).

Normal breath sounds are quiet and not easily heard without a stethoscope. Airflow has little disturbance, moving easily in laminar flow. When listening over smaller airways, these soft sounds are called 'vesicular'. They are louder during inspiration, where there is greater airflow (Bohadana et al., 2014; Boucher et al., 2013; Nagasaka, 2012; Sarkar et al., 2015).

Normal bronchial lung sounds are slightly louder during expiration. They are best heard over larger airways between the scapulae and the apices or anteriorly over

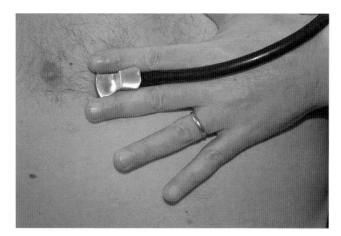

Figure 2.8.6 Holding a chest piece

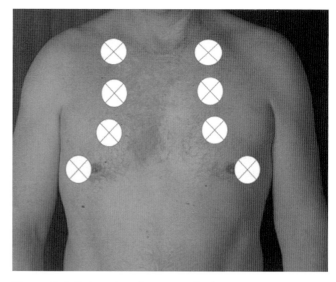

Figure 2.8.8 Anterior chest auscultation

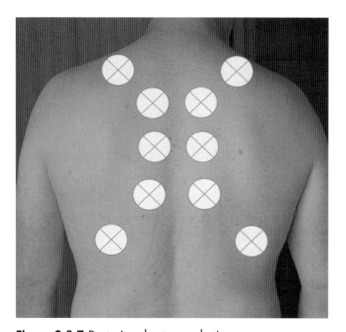

Figure 2.8.7 Posterior chest auscultation

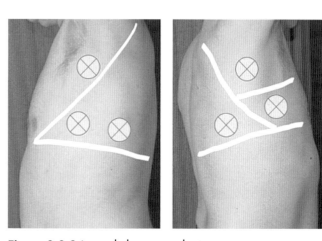

Figure 2.8.9 Lateral chest auscultation

the manubrium. The higher pitched sound is air moving through a tube, with a pause separating inspiration and expiration (Bohadana et al., 2014; Boucher et al., 2013; Nagasaka, 2012; Sarkar et al., 2015).

Auscultation

Auscultate the anterior, posterior and lateral chest locations to assess all the lobes. Some respiratory sounds will be audible throughout all lung fields, while others will be audible only within specific lobes.

Posterior chest

Begin at the mid-clavicular line above the scapula. Move downwards, comparing each side at each level. The next two or three locations should be relatively medial to avoid listening over the scapula where lung sounds are not heard. Once below the scapula, move mid-clavicular again to complete the posterior chest. This may require four to seven levels, depending on the patient's chest size (Fig. 2.8.7).

Anterior chest

Begin at clavicle level, working downwards in the mid-clavicular line. At the lower rib margin, move the stethoscope laterally. For each level, listen to both sides before moving down. This may require three to six levels, depending on the patient's chest size (Fig. 2.8.8).

Lateral chest

Auscultate the left and right lateral chest lobes. The patient's arm may need to be pushed forwards or raised for access (Fig. 2.8.9).

Clinical skill assessment process

The following section outlines the clinical skill assessment tools that should be used to determine a student's ability to demonstrate accurate chest auscultation.

1. Clinical Skill Work Instruction
2. Formative Clinical Skill Assessment (F-CSAT)
3. Performance Improvement Plan (PIP)
4. Summative Clinical Skill Assessment (S-CSAT)
(5. Direct Observation of Procedural Skills (DOPS) – see Chapter 1.1)

Clinical Skill Work Instruction

Equipment and resources: Standardised patient with anterior, lateral and posterior chest exposed to skin; stethoscope with diaphragm suited to chest auscultation; disposable gloves; method of documenting the results

Associated Clinical Skills: Infection control; Communication; Consent; Assessment of respiratory rate and rhythm; Assessment of work of breathing

Chest auscultation

Activity	Critical Action	Rationale
Prepare patient	Position patient sitting upright. If necessary, this assessment can be performed supine and rolling patient laterally.	To allow access to all lung fields.
	Sufficiently remove upper body garments to allow entire chest access. Minimise exposure throughout.	Allows for environment and dignity. Clothing can reduce sounds or cause interfering ones.
Prepare stethoscope for use	The setting should be quiet without extra noise.	To enhance audibility.
	Place earpieces into each ear with the tips pointing slightly towards the nose.	Provides seal and aligns with ear canal.
	Gently tap diaphragm for sound. Adjust for diaphragm in use.	Ensures the active side is against the skin.
	Warm diaphragm by holding it in a hand for a few seconds.	Patient comfort.
	Hold the chest piece with the diaphragm between the first two fingers. The fingers and thumb should not touch the diaphragm edges or patient's skin.	To minimise sound caused by assessor's fingers while allowing the application of downward pressure.
Auscultate sounds	Instruct patient to breathe normally through an open mouth throughout and to not speak.	Maximises airflow and reduces sounds made by the lips.
	Stand behind patient and place diaphragm against posterior chest on upper left or right side. The patient may be leant slightly forwards.	To ensure apex of each lung is included.
	Move down chest listening left to right, with one breath for each point during inspiration and expiration. Move downwards between four to seven levels until lung base is reached.	Allows sounds from same level to be compared.
	Stand in front of patient and repeat process on the anterior chest. Repeat apex to base assessment from mid-clavicular line to lung base at three to six levels. Move more laterally towards the lower chest margin.	To listen over all lung fields.
	Auscultate left and right lateral chest in at least three positions each side: sub-axilla, anterior lower chest margin, posterior lower chest margin. May have to move arm forwards or upwards for access.	
Clarify sounds	Where abnormal sounds are heard, have the patient cough briefly. Repeat auscultation process.	To clear secretions and open collapsed airways.
Report	Accurately document/hand over findings, including abnormal sounds and differences between left and right lung regions.	Accurate record kept and continuity of patient care.

Formative Clinical Skill Assessment (F-CSAT)

Equipment and resources: Standardised patient with anterior, lateral and posterior chest exposed to skin; stethoscope with diaphragm suited to chest auscultation; disposable gloves; method of documenting the results

Associated Clinical Skills: Infection control; Communication; Consent; Assessment of respiratory rate and rhythm; Assessment of work of breathing

Staff/Student being assessed: _____

Chest auscultation

Activity	Critical Action	Participant Performance				
Prepares patient	Positions patient upright or lateral if unable.	0	1	2	3	4
	Removes upper garments to access chest.	0	1	2	3	4
Prepares stethoscope for use	Ensures scene is quiet where possible.	0	1	2	3	4
	Places earpieces into ears, with tips facing forwards.	0	1	2	3	4
	Ensures diaphragm chest piece is ready for use.	0	1	2	3	4
	Warms diaphragm in advance.	0	1	2	3	4
	Holds chest piece between first and second fingers.	0	1	2	3	4
Auscultates sounds	Instructs patient to breathe normally through an open mouth.	0	1	2	3	4
	Stands behind patient for auscultation.	0	1	2	3	4
	Auscultates posterior chest from apex on one side, comparing each side to the other at that level. Moves downward four to seven levels until bases reached.	0	1	2	3	4
	Moves to front of patient and repeats auscultation, one side to the other, top to bottom, three to six levels until bases reached.	0	1	2	3	4
	Auscultates left and right lateral chest in at least three positions each side: sub axilla, anterior lower chest margin, posterior lower chest margin. Moves patient's arm forwards or upwards for access.	0	1	2	3	4
Clarifies sounds	Where abnormal sounds are heard, has patient cough briefly. Repeats auscultation process.	0	1	2	3	4
Reports	Accurately documents/hands over the findings.	0	1	2	3	4

Standard Achieved: (please circle one)

Competent (C)   Not Yet Competent* (NYC)

Staff/Student Name: _____

Assessor (please print name): _____

Signed (Assessor): _____

Date of Assessment: _____

Comments:

*If Not Yet Competent (NYC) a PIP needs to be completed and a repeat of the F-CSAT

Formative Clinical Skill Assessment (F-CSAT) Key

Skill level	Standard of procedure	Quality of performance	Outcome	Level of assistance required
4 Safe for unsupervised practice	Safe Accurate Behaviour is appropriate to context	Confident Accurate Expedient	Achieved intended outcome	No supporting cues* required
3 Requires supervision	Safe Accurate Behaviour is appropriate to context	Confident Accurate Takes longer than required	Achieved intended outcome	Requires occasional supportive cues*
2 Requires assistance	Safe Accurate Behaviour generally appropriate to context	Lacks certainty	Would not have achieved outcome without support	Requires frequent verbal and occasional physical directives in addition to supportive cues*
1 Requires direction	Safe only with guidance Not completely accurate	Unskilled Inefficient	Would not have achieved outcome without support	Requires continuous verbal and frequent physical directive cues*
0 Unsafe	Unsafe Unable to demonstrate behaviour Lack of insight into behaviour appropriate to context	Unskilled	Would not have achieved outcome	Requires continuous verbal and continuous physical directive cues*

*Refers to physical directives or verbal supportive cues

Performance Improvement Plan (PIP)

Please document the agreed education plan and completion timelines for areas assessed as less than 4.

This plan should be presented to assessor prior to commencement of summative assessment.

Where was supervisor support required?	Student summary of deficit. (Why was there a problem?)	Improvement Plan	Completed (Y/N)

Staff /Student Name: _____

Staff/Student Signature: _____

Educator Name: _____

Educator Signature: _____

Summative Clinical Skill Assessment (S-CSAT)

Equipment and resources: Standardised patient with anterior, lateral and posterior chest exposed to skin; stethoscope with diaphragm suited to chest auscultation; disposable gloves; method of documenting the results

Associated Clinical Skills: Infection control; Communication; Consent; Assessment of respiratory rate and rhythm; Assessment of work of breathing

Staff/Student being assessed: _____

- Completed Formative Clinical Skill Assessment (F-CSAT): **YES**   **NO**
- Completed Performance Improvement Plan (PIP): **YES**   **NO**   **N/A**

Chest auscultation

Activity	Critical Action	Achieved Without Direction	
Prepares patient	Positions patient upright or lateral if unable.	NO	YES
	Removes upper garments to access chest.	NO	YES
Prepares stethoscope for use	Ensures scene is quiet where possible.	NO	YES
	Places earpieces into the ear, with tips facing forwards.	NO	YES
	Ensures diaphragm chest piece side is ready for use.	NO	YES
	Ensures diaphragm is warmed in advance.	NO	YES
Auscultates sounds	Holds chest piece correctly between first and second fingers.	NO	YES
	Instructs patient to breathe normally through an open mouth.	NO	YES
	Stands behind patient for auscultation.	NO	YES
	Auscultates posterior chest from apex on one side, comparing each side to the other at that level. Moves downwards four to seven levels until bases reached.	NO	YES
	Moves to front of patient and repeats auscultation process, one side to the other, top to bottom, three to six levels until bases reached and no further sound heard.	NO	YES
	Auscultates left and right lateral chest in at least three positions each side: sub axilla, anterior lower chest margin, posterior lower chest margin. Moves patient's arm forwards or upwards for access.	NO	YES
Clarifies sounds	Where abnormal sounds are heard, has the patient cough briefly. Repeats the auscultation process.	NO	YES
Reports	Accurately documents/hands over the findings.	NO	YES

Clinical findings

Abnormal lung sounds provide clues to disease, as they result from upper or lower airway problems. Some, such as crackles, are intermittent. Others, such as wheezes, are more continuous. Some sounds are amplified, others quiet, and some may be audible near the mouth without a stethoscope (Bohadana et al., 2014; Sarkar et al., 2015).

Chest auscultation is often accompanied by other assessment methods, including visual inspection, percussion or fremitus, to aid differentiation.

Upper airway sounds

Stertor

Stertor is produced by a narrowing of the airway in the pharynx above the larynx, distinguishing it from stridor. It is turbulent airflow heard by placing an ear close to the patient's mouth or auscultation over the neck.

Described as snoring, stertor is caused by the uvula and soft palate muscles relaxing, vibrating with the inward airflow and being drawn towards the glottis. They move away on expiration, making stertor mostly inspiratory. It is low-pitched, which also distinguishes it from stridor.

Stridor

Stridor is a high-pitched, almost whistling noise that is usually heard on inspiration. If severe, it may also be heard on expiration. As it is caused by obstruction in or near the larynx, it is best heard over the neck (Bohadana et al., 2014; Sarkar et al., 2015). It can be mistaken for wheeze.

The causes of stridor include cancerous lesions, vocal cord spasm, inflammation such as croup and foreign body obstruction.

Lower airway sounds

Wheeze

Wheezing is high-pitched whistling from air passing through narrowed lower airways, commonly caused by asthma, anaphylaxis, smoke inhalation or inflammation.

Initially, stronger inspiratory muscles drag air into the alveoli past the obstruction. As air escapes during expiration, there is less expiratory force. Bronchioles collapse, producing turbulent airflow and expiratory wheeze and prolonging the expiratory phase (Bohadana et al., 2014; Nagasaka, 2012; Sarkar et al., 2015).

More severe narrowing of the airways reduces airflow further. Wheeze may become audible during inspiration, be little more than a high-pitched squeak or produce no audible sounds. Subsequent improvements in the patient's condition may improve airflow, making wheezing more audible.

Wheezing is commonly heard throughout all lung fields but may be limited to a smaller area if mucus or infection irritate nearby bronchioles.

Crackles

Crackles are loud popping sounds as collapsed airways open during inspiration. Crackles are divided into coarse- or fine-sounding (Bohadana et al., 2014; Sarkar et al., 2015).

Inside the alveoli is a surfactant coating that decreases surface tension, maintaining partial inflation at the end of expiration. This can be washed out by fluid, particularly pulmonary oedema, causing collapse. Alveolar crackles are fine, brief, high-pitched popping sounds at the end of inspiration as the alveoli reinflate.

Infected or mucus-filled bronchioles can collapse on expiration as the upper airway pressure holding them open escapes. Reopening with inspiration produces coarse, lower pitched crackles, which are heard during mid inspiration.

The location of crackles can vary and include select lobes and one or both lungs. Fine crackles can vary from bases only to all lung fields, though the levels in each lung are typically equal in normal posture.

Sometimes crackles can be cleared by asking the patient to cough before re-auscultation.

Pleural friction rub

Pleural friction rub occurs when the pleural and visceral pleural layers move over each other during breathing.

If inflamed, or without natural lubricant for smooth movement, rubbing may be heard during inspiration and expiration (Bohadana et al., 2014; Sarkar et al., 2015).

Amplified lung sounds: consolidation

Sound transmits more efficiently through liquid than through air. Lungs filled by fluid consolidation, such as pneumonia, transmit sound more efficiently than air-filled alveoli (bronchophony) (Sarkar et al., 2015).

Quiet lung sounds

Pleural effusion

Pleural effusion is abnormal fluid in the pleural space. It reduces lung expansion and airflow, causing dullness when auscultated. This can extend over one or both lungs.

Emphysema

Emphysematous lungs have enlarged alveoli and destruction of the surrounding connective tissue. Airflow reduces with reduced chest recoil, producing quieter vesicular sounds throughout.

Pneumothorax

Pneumothorax involves air in the pleural space. The affected lung is pressed inwards, reducing lung size and the airflow within. Auscultation over the affected area provides no audible sounds. Pneumothorax occurs typically at the apices first, extending downwards and increasing the lung area affected (MacDuff et al., 2010; Noppen, 2010).

Lobectomy

When one or more lung lobes have been removed, there is no sound over that area. Typically, there is a visible surgical scar.

PRACTICE TIP!

Identifying sounds during auscultation is not always easy. Frequent regular practice is needed to increase your experience in applying the correct methods and interpretation. Being familiar with the sounds of normal chests assists when listening to occasional abnormal sounds.

PRACTICE TIP!

Chest sounds can increase or decrease with airflow changes. This might reflect increased air entry and an improvement in the patient's condition. Alternatively, noise reduction might mean airflow reduction and a deterioration in the patient's condition. Consider all findings in the context of the patient's overall condition.

PRACTICE TIP!

Chest sounds are qualitative and provide clues to presenting problems. The results of auscultation must always be considered within the context of the patient's history and the respiratory assessment findings.

PRACTICE TIP!

Where possible, move away anyone who is not needed, or alternatively move the patient to a place of privacy. While leaving on basic clothing items such as a bra is acceptable, chest auscultation is unreliable when performed over clothing.

TEST YOUR KNOWLEDGE QUESTIONS

1. **Define the term auscultation.**
   Auscultation means listening for sounds.

2. **What are two ways to hear breathing sounds?**
   Sounds can be heard near the mouth by unaided ear or heard using a stethoscope over the chest.

3. **What are two broad types of normal breathing sounds?**
   Bronchial and vesicular.

4. **What two abnormal breath sounds are produced in the upper airway?**
   Stertor can occur above the glottis; stridor can occur within or just below the larynx.

5. **What is the functional difference between the bell and the diaphragm?**
   The bell is for lower frequency sounds, such as heart murmurs and bowel sounds; the diaphragm is for higher frequency sounds, including lung and normal heart sounds.

6. **What are crackles and when are they heard?**
   Crackles are collapsed small airways popping open again during inspiration. Coarse crackles are bronchioles opening late in inspiration; fine crackles are alveoli opening at the end of inspiration.

7. **How is a wheeze formed and when does it occur?**
   Wheezing occurs when bronchioles narrow, reducing airflow through them and creating turbulence. Although it initially occurs during expiration, wheezing can also occur during inspiration if airflow worsens.

8. **Do louder respiratory sounds mean the problem is more severe?**
   Not necessarily. Louder sounds than normal may be more severe. However, initial poor airflow might produce quiet sounds. Increasing sounds may indicate improving airflow. Some problems are recognised by reduced airflow and a lack of sound.

9. **Why is the chest auscultated at as many as 18 points?**
   To ensure all lobes of both lungs are adequately assessed over the anterior, posterior and lateral chest.

10. **What important details must be considered when fitting stethoscope earpieces into the ears?**
    They must angle slightly towards the nose, to align with the direction of the ear canal.

References

Bohadana, A., Izbicki, G., Kraman, S.S., 2014. Fundamentals of lung auscultation. *New England Journal of Medicine*, 370(8), 744–751.

Boucher, N., Prystupa, A., Witczak, A., Walczak, E., Dzida, G., Panasiuk, L., 2013. Lung auscultation – identification of common lung sound abnormalities and associated pathologies. *Journal of Preclinical and Clinical Research*, 7(1).

MacDuff, A., Arnold, A., Harvey, J., 2010. Management of spontaneous pneumothorax: British Thoracic Society pleural disease guideline 2010. *Thorax*, 65(Suppl 2), ii18–31.

Nagasaka, Y., 2012. Lung sounds in bronchial asthma. *Allergology International*, 61(3), 35–63.

Noppen, M., 2010. Spontaneous pneumothorax: epidemiology, pathophysiology and cause. *European Respiratory Review*, 19(117), 217–219.

Sarkar, M., Madabhavi, I., Niranjan, N. and Dogra, M., 2015. Auscultation of the respiratory system. *Annals of Thoracic Medicine*, 10(3), 158.

Bibliography

McCance, K.L. and Huether, S.E., 2015. *Pathophysiology: the biologic basis for disease in adults and children*. Sydney: Elsevier.

2.9 | Assessment of speech

Jeff Kenneally

Chapter objectives

At the end of this chapter the reader will be able to:

1. Describe the rationale for assessing speech during respiratory assessment
2. Demonstrate the method of assessing speech quality and quantity
3. Accurately report on the assessment findings
4. Identify pathologies associated with abnormal respiratory speech

Resources required for this assessment

- Patient able to respond to questioning
- Method of documenting the results

Skill matrix

This assessment requires:

- Infection control (CS 1.3)
- Communication (CS 1.5)
- Consent (CS 1.6)
- Assessment of respiratory rate and rhythm (CS 2.6)
- Assessment of work of breathing (CS 2.7)

This assessment is a component of:

- Patient assessment (Chapter 2)

Introduction

Respiratory assessment is largely based on subjective observations. Combinations of findings can be performed together to increase objectivity.

The ability to speak is linked to numerous body systems, including respiratory and neurological. It is useful in assessing respiratory effectiveness as it provides an indication of tidal volume and the degree of respiratory distress.

This chapter discusses speech assessment.

Anatomy and physiology

Speech results from four discernible steps: higher brain functions, the act of breathing, phonation and articulation.

Higher brain function processes language and determines what is to be said. This is transformed into cortex motor functions to draw air into the lungs. The expired airflow produces phonation within the larynx, and then articulation forms speech. Respiration provides the energy source for speech to occur.

As air exits the lungs it passes through trachea, larynx and pharynx. The larynx is important for the first part of speech formation: phonation. It is made up of several connected cartilages that, when moved, cause changes in the vocal cords (also known as vocal folds). The two cords are stretched across the larynx, attached by muscles, with the glottis between. Air pressure variations below the cords force them open which, along with their elastic capacity, causes them to vibrate and produce sounds.

The sound formed in the larynx can then be further modified through upper airway alterations, including the connection between oropharynx and nasopharynx, soft palate and movements of the tongue, jaw and lips. This is the process of articulation, converting phonation sound into understandable speech.

Airflow is produced through diaphragm and external intercostal muscle action expanding the chest and drawing air inwards. In reverse, air escapes the lungs through passive chest recoil, with some assistance from the internal intercostal and abdominal muscles. Resistance to airflow can come from upper airway obstruction such as croup or lower airway restriction including chronic obstructive pulmonary disease (COPD) and asthma.

Respiratory distress decreases tidal volume and distorts normal blood gases. This increases the need to breathe faster and reduces the ability for speech.

Clinical rationale

Speech is a product of multiple body system interactions, allowing it to be used for patient assessment in many different contexts, including respiratory, perfusion, conscious state and mental state assessments. During assessment, speech must be considered in regard to mechanical difficulties such as from traumatic injury or oedema; difficulties due to respiratory illness; an inability due to altered consciousness and impaired ability to cooperate; and, finally, impairment from mental illness.

Respiratory assessment and speech

Speech is an important component of respiratory assessment and is considered from two different aspects. The first is quantitative assessment. This considers duration of speech, including the number of words before a new breath is required. The other is qualitative assessment. This considers what is said and looks at such things as orientation, confusion or inappropriateness.

Speech requires expiratory airflow for phonation to occur. The greater the continuous airflow, the greater the phonation possible. Normally, full sentences can be spoken with one breath. This is the benchmark of normal speech: full and continuous speech of a sentence without interruption by another breath. This is the quantitative assessment (Binazzi et al., 2011; Gondos et al., 2017; Gupta et al., 2010).

Respiratory difficulty typically comes from either obstructed air entry to the lungs or increased resistance to exhaled airflow (Binazzi et al., 2011; Quinn and Coons, 2011). Expiratory reserve volume is reduced and blood gas is deranged, marked by hypoxemia and/or hypercapnia. A reduction in reserve volume and airflow resistance causes a reduction in peak and total exhaled airflow for phonation. If the patient is unable to maintain sufficient airflow, the duration of speech shortens notably. Further, inadequate alveolar ventilation increases the impetus to breathe again more quickly than usual. A shorter time between breaths means a shorter time for phonation (Binazzi et al., 2011; Gondos et al., 2017).

The greater the respiratory difficulty, the greater the adverse impact on speech (Bailey and Hoit, 2002; Gondos et al., 2017; Hoit et al., 2011). Conversely, increased attempts to speak impact adversely on respiratory difficulty and the feeling of breathlessness. This is significant, as it is important that any assessment does not worsen the patient's condition or increase their discomfort. Not only will some people have difficulty speaking effectively during respiratory distress, but this discomfort can create their unwillingness to attempt phonation (Binazzi et al., 2011).

Speech is also a reflection of adequate brain function. This, in turn, relies on several variables, including sufficient oxygen delivery, carbon dioxide removal, glucose delivery and cerebral perfusion. A change in any of these can result in impaired brain function manifested as a range of conscious-state changes, including anxiousness, irritability, delirium, agitation, drowsiness, confusion or stupor. This is the qualitative aspect of breathing.

In addition to being unable to provide normal phonation, altered mentation during respiratory difficulty can cause speech changes (Bailey and Hoit, 2002; Hoit et al., 2011). This includes confused responses such as disorientation to person, time or place, as well as an inability to recall events effectively. Anxiety and agitation can result from altered brain function, including blood gas and glucose abnormality. Verbal responses can be inappropriate and have little relationship to the original question or theme of conversation. Finally, speech can be incomprehensible, with nothing being discernible to the listener. These incomprehensible sounds must be differentiated from abnormal respiratory sounds such as stridor or snoring.

Speech is assessed for quality as well as quantity. An important cause of change in speech quality is during mental impairment. This can change speech patterns as significantly as physical impairment.

The assessment of mental state considers speech and the brain's ability to manage lucid and rational thought processes. Abnormalities can be looked for in the quality of what is said (Bailey and Hoit, 2002; Hoit et al., 2011).

While not exhaustive, speech quality assessments consider how fast the patient speaks, the volume of their speech and vocal tone, which may range from flat affect or monotonous through to excited or agitated, bizarre thought patterns, including delusions, hallucinations or irrational thoughts.

Since agitated conversation can arise from physical and mental impairment, this finding must be considered as part of the overall assessment and in context.

Before a speech assessment is made, it must be clear that the patient is able to communicate without any pre-existing impediment. They must be able to hear, understand the language spoken and be able to normally reply. Any interference from a hearing impairment, language barrier or chronic aphasia/dysphasia impacts on the patient's ability to speak, and alternatives should be found to overcome these challenges in such cases.

To assess speech, a balance must be found between requesting the patient to speak and not causing an increase in breathing difficulty or discomfort (Binazzi et al., 2011). To assess for the *quantity* of speech, any question can be asked that requires lengthy response. Alternatively, the patient can be asked to count from one onwards to see how many words they can say before the next breath is required.

When assessing for *quality* of speech, the answers provided to the questions asked should be specific and relevant. Standard questions are therefore required, particularly during conscious state and mental state assessment, so that the quality of the answer can be considered.

One standard approach is to ask the patient to state their name, what the day/date/or time is and where they currently are located. Disorientation to person, time and place is an indicator of confusion. The specific nature of the questioning can help identify inappropriate responses when they do not relate to what is asked.

Clinical skill assessment process

The following section outlines the clinical skills assessment tools that should be used to determine a student's ability to demonstrate accurate speech assessment.
1. Clinical Skill Work Instruction
2. Formative Clinical Skill Assessment (F-CSAT)
3. Performance Improvement Plan (PIP)
4. Summative Clinical Skill Assessment (S-CSAT)
(5. Direct Observation of Procedural Skills (DOPS) – see Chapter 1.1)

Clinical Skill Work Instruction

Equipment and resources: Patient able to respond to questioning; method of documenting results

Associated Clinical Skills: Infection control; Communication; Consent; Assessment of respiratory rate and rhythm; Assessment of work of breathing

Speech assessment

Activity	Critical Action	Rationale
Prepare patient	Assessing speech can be performed with the patient in any position.	
	Clarify that the patient can understand your spoken language and has no hearing impairment or pre-existing aphasia/dysphasia. If necessary, use an appropriate alternative method of communication, including an interpreter.	If you are assessing the patient responses to any questioning, they must be able to understand the question.
	Inform the patient you are going to ask them a series of questions as part of normal examination.	The questions may seem odd to the patient.
Assess speech quality	Ask the patient's name. Note correctness, drowsiness, disorientation, inappropriateness or incomprehensibleness.	These first three questions are part of a conscious state assessment but will provide information about speech ability. Asking their name ascertains orientation to person.
	Ask where they are. Note correctness, drowsiness, disorientation, inappropriateness or incomprehensibleness.	Asking where they are ascertains orientation to place.
	Ask what the time, day and date are. Note correctness, drowsiness, disorientation, inappropriateness or incomprehensibleness.	Asking what the time, day and date are ascertains orientation to time.
Assess speech quantity	Ask the patient to count from one onwards, making note of what number they reach before the need to take another breath arises.	Assesses speech quantity.
Report	Accurately document/hand over findings, including any abnormality detected.	Continuity of care.

Formative Clinical Skill Assessment (F-CSAT)

Equipment and resources: Patient able to respond to questioning; method of documenting results

Associated Clinical Skills: Infection control; Communication; Consent; Assessment of respiratory rate and rhythm; Assessment of work of breathing

Staff/Student being assessed: _____

Speech assessment

Activity	Critical Action	Participant Performance				
Prepares patient	Acknowledges assessing speech can be performed with the patient in any position.	0	1	2	3	4
	Clarifies that the patient can understand the spoken language and has no hearing impairment or pre-existing aphasia/dysphasia. If necessary, uses an appropriate alternative method of communication, including an interpreter.	0	1	2	3	4
	Informs patient of a series of questions to be asked as part of normal examination.	0	1	2	3	4
Assesses speech quality	Asks the patient's name. Notes correctness, drowsiness, disorientation, inappropriateness or incomprehensibleness.	0	1	2	3	4
	Asks the patient where they are. Notes correctness, drowsiness, disorientation, inappropriateness or incomprehensibleness.	0	1	2	3	4
	Asks what the time, day and date are. Notes correctness, drowsiness, disorientation, inappropriateness or incomprehensibleness.	0	1	2	3	4
Assesses speech quantity	Asks the patient to count from one onwards, making note of what number they reach before the need to take another breath arises.	0	1	2	3	4
Reports	Accurately documents/hands over findings, including any abnormalities noted.	0	1	2	3	4

Standard Achieved: (please circle one)

Competent (C)   Not Yet Competent* (NYC)

Staff/Student Name: _____

Assessor (please print name)**:** _____

Signed (Assessor)**:** _____

Date of Assessment: _____

Comments:

*If Not Yet Competent (NYC) a PIP needs to be completed and a repeat of the F-CSAT

Formative Clinical Skill Assessment (F-CSAT) Key

Skill level	Standard of procedure	Quality of performance	Outcome	Level of assistance required
4 Safe for unsupervised practice	Safe Accurate Behaviour is appropriate to context	Confident Accurate Expedient	Achieved intended outcome	No supporting cues* required
3 Requires supervision	Safe Accurate Behaviour is appropriate to context	Confident Accurate Takes longer than required	Achieved intended outcome	Requires occasional supportive cues*
2 Requires assistance	Safe Accurate Behaviour generally appropriate to context	Lacks certainty	Would not have achieved outcome without support	Requires frequent verbal and occasional physical directives in addition to supportive cues*
1 Requires direction	Safe only with guidance Not completely accurate	Unskilled Inefficient	Would not have achieved outcome without support	Requires continuous verbal and frequent physical directive cues*
0 Unsafe	Unsafe Unable to demonstrate behaviour Lack of insight into behaviour appropriate to context	Unskilled	Would not have achieved outcome	Requires continuous verbal and continuous physical directive cues*

Refers to physical directives or verbal supportive cues

Performance Improvement Plan (PIP)

Please document the agreed education plan and completion timelines for areas assessed as less than 4.

This plan should be presented to assessor prior to commencement of summative assessment.

Where was supervisor support required?	Student summary of deficit. (Why was there a problem?)	Improvement Plan	Completed (Y/N)

Staff/Student Name: _____

Staff/Student Signature: _____

Educator Name: _____

Educator Signature: _____

Summative Clinical Skill Assessment (S-CSAT)

Equipment and resources: Patient able to respond to questioning; method of documenting results

Associated Clinical Skills: Infection control; Communication; Consent; Assessment of respiratory rate and rhythm; Assessment of work of breathing

Staff/Student being assessed: _____

- Completed Formative Clinical Skill Assessment (F-CSAT): **YES** **NO**
- Completed Performance Improvement Plan (PIP): **YES** **NO** **N/A**

Speech assessment

Activity	Critical Action	Achieved Without Direction	
Prepares patient	Acknowledges assessing patient speech can be performed with the patient in any position.	NO	YES
	Clarifies that the patient can understand the spoken language and has no hearing impairment or pre-existing aphasia/dysphasia. If necessary, uses an appropriate alternative method of communication, including an interpreter.	NO	YES
	Informs patient of a series of questions to be asked as part of normal examination.	NO	YES
Assesses speech quality	Asks the patient what their name is. Notes correctness, drowsiness, disorientation, inappropriateness or incomprehensibleness.	NO	YES
	Asks the patient where they are. Notes correctness, drowsiness, disorientation, inappropriateness or incomprehensibleness.	NO	YES
	Asks what the time, day and date are. Notes correctness, drowsiness, disorientation, inappropriateness or incomprehensibleness.	NO	YES
Assesses speech quantity	Asks the patient to count from one onwards, making note of what number they reach before the need to take another breath arises.	NO	YES
Reports	Accurately documents/hands over findings, including any abnormality detected.	NO	YES

Standard Achieved: (please circle one)

Competent (C)   Not Yet Competent* (NYC)

Staff/Student Name: _____

Assessor (please print name): _____

Signed (Assessor): _____

Date of Assessment: _____

Comments:

*If Not Yet Competent (NYC) a PIP needs to be completed and a repeat of the F-CSAT

Clinical findings

Reasons for speech variations include chronic changes in respiration or lung function, restrictions on the ability to speak, mechanical impairment, impaired hearing or understanding, acute confusion and mental illness.

Chronic breathing difficulty

Chronic speech changes must be considered as baseline for any change in patient presentation. In some cases, patients may normally have difficulty with either the quality or quantity of their speech. Chronic lung disorders such as COPD can cause reduced phonation, so deterioration is comparable only to the patient's normal (Binazzi et al., 2011). Make use of the patient's friends/family when assessing what constitutes normal ability for the patient.

Dysphasia/aphasia

It is difficult to assess speech if the patient is normally unable to speak or only with considerable difficulty. Stroke is renowned for chronic aphasia/dysphasia. Other conditions that may cause this include acquired and congenital brain injuries, injury to or polyp growth on the vocal cord, or chronic respiratory muscle weakness.

Mechanical impairment

Facial injury, particularly of the jaw, could render a person unable to speak even if they want and attempt to do so. Oedema, such as from anaphylaxis, can cause similar difficulty.

Impaired hearing/understanding

If a patient cannot hear questions, or cannot understand the language spoken, they may not answer. It is possible the patient may speak regardless, in which case some interpretation of speech quantity may be possible. Family members or interpreters may be useful for interpreting quality and variations from the patient's normal.

Acute delirium/agitation/confusion

Any condition, respiratory or otherwise, that causes confusion or agitation can cause an inappropriate response. This will adversely impact on the quality of answers to questions, making it useful in recognising an underlying problem, including from traumatic and metabolic causes. Ask multiple specific questions to determine if the patient is generally confused about things they should know.

Full sentences can still be possible where confused or inappropriate answers are caused by acute delirium, still allowing quantitative speech assessment.

Mental illness

Acute mental illness shares some similarity with acute delirium/agitation. The qualitative assessment may vary, with the answers given being different from those expected. These answers may or may not be normal for the patient and may therefore require clarification, if possible, from family or friends.

Dissociation between answers and questions might make qualitative assessment difficult; the extent of dissociation might provide the detail in assessing for the presence of mental illness.

Quantitative assessment may remain useful if the patient continues to speak. Though they may not obey any instruction to count from one onwards, the length of their sentences may still be assessable.

PRACTICE TIP!

Exposure to respiratory transmitted infection can be enhanced by immediate proximity. If you are required to be close to the patient, use respiratory protection such as a P2-rated mask.

PRACTICE TIP!

To gain the patient's full cooperation when asking standard questions to determine speech quality, it may be helpful to explain why you are asking seemingly odd questions.

PRACTICE TIP!

When assessing speech quantity, first establish the normal expected baseline. Chronic respiratory illnesses may vary this considerably, making any individual assessment misleading.

PRACTICE TIP!

When assessing speech quantity, avoid asking too many questions. Patients in respiratory difficulty are limited in how many words they can speak. Further demand on them to speak can increase their difficulty.

TEST YOUR KNOWLEDGE QUESTIONS

1. **What are the four discernible steps of speaking?**
   Higher brain functions to determine speech; the act of breathing; phonation in the larynx; articulation as sounds are refined.

2. **What are two assessable parameters for considering speech?**
   Quantitative measures such as speech duration and number of words able to be spoken; qualitative measures such as orientation, confusion or inappropriate speech and thought processes.

3. **What is the benchmark for normal speech?**
   Full and continuous speech of a sentence without interruption by another breath. The qualitative benchmark for normal speech is oriented to person/time/place.

4. **What must be clear to a clinician before assessing any patient's speech?**
   The patient can communicate without pre-existing impediment, including hearing, language spoken and ability to reply.

5. **How does chronic respiratory difficulty impact speech assessment?**
   Chronic illness may cause chronic difficulty speaking altering the 'normal' baseline, making all further assessment comparable to this new standard.

6. **List two reasons, other than impaired phonation, for why a patient may not be able to speak.**
   Aphasia caused by stroke; facial injury impairing speech.

7. **What is required from the assessor to accurately determine speech quality?**
   Ask standard questions to determine if the patient knows their name, the time/day/date and where they are located.

8. **What is the standard question to ask for assessing speech quality?**
   Ask the patient to count from one onwards to see how many words they can speak before the next breath.

9. **Why is quantity of speech commonly reduced during respiratory difficulty?**
   Respiratory illness typically reduces expiratory airflow from either reduced inspiratory volume or resistance to air escape on expiration.

10. **What problems can cause acute or chronic changes in speech quality?**
    Changes in brain function controlling speech, such as stroke; changes in phonation/articulation ability, such as from facial trauma or airway illness: acute delirium or agitation; mental illness.

References

Bailey, E.F. and Hoit, J.D., 2002. Speaking and breathing in high respiratory drive. *Journal of Speech, Language, and Hearing Research*, 45(1), 89–99.

Binazzi, B., Lanini, B., Romagnoli, I., Garuglieri, S., Stendardi, L., Bianchi, R., Gigliotti, F. and Scano, G., 2011. Dyspnea during speech in chronic obstructive pulmonary disease patients: effects of pulmonary rehabilitation. *Respiration*, 81(5), 379–385.

Hoit, J.D., Lansing, R.W., Dean, K., Yarkosky, M., Lederle, A., 2011. Nature and evaluation of dyspnea in speaking and swallowing. In *Seminars in speech and language 2011* (Volume 32, No. 1). New York: Thieme Medical Publishers, pp. 5–20.

Gondos, T., Szabó, V., Sárkány, Á., Sárkány, A., Halász, G., 2017. Estimation of the severity of breathlessness in the emergency department: a dyspnea score. *BMC Emergency Medicine*, 17(1), 13.

Gupta, J.K., Lin, C.H., Chen, Q., 2010. Characterizing exhaled airflow from breathing and talking. *Indoor Air*, 20(1), 31–39.

Quinn, T.J., Coons, B.A., 2011. The Talk Test and its relationship with the ventilatory and lactate thresholds. *Journal of Sports Sciences*, 29(11), 1175–1182.

Bibliography

Craft, J., Gordon, C., Huether, S.E., McCance, K.L. and Brashers, V.L., 2015. *Understanding pathophysiology (ANZ adaptation)*. Sydney: Elsevier.

McCance, K.L. and Huether, S.E., 2015. *Pathophysiology: the biologic basis for disease in adults and children*. Sydney: Elsevier.

2.10 | Pulse oximetry

Jeff Kenneally

Chapter objectives

At the end of this chapter the reader will be able to:

1. Describe the rationale for assessing oxygen saturation with pulse oximetry
2. Demonstrate the method of using pulse oximetry
3. Accurately report on the findings of assessment
4. Identify limitations with using pulse oximeter

Resources required for this assessment

- Standardised patient with detectable pulse
- Pulse oximetry device
- Disposable gloves
- Method of documenting results

Skill matrix

This assessment requires:

- Infection control (CS 1.3)
- Communication (CS 1.5)
- Consent (CS 1.6)

This assessment is a component of:

- Patient assessment (Chapter 2)

Introduction

Assessment of respiratory status includes subjective physical observation and auscultation and objective and quantifiable measurement using pulse oximetry.

Pulse oximetry is non-invasive, and usually accurate, estimation of arterial oxygen saturation. The devices in common use are so widespread and reliable that this measurement is frequently considered another vital sign (Chan et al., 2013). It can allow continued monitoring to provide early clues to improvement or deterioration and guide the administration of supplemental oxygen therapy, and may reduce the need for arterial blood analysis.

Although there are no contraindications for use, pulse oximetry has limitations that are important to understand.

This chapter discusses assessment of pulse oximetry.

Anatomy and physiology

Inspired oxygen depends on the proportion of total gas volume. Air contains 21% oxygen and typical atmospheric air pressure is 760 mmHg. The oxygen partial pressure of inspired air is a fraction of total pressure.

$$21\% \text{ of } 760\,\text{mmHg} = 160\,\text{mmHg denoted as } pO_2$$

Alveoli oxygen partial pressure changes with each ventilation. Oxygen diffuses between pulmonary capillaries, producing arterial partial pressures, which are denoted paO_2.

Almost all oxygen is circulated attached to haemoglobin, with only about 0.3% dissolved in plasma (paO_2). The percentage of arterial haemoglobin combined with oxygen is referred to as oxygen saturation and denoted SaO_2.

Clinical rationale

Pulse oximetry is applied to highly vascular areas such as fingers and earlobes. To a lesser extent, the nose and forehead can be used and sometimes the foot or toes in smaller children (Fouzas et al., 2011).

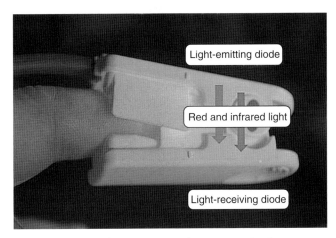

Figure 2.10.1 Light-emitting and receiving diode

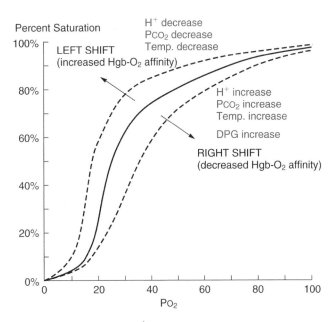

Figure 2.10.2 Oxygen dissociation curve
Oxyhaemoglobin dissociation curve. DPG, diphosphoglycerate.
Source: *Elsevier, 2016, Essential surgical procedures (Chapter 65, Figure 65-4-1), Elsevier.*

Some red and some infrared wavelengths of light can readily penetrate human tissue (Chan et al., 2013) (Fig. 2.10.1). Oxyhaemoglobin and deoxyhaemoglobin absorb this light differently. Pulse oximetry involves either a light-emitting diode transmitting beams of light that are received by a second diode facing the first, or an alternative probe design that attaches flat to the skin and measures reflected light rather than transmitted light (Chan et al., 2013). The light-emitting probe can be either reusable or adhesive single use.

When this light transmits through human tissue, such as a finger, some is absorbed by oxyhaemoglobin, deoxyhaemoglobin and tissue generally. The pulse oximeter measures changes in light absorption when a pulse wave arrives, allowing estimation of arterial levels of oxygen saturation (Milner and Mathews, 2012). These readings approximate what is happening with blood oxygen levels and not the actual arterial blood oxygen partial pressure (paO$_2$). It provides a percentage figure based on comparing oxygen-bound arterial haemoglobin with the less bound haemoglobin returning in venous blood. A percentage figure is only a relative comparison and not an absolute quantitative value for available oxygen (Pretto et al., 2014). Changes in haemoglobin totals can alter absolute values but not the percentage.

Pulse oximetry must detect arterial pulse waves to determine any difference and will not work where there is very low blood flow (Chan et al., 2013; Pretto et al., 2014).

This capillary/cellular level is where oxygen detaches, or dissociates, from haemoglobin for metabolic use. A graphical depiction of oxyhaemoglobin dissociation shows the relationship between paO$_2$ and the oxygen saturation this relates to (see Fig. 2.10.2).

A significant decrease in oxygen partial pressure in arterial blood can be tolerated while still maintaining a high percentage of saturated haemoglobin. However, there is a point at which the lowering of arterial partial oxygen pressure results in a sharp decline in saturated haemoglobin.

Numerous factors influence haemoglobin's affinity for oxygen. Blood becoming acidotic (lowered pH),

whether respiratory or metabolic, and increases in body temperature decrease its affinity. In contrast, circulatory alkalosis (increased pH) and lower body temperature increases affinity. When these parameters are normal, breathing air at sea level pressure should produce an oxygen saturation reading of 94–99% in healthy adults and ≥97% in children. Pulse oximetry values below 94% reflect hypoxaemia in healthy adult patients at sea level. However, newborns can return significantly lower readings, and values of 85% at birth are expected.

Pulse oximeter readings typically show a series averaged out over 10–20 seconds, causing a slight delay, but the results are consistent.

Devices vary in complexity, ranging from devices little bigger than a match box that clip to the finger to those integrated into larger monitoring devices (Milner and Mathews, 2012). Commonly, devices include numerical oxygen saturation value and pulse rate. Some devices include a plethysmogram, which depicts rise and fall waveform as arterial pulses are detected (Fig. 2.10.3).

Factors that reduce inspired oxygen partial pressure can reduce oxygen saturation quickly. This happens with increasing altitude. Even in normal pressurised flight, reduced cabin air pressures can cause normal oxygen saturation to reduce to 92% or less. This can be a critical factor during patient retrieval by air transport.

Clinical skill assessment process

The following section outlines the clinical skill assessment tools that should be used to determine a student's ability to demonstrate accurate assessment of oxygen saturation using pulse oximetry.

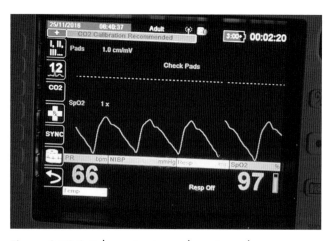

Figure 2.10.3 Pulse oximetry, pulse rate and plethysmogram reading

1. Clinical Skill Work Instruction
2. Formative Clinical Skill Assessment (F-CSAT)
3. Performance Improvement Plan (PIP)
4. Summative Clinical Skill Assessment (S-CSAT)
(5. Direct Observation of Procedural Skills (DOPS) – see Chapter 1.1)

Clinical Skill Work Instruction

Equipment and resources: Standardised patient with detectable pulse; pulse oximetry device; disposable gloves; method of documenting the results

Associated Clinical Skills: Infection control; Communication; Consent

Pulse oximetry

Activity	Critical Action	Rationale
Prepare equipment	Turn on pulse oximeter device. Ensure probe is attached and device operational and ready for use.	Device runs through internal checks for operation.
Prepare patient	Pulse oximetry can be assessed in any position, including upright, supine or lateral.	Patient position has no impact on reading.
	Explain procedure to the patient and obtain their consent.	Requires cooperation.
	Identify body part for probe attachment, including fingers, earlobes, forehead, or infant foot or. Selection depends on convenience and device used.	Choose a place that is easily visible and accessible and where device is unlikely to be dislodged.
	Where blood pressure and pulse oximetry are being evaluated concurrently, select different limbs if possible.	Sphygmomanometer inflation will interfere with blood flow.
	Ensure the chosen body part has adequate warmth and colour.	Sufficient circulation is required to obtain a reliable reading.
	Where a finger is chosen, it is preferable to select one without nail polish; otherwise, removal of polish is recommended.	Dark nail polish colours can impair light transmission and reduce readings slightly.
	If body part is dirty or blood contaminated, clean before use.	For device accuracy and hygiene purposes.

Pulse oximetry continued

Activity	Critical Action	Rationale
Assess pulse oximetry	Attach probe to selected body part. Probe size (paediatric or adult) should match patient size and body part. The body part should fit neatly into the probe.	Using the correct size provides the most accurate reading.
	Allow 5–10 seconds for the reading to stabilise. Depending on device, the pulse rate and pulse quality readings indicate if the reading is reliable.	Allows time for device to identify pulse quality.
	If a reliable reading cannot be obtained, verify correct position of body part inside the probe. If it is correct, consider an alternative body part. To verify device functionality, attach probe to your own finger for comparison.	Cold or poorly perfused peripheral body parts may be unreliable for gaining readings.
	When evaluation is complete, wipe reusable probes with an alcohol or other suitable disinfectant product. If necessary, wipe cables to remove contamination as well.	To maintain infection control.
Report	Accurately document/hand over findings.	Accurate record kept and continuity of patient care.

Formative Clinical Skill Assessment (F-CSAT)

Equipment and resources: Standardised patient with detectable pulse; pulse oximetry device; disposable gloves; method of documenting the results

Associated Clinical Skills: Infection control; Communication; Consent

Staff/Student being assessed: _____

Pulse oximetry

Activity	Critical Action	Participant Performance				
Prepares equipment	Turns on pulse oximeter device. Ensures probe is attached and device is operational and ready for use.	0	1	2	3	4
Prepares patient	Recognises that patient pulse oximetry can be assessed in any position, including upright, supine or lateral.	0	1	2	3	4
	Explains procedure to patient and obtains their consent.	0	1	2	3	4
	Identifies body part to be used for probe attachment, including fingers, earlobes, forehead, or infant foot or toes. Selection depends on convenience and device used.	0	1	2	3	4
	Where blood pressure and pulse oximetry are being evaluated concurrently, selects different limbs if possible.	0	1	2	3	4
	Ensures warmth and colour of body part chosen are adequate.	0	1	2	3	4
	Where a finger is chosen, prefers to select one without nail polish, or otherwise removes polish from fingernail if possible.	0	1	2	3	4
	If body part is dirty or contaminated by blood, cleans before use.	0	1	2	3	4

Pulse oximetry continued

Activity	Critical Action	Participant Performance				
Assesses pulse oximetry	Attaches probe to selected body part. Probe size matches patient size and body part. The body part fits neatly into probe.	0	1	2	3	4
	Allows 5–10 seconds for reading to stabilise. Depending on device, the pulse rate and pulse quality readings indicate whether reading is reliable.	0	1	2	3	4
	If a reliable reading cannot be obtained, verifies correct position of body part inside probe. If correct, considers alternative body part. To verify device functionality, attaches probe to own finger for comparison.	0	1	2	3	4
	When evaluation is complete, wipes reusable probe with an alcohol or other suitable disinfectant product. If necessary, wipes cables to remove contamination as well.	0	1	2	3	4
Reports	Accurately documents/hands over findings.	0	1	2	3	4

Standard Achieved: (please circle one)

Competent (C)   Not Yet Competent* (NYC)

Staff/Student Name: _____

Assessor (please print name)**:** _____

Signed (Assessor)**:** _____

Date of Assessment: _____

Comments:

*If Not Yet Competent (NYC) a PIP needs to be completed and a repeat of the F-CSAT

Formative Clinical Skill Assessment (F-CSAT) Key

Skill level	Standard of procedure	Quality of performance	Outcome	Level of assistance required
4 Safe for unsupervised practice	Safe Accurate Behaviour is appropriate to context	Confident Accurate Expedient	Achieved intended outcome	No supporting cues* required
3 Requires supervision	Safe Accurate Behaviour is appropriate to context	Confident Accurate Takes longer than required	Achieved intended outcome	Requires occasional supportive cues*
2 Requires assistance	Safe Accurate Behaviour generally appropriate to context	Lacks certainty	Would not have achieved outcome without support	Requires frequent verbal and occasional physical directives in addition to supportive cues*

Skill level	Standard of procedure	Quality of performance	Outcome	Level of assistance required
1 Requires direction	Safe only with guidance Not completely accurate	Unskilled Inefficient	Would not have achieved outcome without support	Requires continuous verbal and frequent physical directive cues*
0 Unsafe	Unsafe Unable to demonstrate behaviour Lack of insight into behaviour appropriate to context	Unskilled	Would not have achieved outcome	Requires continuous verbal and continuous physical directive cues*

*Refers to physical directives or verbal supportive cues

Performance Improvement Plan (PIP)

Please document the agreed education plan and completion timelines for areas assessed as less than 4.

This plan should be presented to assessor prior to commencement of summative assessment.

Where was supervisor support required?	Student summary of deficit. (Why was there a problem?)	Improvement Plan	Completed (Y/N)

Staff/Student Name: _____

Staff/Student Signature: _____

Educator Name: _____

Educator Signature: _____

Summative Clinical Skill Assessment (S-CSAT)

Equipment and resources: Standardised patient with detectable pulse; pulse oximetry device; disposable gloves, Method of documenting the results

Associated Clinical Skills: Infection control; Communication; Consent

Staff/Student being assessed: _____

- Completed Formative Clinical Skill Assessment (F-CSAT):   **YES**   **NO**

- Completed Performance Improvement Plan (PIP):   **YES**   **NO**   **N/A**

Pulse oximetry

Activity	Critical Action	Achieved Without Direction	
Prepares equipment	Turns on pulse oximeter device. Ensures probe is attached and device is operational and ready for use.	NO	YES
Prepares patient	Recognises that patient pulse oximetry can be assessed in any position, including upright, supine or lateral.	NO	YES
	Explains procedure to patient and obtains their consent.	NO	YES
	Identifies body part to be used for probe attachment, including fingers, earlobes, forehead, or infant foot or toes. Selection depends on convenience and device being used.	NO	YES
	Where blood pressure and pulse oximetry are being evaluated concurrently, selects different limbs if possible.	NO	YES
	Ensures warmth and colour of body part chosen are adequate.	NO	YES
	Where a finger is chosen, prefers to select one without nail polish, or otherwise removes polish from fingernail if possible.	NO	YES
	If body part is dirty or contaminated by blood, cleans before use.	NO	YES
Assesses pulse oximetry	Attaches probe to selected body part. Probe matches patient size and body part. The body part fits neatly into probe.	NO	YES
	Allows 5–10 seconds for reading to stabilise. Depending on device, pulse rate and pulse quality readings indicate whether reading is reliable.	NO	YES
	If a reliable reading cannot be obtained, verifies correct position of body part inside probe. If it is correct, considers an alternative body part. To verify device functionality, attaches probe to own finger for comparison.	NO	YES
	When evaluation is complete, wipes reusable probe with an alcohol or other suitable disinfectant product. If necessary, wipes cables to remove contamination as well.	NO	YES
Reports	Accurately documents/hands over findings.	NO	YES

Standard Achieved: (please circle one)

Competent (C)   Not Yet Competent* (NYC)

Staff/Student Name: _____

Assessor (please print name)**:** _____

Signed (Assessor)**:** _____

Date of Assessment: _____

Comments:

*If Not Yet Competent (NYC) a PIP needs to be completed and a repeat of the F-CSAT

Clinical findings

The safe and effective use of pulse oximetry relies on key factors, including sufficient haemoglobin and adequate pulse strength, to differentiate arterial and venous flow.

Interfering factors include changes in haemoglobin presentations, fingernail polish, skin colour, ambient light and electromagnetic energy. Further, pulse oximetry discusses only oxygen saturation, without considering carbon dioxide values.

Low oxygen saturation

Pulse oximetry readings are determined using an algorithm that converts light transmission (or reflection) to voltages then ratios of arterial versus venous readings. This is only reliable down to a saturation reading of about 70%. Readings below this may not be accurate (Pretto et al., 2014). However, this should not be a problem since poor readings will correlate with other physical signs of respiratory distress or clinical pathology. Clinicians should use all assessable factors so that they are able to recognise an unwell patient and implement corrective strategies regardless of any inaccuracy in pulse oximetry readings.

Some conditions, particularly chronic obstructive pulmonary disease (COPD), can produce chronic failures in ventilation, gas exchange and hence circulating oxygen and carbon dioxide levels. Finding low oxygen saturation should prompt consideration of what might be a normal lower pulse oximetry level in such specific patients.

Adequate detectable pulse wave

An arterial pulse wave must be detectable by the diode wavelengths for the device to calculate oxyhaemoglobin (Chan et al., 2013). Poor tissue perfusion causes incorrect or no reading at all to be produced. This might be from hypothermia or hypotension, or when the pulse rate is so fast that there is inadequate time for ventricular filling (Chan et al., 2013).

Wherever possible, pulse oximetry should be measured on a different limb from that being used for blood pressure measurement or tourniquet application. Both of these interfere with blood flow and hence oxygen saturation readings.

Anaemia

Reduced haemoglobin levels adversely impact the actual amount of oxygen that can be carried but not the relative proportion. As such, the anaemic patient might have normal oxygen saturation readings yet have reduced actual oxygen circulation. Readings must be interpreted with this in mind.

Carbon monoxide poisoning

Carbon monoxide is a common product of hydrocarbon combustion, which is found as a pollutant in cigarette smoke, combustion heating in homes and motor vehicle exhaust, and is even produced naturally in small quantities during haemoglobin destruction.

Inhaled carbon monoxide diffuses into the blood with 240 times greater affinity to attach to haemoglobin than oxygen. The product is carboxyhaemoglobin and it displaces oxygen from haemoglobin.

For pulse oximetry, this is critical. The diode light wavelengths are also absorbed by carboxyhaemoglobin, meaning a normal pulse oximeter cannot differentiate between oxygen or carbon monoxide attached to haemoglobin. Where carbon monoxide poisoning is suspected, pulse oximetry values cannot be relied on and are misleading (Chan et al., 2013; Feiner et al., 2010).

Methemoglobinemia

Methemoglobin is a form of haemoglobin resulting from iron oxidising from normal Fe^{2+} to Fe^{3+}. This form usually makes up only a very small percentage of total body haemoglobin. Certain genetic deficiencies and exposure to some chemicals can result in increased amounts of methemoglobin, as can nitrate drug use and some antibiotic administration.

Increased methemoglobin reduces oxygen-carrying capacity, creating the potential for cyanosis to occur even in normal paO_2. Importantly, methemoglobin causes abnormal absorption of transmitted light beams, leading to falsely low SpO_2 readings (Chan et al., 2013; Pretto et al., 2014; Verhovsek et al., 2010).

Sulphhaemoglobinemia is a similar condition to methemoglobinemia but with a sulphur atom involved (Chan et al., 2013; Verhovsek et al., 2010).

Venous pulsations

Venous blood does not usually pulse. Clearly, pulse oximetry relies on differences produced by arterial pulse waves. If the light-emitting probe is attached too tightly, it can cause venous pulsations to occur and adversely affect readings. It is usually adhesive finger probes that cause this (Chan et al., 2013; Fouzas et al., 2011).

Fingernail polish

Light transmission can be adversely affected by fingernail polish, particularly darker colours of black, blue and brown (Chan et al., 2013). It is unclear whether there is any clinically significant reduction in reading. Red nail polish is considered least likely to create false readings (Yont et al., 2014).

Skin colour is not associated with inaccuracy of pulse oximetry at higher readings. Very dark skin can cause a small variation in readings as levels drop below 90%. The skin colouration caused by jaundice is not associated with varying readings.

Oxygen not carbon dioxide

An important limitation is that oxygen delivery is only part of ventilation. Any reading must be assessed in the context of the patient's presentation and their ability to remove carbon dioxide (Pretto et al., 2014).

Pulse oximetry provides information related only to oxygen and not to carbon dioxide (Arakawa et al., 2013;

Fouzas et al., 2011; Pretto et al., 2014; Sivilotti et al., 2010). There are situations in which oxygen saturation reading can mislead on overall patient condition.

Supplementary oxygen therapy can raise the oxygen saturation reading. This may restore an acceptable or even normal oxygen saturation reading despite hypoventilation (Sivilotti et al., 2010). In such settings, this restoration will not affect carbon dioxide removal (Arakawa et al., 2013). Hypoventilation cannot be corrected with supplemental oxygen therapy alone, even if oxygen saturation can be.

Gas trapping diseases such as asthma can also cause this mismatch. This situation is also one of hypoventilation reducing carbon dioxide removal from the blood and alveoli. When managing asthma and COPD, pulse oximetry provides no clues to rising carbon dioxide levels (Fouzas et al., 2011).

Bright ambient light

Some pulse oximetry devices may be adversely affected by bright ambient light making them unable to provide an accurate reading. If this is thought to be the cause of poor sensing, remove the patient to a darker environment or cover the probe and body part with a towel or blanket.

Electromagnetic interference

Pulse oximetry devices may be adversely affected by electromagnetic interference produced by electrical equipment including defibrillators, cellular telephones, radio equipment and some domestic electrical appliances. If this is thought to be the cause of an inability to gain a reliable reading, consider moving the patient away from the source of interference or remove or disconnect the electrical equipment (Fouzas et al., 2011).

PRACTICE TIP!

Use specific paediatric probes for the child patient. Adult probes may be too large and not fit child body parts. If the child's fingers are too small for the purpose, the probe may fit the large toe.

PRACTICE TIP!

Pulse oximetry provides information pertaining only to oxygen saturation. This number on its own is insufficient for complete assessment of the severity of the patient's condition. The reading must be assessed in the context of other vital signs and the patient's suspected clinical condition.

PRACTICE TIP!

There are numerous situations where pulse oximetry can provide erroneous or misleading information. Pulse oximetry provides accurate information but within the confines of these limitations.

PRACTICE TIP!

The finger is the most commonly used body part for attaching pulse oximetry probes. Where a reading cannot be obtained, assess the correct placement of the finger within the probe and move the probe to other fingers in turn before gently warming the finger and repeating the test. For verification, test your own finger to ensure the device is working effectively.

TEST YOUR KNOWLEDGE QUESTIONS

1. **What is the unit measure of a pulse oximeter reading?**
    The percentage of arterial oxygen saturation.

2. **What is the normal range of oxygen saturation for most patients?**
    SpO_2 = 94 to 99%

3. **Below what reading do pulse oximetry readings typically become unreliable?**
    SpO_2 = 70%

4. **What happens to the partial pressure of arterial oxygen at saturation levels below 94%?**
    The paO_2 level drops sharply below this lower limit of normal. Above that, a small change in SpO_2 reflects only a small change in paO_2. Below 94%, a small change in SpO_2 reflects a much larger decline in paO_2 and patient deterioration.

5. **What significant factors interfere with the production of a detectable pulse wave?**
    Poor peripheral blood flow to the body part the probe is attached to, or reduced peripheral blood flow such as caused by hypothermia, hypotension, a rapid pulse leaving insufficient time for ventricular filling or by the occlusive pressure of an inflated sphygmomanometer or tourniquet.

6. **What is the usual body part used for attaching a pulse oximetry probe?**
    The finger is most commonly used, followed by the earlobes and large toes.

7. **What effect does carbon monoxide have on pulse oximetry?**
    Pulse oximeters cannot distinguish between carboxyhaemoglobin and oxyhaemoglobin, so patients exposed to the gas can be hypoxemic yet still have acceptable readings.

8. **How does oxygen saturation relate to arterial oxygen partial pressure (paO_2)?**
    Saturation readings approximate oxygen bound to haemoglobin. They can be plotted on an oxyhaemoglobin graph to depict the relationship with paO_2, which relates to plasma dissolved oxygen.

9. **What effect does anaemia have on pulse oximetry?**
    It allows for haemoglobin to be fully oxygen bound and indicates high saturation even though total oxygen levels are lower than adequate.

10. **How should pulse oximetry be used during asthma episodes?**
    CO_2 retention is the greater problem, with many patients being able to maintain acceptable pulse oximetry even when they are in severe distress. Relying on pulse oximetry alone can be misleading.

References

Arakawa, H., Kaise, M., Sumiyama, K., Saito, S., Suzuki, T. and Tajiri, H., 2013. Does pulse oximetry accurately monitor a patient's ventilation during sedated endoscopy under oxygen supplementation? *Singapore Medical Journal*, 54(4), 212–215.

Chan, E.D., Chan, M.M. and Chan, M.M., 2013. Pulse oximetry: understanding its basic principles facilitates appreciation of its limitations. *Respiratory Medicine*, 107(6), 789–799.

Feiner, J.R., Bickler, P.E. and Mannheimer, P.D., 2010. Accuracy of methemoglobin detection by pulse CO-oximetry during hypoxia. *Anesthesia & Analgesia*, 111(1), 143–148.

Fouzas, S., Priftis, K.N. and Anthracopoulos, M.B., 2011. Pulse oximetry in pediatric practice. *Pediatrics*, 128(4), 740–752.

Milner, Q.J. and Mathews, G.R., 2012. An assessment of the accuracy of pulse oximeters. *Anaesthesia*, 67(4), 396–401.

Pretto, J.J., Roebuck, T., Beckert, L. and Hamilton, G., 2014. Clinical use of pulse oximetry: official guidelines from the Thoracic Society of Australia and New Zealand. *Respirology*, 19(1), 38–46.

Sivilotti, M.L., Messenger, D.W., van Vlymen, J., Dungey, P.E. and Murray, H.E., 2010. A comparative evaluation of capnometry versus pulse oximetry during procedural sedation and analgesia on room air. *Canadian Journal of Emergency Medicine*, 12(05), 397–404.

Verhovsek, M., Henderson, M., Cox, G., Luo, H.Y., Steinberg, M.H. and Chui, D.H., 2010. Unexpectedly low pulse oximetry measurements associated with variant hemoglobins: a systematic review. *American Journal of Hematology*, 85(11), 882–885.

Yont, G.H., Korhan, E.A. and Dizer, B., 2014. The effect of nail polish on pulse oximetry readings. *Intensive and Critical Care Nursing*, 30, 111–115.

Bibliography

Craft, J., Gordon, C., Huether, S.E., McCance, K.L. and Brashers, V.L., 2015. *Understanding pathophysiology (ANZ adaptation)*. Sydney: Elsevier.

McCance, K.L. and Huether S.E., 1990. *Pathophysiology: the biologic basis for disease in adults and children*. Sydney: Elsevier.

2.11 | Spirometry

Jeff Kenneally

Chapter objectives

At the end of this chapter the reader will be able to:

1. Describe the rationale for assessing peak exploratory flow rate (PEFR)
2. Demonstrate the method of assessing PEFR
3. Accurately report on assessment findings
4. Identify PEFR contraindications and precautions

Resources required for this assessment

- Suitable patient to perform the test
- PEFR measuring device
- Disposable gloves
- Method of documenting the results

Skill matrix

This assessment requires:
- Infection control (CS 1.3)
- Communication (CS 1.5)
- Consent (CS 1.6)
- Assessment of respiratory rate and rhythm (CS 2.6)
- Assessment of work of breathing (CS 2.7)

This assessment is a component of:
- Patient assessment (Chapter 2)

Introduction

The assessment of anyone with respiratory difficulty is important for diagnosis and to determine severity and appropriate therapy.

Though prehospital assessment tools are frequently rudimentary, spirometry can be a useful tool. Spirometry devices are cheap but reliable, suited to quick use and able to add benefit to patient assessment. It is important to understand their effective use, appropriate indications and contraindications. This chapter discusses these concepts.

Anatomy and physiology

Increased physiological need, such as in illness or physical exertion, alters oxygen consumption and carbon dioxide production. To accommodate this, the air volume moved over time changes through alterations to breathing rate and depth.

Typical lung capacities are outlined in Fig. 2.11.1.

Increasing inspiratory muscle work can significantly increase breath volume. Maximum inspiration volume is the inspiratory capacity, including tidal volume, plus the larger inspiratory reserve.

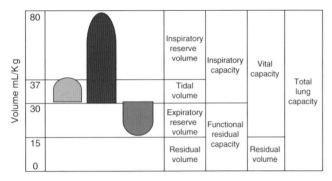

Figure 2.11.1 Lung volumes

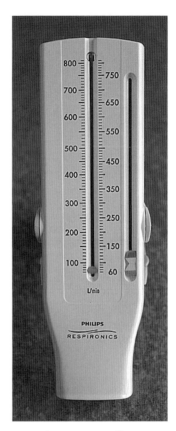

Figure 2.11.2 A peak expiratory flow meter

Expiration removes carbon dioxide. It is normally passive, relying on chest recoil for outward airflow. At the end of normal tidal volume expiration, a large amount of air remains in the lungs. This remaining air can be pushed out using abdominal muscle contraction and internal intercostal muscles to increase the force of expiration. This extra expiration is respiratory reserve volume. A maximum volume can be forced out, leaving some residual volume trapped within the lungs. Together, the reserve and residual volumes form the functional residual capacity.

Forced vital capacity volume (FVC) is the maximum inspiration taken then exhaled to maximum expiration, typically measured in litres (Koegelenberg et al., 2013).

Producing these lung values varies with airway diameter and reactivity, lung structure and chest compliance. Bronchospasm, inflammation and alveolar and supportive connective tissue disorder all adversely impact on functional lung values.

The key determinants of ventilation are the actual volume of the chest and lungs, the musculoskeletal structure of the chest and the capability of the respiratory muscles. The size, sex and age of the patient can strongly influence variations in normal values.

Clinical rationale

Breathing assessment is a largely subjective observation. Spirometry provides quantitative information that can identify early and small airway changes, allowing self-monitoring or evaluation of therapy effectiveness.

Spirometry is a non-invasive lung function test measuring flow of air over time, and is easy to perform. It can be done with complex devices that require calibration or smaller, limited (but still useful) devices for patient use (Mishra et al., 2013) (see Fig. 2.11.2).

Spirometry values must be compared to known standards or previous results, and assessed in context, in order to be useful (Koegelenberg et al., 2013).

FVC is the most basic spirometry measurement. The length of exhalation time can vary, even if the patient is asked to blow out as quickly as possible. When measuring FVC, the total value is sought (Koegelenberg et al., 2013).

If the exhalation time is specified, the forced expiratory volume (FEV) expelled can be measured for that duration.

The duration is denoted after the initials; for example, forced expiration for 1 second is denoted FEV_1, usually referring to the first second of expiration (Koegelenberg et al., 2013). FEV values taken at intervals can show improvement or trends in the response to therapy.

Typically, FEV values are compared to known average results in the community. Most people can exhale within +/−20% of the average population FEV value. Key criteria for the patient and that community must be known, including age, sex, body size and race. Results are only effective if they are compared to similar people (Koegelenberg et al., 2013).

The FEV values can be compared to known standards such as FVC. If FVC is the best any patient can do, FEV will be a fraction of that amount. Typically, FEV_1 is around 75% of the FVC. If the tested FEV is compared to a known FVC benchmark, this ratio may change.

With more complex spirometry devices, multiple analyses of lung volumes and lung function can be determined, many of which relate to airflow from the lungs. However, complex assessment is not suited to emergency management. Arguably, the most useful spirometry assessment is the peak expiratory flow rate (PEFR).

Peak expiratory flow rate (PEFR)

Gas moves from higher to lower pressure areas, flowing as volume over a time:

$$\text{Flow of gas} = \text{Volume of gas}/\text{Time taken}$$

Peak expiratory flow is the maximum gas flow rate achievable during expiration. Peak flow occurs early in forced expiration and is not the total volume exhaled. To be reliable and comparable, it must be performed in a standardised manner (Koegelenberg et al., 2013).

A maximum inspiration is taken before the test, followed by exhaling forcefully for as long as possible. Airflow is usually measured in litres per minute or litres per second (Koegelenberg et al., 2013).

Measuring PEFR is simple but requires attention to detail in order for it to be accurate. The correct position of the patient is important, allowing air to move in and out of the chest without interference. Sitting or standing with the chest upright is best; sitting is arguably safer, since forced expiration can occasionally cause light-headedness (Koegelenberg et al., 2013).

The patient should uncross their legs and place their feet flat on the floor, allowing unrestricted diaphragm and abdominal muscle movement. Loosen restrictive clothing (Koegelenberg et al., 2013).

The mouth is a factor in airflow. Leave dentures fitted into the mouth where possible.

If the PEFR has a disposable mouthpiece, attach a new one. Set the sliding marker scale to zero.

Using a peak flow meter can be challenging during breathing difficulty. Ensure there is nothing in the mouth that can be choked on. The tongue must be kept away from the mouthpiece to avoid obstruction; advise the patient of this. Wrap the mouth around the mouthpiece (Fig. 2.11.3). Some may need a nose clip to ensure maximum airflow comes from the mouth.

Some patients close their glottis during the attempt. This happens when bearing down during such actions as the Valsalva manoeuvre. No air can escape, despite the force of the respiratory muscles interfering with measurement.

The patient takes a deep breath before placing the mouthpiece in their mouth. Forceful maximal expiration follows immediately to empty the lungs, with the patient blowing as hard and long as possible. If necessary, several smaller breaths can be taken beforehand, in preparation for the longer breath. Note the reading when the test is completed.

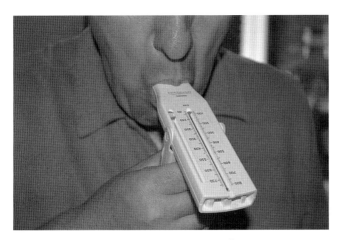

Figure 2.11.3 Using a peak expiratory flow meter

When using more complex spirometry devices, this same method can be used for measuring FVC and FEV. Key variables include age, height, gender and race (Koegelenberg et al., 2013; Mishra et al., 2013; Coates et al., 2013).

Lung function results increase through childhood to a maximum at about 25–35 years old before declining again (Mishra et al., 2013; Sillanpää et al., 2014). Aging brings an increase in airway and lung disease, decreased respiratory muscle effectiveness, chest compliance and recoil. Adult males typically have larger chest and lung volume than females, making gender an important criterion. Child gender variations are not so pronounced (Mishra et al., 2013; Stanojevic et al., 2009; Jat, 2013).

Height is a major variation point; taller people have bigger lungs. Lung function charts have different standard curves for different patient heights (Koegelenberg et al., 2013; Coates et al., 2013).

Increased weight increases difficulty in expanding the lungs and reduces abdominal muscle influence during expiration. Obesity reduces the results of lung function (Mishra et al., 2013; Coates et al., 2013; Banerjee et al., 2014).

Race can influence lung function. Some Asian, African and Indian people have a relatively smaller chest size. This is a less commonly acknowledged criterion that is often not allowed for (Mishra et al., 2013; Banerjee et al., 2014).

The patient may need encouragement to use the device correctly and achieve maximal expiration. To improve the test's reliability, perform it three times, selecting the best result rather than the average. This is most indicative of lung function, as smaller values are less accurate (Koegelenberg et al., 2013). Deep inspiration and forced expiration can temporarily change small airway diameters and alter PEFR, so allow at least 30 seconds between attempts.

PEFR meters are available in two broad types. Low-range meters with flow rates of approximately 0–300 L/min are designed for smaller airflows, such as those of smaller children. The larger variety with a flow rate up to 800 L/min is designed for bigger patients (Koegelenberg et al., 2013).

Indications

Spirometry helps identify reduced expiration capacity. Maintained or reduced FVC, but with notably reduced FEV and PEFR, suggests obstructive lung disease. In such cases, air enters the lungs but cannot easily be exhaled again. Obstructive diseases include asthma, chronic bronchitis, emphysema and cystic fibrosis (Koegelenberg et al., 2013; Drummond et al., 2012; Marcus et al., 2015; Allison et al., 2014).

Restrictive problems cause difficulty inspiring. These reduce FVC but maintain FEV and PEFR. There is less air in the lungs, but it is not trapped and can be expelled comparatively easily. Causes include obesity, lung oedema, empyema and pleural effusions (Koegelenberg et al., 2013; Marcus et al., 2015).

Asthma

Asthma transiently narrows airways, adversely impacting PEFR during attacks. Spirometry can provide an early warning of deterioration as part of patient asthma management plans, help identify the severity of the asthma and guide effective therapy. However, spirometry does not wholly replace other respiratory assessment (Coates et al., 2013; Allison et al., 2014).

COPD

Emphysema is characterised by alveolar reduction and the destruction of the surrounding connective tissue. Chronic bronchitis involves inflammation of the lower airway. Both reduce expiratory airflow (Arne et al., 2010).

COPD produces normal or reduced FVC but notably reduced FEV. This can be due to aging, so variations must be supported with patient history, symptoms and other physical assessment for diagnosis (Drummond et al., 2012; Allison et al., 2014; Arne et al., 2010).

Other indications

Spirometry can be used to assess the occupational risk of developing airway disease, including chemical, dust and fume exposure. It can help evaluate the patient's fitness and suitability for particular activities, such as anaesthetic risk before surgery or working under difficult atmospheric conditions, including underwater diving. It can also be used for assessment following injury or exposure, to guide legal and public health matters (Redlich et al., 2014).

Clinical skill assessment process

The following section outlines the clinical skill assessment tools that should be used to determine a student's ability to demonstrate safe and accurate assessment of spirometry.
1. Clinical Skill Work Instruction
2. Formative Clinical Skill Assessment (F-CSAT)
3. Performance Improvement Plan (PIP)
4. Summative Clinical Skill Assessment (S-CSAT)
(5. Direct Observation of Procedural Skills (DOPS) – see Chapter 1.1)

Clinical Skill Work Instruction

Equipment and resources: Patient; PEFR measuring device; disposable gloves; method of documenting the results

Associated Clinical Skills: Infection control; Communication; Consent; Assessment of respiratory rate and rhythm; Assessment of work of breathing

Spirometry

Activity	Critical Action	Rationale
Prepare equipment	Attach new mouthpiece to the meter. Ensure sliding marker scale is set at 0.	For infection control and correct measurement of PEFR.
Prepare patient	Position the patient sitting upright, with feet flat on the floor. Uncross their legs, with no diaphragm or abdominal muscle restriction. Allow standing if preferred. Ensure patient cannot fall if they become light-headed during the procedure.	To allow maximum inhalation and exhalation without physical interference.
	Loosen or remove restrictive clothing.	To allow full chest expansion.
	Explain the use of the peak flow meter if the patient is unfamiliar with it. Encourage correct use during testing.	To ensure understanding and most effective result.
	Remove foreign material from inside the patient's mouth.	To avoid choke hazard.
	Advise patient to keep their tongue away from the mouthpiece throughout procedure.	The tongue can obstruct airflow through the meter.

Spirometry continued

Activity	Critical Action	Rationale
Perform test	Have the patient take a deep breath immediately prior to testing.	To allow for maximum expiration.
	Have them place their mouth around the mouthpiece, holding it tightly between the lips. If the patient prefers, attach nose clip to ensure all airflow is from the mouth.	To ensure there is no air leakage and that patient exhales fully through mouth.
	Have the patient exhale fast and continuously into the flow meter device for as long as they can.	Peak flow rate is measured early, so forceful expiration is required.
	Note result by inspecting the slide scale on the meter.	To understand patient's PEFR.
	Carefully monitor throughout for adverse response.	Lung function testing is arduous.
	Allow at least 30 seconds for the patient to rest. If able, repeat the test two more times and note all results.	To allow sufficient recovery time between attempts.
	Select the best of the measured values.	Record as PEFR.
	Dispose of single-use items and clean unit for reuse.	For infection control.
Report	Accurately document/hand over findings.	Accurate record kept and continuity of patient care.

Formative Clinical Skill Assessment (F-CSAT)

Equipment and resources: Patient; PEFR measuring device; disposable gloves; method of documenting the results

Associated Clinical Skills: Infection control; Communication; Consent; Assessment of respiratory rate and rhythm; Assessment of work of breathing

Staff/Student being assessed: _____

Spirometry

Activity	Critical Action	Participant Performance				
Prepares equipment	Attaches new mouthpiece to the meter. Ensures sliding marker scale set at 0.	0	1	2	3	4
Prepares patient	Ensures correct sitting position for patient. Allows standing if preferred. Ensures patient cannot fall if they become light-headed during the procedure.	0	1	2	3	4
	Loosens or removes restrictive clothing.	0	1	2	3	4
	Explains peak flow meter use if the patient is unfamiliar with it. Encourages correct use during testing.	0	1	2	3	4
	Has patient remove foreign material from inside their mouth.	0	1	2	3	4
	Advises patient to keep their tongue away from the mouthpiece at all times.	0	1	2	3	4

Spirometry continued

Activity	Critical Action	Participant Performance				
Performs test	Has patient take a deep breath immediately prior to the test.	0	1	2	3	4
	Has them place their mouth around the mouthpiece holding it tightly between the lips. If patient prefers, attaches a nose clip.	0	1	2	3	4
	Has the patient exhale fast and continuously into the flow meter device for as long as they can.	0	1	2	3	4
	Notes result by inspecting slide scale on the meter.	0	1	2	3	4
	Carefully monitors throughout for adverse response.	0	1	2	3	4
	Allows at least 30 seconds for patient to rest. If able, repeats test two more times and notes all results.	0	1	2	3	4
	Selects best of the measured values.	0	1	2	3	4
	Disposes of single-use items and cleans unit for reuse.	0	1	2	3	4
Reports	Accurately documents/hands over findings.	0	1	2	3	4

Standard Achieved: (please circle one)

Competent (C)   Not Yet Competent* (NYC)

Staff/Student Name: _____

Assessor (please print name): _____

Signed (Assessor): _____

Date of Assessment: _____

Comments:

*If Not Yet Competent (NYC) a PIP needs to be completed and a repeat of the F-CSAT

Formative Clinical Skill Assessment (F-CSAT) Key

Skill level	Standard of procedure	Quality of performance	Outcome	Level of assistance required
4 Safe for unsupervised practice	Safe Accurate Behaviour is appropriate to context	Confident Accurate Expedient	Achieved intended outcome	No supporting cues* required
3 Requires supervision	Safe Accurate Behaviour is appropriate to context	Confident Accurate Takes longer than required	Achieved intended outcome	Requires occasional supportive cues*
2 Requires assistance	Safe Accurate Behaviour generally appropriate to context	Lacks certainty	Would not have achieved outcome without support	Requires frequent verbal and occasional physical directives in addition to supportive cues*

Skill level	Standard of procedure	Quality of performance	Outcome	Level of assistance required
1 Requires direction	Safe only with guidance Not completely accurate	Unskilled Inefficient	Would not have achieved outcome without support	Requires continuous verbal and frequent physical directive cues*
0 Unsafe	Unsafe Unable to demonstrate behaviour Lack of insight into behaviour appropriate to context	Unskilled	Would not have achieved outcome	Requires continuous verbal and continuous physical directive cues*

*Refers to physical directives or verbal supportive cues

Performance Improvement Plan (PIP)

Please document the agreed education plan and completion timelines for areas assessed as less than 4.

This plan should be presented to assessor prior to commencement of summative assessment.

Where was supervisor support required?	Student summary of deficit. (Why was there a problem?)	Improvement Plan	Completed (Y/N)

Staff/Student Name: _____

Staff/Student Signature: _____

Educator Name: _____

Educator Signature: _____

Summative Clinical Skill Assessment (S-CSAT)

Equipment and resources: Patient; PEFR measuring device; disposable gloves; method of documenting the results

Associated Clinical Skills: Infection control; Communication; Consent; Assessment of respiratory rate and rhythm; Assessment of work of breathing

Staff/Student being assessed: _____

- Completed Formative Clinical Skill Assessment (F-CSAT):   **YES   NO**

- Completed Performance Improvement Plan (PIP):   **YES   NO   N/A**

Spirometry

Activity	Critical Action	Achieved Without Direction	
Prepares equipment	Attaches new mouthpiece to the meter. Ensures sliding marker set at 0.	NO	YES
Prepares patient	Ensures correct sitting position for patient. Allows standing if preferred. Ensures patient cannot fall if they become light-headed during the procedure.	NO	YES
	Loosens or removes restrictive clothing.	NO	YES
	Explains peak flow meter use if the patient is unfamiliar with it. Encourages correct use during testing.	NO	YES
	Has patient remove foreign material from inside their mouth.	NO	YES
	Advises patient to keep their tongue away from the mouthpiece throughout.	NO	YES
Performs test	Has patient take a deep breath immediately prior to the test.	NO	YES
	Has them place their mouth around the mouthpiece holding it tightly between the lips. If patient prefers, attaches a nose clip.	NO	YES
	Has the patient exhale fast and continuously into the device for as long as they can.	NO	YES
	Notes result by inspecting the slide scale on the meter.	NO	YES
	Carefully monitors throughout procedure for adverse response.	NO	YES
	Allows at least 30 seconds for patient to rest. If able, repeats test two more times and notes all results.	NO	YES
	Selects best value for use.	NO	YES
	Disposes of single-use items and cleans unit for reuse.	NO	YES
Reports	Accurately documents/hands over the findings.	NO	YES

Standard Achieved: (please circle one)

Competent (C)   Not Yet Competent* (NYC)

Staff/Student Name: _____

Assessor (please print name)**:** _____

Signed (Assessor)**:** _____

Date of Assessment: _____

Comments:

*If Not Yet Competent (NYC) a PIP needs to be completed and a repeat of the F-CSAT

Clinical findings

Inability to gain effective patient compliance

Where reliable readings cannot be produced, it may have to be accepted that this test cannot be used. Coughing or breathlessness can cause difficulty the patient cannot overcome.

Small children may not be able to understand or cooperate with instructions or perform properly (Stanojevic et al., 2009; Jat, 2013).

Some adult patients may not be able to understand or cooperate, including those who are agitated, sedated or experiencing altered consciousness. This can be associated with increased respiratory difficulty, hypoxia and hypercapnia.

Procedural complications

PEFR assessment can cause a rise in transient intrathoracic pressure. This could turn a pneumothorax into a tension pneumothorax. Similarly, spirometry should be avoided where lung injury could be worsened by stretching. Haemoptysis could indicate such an injury (Coates et al., 2013).

Forced expiration involves the use of the abdominal muscles to raise intra-abdominal pressure. This can raise intra-aortic pressure, which is problematic for aortic aneurysm. It can cause bleeding where recent chest or abdomen surgery is present (Coates et al., 2013).

Raised intrathoracic pressure can impede superior venous return, causing problems for cerebral aneurysm, stroke or recent neurosurgery. Intraocular pressure can rise, adversely affecting recent eye surgery or glaucoma (Coates et al., 2013).

Increased airway pressure can raise sinus and middle ear pressure, causing pain and potential eardrum rupture following recent sinus surgery (Coates et al., 2013).

Spirometry can be physically demanding, particularly for those with cardiovascular risks. Recent myocardial infarction, significant coronary artery disease or heart failure can be compromised by test strain. Changes in intrathoracic pressure and venous return can impact on cardiac rhythm and blood pressure. Patients with hypotension or hypertension may suffer acute symptoms from sudden changes in blood pressure (Coates et al., 2013).

Vomiting and diarrhoea can be problematic during spirometry. Vomiting precludes the use of spirometry tests, while an increase in intra-abdominal pressure can cause temporary loss of bowel control (Coates et al., 2013).

PRACTICE TIP!

It is important to position the patient correctly and perform the test over several attempts. The assessor should instruct and encourage the patient throughout.

PRACTICE TIP!

Some patients routinely perform spirometry at home to evaluate early signs of worsening obstruction. Ask if they self-test and whether there has been deterioration in their PEFR.

PRACTICE TIP!

Repeated deep breathing can cause problems including dizziness and even collapse. Carefully monitor the patient before and during the assessment, ensuring they are sitting safely throughout.

PRACTICE TIP!

Any spirometry device is a potential source of infection. Disposable mouthpieces should be attached new, and disposed of after use. Patients with active and contagious respiratory illnesses could be too great an infective risk for spirometry.

TEST YOUR KNOWLEDGE QUESTIONS

1. **Define peak expiratory flow.**
   Peak expiratory flow is the maximum airflow achievable during expiration occurring early in forced expiration.

2. **What is spirometry value compared to?**
   Known large equivalent population standards or previous patient results. This allows appreciation of normal expectations and how this reading varies.

3. **How does the patient's weight influence spirometry testing?**
   Weight increases difficulty expanding the lungs and reduces abdominal muscle influence in forcing expiration. Obesity reduces spirometry results.

4. **Why should spirometry be repeated before accepting any value?**
   Repeated testing assesses the ability to reproduce a result and identifies the best result possible, as lesser values are inaccurate.

5. **List two reasons why a patient may not cooperate with spirometry.**
   Small children (<5–6 years old) may not understand or cooperate with instructions; some adults may also not understand or cooperate, including those with altered consciousness or who are sedated.

6. **What is the best position for a person to perform spirometry?**
   Airflow is maximised with the chest upright and unimpeded, either sitting or standing, legs uncrossed and feet flat.

7. **How does age affect spirometry results?**
   Results increase through childhood, to a maximum at about 25–35 years old, before declining again with age.

8. **Is spirometry a critical tool for patient assessment?**
   No. Clues to changes in illness severity and condition are obtainable from usual assessment and pulse oximetry.

9. **How should the patient prepare their lungs before spirometry?**
   Several smaller rapid breaths can be taken just before a maximal inspiration. This full breath maximises the forced vital capacity.

10. **What patient guidance might be required during spirometry testing?**
    Keep the tongue away from the mouthpiece; maintain a good seal with the lips; blow as hard and as long as possible.

References

Allison, R., Andrews, S., Jain, R., Van Gundy, K.P., Peterson, M.W. and Jain, V.V., 2014. Overdiagnosis of severe asthma and COPD in the setting of underutilization of spirometry. In *B43 COPD: Screening and diagnostic tools*. New York: American Thoracic Society, pp. A2972–A2972.

Arne, M., Lisspers, K., Ställberg, B., Boman, G., Hedenström, H., Janson, C. and Emtner, M., 2010. How often is diagnosis of COPD confirmed with spirometry? *Respiratory Medicine*, 104(4), 550–556.

Banerjee, J., Roy, A., Singhamahapatra, A., Dey, P.K., Ghosal, A. and Das, A., 2014. Association of body mass index (BMI) with lung function parameters in non-asthmatics identified by spirometric protocols. *Journal of Clinical and Diagnostic Research*, 8(2), 12.

Coates, A.L., Graham, B.L., McFadden, R.G., McParland, C., Moosa, D. and Provencher, S., 2013. Spirometry in primary care. *Canadian Respiratory Journal*, 20(1), 13–22.

Drummond, M.B., Hansel, N.N., Connett, J.E., Scanlon, P.D., Tashkin, D.P. and Wise, R.A., 2012. Spirometric predictors of lung function decline and mortality in early chronic obstructive pulmonary disease. *American Journal of Respiratory and Critical Care Medicine*, 185(12), 1301–1306.

Jat, K.R., 2013. Spirometry in children. *Primary Care Respiratory Journal*, 22, 221–229.

Koegelenberg, C.F., Swart, F. and Irusen, E.M., 2013. Guideline for office spirometry in adults, 2012. *South African Medical Journal*, 103(1), 52–61.

Marcus, B.S., McAvay, G., Gill, T.M. and Vaz Fragoso, C.A., 2015. Respiratory symptoms, spirometric respiratory impairment, and respiratory disease in middle-aged and older persons. *Journal of the American Geriatrics Society*, 63(2), 251–257.

Mishra, J., Mishra, S., Satpathy, S., Manjareeka, M., Nayak P.K. and Mohanty, P., 2013. Variations in PEFR among males and females with respect to anthropometric parameters. *IOSR Journal of Dental and Medical Sciences*, 5, 47–50.

Redlich, C.A., Tarlo, S.M., Hankinson, J.L., Townsend, M.C., Eschenbacher, W.L., Von Essen, S.G., Sigsgaard, T. and Weissman, D.N., 2014. Official American Thoracic Society technical standards: spirometry in the occupational setting. *American Journal of Respiratory and Critical Care Medicine*, 189(8), 983–993.

Stanojevic, S., Wade, A., Cole, T.J., Lum, S., Custovic, A., Silverman, M., Hall, G.L., Welsh, L., Kirkby, J., Nystad, W. and Badier, M., 2009. Spirometry centile charts for young Caucasian children: the Asthma UK Collaborative Initiative. *American Journal of Respiratory and Critical Care Medicine*, 180(6), 547.

Sillanpää, E., Stenroth, L., Bijlsma, A.Y., Rantanen, T., McPhee, J.S., Maden-Wilkinson, T.M., Jones, D.A., Narici, M.V., Gapeyeva, H., Pääsuke, M. and Barnouin, Y., 2014. Associations between muscle strength, spirometric pulmonary function and mobility in healthy older adults. *Age*, 36(4), 9667.

Bibliography

Craft, J., Gordon, C., Huether, S.E., McCance, K.L. and Brashers, V.L., 2015. *Understanding pathophysiology (ANZ adaptation)*. Sydney: Elsevier.

McCance, K.L. and Huether, S.E., 1990. *Pathophysiology: the biologic basis for disease in adults and children*. Sydney: Elsevier.

2.12 | Assessment of cranial nerve function

Elizabeth Goble

Chapter objectives

At the end of this chapter the reader will be able to:

1. List the cranial nerves
2. Describe the cranial nerve function
3. Perform a cranial nerve examination

Resources required for this assessment

- Standardised patient
- Penlight torch
- Tongue depressor
- Disposable gloves
- Clinical waste bag
- Method of documenting the results

Skill matrix

This assessment requires:

- Infection control (CS 1.3)
- Communication (CS 1.5)
- Consent (CS 1.6)

This assessment is a component of:

- Patient assessment (Chapter 2)

Introduction

The cranial nerves are important in everyday functioning, and any injury or insult to them impacts on morbidity and recovery. Although they are considered peripheral nerves, assessment of them provides insight into brain function. This chapter considers cranial nerve assessment.

Anatomy and physiology

The nervous system has two fundamental levels of organisation. The central nervous system (CNS), consisting of brain and spinal cord, has significant influence on mental status and cognitive ability. The peripheral nervous system (PNS) includes the cranial and spinal nerves.

There are 12 pairs of cranial nerves located on the ventral surface of the brain. They are unique in that they transport information directly to the brain without passing through the spinal cord. They are responsible for several sensory and motor functions, primarily those relating to the face and head. Cranial nerves are always referred to

using roman numerals with their individual functions (see Table 2.12.1).

Clinical rationale

The cranial nerves are responsible for several activities essential in day-to-day functioning, including sensory abilities (smell I, sight II and III, hearing VIII, taste VII and IX) and motor capacities (eye movement III, IV and VI, head movement XI, speaking X and XII, swallowing V, IX and X) (Fig. 2.12.1). They are clinically important because, although officially part of the PNS, they can indicate an underlying CNS injury.

Assessment of three main functions – eye, facial and swallow ability – can provide insight into localised nerve injury or, of more concern, CNS dysfunction.

The optic nerve (II) is more accurately a cranial nerve. It transmits light impulses from the retina, through an optic chiasma then on to the visual cortex. Motor function impulses are returned to control the pupil and regulate the amount of light entering the eye. The chiasma allows for

Table 2.12.1 Summary of cranial nerve modality, conduction direction and function.

Cranial Nerves	Modality	Classic Modality	↔	Function
I (Olfaction)	Special sensory	SVA	A	Smell
II (Optic)	Special sensory	SSA	A	Vision
III (Oculomotor)	Parasympathetic motor	GVE	E	Parasympathetic control of eye muscles
	Somatic motor	GSE	E	
IV (Trochlear)	Somatic motor	GSE	E	Motor control of eye muscles
V (Trigeminal)	Somatic sensory	GSA	A	Touch from face
	Branchial motor	SVE	E	Motor control of mastication
VI (Abducens)	Somatic motor	GSE	E	Control of muscles of the eyes
VII (Facial)	Somatic sensory Visceral sensory	GSA	A	Touch from ear
		SVA	A	Taste
	Parasympathetic motor Branchial motor	GVE	E	Parasympathetic control of oral/nasal/tongue glands
		SVE	E	Muscles of the face
VIII (Vestibulocochlear)	Somatic sensory	SSA	A	Balance/hearing
IX (Glossopharyngeal)	Somatic sensory	GSA	A	Sensation from the tongue
	Visceral sensory	SVA/GVA	A	Sensation from the carotid body and sinus; taste
	Parasympathetic motor	GVE	E	Parasympathetic control of glands and mucosa
	Branchial motor	SVE	E	Control of facial muscles
X (Vagus)	Somatic sensory	GSA	A	Touch from the ear
	Visceral sensory	SVA/GVA	A	Taste; sensory information from the pharynx, larynx, abdomen, heart
	Parasympathetic motor	GVE	E	Parasympathetic control of smooth muscle and glands in the body and throat
	Branchial motor	SVE	E	Motor control of the pharynx and larynx
XI (Accessory)	Branchial/Somatic motor	SVE	E	Control of sternocleidomastoid and trapezius muscles
XII (Hypoglossal)	Somatic motor	GSE	E	Muscles of the tongue

The modality describes the type of information each nerve conducts. Classic modality are the designations given by anatomists: SVA – special visceral afferent; SSA – special sensory afferent; GSA – general sensory afferent; SVE – special visceral efferent; GVE – general visceral efferent; GSE – general sensory efferent; A – afferent; E – efferent. Cranial nerves that contain at least a major afferent branch are bolded.

Source: Adair D., Truong D., Esmaeilpour Z., Gebodh N., Borges H., Ho L., Bremner J. D., Badran B. W., Napadow V., Clark V. P., Bikson M., 2020, Electrical stimulation of cranial nerves in cognition and disease, Brain Stimulation, 13(3), Table 1, 717–750.

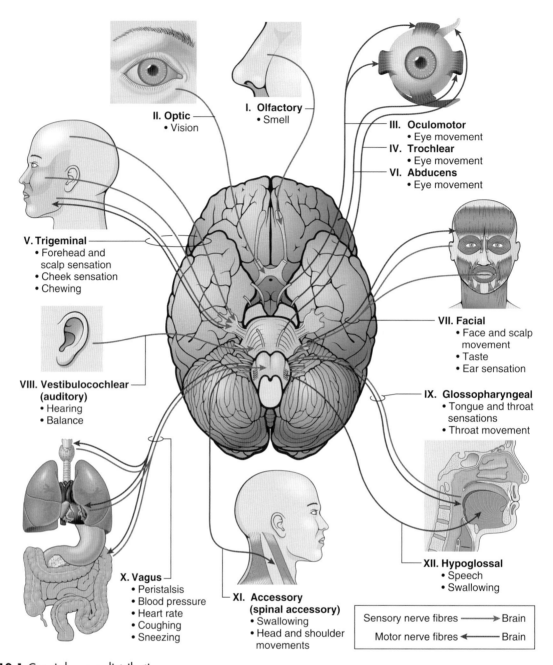

Figure 2.12.1 Cranial nerve distribution

Cranial nerves (I to XII) leading from the base of the brain and showing the parts of the body they affect. Sensory or afferent nerves carry messages towards the brain; motor or efferent nerves carry messages from the brain to muscles and organs. Some nerves (mixed) carry both sensory and motor fibres. Don't try to memorise this figure! Just get the big picture: cranial nerves carry messages to and from the brain to all parts of head and neck and also (in the case of the vagus nerve) to other parts of the body.

Source: *Davi-Ellen, C., 2017, The language of medicine, 11th edn, (Figure 10-2), Saunders.*

crossover of impulse, meaning what affects one eye will normally affect the other (Lueck, 2004). Any blockage of impulse leads to loss of pupil control and dilation.

Clinical skill assessment process

The following section outlines the clinical skill assessment tools that should be used to determine a student's ability to demonstrate accurate assessment of cranial nerves.

1. Clinical Skill Work Instruction
2. Formative Clinical Skill Assessment (F-CSAT)
3. Performance Improvement Plan (PIP)
4. Summative Clinical Skill Assessment (S-CSAT)
(5. Direct Observation of Procedural Skills (DOPS) – see Chapter 1.1)

Clinical Skill Work Instruction

Equipment and resources: Standardised patient; penlight torch; tongue depressor; disposable gloves; method of documenting results

Associated Clinical Skills: Infection control; Communication; Consent

Assessment of cranial nerve function

Activity	Critical Action	Rationale
Prepare patient	Patient can stand, sit or lie. Explain assessment to patient.	Patient cooperation is required.
Oculomotor exam (CN III)	Assess both eyes. Note pupillary size, shape and position. Note symmetry of both eyelids.	Deviation of one eye can indicate lesion, insult or injury.
Pupillary reactivity (CN III)	Right eye: With patient looking straight ahead, move the torch beam from beyond the right side of the patient's face towards but not directly into the right pupil for 0.5–1 second. Note reactivity. Left eye: Repeat process while shining light into the left pupil.	Testing involuntary reaction to light exposure. Both pupils should react when a light is shone into one pupil. Pupil should constrict briskly at least 1 mm. Record as reactive, sluggish or non-reactive.
Extraocular movements (CN III, IV, VI)	Ask the patient to look at the paramedic's finger held 30–40 cm away from the patient's face and follow it with their gaze. Move the finger in four directions (up, right, down, left) and then down towards nose where eyes both look inwards.	To identify abnormalities in facial muscles or applicable cranial nerves.
Facial nerve (CN VII)	Ask patient to smile, frown and/or raise their eyebrows. Look for asymmetry, weakness or marked differences in facial wrinkles (e.g. flattening of the nasolabial fold).	Lesions can result in hemifacial paralysis.
Glossopharyngeal, vagus and hypoglossal nerves (CN IX, X, XII)	Ask patient to open their mouth and say 'Ahh' or 'Ha-ha'. Note elevation of the palate and check for deviation of the uvula. Optionally, the gag reflex can be checked by stimulating back of throat with tongue depressor.	To assess tongue and swallowing muscles and nerves. **This should not be attempted in patients experiencing altered consciousness.**
Olfactory nerve (I)	Ask the patient if they have noted any alterations in smell or taste.	Also assesses nerves VII and IX for taste.
Report	Document/hand over pupillary responses and any abnormal findings.	Accurate record keeping and continuity of care.

Source: *Adapted from Martini et al., 2015.*

Formative Clinical Skill Assessment (F-CSAT)

Equipment and resources: Standardised patient; penlight torch; tongue depressor; disposable gloves; method of documenting results

Associated Clinical Skills: Infection control; Communication; Consent

Staff/Student being assessed: _____

Assessment of cranial nerve function

Activity	Critical Action	Performance				
Prepares patient	Patient can stand, sit or lie. Explains assessment to patient.	0	1	2	3	4
Oculomotor exam (CN III)	Looks at both eyes. Notes pupil size, shape and position. Notes eyelid symmetry.	0	1	2	3	4
Pupillary reactivity (CN III)	Right eye: With patient looking straight ahead, moves penlight torch beam correctly towards right pupil for 0.5–1 second. Notes reactivity. Left eye: Repeats process shining light into the left pupil.	0	1	2	3	4
Extraocular movements (CN III, IV, VI)	Has patient look at paramedic's finger held 30–40 cm away from their face and follow it with their gaze. Moves finger in four directions then down towards nose where eyes both look inwards.	0	1	2	3	4
Facial nerve (CN VII)	Has patient smile, frown and/or raise their eyebrows. Looks for asymmetry, weakness or marked differences in facial wrinkles.	0	1	2	3	4
Glossopharyngeal, vagus and hypoglossal nerves (CN IX, X, XII)	Has patient open their mouth and say 'Ahh' or 'Ha-ha'. Notes elevation of palate and checks for uvula deviation. Considers checking gag reflex by stimulating back of throat with tongue depressor.	0	1	2	3	4
Olfactory nerve (I) and (VII and IX)	Asks patient if they have noted any alterations in smell or taste.	0	1	2	3	4
Reports	Documents/hands over pupillary responses and any abnormal findings.	0	1	2	3	4

Source: *Adapted from Martini et al., 2015.*

Standard Achieved: (please circle one)

Competent (C)   Not Yet Competent* (NYC)

Staff/Student Name: _____

Assessor (please print name)**:** _____

Signed (Assessor)**:** _____

Date of Assessment: _____

Comments:

*If Not Yet Competent (NYC) a PIP needs to be completed and a repeat of the F-CSAT

Formative Clinical Skill Assessment (F-CSAT) Key

Skill level	Standard of procedure	Quality of performance	Outcome	Level of assistance required
4 Safe for unsupervised practice	Safe Accurate Behaviour is appropriate to context	Confident Accurate Expedient	Achieved intended outcome	No supporting cues* required
3 Requires supervision	Safe Accurate Behaviour is appropriate to context	Confident Accurate Takes longer than required	Achieved intended outcome	Requires occasional supportive cues*

Skill level	Standard of procedure	Quality of performance	Outcome	Level of assistance required
2 Requires assistance	Safe Accurate Behaviour generally appropriate to context	Lacks certainty	Would not have achieved outcome without support	Requires frequent verbal and occasional physical directives in addition to supportive cues*
1 Requires direction	Safe only with guidance Not completely accurate	Unskilled Inefficient	Would not have achieved outcome without support	Requires continuous verbal and frequent physical directive cues*
0 Unsafe	Unsafe Unable to demonstrate behaviour Lack of insight into behaviour appropriate to context	Unskilled	Would not have achieved outcome	Requires continuous verbal and continuous physical directive cues*

Refers to physical directives or verbal supportive cues

Performance Improvement Plan (PIP)

Please document the agreed education plan and completion timelines for areas assessed as less than 4.

This plan should be presented to assessor prior to commencement of summative assessment.

Where was supervisor support required?	Student summary of deficit. (Why was there a problem?)	Improvement Plan	Completed (Y/N)

Staff/Student Name: _____

Staff/Student Signature: _____

Educator Name: _____

Educator Signature: _____

Summative Clinical Skill Assessment (S-CSAT)

Equipment and resources: Standardised patient; penlight torch; tongue depressor; disposable gloves; method of documenting results

Associated Clinical Skills: Infection control; Communication; Consent

Staff/Student being assessed: _____

- Completed Formative Clinical Skill Assessment (F-CSAT):   **YES**   **NO**

- Completed Performance Improvement Plan (PIP):   **YES**   **NO**   **N/A**

Assessment of cranial nerve function

Activity	Critical Action	Achieved Without Direction	
Oculomotor exam (CN III)	Looks at both eyes. Notes pupillary size, shape and position. Notes symmetry of both eyelids.	NO	YES
Pupillary reactivity (CN III)	Right eye: With patient looking straight ahead, moves penlight torch beam correctly towards right pupil for 0.5–1 second. Notes reactivity. Left eye: Repeats process shining light into the left pupil.	NO	YES
Extraocular movements (CN III, IV, VI)	Has patient look at paramedic's finger held 30–40 cm away from their face and follow it with their gaze. Moves finger in four directions then down towards nose where eyes both look inwards.	NO	YES
Facial nerve (CN VII)	Asks patient to smile, frown and/or raise their eyebrows. Looks for asymmetry, weakness or marked differences in facial wrinkles (e.g. flattening of the nasolabial fold).	NO	YES
Glossopharyngeal, vagus and hypoglossal nerves (CN IX, X, XII)	Asks patient to open their mouth and say 'Ahh' or 'Ha-ha'. Notes elevation of the palate and checks for uvula deviation. Considers checking gag reflex by stimulating back of throat with tongue depressor.	NO	YES
Olfactory nerve (I) and (VII and IX)	Asks the patient if they have noted any alterations in smell or taste.	NO	YES
Reports	Documents/hands over pupillary responses and any abnormal findings.	NO	YES

Source: *Adapted from Martini et al., 2015.*

Standard Achieved: (please circle one)

Competent (C)   Not Yet Competent* (NYC)

Staff/Student Name: _____

Assessor (please print name)**:** _____

Signed (Assessor)**:** _____

Date of Assessment: _____

Comments: _____

*If Not Yet Competent (NYC) a PIP needs to be completed and a repeat of the F-CSAT

Clinical findings

Pupils (II and III)

Pupil response is reported as response of each pupil to light. Pupillary reaction speed is recorded as brisk (normal), sluggish or non-reactive (Pollak, 2009; Campbell, 2005). Sluggish/absent responses can indicate a rise in intracranial pressure (ICP) or brain injury. Tumour or haemorrhage places pressure on the oculomotor nerve (III). Decreased impulse to the iris sphincter muscle causes it to dilate until it is non-reactive. Although initially on the affected side, continued compression involves both pupils and is ominous (Barrow, 1992; Greaves et al., 2006; Clusmann et al., 2001).

Size is frequently recorded in millimetres (mm) with a range of 1.5–8 mm (normal is between 3 and 5 mm), though it can simply be called normal, dilated or pinpoint. Pupils are usually equal in size, although a 1 mm discrepancy can be normal (Campbell, 2005; Clark et al., 2006). Variations in size can suggest tumour, stroke, migraine, trauma or injury to oculomotor nerve (III) or iris (Lim et al., 2007; Lueck, 2004; Campbell, 2005).

Brainstem haemorrhage or tumour, particularly in the pons, can produce bilateral pinpoint pupils (Balci et al., 2005). Pons dysfunction can also cause ocular 'bobbing' (sudden downward pupil movement before slowly returning to the original position) and nystagmus (biphasic involuntary and oscillatory eyeball motion) (Warlow et al., 2001; Serra and Leigh, 2002).

The actions of some drugs can affect pupil size, since iris muscles have parasympathetic and sympathetic innervation. Atropine, adrenaline and amphetamines can dilate the pupil, while opiates and organophosphates constrict it (Campbell, 2005). Hypoxia adversely affects the retina, reducing its capacity to transmit via the optic nerve (II) and leading to vasodilation (Wilson et al., 2008).

Pupil shape can be round (normal), irregular or oval. Oval pupils can indicate cranial nerve III compression and a rise in ICP (Levin and Arnold, 2005).

Other pupil and eye abnormalities not particularly related to cranial nerve function may be noted and should be included in reporting. These include the following:

- *Coloboma*, though not related to cranial nerve function, is a congenital eye defect commonly referred to as 'keyhole' given its distinctive pupil appearance.
- *Pupil direction* is typically towards the midline. The gaze may be drawn away by hemispheric or brainstem lesion or during seizures, and this is frequently serious (Fisher, 2009; Bradley et al., 2004).
- *Strabismus*, also known as 'lazy eye' and 'cross eyes', sees one or both eyes turned in almost any direction from the midline. It is frequently observed in children.
- *Cataracts* appear as cloudiness of the eye lens and vary from slight to completely opaque. The progression of disease is gradual with age (Mitchell et al., 1996).
- *Glaucoma* may cause the pupil of the affected eye to be cloudy, dilated and unreactive to light (Goldberg et al., 2002; Mitchell et al., 1997; Mitchell et al., 1996).
- *Conjunctivitis* is a red inflammation under the eyelid or even the entire eye around the iris.
- *Hyphema* is visible bleeding between the cornea and iris as a result of traumatic eye injury.

Facial muscle weakness (VII)

The two most common causes of facial muscle weakness are stroke and Bell's palsy of the facial nerve (VII). Asymmetry of the cheeks can be observed, with an inability to smile properly, close both eyes, bare the teeth or inflate the cheek on the affected side (Davis and Gilhooley, 2016; Gilden, 2004; Konecny et al., 2014; Sands et al., 2016).

Smell/taste alteration (I, VII, IX)

Abnormal smell or taste is not a disease in its own right but rather a sign of some other disease. Changes in smell and taste accompany aging, sinonasal problems, head/facial injury causing cranial nerve damage, stroke and neurodegenerative disorders (Dutta et al., 2013; Kesari, 2010; Malaty and Malaty, 2013; Martínez et al,. 2017; Shiue, 2015; Wehling et al., 2015). These changes are often poorly understood and can be acute or progressive. Olfactory sensations can be stimulated as part of an aura associated with seizures and migraine (Liu et al., 2017; Mainardi et al., 2017; Savage et al., 2017). The ability to detect phantom smells that are not actually present is not well understood and not related to normal olfactory degeneration (Sjölund et al., 2017).

PRACTICE TIP!

Bright ambient light can make the assessment of pupils challenging, as they are naturally pinpoint and unreactive in this environment. In such cases, reverse the assessment by covering both eyes for several seconds to allow the pupils to dilate without light stimulus. If only one eye is covered, the pupils will remain pinpoint from light stimulation to the other eye. Remove one hand and note the pupil size and reaction observed. Recover the eye and repeat for the other.

PRACTICE TIP!

External eye examination must occur first. Bruising and swelling are common from traumatic and medical causes. If the eye can be opened by the patient or with minimal assistance, this is acceptable, though they should not force against any major swelling.

PRACTICE TIP!

Cranial nerve changes typically are late or ominous signs. Their finding usually suggests urgency, particularly if a major neurological event is considered the cause.

TEST YOUR KNOWLEDGE QUESTIONS

1. **How many cranial nerves are there and from where do they arise?**
   There are 12 pairs of cranial nerves, arising from the brain itself.

2. **Which three main cranial nerve functions are usually assessed?**
   Eye; facial; swallow ability.

3. **What are two main cranial nerve assessments of the eyes?**
   Motor control to have the eye follow a finger; pupil response to light.

4. **What are the two most common causes of facial muscle weakness?**
   Stroke; Bell's palsy of the facial nerve.

5. **What signs can suggest facial muscle weakness?**
   Cheek asymmetry can be observed with inability to smile properly, close both eyes, bare teeth or inflate the cheek on the affected side.

6. **What can be observed when impulses between eye and brain are interrupted?**
   Pupil dilation occurs.

7. **How is pupil size normally recorded?**
   In millimetres or as normal, dilated or pinpoint.

8. **What reactivity speeds are noted for pupils?**
   Brisk (normal), sluggish or non-reactive.

9. **Which cranial nerve assessment should not be attempted during altered consciousness?**
   Swallowing/tongue reflexes.

10. **How can pupils be assessed in bright ambient light?**
    Reverse the assessment by covering both eyes for several seconds, then uncovering each to allow light entry and noting pupil reactions.

References

Balci, K., Asil, T., Kerimoglu, M., Celik Y. and Utku, U., 2005. Clinical and neuroradiological predictors of mortality in patients with primary pontine hemorrhage. *Clinical Neurology and Neurosurgery*, 108(1), 36–39.

Barrow, D., 1992. *Complications and sequelae of head injury.* Minnesota: American Association of Neurology, p. 119.

Bradley, W., Daroff, R., Fenichel, G. and Jankovic, J., 2004. *Neurology in clinical practice – principles of diagnosis and management.* 4th edn. Oxford: Butterworth Heinemann, p. 715.

Campbell, W. (ed.), 2005. *DeJong's the neurologic examination.* Philadelphia: Lippincott Williams & Wilkins, p. 164.

Clark, A., Clarke, T., Gregson, B., Hooker, P. and Chambers, I., 2006. Variability in pupil size estimation. *Emergency Medicine Journal*, 23(6), 440–441.

Clusmann, H., Schaller, C. and Schramm, J., 2001. Fixed and dilated pupils after trauma, stoke and previous intracranial surgery: management and outcome. *Journal of Neurology, Neurosurgery and Psychiatry*, 71, 175–181.

Davis, A. and Gilhooley, M.J., 2016. Bell's palsy. *InnovAiT*, 9(2), 93–98.

Dutta, T.M., Josiah, A.F., Cronin, C.A., Wittenberg, G.F. and Cole, J.W., 2013. Altered taste and stroke: a case report and literature review. *Topics in Stroke Rehabilitation*, 20(1), 78–86.

Fisher, M. (ed.), 2009. Stroke part 2: clinical manifestations and pathogensis. *Handbook of clinical neurology* (Chapter 29). New York: Elsevier, pp. 583–586.

Gilden, D.H., 2004. Bell's palsy. *New England Journal of Medicine*, 351(13), 1323–1331.

Goldberg, I., Graham, S.L. and Healey, P.R., 2002. Primary open-angle glaucoma. *Medical Journal of Australia*, 177(10), 535–536.

Greaves, I., Porter, K., Hodgetts, T. and Woollard, M., 2006. *Emergency care: a textbook for paramedics*, 2nd edn. London: Elsevier, p. 239.

Kesari, S., 2010. Disturbances of smell and taste. In Mushlin, S. and Greene, H. (eds), *Decision making in medicine*, 3rd edn. St Louis: Mosby Elsevier, pp. 458–459.

Konecny, P., Elfmark, M., Horak, S., Pastucha, D., Krobot, A., Urbanek, K. and Kanovsky, P., 2014. Central facial paresis and its impact on mimicry, psyche and quality of life in patients after stroke. *Biomedical Papers*, 158(1), 133–137.

Levin, L. and Arnold, A. 2005 *Neuro-opthalmology: the practical guide.* New York: Thieme, p. 11.

Lim, A., Constable, I. and Wong, T., 2007. *Colour atlas of opthalmology*, 5th edn. Singapore: World Scientific Publishing Co.

Liu, Y., Guo, X.M., Wu, X., Li, P. and Wang, W.W., 2017. Clinical analysis of partial epilepsy with auras. *Chinese Medical Journal*, 130(3), 318.

Lueck, A. (ed.), 2004. *Functional vision: a practitioner's guide to evaluation and intervention.* Arlington County: AFB Press, p.160.

Mainardi, F., Rapoport, A., Zanchin, G. and Maggioni, F., 2017. Scent of aura? Clinical features of olfactory hallucinations during a migraine attack (OHM). *Cephalalgia*, 37(2), 154–160.

Malaty, J. and Malaty, I.A., 2013. Smell and taste disorders in primary care. *American Family Physician*, 88(12), 852–859.

Martínez, N.A., Carrillo, G.A., Alvarado, P.S., García, C.M., Monroy, A.V. and Campos, F.V., 2017. Clinical importance of olfactory function in neurodegenerative diseases. Revista Médica del Hospital General de México.

Martini, F.H., Nath, J.L. and Bartholomew, E.F., 2015. *Fundamentals of anatomy and physiology.* Essex: Pearson.

Mitchell, P., Smith, W., Attebo, K. and Healey, P.R., 1996. Prevalence of open-angle glaucoma in Australia: the Blue Mountains Eye Study. *Ophthalmology*, 103, 1661–1669.

Mitchell, P., Smith, W. and Chey, T., 1997. Open-angle glaucoma and diabetes: the Blue Mountains Eye Study. *Ophthalmology*, 104, 712–718.

Pollak, A. (ed.), 2009. *Critical care transport.* Sudbury: Jones and Bartlett, p. 117.

Sands, K.A., Shahripour, R.B., Kumar, G., Barlinn, K., Lyerly, M.J., Haršány, M., Cure, J., Yakov, Y.L., Alexandrov, A.W. and Alexandrov, A.V., 2016. Acute isolated central facial palsy as manifestation of middle cerebral artery ischemia. *Journal of Neuroimaging*, 26(5), 499–502.

Savage, S.A., Butler, C.R., Milton, F., Han, Y. and Zeman, A.Z., 2017. On the nose: olfactory disturbances in patients with transient epileptic amnesia. *Epilepsy & Behavior*, 66, 113–119.

Serra, A. and Leigh, R.J., 2002. Diagnostic value of nystagmus: spontaneous and induced ocular oscillations. *Journal of Neurology, Neurosurgery, and Psychiatry*, 73(6), 615–618.

Shiue, I., 2015. Adult taste and smell disorders after heart, neurological, respiratory and liver problems: US NHANES, 2011–2012. *International Journal of Cardiology*, 179, 46–48.

Sjölund, S., Larsson, M., Olofsson, J.K., Seubert, J. and Laukka, E.J., 2017. Phantom smells: prevalence and correlates in a population-based sample of older adults. *Chemical Senses*, 42(4), 309–318.

Warlow, C.P., Dennis, M.S., van Gijn, J., Hankey, G.J., Sandercock, P.A., Bamford, J.M. and Wardlaw, J.M., 2001. *Stroke: a practical guide to management.* New Jersey: Wiley-Blackwell.

Wehling, E., Naess, H., Wollschlaeger, D., Hofstad, H., Bramerson, A., Bende, M. and Nordin, S., 2015. Olfactory dysfunction in chronic stroke patients. *BMC Neurology*, 15(1), 199.

Wilson, M., Edsell, M., Imray, C. and Wright, A. 2008. Changes in pupil dynamics at high altitude – an observational study using a handheld pupillometer. *High Altitude Medicine & Biology*, 9, 319–325.

2.13 | Assessment of motor and sensory nerve function

Elizabeth Goble

Chapter objectives

At the end of this chapter the reader will be able to:

1. Describe the anatomy of the sensory and motor nervous system
2. Perform a sensory and motor nerve assessment
3. Document results of sensory and motor function

Resources required for this assessment

- Standardised patient
- Disposable gloves
- Cotton swab
- Clinical waste bag
- Method of documenting results

Skill matrix

This assessment requires:

- Infection control (CS 1.3)
- Communication (CS 1.5)
- Consent (CS 1.6)

This assessment is a component of:

- Patient assessment (Chapter 2)

Introduction

Sensory nerves carry information from sensory receptors in the peripheral nervous system (PNS) to the brain for interpretation and subsequent action.

The motor nervous system is responsible for all muscle contraction and hormone release, and its integrity and functionality are of profound importance. Evaluation of motor function is important for identifying injury and mitigating the repercussions of traumatic injury.

This chapter discusses the PNS anatomy, physiology and sensory and motor nerve assessment.

Anatomy and physiology

The nervous system has three fundamental levels of organisation: the central nervous system (CNS), consisting of brain and spinal cord; the PNS, which includes 12 pairs of cranial nerves, 31 pairs of spinal nerves from each spinal cord segment (8 cervical, 12 thoracic, 5 lumbar, 5 sacral and 1 coccygeal) (Fig. 2.13.1); and the autonomic nervous

system (ANS). The third level is the parasympathetic and sympathetic nervous divisions of the ANS.

The CNS and PNS incorporate sensory and motor neurons. Sensory neurons are called afferent nerves and carry sensory signals such as pain, pressure and temperature to the spinal cord or brain.

The sensory nervous system identifies and interprets sensory information collected from the internal and external environment by specialised receptors. There are several sensory receptors: those for perceiving information from the special senses such as sight (photoreceptors) and smell/taste (chemoreceptors), and others including nociceptors (pain), thermoreceptors (hot/cold temperatures), proprioceptors (stretch receptors in muscles that identify joint position and keep balance) and mechanoreceptors (hearing, movement, tension and pressure – sharp/dull).

Sensory impulses are transmitted via sensory nerves connecting with the spinal cord segments. Each segment corresponds to body surface regions called dermatomes (Fig. 2.13.2).

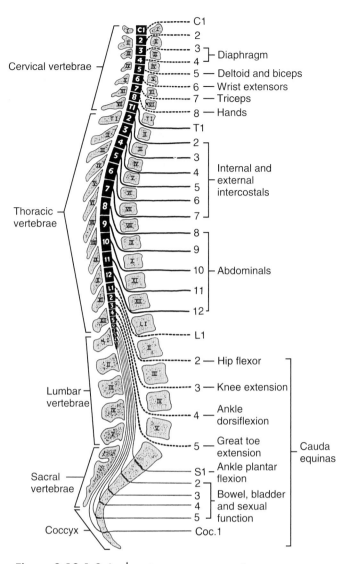

Cervical vertebrae

- C1
- 2
- 3 ⎤ Diaphragm
- 4 ⎦
- 5 — Deltoid and biceps
- 6 — Wrist extensors
- 7 — Triceps
- 8 — Hands
- T1

Thoracic vertebrae

- 2
- 3
- 4 ⎤ Internal and external intercostals
- 5
- 6
- 7
- 8
- 9
- 10 ⎤ Abdominals
- 11
- 12 ⎦
- L1

Lumbar vertebrae

- 2 — Hip flexor
- 3 — Knee extension
- 4 — Ankle dorsiflexion
- 5 — Great toe extension
- S1 — Ankle plantar flexion
- 2
- 3 ⎤ Bowel, bladder and sexual function
- 4
- 5 ⎦

Cauda equinas

Sacral vertebrae

Coccyx

- Coc.1

Figure 2.13.1 Spinal motor nerve segments

Spinal nerves emerging from the spinal cord through the intervertebral foramina and muscle movements that evaluate specific levels of spinal nerve function.

Source: *McQuillan, K.A. and Flynn Makic, M.B., 2020,* Trauma nursing from resuscitation through rehabilitation, *5th edn (Figure 19.9), Elsevier.*

Information is transmitted to the brain through the thalamus to specific processing regions of the cortex depending on the receptor activated, including the auditory, visual and somatosensory regions.

Motor neurons are efferent nerves, with pathways always conducted via two neurons connecting with the target muscle. They can be separated into two categories – upper motor neurons (UMNs) and lower motor neurons (LMNs) – determined by the location of the cell body within the nerve. The cell body of an UMN is located in the cortex or brainstem and crosses over to the opposite side of the spinal cord (decussates) before terminating on the LMN. The LMN cell body is located in the ventral horn of the spinal cord and its axon runs down the same side of the spinal cord before terminating on the target muscle.

PNS motor nerves can be further categorised by level of conscious control. The somatic nervous system controls muscles under voluntary control. This involves all skeletal movement, including muscles of the head and neck controlled by the 12 pairs of cranial nerves. Motor nerves transmit impulses away from the CNS to the effectors (muscle fibres or glands), which stimulate muscle contraction or hormone release.

The ANS innervates all smooth muscles and glands not under voluntarily control, including the heart and peristaltic gut smooth muscle (Fig. 2.13.3). Sympathetic nerves innervate primarily from thoracic and first lumbar vertebrae and are responsible for preparing the body for action/attention. The parasympathetic nerves originate from the cervical and lumbar/sacral spine and are most active during rest and digestion (Craft et al., 2015; McCance and Huether, 2015, Martini et al., 2015; Noback et al., 1991).

Clinical rationale

Sensory nerve assessment is necessary to determine the integrity of the spinal cord after insult/injury. The initial prehospital neurological assessment does not require precision when determining the exact point of compromise; it is important for determining the aetiology of acute conditions or the extent of traumatic injury. The assessment is generally subjective as it relies on patient reports.

Sensation can be assessed by comparing light touch, such as from a cotton swab, and a gentle pricking effect from the hard swab end, or even a blunt medication drawing-up needle tip or pen.

The motor nerve examination is more objective, as motor function can be reviewed by determining the integrity of the automatic reflexes and other observable states such as tone, strength, positioning and coordination (Cameron et al., 2009; Wolfson et al., 2009).

Motor and sensory nerves run the length of the spinal cord in different tracts. Injury or compromise can impact on some or all tracts, potentially causing varying changes in movement and/or sensation.

Clinical skill assessment process

The following section outlines the clinical skill assessment tools that should be used to determine a student's ability to demonstrate accurate assessment of motor and sensory function.

1. Clinical Skill Work Instruction
2. Formative Clinical Skill Assessment (F-CSAT)
3. Performance Improvement Plan (PIP)
4. Summative Clinical Skill Assessment (S-CSAT)
(5. Direct Observation of Procedural Skills (DOPS) – see Chapter 1.1)

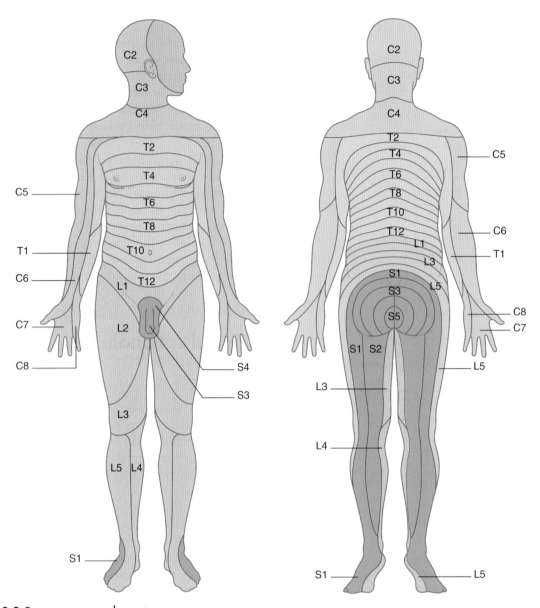

Figure 2.13.2 Somatosensory dermatomes

Source: *Mtui, E., Dockery, P. and Gruener, G., 2016,* Fitzgerald's clinical neuroanatomy and neuroscience, *7th edn (Figure 14.13), Elsevier.*

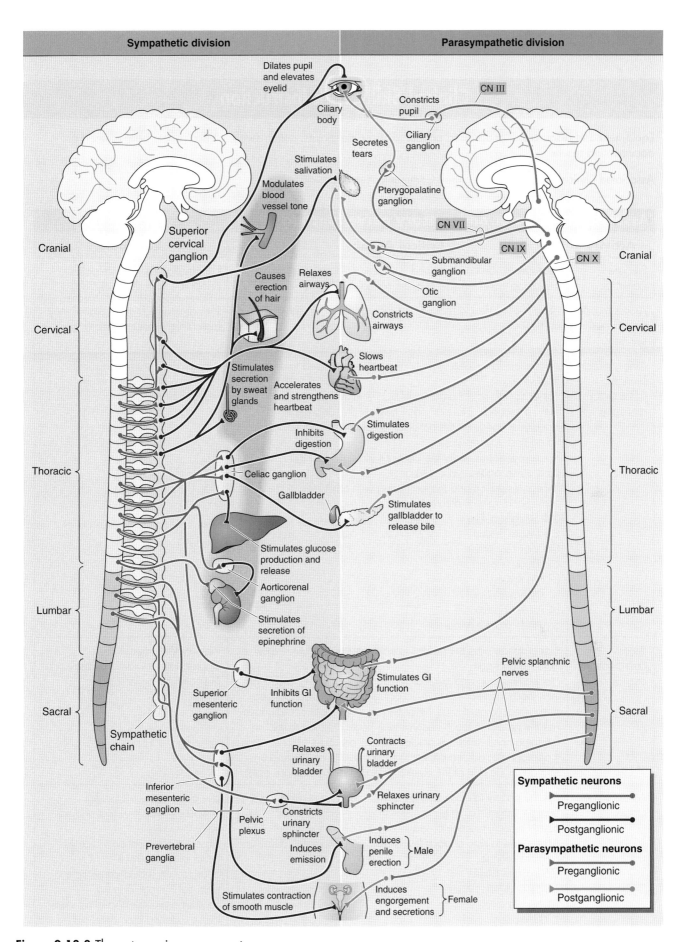

Sympathetic division | **Parasympathetic division**

Dilates pupil and elevates eyelid
Ciliary body
Constricts pupil — CN III
Ciliary ganglion
Secretes tears
Stimulates salivation
Pterygopalatine ganglion
Modulates blood vessel tone
Superior cervical ganglion
Cranial
CN VII
CN IX
Submandibular ganglion
CN X
Otic ganglion
Cranial

Causes erection of hair
Relaxes airways
Constricts airways
Cervical
Cervical

Stimulates secretion by sweat glands
Slows heartbeat
Accelerates and strengthens heartbeat
Inhibits digestion
Stimulates digestion
Celiac ganglion
Gallbladder
Stimulates gallbladder to release bile
Thoracic
Thoracic

Stimulates glucose production and release
Aorticorenal ganglion
Stimulates secretion of epinephrine
Lumbar
Lumbar

Superior mesenteric ganglion
Inhibits GI function
Stimulates GI function
Pelvic splanchnic nerves
Sympathetic chain
Sacral
Sacral

Inferior mesenteric ganglion
Pelvic plexus
Prevertebral ganglia
Relaxes urinary bladder
Constricts urinary sphincter
Induces emission
Contracts urinary bladder
Relaxes urinary sphincter
Induces penile erection — Male
Stimulates contraction of smooth muscle
Induces engorgement and secretions — Female

Sympathetic neurons
Preganglionic
Postganglionic
Parasympathetic neurons
Preganglionic
Postganglionic

Figure 2.13.3 The autonomic nervous system

Organisation of the sympathetic and parasympathetic divisions of the ANS. The left panel shows the sympathetic division. The cell bodies of sympathetic preganglionic neurons are in the intermediolateral column of the thoracic and lumbar spinal cord (T1–L3). Their axons project to paravertebral ganglia (the sympathetic chain) and prevertebral ganglia. Postganglionic neurons therefore have long projections to their targets. The right panel shows the parasympathetic division. The cell bodies of parasympathetic preganglionic neurons are either in the brain (midbrain, pons, medulla) or in the sacral spinal cord (S2–S4). Their axons project to ganglia very near (or even inside) the end organs. Postganglionic neurons therefore have short projections to their targets.

Source: Boron, W.F. and Boulpaep, E.L., 2017, Medical physiology, 3rd edn (Figure 14-4), Elsevier.

Clinical Skill Work Instruction

Equipment and resources: Standardised patient; disposable gloves; cotton swab; clinical waste bag; method of documenting results

Associated Clinical Skills: Infection control; Communication; Consent

Assessment of motor and sensory nerve function

Activity	Critical Action	Rationale
Prepare patient	Assessment can be performed with patient in any position. Explain to patient nature of examination.	Explanation assists with patient cooperation and anxiety.
Assess muscle tone/size/ symmetry	Note tone of muscle groups and record it: flaccid, spasticity, rigidity.	Loss of muscle mass (atrophy) may indicate chronic conditions.
Assess muscle strength: gross motor assessment	Ask patient to squeeze your fingers with each hand to assess any weakness. Ask patient to hold their arms at 90° with their palms up for 10–15 seconds. Note any downwards drift or pronation. Place your hands on the patient's forearms. Ask patient to push up against your resistance. Place your hands under the patient's forearms. Ask patient to push down against your resistance. Repeat resistance and motion testing with other muscle groups corresponding with different spinal cord segments: C4 Shrug shoulder C5 Elbow flexion C6 Wrist extension C7 Elbow extension L2 Hip flexion L3 Knee extension L4 Ankle dorsiflexion S1 Ankle plantar flexion	Alterations in strength against resistance or movement may indicate brain or spinal cord insult.
Assess coordination/ control	If appropriate, ask the patient to walk and then return. Observe balance and gait. Hold a finger up and ask the patient to touch it with their finger then touch their nose. Move your finger to a different position and repeat as quickly as the patient is able. Note coordination. Ask the patient to touch each of their fingers to their thumb on the same hand in turn as quickly as they are able. If appropriate, ask the patient to slide the heel of one foot up and down the shin of the other leg as quickly as they are able.	Inability to demonstrate appropriate coordination may indicate cerebellar insult.
Assess sense of touch	Ask the patient to close their eyes and identify where they are being touched. Touch patient skin in series with sharp point to assess sensory function of sequential spinal cord segments. Assess side to side at each level, working proximal to distal: Patient forehead C6 Dorsum thumb C8 Dorsum little finger T4 Nipple level T10 Umbilical level T12 Groin L1 Anterior thigh L3 Inner knee L5 Dorsum foot at third metatarsal S1 Lateral heel (calcaneus)	Eye closing ensures patient describes what they feel and not what they see. Absence of sensation indicates brain or spinal insult. Sharp touch should cause light pain but not cause injury. Forehead provides baseline since this is supplied by cranial not spinal nerves.

Assessment of motor and sensory nerve function continued

Activity	Critical Action	Rationale
Assess perception	Repeat the touch process, randomly alternating using sharp end and dull end of the cotton swab.	Light and sharp touch sensation might vary.
Assess sense of pain	If sensory perception is compromised, determine response to deeper pain (e.g. squeeze a fingernail, apply pressure to sternum, push supraorbital notch).	To determine if there is any sensory response at all.
Report	Accurately document/hand over findings.	Accurate record kept and continuity of patient care.

Source: *Adapted from Roberts et al., 2017; Zhang et al., 2017.*

Formative Clinical Skill Assessment (F-CSAT)

Equipment and resources: Standardised patient; disposable gloves; cotton swab; clinical waste bag; method of documenting results

Associated Clinical Skills: Infection control; Communication; Consent

Staff/Student being assessed: _____

Assessment of motor and sensory nerve function

Activity	Critical Action	Performance				
Assesses muscle tone/size/symmetry	Notes tone of muscle groups and records: flaccid, spasticity, rigidity.	0	1	2	3	4
Assesses muscle strength: gross motor assessment	Has patient squeeze assessor fingers with each hand to determine any weakness. Has patient hold their arms at 90° with palms up for 10–15 seconds. Notes any downward drift or pronation. Places hands on patient's forearms. Has patient push up against resistance. Places hands under patient's forearms. Has patient push down against resistance. Repeats resistance and range of motion testing with other muscle groups to assess spinal cord segments (shoulders, elbows, wrists, hips, knees, feet).	0	1	2	3	4
Assesses coordination/control	If appropriate, has patient walk away and return. Observes balance and gait. Holds finger up and has patient touch it with their finger then touch their nose. Moves finger to a different position and repeats as quickly as patient able. Notes coordination. Has patient touch each of their fingers to their thumb on the same hand in turn as quickly as they are able. If appropriate, has patient slide heel of one foot up and down shin of the other leg as quickly as they are able.	0	1	2	3	4
Assesses sense of touch	Has patient close their eyes and identify where they are being touched. Touches patient's skin in multiple places in series, left and right, using sharp end of cotton swab.	0	1	2	3	4
Assesses perception	Repeats touch process randomly, alternately using sharp and dull cotton swab end.	0	1	2	3	4
Assesses sense of pain	If sensory perception has been compromised, determines response to deeper pain.	0	1	2	3	4
Reports	Accurately documents/hands over findings.	0	1	2	3	4

Source: *Adapted from Roberts et al., 2017; Zhang et al., 2017.*

Standard Achieved: (please circle one)

Competent (C)   Not Yet Competent* (NYC)

Staff/Student Name: _____

Assessor (please print name)**:** _____

Signed (Assessor)**:** _____

Date of Assessment: _____

Comments:

*If Not Yet Competent (NYC) a PIP needs to be completed and a repeat of the F-CSAT

Formative Clinical Skill Assessment (F-CSAT) Key

Skill level	Standard of procedure	Quality of performance	Outcome	Level of assistance required
4 Safe for unsupervised practice	Safe Accurate Behaviour is appropriate to context	Confident Accurate Expedient	Achieved intended outcome	No supporting cues* required
3 Requires supervision	Safe Accurate Behaviour is appropriate to context	Confident Accurate Takes longer than required	Achieved intended outcome	Requires occasional supportive cues*
2 Requires assistance	Safe Accurate Behaviour generally appropriate to context	Lacks certainty	Would not have achieved outcome without support	Requires frequent verbal and occasional physical directives in addition to supportive cues*
1 Requires direction	Safe only with guidance Not completely accurate	Unskilled Inefficient	Would not have achieved outcome without support	Requires continuous verbal and frequent physical directive cues*
0 Unsafe	Unsafe Unable to demonstrate behaviour Lack of insight into behaviour appropriate to context	Unskilled	Would not have achieved outcome	Requires continuous verbal and continuous physical directive cues*

*Refers to physical directives or verbal supportive cues

Performance Improvement Plan (PIP)

Please document the agreed education plan and completion timelines for areas assessed as less than 4.

This plan should be presented to assessor prior to commencement of summative assessment.

Where was supervisor support required?	Student summary of deficit. (Why was there a problem?)	Improvement Plan	Completed (Y/N)

Staff/Student Name: _____

Staff/Student Signature: _____

Educator Name: _____

Educator Signature: _____

Summative Clinical Skill Assessment (S-CSAT)

Equipment and resources: Standardised patient; disposable gloves; cotton swab; clinical waste bag; method of documenting results

Associated Clinical Skills: Infection control; Communication; Consent

Staff/Student being assessed: _____

- Completed Formative Clinical Skill Assessment (F-CSAT): **YES   NO**

- Completed Performance Improvement Plan (PIP): **YES   NO   N/A**

Assessment of motor and sensory nerve function

Activity	Critical Action	Achieved Without Direction	
Assesses muscle tone/size/symmetry	Notes tone of muscle groups and records: flaccid, spasticity, rigidity.	NO	YES
Assesses muscle strength: gross motor assessment	Has patient squeeze fingers with each hand to determine any weakness. Has patient hold their arms at 90° with palms up for 10–15 seconds. Notes any downward drift or pronation. Places hands on patient's forearms. Has patient push up against resistance. Places hands under the patient's forearms. Has patient push down against resistance. Repeats resistance and range of motion testing with other muscle groups to assess spinal cord segments (fingers, wrists, elbows, shoulders, knees, feet).	NO	YES

Assessment of motor and sensory nerve function continued

Activity	Critical Action	Achieved Without Direction	
Assesses coordination/ control	If appropriate, has patient walk away and return. Observes balance and gait. Holds finger up and has patient touch it with their finger and then touch their nose. Moves finger to a different position and repeats as quickly as the patient is able. Notes coordination. Has patient touch each of their fingers to their thumb on the same hand in turn as quickly as they are able. If appropriate, has patient slide heel of one foot up and down shin of the other leg as quickly as able.	NO	YES
Assesses sense of touch	Has patient close their eyes and identify where they are being touched. Touches patient's skin in multiple locations in series, left to right, using the sharp end of a cotton swab.	NO	YES
Assesses perception	Repeats the touch process randomly, alternately using sharp end and dull end of the cotton swab.	NO	YES
Assesses sense of pain	If sensory perception has been compromised, determines response to deeper pain.	NO	YES
Reports	Accurately documents/hands over findings.	NO	YES

Source: *Adapted from Roberts et al., 2017; Zhang et al., 2017.*

Standard Achieved: (please circle one)

Competent (C)   Not Yet Competent* (NYC)

Staff/Student Name: _____

Assessor (please print name)**:** _____

Signed (Assessor)**:** _____

Date of Assessment: _____

Comments:

*If Not Yet Competent (NYC) a PIP needs to be completed and a repeat of the F-CSAT

Clinical findings

Motor function

Motor function can provide differing results, including tone (from flaccid to tensed rigid or spasticity) and strength (from slight weakness (-paresis) to complete paralysis (-plegia)). Strength results include deliberate but weak movement, movement against gravity, movement against assessor resistance and normal movement (Roberts et al., 2017).

A lack of movement might be observed for other reasons, including pain or injury where the inability or unwillingness is not caused by nerve dysfunction. This should be noted in the results.

Sensation

The patient may have no sensation at all or may be unable to differentiate sharp from dull. Sensation may be altered in a variety of ways, including sensation loss, numbness, pain, tingling or even hypersensitivity. This may be normal (Roberts et al., 2017), but problems can be due to peripheral or central causes.

Alterations in motor and sensory activity can be bilateral or unilateral, varying with the extent of cord injury.

Spinal segment limitations

High cervical segments (C2–C4), most thoracic segments (T2–L1) and most sacral segments (S2–S5) cannot be assessed through limb motor function (Schuld et al., 2015).

PRACTICE TIP!

The answer to a single question such as 'Can you feel this?' is sufficient to commence gathering information on several neurological sources at once, including level of consciousness (midbrain and brainstem structures), hearing (CN VIII), comprehension (cerebral cortex) and speech (motor function). Develop a routine that elicits the greatest amount of information while asking the least questions, thus enhancing the speed with which a thorough neurological assessment can be completed.

PRACTICE TIP!

Motor and sensory assessment can be performed as a stand-alone evaluation or incorporated in with other progressive physical assessments for injuries and abnormalities.

PRACTICE TIP!

A thorough emergency neurological examination can reveal subtle changes. Distracting injuries, altered consciousness and scene noise can all adversely impact on reliability.

TEST YOUR KNOWLEDGE QUESTIONS

1. **How many pairs of nerves comprise the peripheral nervous system and from what part of the spine do they originate?**
   There are 31 pairs of spinal nerves that pass between each vertebra: 8 cervical, 12 thoracic, 5 lumbar, 5 sacral and 1 coccygeal.

2. **Which four body areas are touched to ascertain sensory nerve integrity, and from which spinal region do they emanate?**
   The shoulder and arm are innervated from cervical nerves, the torso by thoracic nerves, the thighs and shins by lumbar nerves and the calves by sacral nerves.

3. **In motor nerve assessment, what is the first action in assessing muscle strength?**
   Ask the patient to squeeze your fingers with each hand to detect weakness.

4. **Why is the forehead/face used as a reference point for motor and sensation assessment?**
   This is controlled by cranial and not spinal nerves.

5. **Why are two levels of sensation compared at the same dermatome locations?**
   The response to light pain and gentle touch might vary.

6. **What devices can be used to elicit light pain response?**
   Hard end of a cotton swab, blunt drawing-up needle, biro point.

7. **What motor strength responses might be provided?**
   Normal movement, movement against resistance, movement against gravity, deliberate but weak movement.

8. **Dermatomes correspond with what part of the nervous system?**
   Spinal cord segments.

9. **Why should the patient close their eyes during sensory assessment?**
   To ensure they describe what they feel and not what they see.

10. **Why is motor function assessment more objective than sensory?**
    Motor function can be observed; sensory function relies on testimony.

References

Cameron, P., Jelinek, G., Kelly, A.-M., Murray, L. and Brown, A.F., 2009. *Textbook of adult emergency medicine*. London: Elsevier.

Craft, J., Gordon, C., Huether, S.E., McCance, K.L. and Brashers, V.L., 2015. *Understanding pathophysiology (ANZ adaptation)*. Sydney: Elsevier.

Martini, F.H., Nath, J.L. and Bartholomew, E.F., 2015. *Fundamentals of anatomy & physiology*. Essex: Pearson.

McCance, K.L. and Huether, S.E., 2015. *Pathophysiology: the biologic basis for disease in adults and children*. Sydney: Elsevier.

Noback, C.R., Strominger, N.L. and Demarest, R.J., 1991. *The human nervous system*. Pennsylvania: Lea & Febige.

Roberts, T.T., Leonard, G.R. and Cepela, D.J., 2017. Classifications in brief: American Spinal Injury Association (ASIA) Impairment Scale, *Clinical Orthopaedics and Related Research*, 475, 1499–1504.

Schuld, C., Franz, S., Van Hedel, H.J.A., Moosburger, J., Maier, D., Abel, R., van de Meent, H., Curt, A., Weidner, N., Rupp, R. and EMSCI study group, 2015. International standards for neurological classification of spinal cord injury: classification skills of clinicians versus computational algorithms. *Spinal Cord*, 53(4), 234.

Wolfson, A.B., Hendey, G.W. and Ling, L.J., 2009. *Clinical practice of emergency medicine*. Philadelphia: Lippincott Williams and Wilkins.

Zhang, J.W., Wang, Q., Wang, X.F., Gao, M.M., Yun, X.P., Wu, H.F. and Hong, Y., 2017. Sensory thresholds at different sites of the foot: a valuable reference for neurologic examinations. *Spinal Cord*, 55(4), 396.

Chapter objectives

At the end of this chapter the reader will be able to:

1. Describe the relevant anatomy of the cognitive nervous system
2. Perform a mental status assessment
3. Accurately assess a patient's mental status

Resources required for this assessment

- Standardised patient
- Hand decontamination agent
- Disposable gloves
- Clinical waste bag
- Method of documenting results

Skill matrix

This assessment requires:

- Infection control (CS 1.3)
- Communication (CS 1.5)
- Consent (CS 1.6)
- Assessment using the modified Glasgow Coma Scale (CS 2.1)
- Assessing the AVPU score (CS 2.2)

This assessment is a component of:

- Patient assessment (Chapter 2)

Introduction

Neurology and its components are of particular concern in emergency medicine. Neurological insult or injury is implicated in over 50% of deaths occurring due to trauma (Cameron et al., 2009). Stroke as an isolated condition is the third leading cause of death in Australia (ABS, 2015). and a leading cause of death among Māori and non-Māori New Zealanders Both the short- and long-term effects of stroke contribute to significant physical, psychological and social limitations. Rapid identification and management can improve morbidity/mortality rates and quality of life.

Several nervous system injuries cause an alteration in consciousness and mental status. This chapter provides the basic anatomy and physiology relating to cognitive function and describes the assessment of mental status.

Anatomy and physiology

The brain is structurally separated into several regions that perform specific functions. The midbrain and brainstem contain structures that process visual and auditory data, relay sensory information and motor responses and take part in autonomic regulation. Above this region is the diencephalon, containing the thalamus, which is the processing centre for sensory information, and the hypothalamus, which is responsible for autonomic functions, hormone production and a level of emotion control. The bulk of the brain surrounding these structures is the cerebrum or cerebral cortex. This entire cortical structure is interconnected to coordinate all conscious thought processes, memory processing and storage, and all skeletal muscular function. The cortex is in turn divided into four functionally separate lobes: the frontal lobe is the control centre for cognition, memory, problem solving, judgment, language and general information processing, along with motor function; the temporal lobe is primarily responsible for auditory processing; the parietal lobe deals with sensory information and visual perception; and the occipital lobe coordinates all other visual processing. Underneath the cortex, behind the brainstem, is the cerebellum, which is involved in coordination, spatial awareness and timing (Martini et al., 2015).

'Mental status' refers to the assessment of the acuity of mind or level of consciousness exhibited, determined by state of awareness and ability to perceive and react appropriately to environmental stimuli. Consciousness is controlled by several brain regions in a coordinated manner, specifically utilising the brainstem and midbrain nuclei (reticular formation, thalamus etc.) and all parts of the cerebral cortex (Bennett, 1997).

Clinical rationale

An examination of mental status is performed to determine cognitive and behavioural functioning as an indication of the integrity of the brain, specifically the cerebral cortex where higher brain functions take place. The most clinically relevant aspects are alertness, orientation to person, place, time and situation, language, reasoning and memory.

Once an alteration in the patient's normal mental status has been established, it is necessary to determine likely causes, since these can dictate or modify any course of treatment. Although altered mental status is common in several psychiatric and emotional conditions, it can also reflect changes in brain function caused by intoxication, infection, injury and certain medical conditions. Alterations can occur rapidly or over hours or days, depending on the aetiology.

A useful mnemonic often used to assist remembering the many possible alternative aetiologies is 'AEIOU TIPS' (Sanello et al., 2018):

A Alcohol or other substance Abuse / Acidosis
E Environmental / Epilepsy / Endocrine
I Infection (meningitis/encephalitis)
O Overdose / Oxygen deficiency
U Underdose / Uraemia (due to kidney failure or congestive cardiac failure)
T Trauma / Tumour
I Insulin (hyper- or hypoglycaemia)
P Psychogenic / Poison
S Stroke / Shock

The approach to mental status assessment must always consider personal risk and safety. Some behavioural abnormalities can lead to unpredictable, aggressive and even violent behaviour. This might be determined from information given during the call or by those at scene, even before the ambulance arrives. It may be necessary to seek personnel support in some cases, to ensure assessment and management of the patient are performed safely.

The mental status assessment is intended to recognise changed and abnormal behaviour rather than to be used for diagnosis. It can be divided into three broad elements: those that are observable; those that can be heard, whether spontaneously or through discussion; and those that require some form of testing. The assessment combines specific tests to assess higher functions, attention and memory. It also considers appearance, behaviour and mood (Finney et al., 2016).

Most mental status testing is performed using a modified form of mental state examination (MSE) or mini-mental state exam (MMSE) (Finney et al., 2016; Folstein et al., 1975; Trzepacz et al., 2015). This typically considers patient cognition, taking into account level of alertness and orientation to surroundings, and the use of structured testing to assess ability to pay attention, concentrate and recall. Results can indicate problems ranging from mental illness and dementia through to acute delirium.

Clinical skill assessment process

The following section outlines the clinical skill assessment tools that should be used to determine a student's ability to demonstrate accurate mental status assessment.

1. Clinical Skill Work Instruction
2. Formative Clinical Skill Assessment (F-CSAT)
3. Performance Improvement Plan (PIP)
4. Summative Clinical Skill Assessment (S-CSAT)
(5. Direct Observation of Procedural Skills (DOPS) – see Chapter 1.1)

Clinical Skill Work Instruction

Equipment and resources: Standardised patient; hand decontamination agent; disposable gloves; clinical waste bag; method of documenting results

Associated Clinical Skills: Infection control; Communication; Consent; Assessment using the Glasgow Coma Scale; Assessing the AVPU score

Mental status assessment

Activity	Critical Action	Rationale
Safety	Consider risk and safety if patient's behaviour appears bizarre or threatening. Don personal protection as appropriate.	Abnormal thinking can lead to unpredictable behaviour. Reports from others may be sufficient for risk assessment.

Observable

Activity	Critical Action	Rationale
Initial approach	When moving towards the patient, note when they open their eyes: spontaneously on approach, on verbal exchange, in response to pain, or no response. Obtain consent to continue if possible.	Eye opening is part of AVPU/GCS and forms part of consciousness-level assessment (see Chapters 2.1 and 2.2).
Behaviour	Note incongruous behaviour, e.g. disproportionate anxiety, threats/violence, pacing, avoidance or excessive eye contact.	Can be hugely varied. Compare to the patient's normal where possible. Look also for muscle tremor, tics, dystonia.
Affect/mood	Note mood and its appropriateness for the context (including predictability). Include depression, mania, withdrawal, euphoria, anxiety.	Mood is what the patient describes feeling. Affect is how that presents to others.
Grooming/ hygiene	Note appropriateness/cleanliness of attire and person for the season/situation. Include cleanliness and odour.	Deterioration may indicate psychological condition or organic brain disorder through failure of self-care. Mania may produce exaggerated dress style or colour.
Level of consciousness	Determine whether the patient is alert, lethargic, obtunded, stuporous or comatose.	Suggests significant impairment and inability to fully cooperate with assessment.

Listenable

Activity	Critical Action	Rationale
Orientation (person/ place/time)	Ask the patient what is their name, where they are, and what day, month and year this is.	Orientation forms part of consciousness-level assessment.
Speech/ language	Assess the quality of the patient's verbal responses: speech rate/ volume, converses appropriately, confused conversation, uses inappropriate words, makes sounds only, no sounds.	Speech also forms part of consciousness-level assessment.
Thought process	Note if there is poor interconnection between thoughts, vague thinking, or patient is easily distracted.	These may be expressed by the patient without any other interaction.
Thought content	Listen for phobias, delusions, preoccupations, hallucinations.	Deviations from reality.
Cognition	Note if there is poor ability to organise thoughts or lack of insight.	May be detected during conversational elements.

Assessable

Activity	Critical Action	Rationale
Circumstances	Determine family support, drug use, socioeconomic status, life stressors.	May prompt acute causes of problems or difficulties faced in recovery.
Memory 1	Ask the patient to remember three unrelated objects and repeat them back to you, e.g. apple, table, coin. Record how many trials it took for them to remember.	Cognitive memory testing.
Cognitive ability	Ask the patient to spell the word 'world' backwards or to take 7 away from 100 as many times as they can.	Cognitive assessment.

Mental status assessment continued

Activity	Critical Action	Rationale
Memory 2	Ask the patient if they can remember the three objects that you asked them to remember earlier.	Further cognitive memory testing.
Self-harm	Ask directly if the patient is considering or has considered self-harm.	Self-harm implies immediate risk to patient.
Report	Accurately document/hand over findings.	Accurate record keeping and continuation of care.

Source: *Adapted from Cameron et al., 2009; Finney et al., 2016.*

Formative Clinical Skill Assessment (F-CSAT)

Equipment and resources: Standardised patient; hand decontamination agent; disposable gloves; clinical waste bag; method of documenting results

Associated Clinical Skills: Infection control; Communication; Consent; Assessment using the Glasgow Coma Scale; Assessing the AVPU score

Staff/Student being assessed: _____

Mental status assessment

Activity	Critical Action	Performance				
Safety	Considers risk and safety if patient's behaviour appears bizarre or threatening. Dons personal protection as appropriate.	0	1	2	3	4
Initial approach	When moving towards the patient, notes when they opened their eyes: spontaneously on approach, on verbal exchange, in response to pain, or no response. Obtains consent to continue if possible.	0	1	2	3	4
Behaviour	Notes incongruous behaviour.	0	1	2	3	4
Affect/mood	Notes mood and its appropriateness for the context.	0	1	2	3	4
Grooming/ hygiene	Notes appropriateness/cleanliness of attire and person for the season/ situation.	0	1	2	3	4
Level of consciousness	Determines if patient is alert, lethargic, obtunded, stuporous or comatose.	0	1	2	3	4
Orientation	Asks the patient what is their name, where they are, and what day, month, and year it is.	0	1	2	3	4
Speech/ language	Notes the quality of the patient's verbal responses.	0	1	2	3	4
Thought process	Notes if there is poor interconnection between thoughts, vague thinking, or patient is easily distracted.	0	1	2	3	4
Thought content	Listens for phobias, delusions, preoccupations, hallucinations.	0	1	2	3	4
Cognition	Notes poor ability to organise thoughts or lack of insight.	0	1	2	3	4
Circumstances	Determines family support, drug use, socioeconomic status, life stressors.	0	1	2	3	4
Memory 1	Asks patient to remember three unrelated objects, e.g. apple, table, coin. Records how many trials it takes to remember correctly.	0	1	2	3	4

Mental status assessment continued

Activity	Critical Action	Performance				
Cognitive ability	Asks patient to spell the word 'world' backwards. Records result.	0	1	2	3	4
Memory 2	Asks patient to recall the three objects they were asked to remember earlier. Records result.	0	1	2	3	4
Self-harm	Asks directly if the patient is considering or has considered self-harm.	0	1	2	3	4
Reports	Accurately documents/hands over findings.	0	1	2	3	4

Source: Adapted from Cameron et al., 2009; Finney et al., 2016.

Standard Achieved: (please circle one)

Competent (C)   Not Yet Competent* (NYC)

Staff/Student Name: _____

Assessor (please print name): _____

Signed (Assessor): _____

Date of Assessment: _____

Comments:

*If Not Yet Competent (NYC) a PIP needs to be completed and a repeat of the F-CSAT

Formative Clinical Skill Assessment (F-CSAT) Key

Skill level	Standard of procedure	Quality of performance	Outcome	Level of assistance required
4 Safe for unsupervised practice	Safe Accurate Behaviour is appropriate to context	Confident Accurate Expedient	Achieved intended outcome	No supporting cues* required
3 Requires supervision	Safe Accurate Behaviour is appropriate to context	Confident Accurate Takes longer than required	Achieved intended outcome	Requires occasional supportive cues*
2 Requires assistance	Safe Accurate Behaviour generally appropriate to context	Lacks certainty	Would not have achieved outcome without support	Requires frequent verbal and occasional physical directives in addition to supportive cues*
1 Requires direction	Safe only with guidance Not completely accurate	Unskilled Inefficient	Would not have achieved outcome without support	Requires continuous verbal and frequent physical directive cues*
0 Unsafe	Unsafe Unable to demonstrate behaviour Lack of insight into behaviour appropriate to context	Unskilled	Would not have achieved outcome	Requires continuous verbal and continuous physical directive cues*

*Refers to physical directives or verbal supportive cues

Performance Improvement Plan (PIP)

Please document the agreed education plan and completion timelines for areas assessed as less than 4.

This plan should be presented to assessor prior to commencement of summative assessment.

Where was supervisor support required?	Student summary of deficit. (Why was there a problem?)	Improvement Plan	Completed (Y/N)

Staff/Student Name: _____

Staff/Student Signature: _____

Educator Name: _____

Educator Signature: _____

Summative Clinical Skill Assessment (S-CSAT)

Equipment and resources: Standardised patient; hand decontamination agent; disposable gloves; clinical waste bag; method of documenting results

Associated Clinical Skills: Infection control; Communication; Consent; Assessment using the Glasgow Coma Scale; Assessing the AVPU score

Staff/Student being assessed: _____

- Completed Formative Clinical Skill Assessment (F-CSAT):   **YES   NO**
- Completed Performance Improvement Plan (PIP):   **YES   NO   N/A**

Mental status assessment

Activity	Critical Action	Achieved Without Direction	
Safety	Considers risk and safety if patient's behaviour appears bizarre or threatening. Dons personal protection as appropriate.	NO	YES
Initial approach	When moving towards the patient, notes when they opened their eyes: spontaneously on approach, on verbal exchange, in response to pain, or no response. Obtains consent to continue if possible.	NO	YES
Behaviour	Notes incongruous behaviour.	NO	YES
Affect/mood	Notes mood and its appropriateness for the context.	NO	YES
Level of consciousness	Determines if patient is alert, lethargic, obtunded, stuporous or comatose.	NO	YES
Orientation	Asks the patient what is their name, where they are, and what day, month and year it is.	NO	YES

Mental status assessment continued

Activity	Critical Action	Achieved Without Direction	
Speech/ language	Notes quality of the patient's verbal responses.	NO	YES
Thought process	Notes if there is poor interconnection between thoughts, vague thinking, or patient is easily distracted.	NO	YES
Thought content	Listens for phobias, delusions, preoccupations, hallucinations.	NO	YES
Cognition	Notes poor ability to organise thoughts or lack of insight.	NO	YES
Circumstances	Determines family support, drug use, socioeconomic status, life stressors.	NO	YES
Memory 1	Asks patient to remember three unrelated objects, e.g. apple, table, coin. Records how many trials it took to remember correctly.	NO	YES
Cognitive ability	Asks patient to spell the word 'world' backwards. Record if correct.	NO	YES
Memory 2	Asks patient to recall the three objects they were asked to remember earlier.	NO	YES
Self-harm	Asks directly if the patient is considering or has considered self-harm.	NO	YES
Reports	Accurately documents/hands over findings.	NO	YES

Source: *Adapted from Cameron et al., 2009; Finney et al., 2016.*

Standard Achieved: (please circle one)

Competent (C)   Not Yet Competent* (NYC)

Staff/Student Name: _____

Assessor (please print name): _____

Signed (Assessor): _____

Date of Assessment: _____

Comments:

*If Not Yet Competent (NYC) a PIP needs to be completed and a repeat of the F-CSAT

Clinical findings

Patient/paramedic interaction

Many of the mental status assessment criteria can be assessed without actually contacting and conversing with the patient. Responses including behaviour, affect/mood, grooming/hygiene and level of consciousness can be assessed from a distance. If the patient is alert, speech/language, orientation and cognitive ability/comprehension may also be discernible.

Behavioural responses can vary considerably. Some presentations can be threatening to the paramedic, including mental illness and medical causes. The latter include hypoxia and hypoglycaemia. Always put safety first and consider de-escalation strategies, withdrawing or even not approaching until an alternative plan is devised.

In turn, the paramedic's demeanour has potential to disturb or aggravate the patient. Ensure you show respect, courtesy and patience, both verbally and non-verbally, and are non-judgmental in your approach.

Any patient testing will require some cooperation. This may not be forthcoming in all acute situations, particularly if consciousness is reduced or a medical cause has impaired the patient's capacity.

PRACTICE TIP!

Patients with long-term deterioration of mental status (Alzheimer's disease, dementia) have often developed their own manner of answering questions that may mask that they cannot remember the answer or perhaps understand the question. Consider answers to several questions in context rather than forming conclusions after a single answer.

PRACTICE TIP!

Gain the patient's permission where possible before conducting a mental status assessment, and appropriately document if the situation required performing the assessment without the patient's approval.

TEST YOUR KNOWLEDGE QUESTIONS

1. **Mental status assessment can be divided into three broad elements. What are they?**
    Those that are observable; those that can be heard; those that require discussion.

2. **What does the mnemonic AEIOU TIPS stand for?**
    A Alcohol or other substance Abuse Acidosis
    E Environmental/Epilepsy/Endocrine
    I Infection (meningitis/encephalitis)
    O Overdose/Oxygen deficiency
    U Underdose/Uraemia
    T Trauma/Tumour
    I Insulin (hyper or hypoglycaemia)
    P Psychogenic/Poison
    S Stroke/Shock

3. **What mental status signs are assessable from observation alone?**
    Behaviour; affect/mood; grooming/hygiene; level of consciousness.

4. **What functions require assessment through questioning?**
    Higher cognitive functions, including memory and attention.

5. **To determine a patient's cognitive ability, what should you ask them to do?**
    Spell the word 'world' backwards or take 7 away from 100 as many times as you can.

6. **When can key scene safety information be determined?**
    At any time, including from the call information or from those at scene, even before the ambulance arrives.

7. **What speech quality options can be determined?**
    Speech rate/volume; appropriate conversation; confused conversation; inappropriate word use; sounds only; no sounds.

8. **What thought processes and content can be assessed?**
    Poor interconnection between thoughts; vague thinking; phobias; delusions; preoccupations; hallucinations; ease of distraction.

9. **What is the best way to determine if a patient is considering or has considered self-harm?**
    Ask them directly.

10. **What grooming/hygiene observations can be made?**
    Note the appropriateness of the patient's attire and person for the season/situation, including cleanliness and odour.

References

ABS (Australian Bureau of Statistics), 2015. *Causes of death, Australia, 2012.* Canberra: Australian Bureau of Statistics.

Bennett, M.R., 1997. *The idea of consciousness.* Amsterdam: Harwood Academic Publishers.

Cameron, P., Jelinek, G., Kelly, A.M., Murray, L. and Brown, A.F.T., 2009. *Textbook of adult emergency medicine.* London: Churchill Livingstone.

Finney, G.R., Minagar, A. and Heilman, K.M., 2016. Assessment of mental status. *Neurologic Clinics*, 34(1), 1–16.

Folstein, M.F., Folstein, S.E. and McHugh, P.R., 1975. 'Mini-mental state': a practical method for grading the cognitive state of patients for the clinician. *Journal of Psychiatric Research*, 12(3), 189–198.

Martini, F.H., Nath, J.L. and Bartholomew, E.F., 2015. *Fundamentals of anatomy and physiology.* New Jersey: Prentice Hall, pp. 538–557.

Sanello, A., Gausche-Hill, M., Mulkerin, W., Sporer, K.A., Brown, J.F., Koenig, K.L., Rudnick, E.M., Salvucci, A.A. and Gilbert, G.H., 2018. Altered mental status: current evidence-based recommendations for prehospital care. *Western Journal of Emergency Medicine*, 19(3), p. 529.

Trzepacz, P.T., Hochstetler, H., Wang, S., Walker, B. and Saykin, A.J., 2015. Relationship between the Montreal Cognitive Assessment and Mini-mental State Examination for assessment of mild cognitive impairment in older adults. *BMC Geriatrics*, 15(1), 107.

Functional capacity assessment

Jeff Kenneally

Chapter objectives

At the end of this chapter the reader will be able to:

1. Describe the rationale for functional capacity assessment (FCA)
2. Demonstrate the method of FCA
3. Accurately report on assessment findings
4. Identify pathologies associated with abnormal functional capacity

Resources required for this assessment

- Patient able to respond to assessment
- Method of documenting results

Skill matrix

This assessment requires:

- Communication (CS 1.5)
- Consent (CS 1.6)

This assessment is a component of:

- Patient assessment (Chapter 2)

Introduction

Functional capacity assessment (FCA) provides a guide to a person's ability to perform daily life activities. It is not specific to any particular disease but can indicate illness or functional decline. Decline reduces quality of life and leads to poor outcomes. Although paramedics do not formally assess functional capacity, they have a unique opportunity to observe and report on the issues identified for ongoing care. This chapter discusses functional capacity prehospital assessment.

Anatomy and physiology

Many higher brain processes, including thinking, planning and problem solving, occur in the cerebral cortex frontal lobe. This is also responsible for motor control, personality and emotions. The parietal lobe has a role in sensory perception, concentration, language comprehension, writing, speech and ability to navigate.

Memory results from multiple central nervous inputs, including the cortex, hippocampus, thalamus and basal nuclei. Declarative memory recalls learned information, such as names and events, and relates to conscious thoughts. Nondeclarative memory recalls skills and experiences, accessing them subconsciously as emotional responses.

Walking allows the performance of daily activities and independent living. The cerebellum receives information from visual and equilibrium inputs and proprioceptors throughout the body to establish body position. This allows it to determine the strength and direction of motor responses from the motor cortex. A functional peripheral nervous system and skeletal muscle are required for the response; steadiness and speed of gait are important measures of the system's overall effectiveness.

Clinical rationale

Many patient assessments are based on the failure of one or more body systems during acute deterioration or an emergency. However, not all deteriorations are acute; many cause long-term lifestyle changes and difficulties, contributing to accidents and injuries. Early recognition and assistance can change the patient's quality of life. Prompts for issues with functional capacity include multiple medical conditions, a decrease in activity or the ability to communicate, or a request for transfer into supported living due to the patient's frailty.

Some changes may be detectable only by assessing the performance of specific tasks, including observing daily activities within the home. Paramedics are frequently the only people to do this, so recognition and reporting are vital. This is easily overlooked during emergency attendance.

The aged are particularly vulnerable to general deterioration as they accumulate comorbidities. Cognitive, physical and functional decline limits the ability to perform activities and avoid future mishap or injury (Jekel et al., 2015; Jyrkka et al., 2011; Millan-Calenti et al., 2010; Peel et al., 2013; Roedl et al., 2016; Vagetti et al., 2014).

Much of this assessment is through observation or simple questioning (Jekel et al., 2015; Oresanya et al., 2014; Partridge et al., 2014; Peel et al., 2013; Roedl et al., 2016). Partners and family members can help with this. Assessment includes:
1. Identifying impediments to basic daily living activities
2. Evaluating the patient's ability to get up from a sitting position
3. Evaluating the patient's gait
4. Establishing if falls occur, how often and the possible causes
5. Assessing for cognitive impairment
6. Assessing for major depressive illness

This assessment has the potential to be difficult and demeaning for the recipient. It is not easy being confronted with decline, so it is important to communicate with respect and provide emotional support throughout.

Uninterrupted communication is important for gathering accurate information. Establish whether there is any hearing or visual impairment to avoid contributing to performance difficulties. Ensure that lighting is adequate and turn off distracting or interfering radio or television. Allow sufficient time for the patient to respond, remembering that taking longer does not always indicate impairment. If using written communication, ensure the print size is suitable.

Activities of daily living

Activities of daily living are divisible three ways (Roedl et al., 2016; Vagetti et al., 2014):
1. *Basic life functions* include dressing/undressing, meal preparation, bathing and toilet activities, operating appliances, including television and telephone, and self-administering medication.
2. *Ordered life functions* include the ability to maintain a clean home, wash clothing and administer basic finances, such as paying bills. These are sacrificed as difficulties increase.

3. *Advanced social activities* include walking out on the street, driving a vehicle, using public transport and going shopping.

An inability to perform ordered life functions and advanced social activities suggests a need for home support (Vagetti et al., 2014). Given that few people observe a person within their own home, report the cleanliness of the home and any difficulties the house itself presents. House modifications, including steps, rails, tap fittings and bathroom appliances, can improve a person's quality of life.

Any restriction of basic life functions is more significant, as it indicates a failure of the person's ability to care for themselves and live independently (Vagetti et al., 2014). A decline can prompt them to avoid requests for assistance for fear of losing their independence. Where possible, assert that alternatives and supports are available to enhance independent living rather than remove it (Vagetti et al., 2014).

Ask the person how they dress, prepare meals and get to the toilet and bath, and what their medication regime is. Ask them about any difficulties they experience, and incorporate into your assessment any information/clarification provided by family members or carers. Observe the patient's use of their kitchen, bathroom and toilet. Ask how they organise their daily finances and about their ability to go shopping. Observe their clothing and the general tidiness of the home.

Ability to stand up, walk, sit down

The ability to stand up, walk and sit down again is easy to assess and observe using the Timed Up and Go (TUG) test (Jacobs and Fox, 2008). Any difficulty in performing these actions will challenge daily activities.

Observe the person rising from a commonly used chair, move a short distance (about 3 m) before turning and sitting down again. Time the action and monitor any difficulties throughout. It is typically achievable in <20 seconds; failure to achieve success in this timeframe suggests a difficulty with normal daily activities and an increased risk of falls.

Make note of the key steps, including the person's ability to sit correctly and move from sitting to standing, their gait, and their ability to turn and sit again (Elsawy and Higgins, 2011).

Gait and falls assessment

Gait and falls assessment is a rudimentary evaluation tool (Peel et al., 2013). The ability to move around defines activities including shopping, social activities, food preparation and basic toilet and bathroom functions.

With age, walking typically becomes slow and difficult. By the age of 80, as many as one in two people has an observable difficulty in walking (Leite Vieira et al., 2013). Contributing factors include arthritis, neuromuscular diseases and balance and coordination difficulties (Leite Vieira et al., 2013). Assistance is often needed, ranging from devices such as frames through to carer support.

A severe complication of gait deterioration is falls, which increase the risk of death and serious injury. Falls impose on carers and emergency services. Preceding medical causes, including syncope, warrant medical assessment.

Assessing gait and falls risk can be through questioning patient and family members/carers and by observation. Ask the person whether they feel unsteady during walking or require assistance to move around. Ask whether they have had falls or felt close to falling. During the standing-walking-sitting assessment, observe their gait (Elsawy and Higgins, 2011).

Cognitive impairment

Cognitive impairment includes difficulty with thinking clearly, communicating thoughts, understanding surrounding events, memory/recall, recognition and orientation. Confusion, agitation and frustrated mood changes can indicate underlying difficulties. The usual cause of cognitive impairment is dementia or depressive mood disorder (Oresanya et al., 2014).

The prevalence of cognitive impairment rises from the age of 60 to almost one in two people after age 90. It causes functional problems including medication compliance and increased caregiver difficulties (Jekel et al., 2015).

Cognitive assessment begins with evaluating the ability to provide basic person, time and place orientation. Ask the person if they can provide their name and state where and when they are. Ask the patient and family/carers if confusion or memory difficulties have been observed.

Challenge further. Place three clearly recognisable but unrelated items in front of the person and have them identify them. Remove the items and then distract the person with a suitable diversion; for example, have them draw the time on a circular clock face. After a minute has passed, ask if they can recall the three items you showed them earlier. Recall of one or no items suggests cognitive impairment, including dementia, while recalling two to three items suggests little if any cognitive impairment (Elsawy and Higgins, 2011).

Depressive illness

Depressive illness is common among the elderly and is frequently observed in residential and aged care settings. Contributing factors include loneliness, alcoholism and the effects of comorbid illnesses. It is a compounding problem, as quality of life can contribute to depression, with mood in turn lowering quality of life and participation (Oresanya et al., 2014).

Depression can be difficult to differentiate from dementia, as there can be overlapping memory or concentration difficulties. Before deciding whether any decline is cognitive or physical, consider mood disorder as the possible cause.

While depression requires professional diagnosis, questioning can indicate whether it may be present. Ask the person if they have been feeling sad or low in mood. If so, is this new or have they been feeling like this for some time? Ask whether they have felt hopelessness or worthlessness, or if they have lost interest in or unable to gain pleasure from life activities. Do they have any other unusual feelings, including anxiety or feeling stressed? Ask family member/carers for their input into these questions too.

Clinical skill assessment process

The following section outlines the clinical skill assessment tools that should be used to determine a student's ability to demonstrate assessment of functional capacity.

1. Clinical Skill Work Instruction
2. Formative Clinical Skill Assessment (F-CSAT)
3. Performance Improvement Plan (PIP)
4. Summative Clinical Skill Assessment (S-CSAT)
(5. Direct Observation of Procedural Skills (DOPS) – see Chapter 1.1)

Clinical Skill Work Instruction

Equipment and resources: Patient able to respond to assessment; method of documenting results

Associated Clinical Skills: Communication; Consent

Functional capacity assessment

Activity	Critical Action	Rationale
Prepare patient	Begin with the patient seated in a chair they normally use.	Assessment includes standing from this position.
	Check the patient can understand your spoken language and has no hearing impairment. If necessary, use alternative communication method, including an interpreter.	Patient must be able to understand questioning.
	Inform the patient that the examination includes a series of routine questions.	The patient needs to be cooperative and at ease. The questions may seem odd.

Functional capacity assessment continued		
Activity	**Critical Action**	**Rationale**
Assess activities of living	Observe ability to undertake basic life functions, including dressing, preparing meals, use bathroom/toilet and self-administer medication. Where possible, have the patient demonstrate part of each activity.	To assess basic living ability.
	Ask patient and family member/carers about difficulties performing any basic life functions.	
	Observe ability for ordered life function, including maintaining home cleanliness, washing clothes and paying bills.	To assess ordered life function.
	Ask patient and family member/carer about ordered life function difficulties.	
	Ask patient and family member/carer if there is any difficulty walking out on the street, driving a vehicle or going shopping.	To assess advanced life function.
Assess standing from sitting and gait (Timed Up and Go)	Commence timing this part of the assessment. From sitting normally in a chair, have the patient rise to standing. Observe any difficulty.	The stand, walk and sit again test should take <20 seconds.
	Observe any gait difficulty walking forwards approximately 3 m from the chair.	
	Have the patient turn and return to the chair. Observe any difficulty.	
	Have them sit back down on the chair. Observe any difficulty. Cease timing.	
	Ask patient and family member/carer about any unsteadiness during walking or if any assistance has been required.	
	Ask patient and family member/carer if there have been any recent falls or feelings of near falling.	
Assess for cognitive impairment	Ask patient and family member/carer if they have observed any patient orientation or memory difficulties.	Ability to recall 0–1 items suggests cognitive impairment. Ability to recall 2–3 items suggests little, if any, cognitive impairment.
	Place three recognisable but unrelated items in front of patient and have them identify them. Remove items from view.	
	Provide suitable distraction. For example, distract the patient by having them draw a simple circular clock face, including drawing the current time.	
	After 1 minute, have them recall the three items observed earlier. Note number of items recalled.	
Assess for depression	Ask patient and family member/carer if patient has been feeling sad, hopeless, worthless or low mood, or has lost interest in/is unable to gain pleasure from life activities. Ask if they have any unusual feelings, including stress or anxiety. Ask what activities interest or entertain them during the day. Establish how long any negative responses have been going on for.	Assists differentiation from cognitive impairment.
Report	Accurately document/hand over findings.	Accurate record kept and continuity of patient care.

Source: *Adapted from Jekel et al., 2015; Oresanya et al., 2014; Partridge et al., 2014; Peel et al., 2013; Roedl et al., 2015.*

Formative Clinical Skill Assessment (F-CSAT)

Equipment and resources: Patient able to respond to assessment; method of documenting results

Associated Clinical Skills: Communication; Consent

Staff/Student being assessed: _____

Functional capacity assessment

Activity	Critical Action	Participant Performance				
Prepares patient	Begins with patient seated in a chair they normally use.	0	1	2	3	4
	Checks that patient can understand spoken language and has no hearing impairment. If necessary, uses alternative communication method, including interpreter.	0	1	2	3	4
	Informs intention to ask a series of routine questions as part of normal examination.	0	1	2	3	4
Assesses activities of basic living	Observes living area for ability to undertake basic life functions. Where possible, has the patient demonstrate part of each activity. Asks patient and family member/carer if there have been any difficulties performing any basic life functions.	0	1	2	3	4
	Observes house for ordered life function activities. Asks patient and family member/carer if there has been any difficulty with ordered life function activities.	0	1	2	3	4
	Asks patient and family member/carer if there has been any difficulty with advanced life function activities.	0	1	2	3	4
Assesses standing from sitting and gait (Timed Up and Go)	Commences timing this part of the assessment. With patient sitting normally in a chair, has them rise to stand. Observes patient gait walking forwards approximately 3 m. Has patient turn and return to the chair. Has patient sit back down on the chair. Observes any difficulties. Ceases timing. Asks patient and family member/carer about any unsteadiness walking or assistance required. Asks patient and family member/carer if there have been any recent falls or feelings of near falling.	0	1	2	3	4
Assesses for cognitive impairment	Asks family member/carer if they have observed any patient orientation or memory difficulties.	0	1	2	3	4
	Places three recognisable but unrelated items in front of the patient and has them identify them. Removes items from view.	0	1	2	3	4
	Provides suitable distraction. For example, distracts the patient by having them draw a simple circular clock face indicating current time.	0	1	2	3	4
	After 1 minute, has patient recall the three items observed earlier. Notes number of items recalled.	0	1	2	3	4
Assesses for depression	Asks patient and family member/carer if patient has been feeling sad, hopeless, worthless or low in mood, or if they have lost interest in or are unable to gain pleasure from life activities. Asks if they have any unusual feelings, including stress or anxiety. Asks what activities interest or entertain them during the day. Establishes duration of any negative responses.	0	1	2	3	4
Reports	Accurately documents/hands over findings.	0	1	2	3	4

Source: *Adapted from Jekel et al., 2015; Oresanya et al., 2014; Partridge et al., 2014; Peel et al., 2013; Roedl et al., 2015.*

Standard Achieved: (please circle one)

Competent (C)   Not Yet Competent* (NYC)

Staff/Student Name: _____

Assessor (please print name)**:** _____

Signed (Assessor)**:** _____

Date of Assessment: _____

Comments:

*If Not Yet Competent (NYC) a PIP needs to be completed and a repeat of the F-CSAT

Formative Clinical Skill Assessment (F-CSAT) Key

Skill level	Standard of procedure	Quality of performance	Outcome	Level of assistance required
4 Safe for unsupervised practice	Safe Accurate Behaviour is appropriate to context	Confident Accurate Expedient	Achieved intended outcome	No supporting cues* required
3 Requires supervision	Safe Accurate Behaviour is appropriate to context	Confident Accurate Takes longer than required	Achieved intended outcome	Requires occasional supportive cues*
2 Requires assistance	Safe Accurate Behaviour generally appropriate to context	Lacks certainty	Would not have achieved outcome without support	Requires frequent verbal and occasional physical directives in addition to supportive cues*
1 Requires direction	Safe only with guidance Not completely accurate	Unskilled Inefficient	Would not have achieved outcome without support	Requires continuous verbal and frequent physical directive cues*
0 Unsafe	Unsafe Unable to demonstrate behaviour Lack of insight into behaviour appropriate to context	Unskilled	Would not have achieved outcome	Requires continuous verbal and continuous physical directive cues*

*Refers to physical directives or verbal supportive cues

Performance Improvement Plan (PIP)

Please document the agreed education plan and completion timelines for areas assessed as less than 4.

This plan should be presented to assessor prior to commencement of summative assessment.

Where was supervisor support required?	Student summary of deficit. (Why was there a problem?)	Improvement Plan	Completed (Y/N)

Staff/Student Name: _____

Staff/Student Signature: _____

Educator Name: _____

Educator Signature: _____

Summative Clinical Skill Assessment (S-CSAT)

Equipment and resources: Patient able to respond to assessment; method of documenting results

Associated Clinical Skills: Communication; Consent

Staff/Student being assessed: _____

- Completed Formative Clinical Skill Assessment (F-CSAT):   **YES   NO**
- Completed Performance Improvement Plan (PIP):   **YES   NO   N/A**

Functional capacity assessment

Activity	Critical Action	Achieved Without Direction	
Prepares patient	Begins with patient seated in a chair they normally use.	NO	YES
	Checks that patient can understand spoken language and has no hearing impairment. If necessary, uses an alternative method of communication, including interpreter.	NO	YES
	Informs intention to ask a series of routine questions as part of normal examination.	NO	YES
Assesses activities of basic living	Observes living area for ability to undertake basic life functions. Where possible, has the patient demonstrate part of each activity. Asks patient and family member/carer if there have been any difficulties performing any basic life functions.	NO	YES
	Observes house for ordered life function activities. Asks patient and family member/carer if there has been any difficulty with ordered life function activities.	NO	YES
	Asks patient and family member/carer if there has been any difficulty with advanced life function activities.	NO	YES

Functional capacity assessment continued

Activity	Critical Action	Achieved Without Direction	
Assesses standing from sitting and gait (Timed Up and Go)	Commences timing this assessment part. With patient sitting normally in a chair, has them rise to stand. Observes patient gait walking forwards approximately 3 m. Has patient turn and return to the chair. Has patient sit back down on the chair. Observes any difficulties. Ceases timing. Asks patient and family member/carer about any unsteadiness walking or assistance required. Asks patient and family member/carer if there have been any recent falls or feelings of near falling.	NO	YES
Assesses for cognitive impairment	Asks family member/carer if they have observed any patient orientation or memory difficulties.	NO	YES
	Places three recognisable but unrelated items in front of the patient and has them identify them. Removes items from view.	NO	YES
	Provides suitable distraction. For example, distracts the patient by having them draw a simple circular clock face indicating current time.	NO	YES
	After 1 minute, has patient recall the three items observed earlier. Notes number of items recalled.	NO	YES
Assesses for depression	Asks patient and family member/carer if patient has been feeling sad, hopeless, worthless or low in mood, or if they have lost interest in or are unable to gain pleasure from life activities. Asks if they have any unusual feelings, including stress or anxiety. Asks what activities interest or entertain them during the day. Establishes duration of any negative responses.	NO	YES
Reports	Accurately documents/hands over findings.	NO	YES

Source: *Adapted from Jekel et al., 2015; Oresanya et al., 2014; Partridge et al., 2014; Peel et al., 2013; Roedl et al., 2015.*

Standard Achieved: (please circle one)

Competent (C)   Not Yet Competent* (NYC)

Staff/Student Name: _____

Assessor (please print name): _____

Signed (Assessor): _____

Date of Assessment: _____

Comments:

*If Not Yet Competent (NYC) a PIP needs to be completed and a repeat of the F-CSAT

Clinical findings

Acute cognitive changes

Cognitive impairment is an observation rather than a specific diagnosis. It must be differentiated from acute consciousness changes including medication effects, illicit drug actions, hypoxia, hypercapnia, hypoglycaemia or infection. These can occur quickly, but are often able to be remedied (Elsawy and Higgins, 2011; Jekel et al., 2015; Oresanya et al., 2014).

Multi-pharmacy

Medication interactions can have a significant influence on functional status. There is often no single oversight over multiple practitioner prescriptions (Elsawy and Higgins, 2011; Jyrkka et al., 2011).

Alcoholism

Alcohol abuse can lead to acute presentations of poor balance, falls and injuries, and reduce the ability for self-care.

Social circumstances

Helpful neighbours, shared family accommodation or live-in carers can partly offset issues with functional capacity (Elsawy and Higgins, 2011).

PRACTICE TIP!

During the assessment, make note of any limitations and difficulties the patient's house provides. A lack of ramps, awkward tap fittings, unsuitable furniture and poorly designed bathrooms are examples of correctable options.

PRACTICE TIP!

When making a functional assessment, explain why you are asking seemingly odd questions to help gain the patient's full cooperation.

PRACTICE TIP!

Where possible, first establish the normal expected baseline for each individual. Acute changes or rapid deteriorations may suggest remediable illness.

PRACTICE TIP!

FCA may not contribute greatly to emergency decision making. However, it can provide information for decisions about recovery, rehabilitation, and changes to avoid the recurrence of injury or illness.

TEST YOUR KNOWLEDGE QUESTIONS

1. **What are the six elements of FCA?**
    Identify: any impediments to basic daily living activities; the ability to get up from sitting position; gait; the occurrence of falls, including how often and any possible cause; cognitive impairment; major depressive illness.

2. **What are the five basic life functions that reflect activities of daily living?**
    Dressing/undressing; meal preparation; bathing/toilet activities; operating appliances, including television and telephone; medication self-administration.

3. **Which ordered life functions can be assessed as activities of daily living?**
    Ability to: maintain house cleanliness; wash clothes; administer basic finances, such as paying bills.

4. **How quickly should a person be able to complete the stand up, walk and sit down test?**
    <20 seconds.

5. **What are three methods by which gait and falls risk can be assessed?**
    Patient questioning; family member/carer questioning; direct observation.

6. **What difficulties are considered in cognitive assessment?**
    The ability to think clearly; communication; thought processes; understanding what is happening around them; memory and recall; recognition; orientation to person, time and place; confusion; agitation; frustrated changes in mood.

7. **How many objects on the three-item recognition test must be recalled to suggest normal cognition?**
    Two to three.

8. **Which clinical problems are difficult to differentiate from depression?**
    Dementia has an overlapping appearance of memory or concentration difficulties. Before deciding whether any decline is cognitive or of a physical nature, mood disorder must be considered.

9. **What are the indications for FCA?**
    Multiple medical conditions impacting on life; a decrease in the normal ability to communicate or be active; any request for a move into supported living due to frailty or advancing age.

10. **What acute cognitive changes should be considered during assessment?**
    Medication side effects; hypoxia; hypercapnia; hypoglycaemia; infection; illicit drug actions.

References

Elsawy, B. and Higgins, K.E., 2011. The geriatric assessment. *American Family Physician*, 83(1), 48–56.

Jacobs, M. and Fox, T., 2008. Using the 'Timed Up and Go/TUG' test to predict risk of falls. *Assisted Living Consult*, 2, 16–18.

Jekel, K., Damian, M., Wattmo, C., Hausner, L., Bullock, R., Connelly, P.J., Dubois, B., Eriksdotter, M., Ewers, M., Graessel, E. and Kramberger, M.G., 2015. Mild cognitive impairment and deficits in instrumental activities of daily living: a systematic review. *Alzheimer's Research & Therapy*, 7(1), 7.

Jyrkkä, J., Enlund, H., Lavikainen, P., Sulkava, R. and Hartikainen, S., 2011. Association of polypharmacy with nutritional status, functional ability and cognitive capacity over a three-year period in an elderly population. *Pharmacoepidemiology and Drug Safety*, 20(5), 514–522.

Leite-Vieira, D.C., Tajra, V., da Cunha, D., Lopes de Farias, D., de Oliveira, A., Teixeira, T.G., Rodrigues-Martins, W., de Oliveira, M. and Prestes, J., 2013. Decreased functional capacity and muscle strength in elderly women with metabolic syndrome. *Clinical Interventions in Aging*, 8, 1377–1386.

Millán-Calenti, J.C., Tubío, J., Pita-Fernández, S., González-Abraldes, I., Lorenzo, T., Fernández-Arruty, T. and Maseda, A., 2010. Prevalence of functional disability in activities of daily living (ADL),

instrumental activities of daily living (IADL) and associated factors, as predictors of morbidity and mortality. *Archives of Gerontology and Geriatrics*, 50(3), 306–310.

Oresanya, L.B., Lyons, W.L. and Finlayson, E., 2014. Preoperative assessment of the older patient: a narrative review. *JAMA*, 311(20), 2110–2120.

Partridge, J.S., Harari, D., Martin, F.C. and Dhesi, J.K., 2014. The impact of pre-operative comprehensive geriatric assessment on postoperative outcomes in older patients undergoing scheduled surgery: a systematic review. *Anaesthesia*, 69(s1), 8–16.

Peel, N.M., Kuys, S.S. and Klein, K., 2013. Gait speed as a measure in geriatric assessment in clinical settings: a systematic review. *The Journals of Gerontology Series A: Biological Sciences and Medical Sciences*, 68(1), 39–46.

Roedl, K.J., Wilson, L.S. and Fine, J., 2016. A systematic review and comparison of functional assessments of community-dwelling elderly patients. *Journal of the American Association of Nurse Practitioners*, 28(3), pp. 160–169.

Vagetti, G.C., Barbosa Filho, V.C., Moreira, N.B., Oliveira, V.D., Mazzardo, O. and Campos, W.D., 2014. Association between physical activity and quality of life in the elderly: a systematic review, 2000–2012. *Revista Brasileira de Psiquiatria*, 36(1), 76–88.

Bibliography

Craft, J., Gordon, C., Huether, S.E., McCance, K.L. and Brashers, V.L., 2015. *Understanding pathophysiology (ANZ adaptation)*. Sydney: Elsevier.

McCance, K.L. and Huether, S.E., 2015. *Pathophysiology: the biologic basis for disease in adults and children*. Sydney: Elsevier.

2.16 | Pain assessment

Joelene Gott and Jeff Kenneally

Chapter objectives

At the end of this chapter the reader will be able to:

1. Describe the rationale for pain assessment
2. Demonstrate assessing pain
3. Accurately report findings

Resources required for this assessment

- Standardised patient
- Hand decontamination agent
- Disposable gloves
- Method of documenting results

Skill matrix

This assessment requires:
- Infection control (CS 1.3)
- Communication (CS 1.5)
- Consent (CS 1.6)

This assessment is a component of:
- Patient assessment (Chapter 2)

Introduction

The International Association for the Study of Pain (IASP, 2018) describes pain as 'an unpleasant sensory and emotional experience associated with actual or potential tissue damage, or described in terms of such damage'. It is important for the body in identifying physical threats, allocating an appropriate level of priority to them and providing a suitable response (Vlaeyen et al., 2016).

Assessing pain can be difficult, as it is individually subjective. It is important to understand the complexities around pain experiences, including emotion, cognition, motivation and prior history.

This chapter discusses paramedic assessment of the patient in pain.

Anatomy and physiology

Pain can be acute or chronic. It is a major reason for paramedic attendance, and the provision of analgesia is one of the most common interventions.

There are different types of pain. *Nociceptive pain* is the most common, produced by noxious stimuli of the peripheral nervous system, including temperature, pressure or injury.

Neuropathic pain, caused by injury or disease of the nervous system itself, feels like it is coming from where the affected nerve innervates. Examples include herpes zoster infections, multiple sclerosis and nerve compression from tumour.

Psychogenic pain is pain that is reported, including severe and persistent pain, but has no apparent underlying pathology.

There are four basic processes in nociception: transduction, transmission, perception and modulation. Nociceptors are distributed in somatic and visceral structures including the skin, muscles, connective tissue, bones, joints, gastrointestinal tract and visceral organs (Wood, 2008).

Pain impulses are transmitted from the site via the spinal cord to the thalamus, cortex and brain, provoking responses. Pain perception becomes a conscious experience, with the affective-motivational, sensory-discriminative, emotional and behavioural components being different for each individual.

Recognising, describing and locating pain varies with origin. *Visceral pain* is 'organ' or internal pain. It is comparatively vague and diffuse, since organs have less innervation and feed into ganglion and multiple spinal cord segments. In effect, the body 'loses' the problem specificity. *Somatic pain* is external and, in contrast to visceral pain, is easily located and describable, as it links directly to a specific spinal cord segment (Noda and Ikusaka, 2012). *Referred pain* is felt in a different part of the body to where the actual problem is.

Interpreting pain then communicating its presence requires sufficient cognitive ability. Small children, intellectually disabled people and those who are cognitively/intellectually impaired can all have difficulty in communicating that they have pain.

Clinical rationale

Pain can be localised or generalised, and mild through to severe. Paramedic variables include context, experience, distractions and bias. The assessment of pain requires clinical judgment, considering multiple patient variables to minimise the potential for error.

History

Begin the pain assessment by asking about the patient's history. Is there known illness or injury (acute or chronic) that could be causing them pain? Has the patient complained of pain? Do they acknowledge they have pain when asked? Patient self-reporting is the most important means of identifying pain (Chow et al., 2016; Garra et al., 2010; Schofield and Abdullah, 2018).

Evaluation

Determine the location of the pain by asking the patient to locate it on their body or, if easier, by pointing to your own body. Children can point to the location on a doll or bear toy. If effective, the patient can simply describe the location of their pain.

Ask whether the pain radiates to any other part of the body, and gain a description of the pain. Also ask the patient about when the pain started; whether there is any known association with the onset of pain; and if anything worsens or aggravates the pain, or, conversely, if there has been any factor that can provide any relief from the pain (Johnson et al., 2015).

Verbal pain score

Determine the severity of pain, where possible, using the patient's own rating. Verbal numerical rating scores are one method (Ismail et al., 2015; Jennings et al., 2009; Lord, 2009) commonly used for emergency triage (Vuille et al., 2018). Have the patient rate their pain numerically, using 0 (no pain) to 10 (the worst pain the patient can

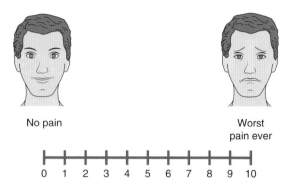

Figure 2.16.1 Visual analogue scale

Instruct the patient to point to the position on the line between the faces to indicate how much pain they are currently feeling. The far left end indicates 'no pain' and the far right end indicates 'worst pain ever'.

Source: *Grantham, H., Boyd, L., Johnson, M. and Eastwood, K., 2015, Paramedic principles and practice ANZ: a clinical reasoning approach (Chapter 28, Figure 28.2), Elsevier.*

imagine) to provide an empirical score that allows you to evaluate the trend and changes in their condition.

Although this method is effective, it can prove difficult to explain to some patients how to use it. An alternative method is to ask the patient to describe the severity of their pain as mild, moderate or severe (the verbal descriptor scale) (Lord, 2009).

However, it is difficult to determine the presence or severity of pain in aphasic patients, and the results are unreliable (de Vries et al., 2017).

Visual analogue scale

One alternative to the verbal pain score is to use an incrementally marked line and ask the patient to point to their pain level (Fig. 2.16.1). This is as effective as verbal scoring (Ismail et al., 2015).

Faces can be added to the line, ranging from a neutral expression to a grimace. The FACES pain scale is designed for use with child patients. It has six faces, ranging from smiling to unhappy/crying (Fig. 2.16.2), with each representing increasing pain. Explain to the child that the first face represents no pain, the last the worst pain they can imagine. In between is 'mild', 'moderate', 'a lot', then 'very bad'. The child selects the pain they feel (Wong and Baker, 1988). To improve the child's understanding of the process, briefly describe what each face might represent.

These methods are less reliable where the patient has a cognitive impairment (Schofield and Abdullah, 2018) and for smaller children, who are unable to understand the directions or the abstract concept of 'the worst possible pain' (Garra et al., 2010).

Physiological signs and behavioural responses do not require active patient input into the assessment. Behavioural responses are useful to correlate with cooperative findings or as an alternative method where there is reduced cooperation, including coma, cognitive impairment, language and age barriers (Lord, 2009).

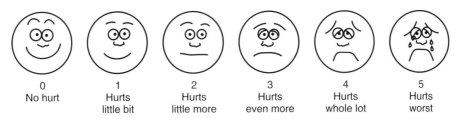

Figure 2.16.2 The FACES pain scale
Source: *Hockenberry M.J. and Wilson, D., 2015,* Wong's nursing care of infants and children, *10th edn, Mosby.*

Table 2.16.1 The PAINAD pain assessment tool

Behaviour	0	1	2	Score
Facial expression	Smiling or neutral	Sad, frowning	Eyes closed, grimacing, wincing	
Body language	Relaxed	Tense, distressed, restless, pacing	Rigid body, fists clenched, knees pulled up posture, localising, guarding, pushing away, striking out	
Breathing independent of vocalisation	Normal	Occasionally laboured or hyperventilating	Noisy laboured breathing and continued hyperventilation	
Negative vocalisation	Normal	Occasional moan/groan	Repeated calling out, loud moaning, crying, troubled	
Consolable	Calm	Distracted or reassured easily by voice/touch	Unable to console or distract	
Total				

Source: *Adapted from Warden et al., 2003.*

Physiological signs

The evaluation of physiological vital signs lacks specificity. Heart rate, blood pressure, respiratory rate and diaphoresis can all be altered by an underlying illness, anxiety or a response to the surrounding stimuli, as well as by pain (Chanques et al., 2014; McGuire et al., 2016). Vital signs do not reliably change with pain, so they are not assessed specifically for that purpose (Arbour et al., 2014; Arbour and Gelinas, 2010; Daoust et al., 2016; Gelinas et al., 2017; Kapoustina et al., 2014; Lord and Woollard, 2010).

Behavioural responses

Despite having common pain processing pathways, individuals present differently. Pain is a dominant cause of the behavioural responses that are usable in assessment, even though these responses lack specificity for pain alone (McGuire et al., 2016; Riddell et al., 2016; Thrane et al., 2016). Facial expressions are particularly reliable signs of pain (Oosterman et al., 2016), and body language/posture is also useful. Undesired behaviour, such as agitation or aggression, may be caused by undiagnosed pain (Malara et al., 2016).

Behavioural features have increased significance where verbal interrogation is not possible or reliable. This is so for infants and cognitively impaired patients who lack understanding of the concepts required to report or describe their pain or use numerical pain scores (Chanques et al., 2014; Georgiou et al., 2015; Jones and Mitchell, 2015; Lichtner et al., 2014; Ngu et al., 2015; Quinn et al., 2015).

Interpreting behavioural observations is most reliable when it is supported by someone who knows the patient, including parents, carers or nurses (Lichtner et al., 2014).

Pain in sedated patients is difficult to assess. It can go unrecognised and unmanaged and be exacerbated by movement or performing procedures. Recognition of pain allows the use of appropriate analgesia instead of further sedation (Chanques et al., 2014; Georgiou et al., 2014).

Numerous comparable pain assessment tools exist. None are universally used, as they all have criteria for behavioural observations (Lichtner et al., 2014; van der Steen et al., 2015). Many have criteria suited to palliative, dementia and end-of-life care that are not necessarily directly translatable to emergency or prehospital care.

Pain Assessment in Advanced Dementia scale

The Pain Assessment in Advanced Dementia (PAINAD) scale (Table 2.16.1) evaluates five behaviours associated with pain and its severity (Fry et al., 2017; Jordan et al., 2011; Warden et al., 2003; Zwakhalen et al., 2006). Each criterion scores 0 for normal, 1 for intermediate and 2 for strong response. The pain scores are 0–1 for no pain, 2–4 for light pain, 5–6 for moderate pain and 7–10 for severe pain (Malara et al., 2016). Though the scale was devised

Table 2.16.2 The FLACC pain scale

Behaviour	0	1	2	Score
Face	Normal expression	Grimacing, frowning	Clenched jaw, quivering chin	
Legs	Normal posture	Restless, uneasy	Kicking, legs drawn	
Activity	Normal activity	Squirming, tense	Arched, rigid	
Cry	Not crying (awake or asleep)	Complaining, crying	Screaming	
Consolable	Content	Reassured by hugging/distraction	Difficult/unable to console	
Total				

Source: *Adapted from Merkel et al., 1997.*

for dementia patients, its utility has been supported in critical-care use (Paulson-Conger et al., 2011).

Other observable changes include interactions and eating habits. Pain can affect mood, energy, enjoyment, activities or sleep (Reid et al., 2015). These criteria are absent from the PAINAD scale, reducing its usefulness at identifying subtle pain signs. However, this is more problematic for the long-term care of non-verbal patients than it is for the short-term needs of paramedics (Herr et al., 2006).

Facial and body language signs are strongly indicative of acute pain in assessing non-communicative critical-care patients (Gelinas et al., 2017; Al Darwish et al., 2016; Chanques et al., 2014; Georgiou et al., 2015; McGuire et al., 2016; Rijkenberg et al., 2015).

FLACC scale

The Faces, Legs, Activity, Cry, Consolable (FLACC) scale (Table 2.16.2) was originally devised to assess pain in smaller children (Merkel et al., 1997). Each feature scores 0 for normal, 1 for intermediate and 2 for intense response (Crellin et al., 2015; Ge et al., 2015; Kochman et al., 2017; McGuire et al., 2016; Pedersen et al., 2015). The total of the scores indicates pain severity (Merkel et al., 1997).

Clinical skill assessment process

The following section outlines the clinical skills assessment tools that should be used to determine a student's ability to demonstrate accurate patient pain assessment.
1. Clinical Skill Work Instruction
2. Formative Clinical Skill Assessment (F-CSAT)
3. Performance Improvement Plan (PIP)
4. Summative Clinical Skill Assessment (S-CSAT)
(5. Direct Observation of Procedural Skills (DOPS) – see Chapter 1.1)

Clinical Skill Work Instruction

Equipment and resources: Standardised patient; hand decontamination agent; disposable gloves; method of documenting results

Associated Clinical Skills: Infection control; Communication; Consent

Pain assessment

Activity	Critical Action	Rationale
Prepare patient	Explain assessment. Gain informed consent. Patient can remain in position of their choice.	Consent and cooperation.
Establish history	Has there been an event likely to cause pain? Does the patient have an illness or injury likely to cause pain? Has the patient been complaining of pain?	Direct evidence of pain presence.
Initial assessment	Is the patient able to provide reliable interaction with verbal questioning? If Yes, move to pain evaluation (visual analogue). If No, move to PAINAD behaviour pain assessment (adult) or FLACC assessment (child).	To determine if patient can cooperate or not in assessment.

Pain assessment continued

Activity	Critical Action	Rationale
Pain evaluation	Question patient: Where is the pain located? Have the patient point to the painful area. Have the patient describe the pain. Does the pain radiate to any other part of the body? Does anything relieve the pain? Does anything aggravate the pain? Are there other signs or symptoms related to the pain or that coincided with its onset? When did the pain start?	Accurate detail of pain presentation.
Verbal pain score	Explain 0–10 pain score: 0 = no pain, 10 = the worst pain imaginable. Have the patient provide the value equalling their pain. If they are unable to do so, have them equate their pain to mild, moderate, severe.	Verbal reporting most reliable provided patient cooperating.
Visual analogue scale	If patient is unable to speak, explain 0–10 pain scale as for the verbal pain score. Have them point to a number on an incrementally marked line to indicate their pain score.	Alternative to verbal reporting also requiring cooperation.
Paediatric visual analogue scale	For the small child, show them the six FACES scale pictures. Explain the meaning of each face to facilitate understanding and response.	Alternative to visual analogue intended for child use.
PAINAD behaviour pain assessment	*Facial expression:* normal = 0, sad/frowning = 1, eyes closed, grimacing, wincing = 2. *Body language:* relaxed = 0, tense, distressed = 1, rigid, fists clenched, knees pulled up, localising, guarding, pushing away, striking out = 2. *Breathing:* normal = 0, occasionally laboured = 1, laboured/hyperventilating = 2. *Negative vocalisation:* normal = 0, occasional moan/groan = 1, repeated calling out, loud moaning, crying, troubled = 2. *Consolable:* calm = 0, distracted, reassured = 1, unable to console = 2.	Behavioural criteria most reliable in those unable to verbalise/cooperate.
FLACC behaviour pain assessment (smaller child)	Observe and score patient responses: *Face:* normal = 0, grimacing/frowning = 1, clenched jaw/quivering chin = 2. *Legs:* normal = 0, restless/uneasy = 1, kicking/legs drawn = 2. *Activity:* normal = 0, squirming/tense = 1, arched/rigid = 2. *Cry:* not crying = 0, complaining/crying = 1, screaming = 2. *Consolable:* content = 0, reassured by hugging/distraction = 1, difficult/unable to console = 2.	Behavioural criteria most reliable in children.
Report	Document/hand over findings, including pain severity.	Accurate record and care continuity.

Source: *Adapted from Johnson et al., 2015.*

Formative Clinical Skill Assessment (F-CSAT)

Equipment and resources: Standardised patient; hand decontamination agent; disposable gloves; method of documenting results

Associated Clinical Skills: Infection control; Communication; Consent

Staff/Student being assessed: _____

Pain assessment

Activity	Critical Action	Performance				
Prepares patient	Explains assessment. Gains informed consent.	0	1	2	3	4
Patient history	Determines whether there has been any event likely to cause pain. Establishes any illness/injury likely to cause pain. Determines if patient has been complaining of pain.	0	1	2	3	4
Initial assessment	Establishes if the patient can provide reliable interaction with verbal questioning. If Yes, moves to pain evaluation. If No, moves to PAINAD (adult) behaviour pain assessment or FLACC (child) assessment.	0	1	2	3	4
Pain evaluation	Questions patient: Where is the pain located? Has them point to the painful area. Has the patient describe the pain. Does the pain radiate to any other part of the body? Does anything relieve the pain? Does anything aggravate the pain? Are there other signs or symptoms related to the pain or that coincided with its onset? When did the pain start?	0	1	2	3	4
Verbal pain score	Has patient quote pain score on 0–10 scale after process has been explained. If unable, has patient quote pain as mild, moderate or severe.	0	1	2	3	4
Visual analogue scale	If patient unable to speak, has them point to 0–10 pain score on incrementally marked line after process has been explained.	0	1	2	3	4
Paediatric visual analogue scale	For small children, uses FACES scale, with child indicating result.	0	1	2	3	4
PAINAD behaviour pain assessment	Observes facial expression, body language, respiratory pattern, negative vocalisation and consolability, scoring 0, 1 or 2 for each. Calculates total.	0	1	2	3	4
FLACC behaviour pain assessment (smaller child)	Observes facial expression, leg, activity, crying and consolability, scoring 0, 1 or 2 depending on result. Calculates total.	0	1	2	3	4
Reports	Documents/hands over findings, including pain severity.	0	1	2	3	4

Source: Adapted from Johnson et al., 2015.

Standard Achieved: (please circle one)

Competent (C)   Not Yet Competent* (NYC)

Staff/Student Name: _____

Assessor (please print name): _____

Signed (Assessor): _____

Date of Assessment: _____

Comments:

*If Not Yet Competent (NYC) a PIP needs to be completed and a repeat of the F-CSAT

Formative Clinical Skill Assessment (F-CSAT) Key

Skill level	Standard of procedure	Quality of performance	Outcome	Level of assistance required
4 Safe for unsupervised practice	Safe Accurate Behaviour is appropriate to context	Confident Accurate Expedient	Achieved intended outcome	No supporting cues* required
3 Requires supervision	Safe Accurate Behaviour is appropriate to context	Confident Accurate Takes longer than required	Achieved intended outcome	Requires occasional supportive cues*
2 Requires assistance	Safe Accurate Behaviour generally appropriate to context	Lacks certainty	Would not have achieved outcome without support	Requires frequent verbal and occasional physical directives in addition to supportive cues*
1 Requires direction	Safe only with guidance Not completely accurate	Unskilled Inefficient	Would not have achieved outcome without support	Requires continuous verbal and frequent physical directive cues*
0 Unsafe	Unsafe Unable to demonstrate behaviour Lack of insight into behaviour appropriate to context	Unskilled	Would not have achieved outcome	Requires continuous verbal and continuous physical directive cues*

*Refers to physical directives or verbal supportive cues

Performance Improvement Plan (PIP)

Please document the agreed education plan and completion timelines for areas assessed as less than 4.

This plan should be presented to assessor prior to commencement of summative assessment.

Where was supervisor support required?	Student summary of deficit. (Why was there a problem?)	Improvement Plan	Completed (Y/N)

Staff/Student Name: _____

Staff/Student Signature: _____

Educator Name: _____

Educator Signature: _____

Summative Clinical Skill Assessment (S-CSAT)

Equipment and resources: Standardised patient; hand decontamination agent; disposable gloves; method of documenting results

Associated Clinical Skills: Infection control; Communication; Consent

Staff/Student being assessed: _____

- Completed Formative Clinical Skill Assessment (F-CSAT):   **YES   NO**

- Completed Performance Improvement Plan (PIP):   **YES   NO   N/A**

Pain assessment

Activity	Critical Action	Achieved	Without Direction
Prepares patient	Explains assessment. Gains informed consent.	NO	YES
Establishes history	Determines whether there has been any event likely to cause pain. Establishes any illness/injury likely to cause pain. Determines if patient has been complaining of pain.	NO	YES
Initial assessment	Establishes if the patient can provide reliable interaction with verbal questioning. If Yes, moves to pain evaluation. If No, moves to PAINAD (adult) behaviour pain assessment or FLACC (child) assessment.	NO	YES

	Pain assessment continued		
Activity	**Critical Action**	**Achieved Without Direction**	
Pain evaluation	Questions patient: Where is the pain located? Has them point to the painful area. Has the patient describe the pain. Does the pain radiate to any other part of the body? Does anything relieve the pain? Does anything aggravate the pain? Are there other signs or symptoms related to the pain or that coincided with its onset? When did the pain start?	NO	YES
Verbal pain score	Has patient quote pain score on 0–10 scale after process has been explained. If unable, has patient quote mild, moderate or severe.	NO	YES
Visual analogue score	If patient unable to speak, has them point to 0–10 pain score on incrementally marked line after process has been explained.	NO	YES
Paediatric visual analogue scale	For small children, uses FACES scale, with child indicating result.	NO	YES
PAINAD behaviour pain assessment	Observes facial expression, body language, respiratory pattern, negative vocalisation and consolability. Scores 0, 1 or 2 for each. Calculates total.	NO	YES
FLACC behaviour pain assessment (smaller child)	Observes facial expression, leg, activity, crying and consolability, scoring 0, 1 or 2 depending on result. Calculates total.	NO	YES
Reports	Documents/hands over findings, including pain severity.	NO	YES

Source: *Adapted from Johnson et al., 2015.*

Standard Achieved: (please circle one)

Competent (C)   Not Yet Competent* (NYC)

Staff/Student: _____

Assessor (please print name)**:** _____

Signed (Assessor)**:** _____

Date of Assessment: _____

Comments:

*If Not Yet Competent (NYC) a PIP needs to be completed and a repeat of the F-CSAT

Clinical findings

Objective versus subjective

The individual personalities of patients can influence pain presentations, creating differences between how patients describe their pain and how they appear affected by it. Some may state they are in great pain but not appear so. Conversely, others may appear to be in significant pain yet describe it less significantly. The paramedic might make a personal interpretation of how much pain the patient is really in, overruling the patient's claims (bias). When assessment findings do not appear to match, they must be reconciled.

Descriptors

Patients may use specific words for their pain, including 'burning', 'sharp', 'stabbing', 'aching', 'indigestion', 'heavy' or 'throbbing'. Use the patient's own words during assessment, as the patient may consider them substitutes for the word 'pain' itself.

PRACTICE TIP!

When using pain scales with self-nominated pain scores, the patient must have sufficient reasoning to be able to understand what the score or face means in the context in which it is being used. This requires the patient to have sufficient maturity or cognitive ability to do so. Invest time to explain the method so as to gain the best result possible.

PRACTICE TIP!

Pain is a very personal experience. Not all pain presentations will be obvious. The best method of discovering a patient is in pain is for them to self-report it. Even if the patient lacks cognitive ability or normal consciousness, any words declaring they are in pain must be considered.

PRACTICE TIP!

Chronic pain assessment is more about clarifying if this is the same problem as the one that already exists. New pain requires a fuller assessment to determine its origin and urgency.

TEST YOUR KNOWLEDGE QUESTIONS

1. **What is the most effective means of identifying whether a patient has pain?**
   The patient's self-reporting that they have pain.

2. **What are the most common questions for pain evaluation?**
   'Where is the pain located?' (have the patient point to the painful area); 'Can you describe the pain?'; 'Does the pain radiate to any other part of the body?'; 'Does anything relieve the pain? Does anything aggravate the pain?'; 'Are there other signs or symptoms related to the pain or that coincided with its onset?'; 'When did the pain start?'.

3. **If the patient is unable to provide reliable interaction with verbal questioning, what should be the paramedic response in order to continue pain assessment?**
   Move to PAINAD behaviour pain assessment (adults) or FLACC assessment (children).

4. **What verbal cooperative methods can describe pain severity?**
   Verbal pain score; verbal descriptor scale.

5. **What non-verbal cooperative methods can describe pain severity?**
   Visual analogue scale; FACES pain scale.

6. **What is the role of physiological vital signs in pain assessment?**
   It is non-specific and not essential.

7. **What are the key behavioural criteria for assessing non-cooperative adults?**
   Breathing; negative vocalisation; facial expression; body language; consolable.

8. **What are the key behavioural criteria for assessing non-cooperative children?**
   FLACC: Faces, Legs, Activity, Cry, Consolability.

9. **What are the most important signs of pain in non-cooperative patients?**
   Facial expressions; body language.

10. **How do you respond if the patient refers to pain by another descriptor term?**
    Use their word to ensure you are both referring to the same thing.

References

Al Darwish, Z.Q., Hamdi, R. and Fallatah, S., 2016. Evaluation of pain assessment tools in patients receiving mechanical ventilation. *AACN Advanced Critical Care*, 27(2), 162–172.

Arbour, C., Choinière, M., Topolovec-Vranic, J., Loiselle, C.G. and Gélinas, C., 2014. Can fluctuations in vital signs be used for pain assessment in critically ill patients with a traumatic brain injury? *Pain Research and Treatment*, doi: 10.1155/2014/175794.

Arbour, C. and Gélinas, C., 2010. Are vital signs valid indicators for the assessment of pain in postoperative cardiac surgery ICU adults? *Intensive and Critical Care Nursing*, 26(2), 83–90.

Chanques, G., Pohlman, A., Kress, J.P., Molinari, N., De Jong, A., Jaber, S. and Hall, J.B., 2014. Psychometric comparison of three behavioural scales for the assessment of pain in critically ill patients unable to self-report. *Critical Care*, 18(5), R160.

Chow, S., Chow, R., Lam, M., Rowbottom, L., Hollenberg, D., Friesen, E., Nadalini, O., Lam, H., DeAngelis, C. and Herrmann, N., 2016. Pain assessment tools for older adults with dementia in long-term care facilities: a systematic review. *Neurodegenerative Disease Management*, 6(6), 525–538.

Crellin, D.J., Harrison, D., Santamaria, N. and Babl, F.E., 2015. Systematic review of the Face, Legs, Activity, Cry and Consolability scale for assessing pain in infants and children: is it reliable, valid, and feasible for use? *Pain*, 156(11), 2132–2151.

de Vries, N.J., Sloot, P.H. and Achterberg, W.P., 2017. Pain and pain assessment in stroke patients with aphasia: a systematic review. *Aphasiology*, 31(6), 703–719.

Daoust, R., Paquet, J., Bailey, B., Lavigne, G., Piette, É., Sanogo, K. and Chauny, J.M., 2016. Vital signs are not associated with self-reported acute pain intensity in the Emergency Department. *Canadian Journal of Emergency Medicine*, 18(1), 19–27.

Fry, M., Arendts, G. and Chenoweth, L., 2017. Emergency nurses' evaluation of observational pain assessment tools for older people with cognitive impairment. *Journal of Clinical Nursing*, 26(9–10), 1281–1290.

Garra, G., Singer, A.J., Taira, B.R., Chohan, J., Cardoz, H., Chisena, E. and Thode, H.C., 2010. Validation of the Wong-Baker FACES pain rating scale in pediatric emergency department patients. *Academic Emergency Medicine*, 17(1), 50–54.

Herr, K., Bjoro, K. and Decker, S., 2006. Tools for assessment of pain in nonverbal older adults with dementia: a state-of-the-science review. *Journal of Pain and Symptom Management*, 31(2), 170–192.

IASP (International Association for the Study of Pain), 2018. Retrieved from: https://www.iasp-pain.org

Ismail, A.K., Ghafar, M.A.A., Shamsuddin, N.S.A., Roslan, N.A., Kaharuddin, H. and Muhamad, N.A.N., 2015. The assessment of acute pain in pre-hospital care using verbal numerical rating and visual analogue scales. *Journal of Emergency Medicine*, 49(3), 287–293.

Ge, X., Tao, J.R., Wang, J., Pan, S.M. and Wang, Y.W., 2015. Bayesian estimation on diagnostic performance of Face, Legs, Activity, Cry, and Consolability and Neonatal Infant Pain Scale for infant pain assessment in the absence of a gold standard. *Pediatric Anesthesia*, 25(8), 834–839.

Gélinas, C., Puntillo, K.A., Levin, P. and Azoulay, E., 2017. The Behavior Pain Assessment Tool for critically ill adults: a validation study in 28 countries. *Pain*, 158(5), 811–821.

Georgiou, E., Hadjibalassi, M., Lambrinou, E., Andreou, P. and Papathanassoglou, E.D., 2015. The impact of pain assessment on critically ill patients' outcomes: a systematic review. *BioMed Research International*, doi: 10.1155/2015/503830.

Jennings, P.A., Cameron, P. and Bernard, S., 2009. Measuring acute pain in the prehospital setting. *Emergency Medicine Journal*, 26(8), 552–555.

Johnson, M., Boyd, L., Grantham, H.J. and Eastwood, K., 2015. *Paramedic principles and practice ANZ* (Chapter 8). Sydney: Harcourt.

Jones, S. and Mitchell, G., 2015. Assessment of pain and alleviation of distress for people living with a dementia. *Mental Health Practice (2014+)*, 18(10), 32.

Jordan, A., Hughes, J., Pakresi, M., Hepburn, S. and O'Brien, J.T., 2011. The utility of PAINAD in assessing pain in a UK population with severe dementia. *International Journal of Geriatric Psychiatry*, 26(2), 118–126.

Kapoustina, O., Echegaray-Benites, C. and Gélinas, C., 2014. Fluctuations in vital signs and behavioural responses of brain surgery patients in the intensive care unit: are they valid indicators of pain? *Journal of Advanced Nursing*, 70(11), 2562–2576.

Kochman, A., Howell, J., Sheridan, M., Kou, M., Ryan, E.E.S., Lee, S., Zettersten, W. and Yoder, L., 2017. Reliability of the Faces, Legs, Activity, Cry, and Consolability Scale in assessing acute pain in the Pediatric Emergency Department. *Pediatric Emergency Care*, 33(1), 14–17.

Lichtner, V., Dowding, D., Esterhuizen, P., Closs, S.J., Long, A.F., Corbett, A. and Briggs, M., 2014. Pain assessment for people with dementia: a systematic review of systematic reviews of pain assessment tools. *BMC Geriatrics*, 14(1), 138.

Lord, B., 2009. Paramedic assessment of pain in the cognitively impaired adult patient. *BMC Emergency Medicine*, 9(1), 20.

Lord, B. and Woollard, M., 2010. The reliability of vital signs in estimating pain severity among adult patients treated by paramedics. *Emergency Medicine Journal*, emj-2009.

Malara, A., De Biase, G.A., Bettarini, F., Ceravolo, F., Di Cello, S., Garo, M., Praino, F., Settembrini, V., Sgro, G., Spadea, F. and Rispoli, V., 2016. Pain assessment in elderly with behavioral and psychological symptoms of dementia. *Journal of Alzheimer's Disease*, 50(4), 1217–1225.

McGuire, D.B., Kaiser, K.S., Haisfield-Wolfe, M.E. and Iyamu, F., 2016. Pain assessment in non-communicative adult palliative care patients. *The Nursing Clinics of North America*, 51(3), 397.

Merkel S.I., Voepel-Lewis, T., Shayevitz, J.R. and Malviya, S., 1997. The FLACC: a behavioural scale for scoring postoperative pain in young children. *Pediatric Nursing*, 23(3).

Ngu, S.S., Tan, M.P., Subramanian, P., Rahman, R.A., Kamaruzzaman, S., Chin, A.V., Tan, K.M. and Poi, P.J., 2015. Pain assessment using self-reported, nurse-reported, and observational pain assessment tools among older individuals with cognitive impairment. *Pain Management Nursing*, 16(4), 595–601.

Noda, K. and Ikusaka, M., 2012. Tips for taking history of pain. *Brain and Nerve (Shinkei Kenkyu No Shinpo)*, 64(11), 1273–1277.

Oosterman, J.M., Zwakhalen, S., Sampson, E.L. and Kunz, M., 2016. The use of facial expressions for pain assessment purposes in dementia: a narrative review. *Neurodegenerative Disease Management*, 6(2), 119–131.

Paulson-Conger, M., Leske, J., Maidl, C., Hanson, A. and Dziadulewicz, L., 2011. Comparison of two pain assessment tools in nonverbal critical care patients. *Pain Management Nursing*, 12(4), 218–224.

Pedersen, L.K., Rahbek, O., Nikolajsen, L. and Møller-Madsen, B., 2015. The revised FLACC score: reliability and validation for pain assessment in children with cerebral palsy. *Scandinavian Journal of Pain*, 9, 57–61.

Quinn, B.L., Seibold, E. and Hayman, L., 2015. Pain assessment in children with special needs: a review of the literature. *Exceptional Children*, 82(1), 44–57.

Reid, M.C., Eccleston, C. and Pillemer, K., 2015. Management of chronic pain in older adults. *BMJ*, 350(7995), 1–10.

Riddell, R.P., Fitzgerald, M., Slater, R., Stevens, B., Johnston, C. and Campbell-Yeo, M., 2016. Using only behaviours to assess infant pain: a painful compromise? *Pain*, 157(8), 1579–1580.

Rijkenberg, S., Stilma, W., Endeman, H., Bosman, R.J. and Oudemans-van Straaten, H.M., 2015. Pain measurement in mechanically ventilated critically ill patients: behavioral pain scale versus critical-care pain observation tool. *Journal of Critical Care*, 30(1), 167–172.

Schofield, P. and Abdulla, A., 2018. Pain assessment in the older population: what the literature says. *Age and Ageing*, 47(3), 324–327.

Thrane, S.E., Wanless, S., Cohen, S.M. and Danford, C.A., 2016. The assessment and non-pharmacologic treatment of procedural pain from infancy to school age through a developmental lens: a synthesis of evidence with recommendations. *Journal of Pediatric Nursing: Nursing Care of Children and Families*, 31(1), e23–e32.

van der Steen, J.T., Sampson, E.L., Van den Block, L., Lord, K., Vankova, H., Pautex, S., Vandervoort, A., Radbruch, L., Shvartzman, P., Sacchi, V. and de Vet, H.C., 2015. Tools to assess pain or lack of comfort in dementia: a content analysis. *Journal of Pain and Symptom Management*, 50(5), 659–675.

Vlaeyen, J.W., Crombez, G. and Linton, S.J., 2016. The fear-avoidance model of pain. *Pain*, 157(8), 1588–1589.

Vuille, M., Foerster, M., Foucault, E. and Hugli, O., 2018. Pain assessment by emergency nurses at triage in the emergency department: a qualitative study. *Journal of Clinical Nursing*, 27(3–4), 669–676.

Warden, V., Hurley, A.C. and Volicer, L., 2003, Development and psychometric evaluation of the Pain Assessment in Advanced Dementia (PAINAD) scale. *Journal of the American Medical Directors Association*, 4(1), 9–15.

Wong, D.L. and Baker, C.M., 1988. Pain in children: comparison of assessment scales. *Pediatric Nursing*, 14(1), 9–17.

Wood, S., 2008. Assessment of pain. *Nursing Times*, 10042–10047.

Zwakhalen, S.M., Hamers, J.P. and Berger, M.P., 2006. The psychometric quality and clinical usefulness of three pain assessment tools for elderly people with dementia. *Pain*, 126(1–3), 210–220.

Bibliography

Curtis, K. and Ramsden, C., 2015. *Emergency and trauma care for nurses and paramedics*. Sydney: Elsevier.

Johnson, M., Boyd, L., Grantham, H.J. and Eastwood, K., 2014. *Paramedic principles and practice ANZ*. Sydney: Harcourt.

McCance, K.L. and Huether, S.E., 2015. *Pathophysiology: the biologic basis for disease in adults and children*. Sydney: Elsevier.

2.17 | Abdominal assessment

Dianne Inglis

Chapter objectives

At the end of this chapter the reader will be able to:

1. Describe the rationale behind abdominal assessment
2. Demonstrate abdominal assessment
3. Accurately report findings

Resources required for this assessment

- Standardised patient or mannequin
- Hand decontamination agent
- Disposable gloves
- Stethoscope
- Method of documenting results

Skill matrix

This assessment requires:

- Infection control (CS 1.3)
- Communication (CS 1.5)
- Consent (CS 1.6)
- Pain assessment (CS 2.16)

This assessment is a component of:

- Patient assessment (Chapter 2)

Introduction

The importance of the abdomen is often overlooked during examination, with priority being given instead to the head, chest and limbs. However, the abdomen is the source of many problems encompassing a number of body systems, including traumatic injury and a diverse range of medical complaints.

This chapter discusses paramedic assessment of the patient abdomen.

Anatomy and physiology

The abdominal cavity contains the digestive organs, including the stomach and small and large intestines, the great vessels of the aorta and vena cava, and the reproductive and urinary organs.

Covering the abdominal content is the peritoneum, which has an inner visceral (organ) lining and an outer parietal abdominal wall lining. Innervation of the parietal and visceral nerves differs. Irritation/inflammation of the parietal layer causes localised pain, tenderness and abdominal wall rigidity, while visceral pain is less specific and frequently harder to locate and describe.

Intestinal peristalsis may be relatively slow but it produces sounds as gas, fluid and digested material move through its lumen. Normal bowel sounds are distinctive while particular diseases can cause detectable abnormalities, including absence or hyperactivity.

The abdomen is relatively large. For ease of describing the location of abnormal findings, there are two ways to divide the abdomen (Baid, 2009). The first is the quadrant method, where the umbilicus forms the centre point and a line is drawn vertically up to the sternum and down to the groin, and another drawn perpendicular from left to right. The four quadrants are the left and right upper and the left and right lower (Fig. 2.17.1). Alternatively, for increased specificity, the abdomen can be divided into nine regions (squares) of equal size (Fig. 2.17.2). The upper three are the left and right hypochondriac at the lower chest margin

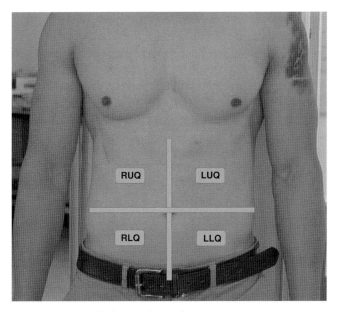

Figure 2.17.1 Abdominal quadrants

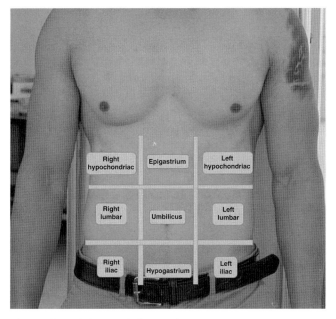

Figure 2.17.2 Nine abdominal regions

separated by the epigastrium. The middle three are the left and right lumbar separated by the central umbilical. The lower three are the left and right iliac separated by the hypogastric region.

Clinical rationale

Abdominal assessment involves different elements that collectively provide findings. The key elements are history, inspection, auscultation, palpation and percussion. The order of these elements is important for comprehensiveness and because some methods impact on others. History taking and a visual inspection are performed first to help relax both the patient and the abdominal musculature.

To ensure the patient's comfort and dignity are maintained, ensure the chest and groin are sufficiently clothed or covered (Fig. 2.17.3).

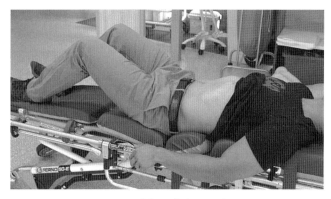

Figure 2.17.3 Positioned for abdominal examination

History

The patient's history includes a record of what has prompted the current call for assistance along with any previous relevant disease. These provide clues to guide further examination.

Ask the patient about:
- any previous illness and compare to this presentation. Is this the same? Is there known diagnosis? Are there precipitating factors including eating or alcohol consumption?
- if there is pain, where it is located and whether it radiates elsewhere. Have them describe the pain. Sharper, well-localised pain suggests a parietal origin while visceral pain is caused by organ distension and inflammation (Al-Chaer and Traub, 2002; Macaluso and McNamara, 2012)
- the severity of the pain (see Chapter 2.16). While this can guide management, it may mislead in terms of the severity of the problem. Severe pain can be from a benign cause, including gas trapped in the bowel, whereas mild pain may be associated with cancer
- the time of onset and duration of illness, previous similar events and their confirmed diagnosis, and any relieving and aggravating factors
- current and typical fluid and food intake: Is the patient still eating and drinking as usual or not?
- any other gastrointestinal abnormalities, including any nausea or vomiting. If vomiting, how many times? This can lead to dehydration or metabolic imbalance. Was the vomitus food, bile or frank or darkened blood?
- bowel movements. What is the usual motion pattern? Have the motions been regular? If not, in what way have they been different from usual? Has there been increased watery motions or decreased motions altogether? If there has been delay since the last motion, how long has it been? How did the motion appear? Did it contain frank or darkened blood? How much? Do motions pass easily or are difficulty and straining normal?
- any possibility of pregnancy (see Chapter 8.1) (not every abdominal issue will be related to gastrointestinal problems). Is there any association with normal menstruation?

- any urinary abnormalities, including frequency, retention, burning, abnormal smell or blood present in the urine.

Inspection

The next part of the assessment is visual inspection. Look for obvious clues, including the patient's preferred posture. Is there any knee/hip flexing in an attempt to relax abdominal muscles? Is the patient rolling around in discomfort or using an arm to guard or rub painful areas?

Position the patient supine and remove sufficient clothing to allow assessment. Slightly flexing the knees can help relax the abdominal wall muscles. Placing the patient's arms by their sides (rather than lifted behind their head) can further relax abdominal muscles. Ensure there is sufficient lighting for the assessment.

Note the general shape of the abdomen, including its size and distension. Is it flat and muscled or curved inwards or outwards? Generalised distension can be from trapped gas/liquid in the bowel, ascites or even obesity. Upper abdominal distension can indicate gastric dilation or pancreatic disease. Lower abdominal distension may indicate pregnancy, uterine or bladder problems.

Look for:
- abnormal protrusion or masses that might indicate underlying growths or hernias. Have the patient take a deep breath and briefly hold it to see if any abnormality appears
- obvious marks, including scars from past surgery or injury. If found, do they correspond with the gathered history? Are the scars new, infected or old?
- visible pulsations that could indicate aortic aneurysm
- visible veins that may present in an emaciated person or where there is portal hypertension
- striae (stretch marks) indicating weight loss, ascites or past pregnancy
- any discolouration, such as blueness, that might indicate underlying bleeding, or the yellow of jaundice
- bruising and abrasions that might suggest injury or trauma
- welts or rash that might indicate immune response.

Any finding should be linked to the patient's history assessment to determine its possible cause.

Auscultation

For this part of the assessment, the patient remains in the same position as for the inspection. Bowel sounds are high pitched, so use the stethoscope diaphragm. These sounds transmit readily, so listening in the middle of each quadrant is sufficient (Karnath and Mileski, 2002).

Normal bowel peristalsis creates gurgling sounds during the period of each minute. Disease can cause these sounds to alter or become absent. Sounds can differ either side of a bowel obstruction (Ching and Tan, 2012; Gu et al., 2010). Early obstruction can increase peristaltic waves, causing an increase in the frequency and loudness of sound. The absence of sounds for a full minute suggests reduced gastrointestinal tract activity, particularly post-

surgery or if infected. If no sounds are heard over 1 minute, continue listening for 3–4 minutes further to be sure. A longer absence of sound is serious (Baid, 2009; Yamaguchi et al., 2006).

Other sounds, including bruits and rubs, may occasionally be audible. Aortic bruits, a 'swishing' sound caused by atherosclerosis reducing blood flow, can be auscultated just superior to the umbilicus. Bruits may also be heard with abdominal aortic aneurysm. Renal artery bruits may be heard just left and right of this location.

Rubs are not commonly present and indicate a inflamed peritoneal surface contacting an underlying organ. Listening for bruits and rub sounds is a more complex form of assessment that is of less value to paramedics for clinical decision making. It requires an understanding of the sounds being listened for.

Palpation

Palpation can stimulate bowel activity, so it should always be performed after auscultation (Baid, 2009).

The patient continues in the same position. Divide the abdomen, using the nine regions for greater specificity, moving sequentially from one to the next. Painful abdominal areas should be palpated last to avoid causing muscle tensing or loss of cooperation.

Initially, gently press the abdominal wall inwards about 1 cm with the finger pads (Fig. 2.17.4). Watch the patient's face as you do so, looking for any grimaces or other signs of discomfort. Crepitus caused by subcutaneous gas or fluid may be palpable.

Light palpation can elicit tenderness with or without pain present. Tenderness suggests peritoneal inflammation/infection. The location helps the paramedic identify the underlying disease through their anatomical understanding of what lies beneath the abdominal wall. A generalised tenderness suggests broader peritoneal involvement.

Tenderness can be described in terms of the depth of palpation (such as light or deep) required to produce any response, its severity and whether it occurred during pressing or release. Release (or rebound) tenderness is

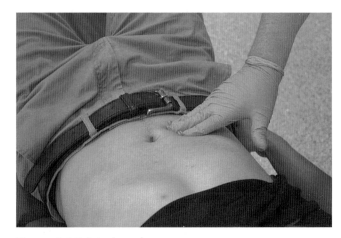

Figure 2.17.4 Light palpation

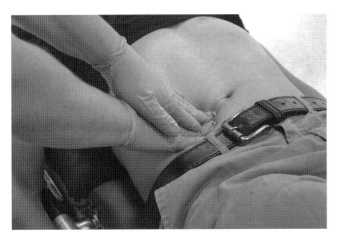

Figure 2.17.5 Deeper palpation

evident as the pressure is slowly removed; note whether discomfort was produced with application or removal.

Follow light pressure with deeper palpation. Place the palm of one hand on the abdominal wall, and then press the other hand over it. The upper hand applies downward pressure, pushing the lower hand fingertips inwards 3–5 cm while simultaneously maintaining a slight circular motion of the fingertips (Fig. 2.17.5). This is more appropriate for palpating masses or specific organs.

Underlying peritoneal infection/inflammation causes involuntary muscle tensing and wall rigidity. Palpation can detect rigidity that is either localised over a region or generalised across the abdomen. The latter is called guarding and can be a voluntary action to protect against pain (Macaluso and McNamara, 2012). To reduce this, provide reassurance and palpate painful areas last.

The liver in the right upper quadrant and spleen (when enlarged) in the left upper can normally be felt just below the costal margins. Have the patient inhale deeply to push them downwards during assessment.

Masses can be felt during palpation, and their size, location and tenderness are assessable.

Percussion

Percussion is most useful where ascites is present.

The patient remains in the same position. Firmly push the middle finger of the non-dominant hand in turn in the middle of each of the nine abdominal regions. With the tip of the middle finger of the dominant hand, sharply tap the pressing finger. The audible sound can be:

- tympanic, the higher pitched sound suggesting that it is air-filled, which is normal over most of the abdomen
- dullness, a flat-pitched sound suggesting fluid, which is normal over an organ or ascites.

Ascites forms where excess fluid is produced within the abdomen or there is a failure of absorption. Where ascites is present, gas-filled intestines create tympany around the umbilicus (when supine). Dullness may be heard towards the flanks, where fluid settles.

Clinical skill assessment process

The following section outlines the clinical skill assessment tools that should be used to determine a student's ability to demonstrate accurate abdominal assessment.

1. Clinical Skill Work Instruction
2. Formative Clinical Skill Assessment (F-CSAT)
3. Performance Improvement Plan (PIP)
4. Summative Clinical Skill Assessment (S-CSAT)
(5. Direct Observation of Procedural Skills (DOPS) – see Chapter 1.1)

Clinical Skill Work Instruction

Equipment and resources: Patient or mannequin; hand decontamination agent; disposable gloves; stethoscope; method of documenting results

Associated Clinical Skills: Infection control; Communication; Consent; Pain assessment

Abdominal assessment

Activity	Critical Action	Rationale
Personal protection	Don PPE as appropriate.	Infection control/minimisation.
Prepare patient	Reassure patient. Explain procedure. Gain consent.	Require patient compliance.
	Lay patient supine with arms by their side and knees supported and slightly flexed.	To relax abdominal muscles.
	Remove sufficient clothing to allow examination. Cover chest and groin for privacy.	Abdominal assessment requires visual exposure.

Abdominal assessment continued

Activity	Critical Action	Rationale
Establish history	Question patient about: • past medical history, including confirmed illness/diagnosis • current events, including onset time and duration, relieving or aggravating factors • pain complaints • eating/drinking patterns • nausea/vomiting • bowel/urinary abnormalities.	To be precise about current and previous known problems. Explore responses with follow-up questions to elicit greater understanding.
Abdominal inspection	Note any limb guarding, knee flexing or positional discomfort evident. Visualise for: • abdominal shape/contour • localised masses/bulges • scars or striae • visible pulsations • discolouration, welts/rashes • bruising or abrasions.	Visible clues of underlying problems.
Auscultation	Warm the stethoscope if cold. Place the diaphragm over the middle of one abdominal quadrant. Listen for up to 1 minute. Repeat for the other quadrants. Note sound heard for pitch and frequency. If nothing is heard, continue to listen in one lower quadrant for 3–4 minutes. Listen just superior to the umbilicus for bruits.	The lumbar region is the best place to hear gurgling bowel sounds. Above the umbilicus is the best location for aortic bruits.
Palpation	Warm hands if cold. Lightly press finger pads of one hand 1 cm into the middle of each of the nine regions in turn while observing patient's face for response. If the patient is complaining of pain, palpate that region last.	To assess for tenderness caused and muscle wall rigidity or guarding.
	Place fingertips of one hand into middle of each of the nine regions, this time with the second hand on top of the fingers, and push downwards 3–5 cm.	Feeling for masses.
Percussion	Press the middle finger of one hand firmly down into one abdominal region. With the other hand, tap sharply several times on the finger, noting if the sound is dull or tympanic. Repeat for each of the other regions.	Seeking air or fluid-filled areas.
Report	Document/hand over abnormal findings.	Accurate record. Continuity of patient care

Formative Clinical Skill Assessment (F-CSAT)

Equipment and resources: Patient or mannequin; hand decontamination agent; disposable gloves; stethoscope; method of documenting results

Associated Clinical Skills: Infection control; Communication; Consent; Pain assessment

Staff/Student being assessed: _____

Abdominal assessment

Activity	Critical Action	Performance				
Personal protection	Dons PPE.	0	1	2	3	4
Prepares patient	Reassures patient. Explains procedure. Gains consent. Lays patient supine with arms by their side and knees supported and slightly flexed. Removes sufficient clothing to allow examination.	0	1	2	3	4
Establishes history	Questions: • past medical history • current events, including onset time/duration, relieving/aggravating factors • pain, nausea/vomiting, bowel/urinary abnormalities, eating/drinking patterns.	0	1	2	3	4
Abdominal inspection	Notes patient's natural position. Visualises abdominal shape/contour and any other abnormalities present.	0	1	2	3	4
Auscultation	Warms stethoscope. Auscultates over each quadrant for up to 1 minute. Notes sound heard. Continues auscultating 3–4 minutes if nothing is heard. Listens just superior to umbilicus.	0	1	2	3	4
Palpation	Warms hands. Lightly palpates each of the nine regions. Repeats using firm palpation.	0	1	2	3	4
Percussion	Presses middle finger into middle of each of the nine regions and taps several times, assessing percussion.	0	1	2	3	4
Reports	Documents/hands over abnormal findings.	0	1	2	3	4

Standard Achieved: (please circle one)

Competent (C)   Not Yet Competent* (NYC)

Staff/Student Name: _____

Assessor (please print name): _____

Signed (Assessor): _____

Date of Assessment: _____

Comments:

*If Not Yet Competent (NYC) a PIP needs to be completed and a repeat of the F-CSAT

Formative Clinical Skill Assessment (F-CSAT) Key

Skill level	Standard of procedure	Quality of performance	Outcome	Level of assistance required
4 Safe for unsupervised practice	Safe Accurate Behaviour is appropriate to context	Confident Accurate Expedient	Achieved intended outcome	No supporting cues* required
3 Requires supervision	Safe Accurate Behaviour is appropriate to context	Confident Accurate Takes longer than required	Achieved intended outcome	Requires occasional supportive cues*
2 Requires assistance	Safe Accurate Behaviour generally appropriate to context	Lacks certainty	Would not have achieved outcome without support	Requires frequent verbal and occasional physical directives in addition to supportive cues*
1 Requires direction	Safe only with guidance Not completely accurate	Unskilled Inefficient	Would not have achieved outcome without support	Requires continuous verbal and frequent physical directive cues*
0 Unsafe	Unsafe Unable to demonstrate behaviour Lack of insight into behaviour appropriate to context	Unskilled	Would not have achieved outcome	Requires continuous verbal and continuous physical directive cues*

*Refers to physical directives or verbal supportive cues

Performance Improvement Plan (PIP)

Please document the agreed education plan and completion timelines for areas assessed as less than 4.

This plan should be presented to assessor prior to commencement of summative assessment.

Where was supervisor support required?	Student summary of deficit. (Why was there a problem?)	Improvement Plan	Completed (Y/N)

Staff/Student Name: _____

Staff/Student Signature: _____

Educator Name: _____

Educator Signature: _____

Summative Clinical Skill Assessment (S-CSAT)

Equipment and resources: Patient or mannequin; hand decontamination agent; disposable gloves; stethoscope; method of documenting results

Associated Clinical Skills: Infection control; Communication; Consent; Pain assessment

Staff/Student being assessed: _____

- Completed Formative Clinical Skill Assessment (F-CSAT):   **YES**   **NO**

- Completed Performance Improvement Plan (PIP):   **YES**   **NO**   **N/A**

Abdominal assessment

Activity	Critical Action	Achieved Without Direction	
Personal protection	Dons PPE.	NO	YES
Prepares patient	Reassures patient. Explains procedure. Gains consent. Lays patient supine with arms by their side and knees supported and slightly flexed. Removes sufficient clothing to allow examination.	NO	YES
Establishes history	Questions: • past medical history • current events including onset/duration, relieving aggravating factors • pain, nausea, vomiting, bowel/urinary abnormalities • eating/drinking patterns.	NO	YES
Abdominal inspection	Notes patient natural position. Visualises abdominal shape/contour and any other abnormalities present.	NO	YES
Auscultation	Warms stethoscope. Auscultates over each quadrant for up to 1 minute. Notes sounds heard. Continues auscultating 3–4 minutes if nothing is heard. Listens just superior to umbilicus.	NO	YES
Palpation	Warms hands. Lightly palpates each of the nine regions. Repeats using firm palpation.	NO	YES
Percussion	Presses middle finger into middle of each of the nine regions and taps several times, assessing percussion.	NO	YES
Reports	Documents/hands over abnormal findings.	NO	YES

Standard Achieved: (please circle one)

Competent (C)   Not Yet Competent* (NYC)

Staff/Student Name: _____

Assessor (please print name)**:** _____

Signed (Assessor)**:** _____

Date of Assessment: _____

Comments:

*If Not Yet Competent (NYC) a PIP needs to be completed and a repeat of the F-CSAT

Clinical findings

Organ assessment

Different organs, including the liver, spleen and kidneys, can be palpated, particularly for enlargement. This is typically outside the scope of paramedic assessment and requires greater specific anatomical knowledge.

Pregnancy

Abdominal size and measurement of fundal height provide information about the stage of pregnancy. Further palpation can determine fetal position.

Other findings

Abdominal complaints do not exist in isolation from other parts of the body. Abdominal assessment is therefore typically conducted as part of a broader assessment for concurrent signs of illness.

Referred pain is where patient discomfort is noted away from the causative source, such as when shoulder-tip pain is felt during gall, liver or splenic disease. Radiated pain is similar, with the patient being unable to locate its source, such as where the pain of acute coronary syndrome presents simultaneously in the chest, arms, neck and epigastrium. These vagaries result from complex and shared visceral nervous innervation into multiple spinal cord segments, making it difficult for the brain to decipher (Borowczyk, 2013; Giamberardino et al., 2010; Giamberardino, 2003; Janig, 2014).

PRACTICE TIP!

Palpate and percuss the abdomen last, leaving any known painful areas to the very last. Bowel activity can increase after palpation. Guarding and a lack of cooperation can ensue if the patient anticipates pain.

PRACTICE TIP!

Always assess the patient's history first to help put them at ease during examination. The patient's cooperation is necessary to allow a comprehensive assessment and avoid guarding, which interferes with it.

PRACTICE TIP!

Abdominal assessment involves part removal of clothing, abdominal visualisation and palpation. This can cause gender or cultural concerns. If your explanation does not prove sufficient, having family members accompany or even changing assessor may be necessary to gain the patient's consent.

TEST YOUR KNOWLEDGE QUESTIONS

1. **What are the five elements of abdominal assessment?**
   History; inspection; auscultation; palpation; and percussion.

2. **What is the ideal position for the patient during abdominal assessment?**
   Supine, with the arms by the side and knees slightly flexed.

3. **What two methods can be used to artificially divide the abdomen for assessment?**
   Four quadrants; nine smaller regions.

4. **What time duration is required to auscultate for bowel sounds?**
   Up to 1 minute in each quadrant; 3–4 minutes further if nothing is heard.

5. **What is light palpation assessing for?**
   Rigidity, guarding and tenderness.

6. **What two sounds can be heard during abdominal percussion?**
   Tympanic sounds indicating air-filled areas; dullness, suggesting fluid-filled areas.

7. **Why is auscultation performed before palpation?**
   Palpation can stimulate bowel activity and so change bowel sounds.

8. **What sounds can be heard during abdominal auscultation?**
   Gurgling sounds, no sounds or artery bruits.

9. **How does deep palpation differ from light?**
   It uses two hands instead of one, pressing in 3–4 cm instead of 1 cm.

10. **What is the difference between rigidity and guarding?**
    Rigidity is localised muscle tension; guarding is generalised tension across the abdomen.

References

Al-Chaer, E.D. and Traub, R.J., 2002. Biological basis of visceral pain: recent developments. *Pain*, 96(3), 221–225.

Baid, H., 2009. A critical review of auscultating bowel sounds. *British Journal of Nursing*, 18(18), 1125.

Borowczyk, J.M., 2013. Visceral referred pain. In Gebhart, G.F. and Schmidt, R.F. (eds), *Encyclopedia of pain*. Berlin/Heidelberg: Springer-Verlag, pp. 4225–4228.

Ching, S.S. and Tan, Y.K., 2012. Spectral analysis of bowel sounds in intestinal obstruction using an electronic stethoscope. *World Journal of Gastroenterology*, 18(33), 4585–4592.

Giamberardino, M..A., 2003. Referred muscle pain/hyperalgesia and central sensitisation. *Journal of Rehabilitation Medicine-Supplements*, 41, 85–88.

Giamberardino, M.A., Affaitati, G. and Costantini, R., 2010. Visceral referred pain. *Journal of Musculoskeletal Pain*, 18(4), 403–410.

Gu, Y., Lim, H.J. and Moser, M.A., 2010. How useful are bowel sounds in assessing the abdomen? *Digestive Surgery*, 27(5), 422–426.

Jänig, W., 2014. Neurobiology of visceral pain. *Schmerz,* 28(3), 233–251.

Karnath, B. and Mileski, W., 2002. Acute abdominal pain. *Hospital Physician*, 38, 45–50.

Macaluso, C.R. and McNamara, R.M., 2012. Evaluation and management of acute abdominal pain in the emergency department. *International Journal of General Medicine*, 5, 789.

Yamaguchi, K., Yamaguchi, T., Odaka, T. and Saisho, H., 2006. Evaluation of gastrointestinal motility by computerized analysis of abdominal auscultation findings. *Journal of Gastroenterology and Hepatology*, 21(3), 510–514.

2.18 | Tympanic temperature recording

Joelene Gott

Chapter objectives

At the end of this chapter the reader will be able to:

1. Describe the rationale for assessing tympanic temperature
2. Demonstrate how to assess tympanic temperature
3. Accurately report on the findings

Resources required for this assessment

- Standardised patient
- Hand decontamination agent
- Disposable gloves
- Clinical waste bag
- Digital tympanic thermometer and probe covers
- Method of documenting the results

Skill matrix

This assessment requires:
- Infection control (CS 1.3)
- Communication (CS 1.5)
- Consent (CS 1.6)

This assessment is a component of:
- Patient assessment (Chapter 2)

Introduction

Accurate temperature measurement is a critical component of paramedic assessment and management of patients, whether they are critically injured or ill or have a minor illness. Humans are homoeothermic, with a core temperature that is regulated regardless of external environmental changes (McCance and Heuther et al., 2015).

Tympanic temperature measurement is the preferred method of measuring someone's temperature in the prehospital emergency setting. It is non-invasive, can be done rapidly and is a very simple measurement to use. This chapter will discuss effective tympanic temperature evaluation.

Anatomy and physiology

Temperature regulation is controlled by the thermoregulatory centres in the hypothalamus. The human body has both peripheral and central thermoreceptors, including in the skin, hypothalamus, abdominal organs and spinal cord. These thermoreceptors send information about the skin and core temperatures to the hypothalamus. If the temperatures are high or low, the hypothalamus responds by triggering heat production, heat conservation or heat loss mechanisms (McCance and Heuther, 2015).

The body's internal temperature regulators can be affected by different factors such as weather, exercise/activity, infection and the body's own circadian rhythm (Levander and Grodzinsky, 2017). However, not all parts of the body maintain the same temperature; for example, the extremities of the body tend to be cooler than the torso (McCance and Heuther, 2015). Core temperature is generally higher than that at the skin.

The tympanic membrane receives blood from the internal carotid artery, which runs very near to the membrane and also supplies the hypothalamus (Gasim et al., 2013; Yeoh et al., 2017). The tympanic membrane is at the distal end of the ear canal, only a short distance from the ear opening.

Clinical rationale

Body temperature can be assessed in various sites, including the mouth (oral), armpit (axillary), rectum and forehead (temporal), with each approximating actual core temperature. Temperature variations between sites are commonly observed.

Rectal temperature

Rectal temperature evaluation instantly raises concerns about patient discomfort and hygiene. The rectal site has a blood flow that is relatively isolated and removed from the central nervous system and core circulation. Temperature changes at this site can lag well behind those of other sites; rectal stool can impact adversely on readings; and there is risk of mucosal injury during insertion of the device (Sund-Levander and Grodzinsky, 2013).

Oral route

The oral route has been the one traditionally used. The mouth receives significant blood supply from the carotid artery, making it reflective of core temperature. However, significant variations can be found between anterior and posterior placement. The route requires some patient cooperation while the reading is taken, during which the patient will have a reduced ability to speak. Readings can be adversely affected by eating, drinking, smoking, chewing and salivation (Sund-Levander and Grodzinsky, 2013).

Axillary site

The axillary site (armpit) is less invasive and unhygienic than the rectal and oral routes but can be more affected by ambient temperature and sweating. It can show a wide variation in the accuracy and reliability of readings, with slight placement differences (Sund-Levander and Grodzinsky, 2013).

Temporal evaluation

Temporal (forehead) evaluation is simple, the least invasive and the most hygienic method of temperature measurement, making it appealing. Conversely, it provides only an estimate of temporal artery temperature and is adversely impacted by sweating, the use of makeup and body oils, moisture, the thickness of subcutaneous fat and bone, and the placement of the device (Sund-Levander and Grodzinsky, 2013).

Tympanic assessment

Tympanic assessment is a suitable and accurate reflection of core temperature, given the blood supply commonality with the hypothalamus (Gasim et al., 2013; Yamakoshi et al., 2013). This includes critically ill hypothermic, normothermic and hyperthermic patients (Bijur et al., 2016; Chue et al., 2012; Flouris and Cheung, 2010; Hasper et al., 2011; Hocker et al., 2012). Its use for assessing children has been shown to be less, but still satisfactorily, reliable (Allegaert et al., 2014; Barnett et al.,

2011; Batra and Goyal, 2013; Jefferies et al., 2011; Paes et al., 2010; Zhen et al., 2015).

Alternative assessment routes can be time-consuming, include patient discomfort, be complex or even create hygiene concerns (Yeoh et al., 2017). In contrast, tympanic assessment is quick, reliable and substantially without any of these concerns (Arslan et al., 2011).

Tympanic measurement works by using an infrared light to detect thermal infrared energy emitted from the tympanic membrane. The critical key is ensuring that the probe is aimed at the membrane during assessment and not at the ear canal itself. The anatomy of the outer ear and ear canal must first be straightened to ensure direct alignment of the probe and membrane.

For adults, the ear typically needs to be tugged superiorly by holding the upper, outer ear and pulling upwards (Fig. 2.18.1). This aligns the ear canal with the outer ear (Temdrup and Rajk, 1992). Lower than accurate readings can be gained if this is not performed (Levander and Grodzinsky, 2017).

Ear canal anatomy varies for children. For infants, the outer ear must be pulled posteriorly to straighten the ear canal (Fig. 2.18.2). For children between 1 year of age and adult age, the ear must be pulled upwards and posteriorly (Fig. 2.18.3).

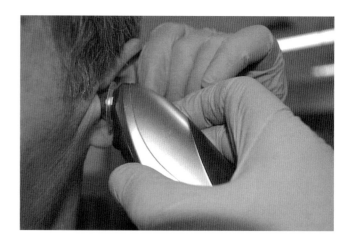

Figure 2.18.1 Straightening the adult ear canal

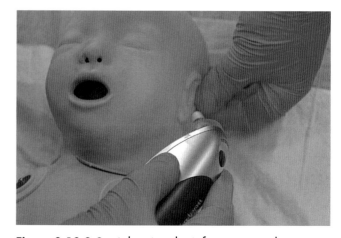

Figure 2.18.2 Straightening the infant ear canal

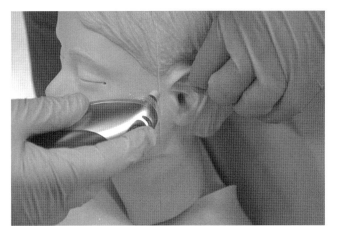

Figure 2.18.3 Straightening the child ear canal

Only with the ear canal straightened can a probe be inserted gently but firmly into the ear. For infection control purposes, a new probe cover should be used each time.

For paramedic use in emergencies, any thermometer must be accurate in assessing a wide range of hypothermic to hyperthermic temperatures (at least 42°C to <30°C).

Clinical skill assessment process

The following section outlines the clinical skill assessment tools that should be used to determine a student's ability to demonstrate accurate measurement of tympanic temperature.

1. Clinical Skill Work Instruction
2. Formative Clinical Skill Assessment (F-CSAT)
3. Performance Improvement Plan (PIP)
4. Summative Clinical Skill Assessment (S-CSAT)
(5. Direct Observation of Procedural Skills (DOPS) – see Chapter 1.1)

Clinical Skill Work Instruction

Equipment and resources: Standardised patient; hand decontamination agent; disposable gloves; clinical waste bag; digital tympanic thermometer and probe covers; method of documenting results

Associated Clinical Skills: Infection control; Communication; Consent

Tympanic temperature recording

Activity	Critical Action	Rationale
Prepare equipment	Identify rationale for performing observation. Gather required equipment.	Assemble all items necessary beforehand.
Personal protection	Don appropriate personal protective equipment (PPE).	To prevent the spread of infection.
Prepare patient	Explain procedure and advise of brief discomfort. Obtain consent.	Patient may be unwilling or 'startle' or 'scare'.
Prepare thermometer	Maintain instrument in a hygienic condition. Attach a new probe cover. Confirm device is in 'ready' mode.	If the device is not used, it may switch off and require a new probe attachment to reset.
Assess temperature	Pull ear to align ear canal, using a technique appropriate to the patient's age. Gently insert probe tip into the ear canal as far as it will go.	Ear alignment is necessary to allow probe to assess tympanic membrane.
	Press activation button to initiate assessment. When reading appears/alarm sounds, remove thermometer from ear. Note reading.	Record reading when device provides it.
Dispose of waste	Dispose of ear probe as clinical waste.	For infection control.
Report	Document measurement and any detected problems.	Accurate record kept and continuity of patient care.

Formative Clinical Skill Assessment (F-CSAT)

Equipment and resources: Standardised patient; hand decontamination agent; disposable gloves; clinical waste bag; digital tympanic thermometer and probe covers; method of documenting results

Associated Clinical Skills: Infection control; Communication; Consent

Staff/Student being assessed: _____

Tympanic temperature recording

Activity	Critical Action	Performance				
Prepares equipment	Identifies rationale for performing observation. Gathers required equipment.	0	1	2	3	4
Personal protection	Dons appropriate PPE.	0	1	2	3	4
Prepares patient	Explains procedure and advises of brief discomfort. Obtains consent.	0	1	2	3	4
Prepares thermometer	Maintains instrument in a hygienic condition. Attaches a new probe cover. Confirms the device is in 'ready' mode.	0	1	2	3	4
Assesses temperature	Pulls ear to align ear canal. Uses technique appropriate to patient's age. Gently inserts probe tip into the ear canal as far as it will go.	0	1	2	3	4
	Presses activation button to initiate assessment. When reading appears/ alarm sounds, removes thermometer from ear. Notes reading.	0	1	2	3	4
Disposes of waste	Disposes of ear probe as clinical waste.	0	1	2	3	4
Reports	Documents measurement and any detected problems.	0	1	2	3	4

Standard Achieved: (please circle one)

Competent (C)   Not Yet Competent* (NYC)

Staff/Student Name: _____

Assessor (please print name): _____

Signed (Assessor): _____

Date of Assessment: _____

Comments:

*If Not Yet Competent (NYC) a PIP needs to be completed and a repeat of the F-CSAT

Formative Clinical Skill Assessment (F-CSAT) Key

	Standard of procedure	Quality of performance	Outcome	Level of assistance required
4 Safe for unsupervised practice	Safe Accurate Behaviour is appropriate to context	Confident Accurate Expedient	Achieved intended outcome	No supporting cues* required
3 Requires supervision	Safe Accurate Behaviour is appropriate to context	Confident Accurate Takes longer than required	Achieved intended outcome	Requires occasional supportive cues*
2 Requires assistance	Safe Accurate Behaviour generally appropriate to context	Lacks certainty	Would not have achieved outcome without support	Requires frequent verbal and occasional physical directives in addition to supportive cues*
1 Requires direction	Safe only with guidance Not completely accurate	Unskilled Inefficient	Would not have achieved outcome without support	Requires continuous verbal and frequent physical directive cues*
0 Unsafe	Unsafe Unable to demonstrate behaviour Lack of insight into behaviour appropriate to context	Unskilled	Would not have achieved outcome	Requires continuous verbal and continuous physical directive cues*

*Refers to physical directives or verbal supportive cues

Performance Improvement Plan (PIP)

Please document the agreed education plan and completion timelines for areas assessed as less than 4.

This plan should be presented to assessor prior to commencement of summative assessment.

Where was supervisor support required?	Student summary of deficit. (Why was there a problem?)	Improvement Plan	Completed (Y/N)

Staff/Student Name: _____

Staff/Student Signature: _____

Educator Name: _____

Educator Signature: _____

Summative Clinical Skill Assessment (S-CSAT)

Equipment and resources: Standardised patient; hand decontamination agent; disposable gloves; clinical waste bag; digital tympanic thermometer and probe covers; method of documenting results

Associated Clinical Skills: Infection control; Communication; Consent

Staff/Student being assessed: _____

- Completed Formative Clinical Skill Assessment (F-CSAT): **YES   NO**
- Completed Performance Improvement Plan (PIP): **YES   NO   N/A**

Tympanic temperature recording

Activity	Critical Action	Achieved Without Direction	
Prepares equipment	Identifies rationale for performing observation. Gathers required equipment.	NO	YES
Personal protection	Dons appropriate PPE.	NO	YES
Prepares patient	Explains procedure and advises of brief discomfort. Obtains consent.	NO	YES
Prepares thermometer	Maintains instrument in a hygienic condition. Attaches a new probe cover. Confirms device is in 'ready' mode.	NO	YES
Assesses temperature	Pulls ear to align ear canal. Uses technique appropriate to patient's age. Gently inserts probe tip into the ear canal as far as it will go.	NO	YES
	Presses activation button to initiate assessment. When reading appears/ alarm sounds, removes thermometer from ear. Notes reading.	NO	YES
Disposes of waste	Disposes of ear probe as clinical waste.	NO	YES
Reports	Documents measurement and detected problems.	NO	YES

Standard Achieved: (please circle one)

Competent (C)   Not Yet Competent* (NYC)

Staff/Student Name: _____

Assessor (please print name): _____

Signed (Assessor): _____

Date of Assessment: _____

Comments:

*If Not Yet Competent (NYC) a PIP needs to be completed and a repeat of the F-CSAT

Clinical findings

Afebrile/normothermic (36.2 °C to 37.5 °C)

Normal adult body temperature reading is maintained between 36.2 and 37.5 degrees Celsius (97.2 to 99.5 degrees Fahrenheit), typically at around 37 °C (98.6 °F). Within this temperature range, the balance between heat loss and heat production is preserved. Heat is lost through radiation, which is affected by the rate of blood flow to the skin's surface, along with evaporation through sweat, convection and conduction. The body's insulation of fat assists in maintaining the body's temperature when exposed to hot and cold environments. Messages sent from the hypothalamus in response to thermoregulatory sensors dictate the physiological pathway to cool or heat the body.

Children tend to have slightly higher body temperatures accompanying their faster metabolism and growth (Levander and Grodzinsky, 2017).

Older adults are less able to detect external temperature and provide physiological adjustment, as there is less muscle for heat production and skin receptors are less effective (Guergova and Dufour, 2011). An altered metabolism and the impact of medication enhance these differences. Older adults typically have a 0.2 °C lower temperature range than other adults (Levander and Grodzinsky, 2017; Lu et al., 2010; Waalen and Buxbaum, 2011).

Females maintain slightly higher body temperature than males by 0.2 °C (Levander and Grodzinsky, 2017). Obesity is similarly associated with a 0.2 °C elevation in temperature, possibly due to the effect of adipose tissue as an inflammatory mediator (Waalen and Buxbaum, 2011).

Temperature readings using a tympanic thermometer are typically slightly lower than core temperature (Table 2.18.1).

Febrile (>37.5 °C)

A patient is febrile when their temperature goes above 37.5 °C and the fever occurs as an acute response to an infection or inflammation within the body. During fever, the thermoregulatory mechanism adjusts to the higher temperature, establishing a new set point that is considered to be helpful in fighting infection (Sullivan and Ferrar, 2011). Peripheral vasoconstriction occurs, causing blood to be shunted towards the body's core to maintain the higher temperature along with metabolic rate increases and shivering (McCance and Heuther, 2015). The equivalent temperature from a non-fever cause is considered far more serious (Sullivan and Ferrar, 2011).

Severe hyperthermia (>40 °C)

Hyperthermia results from a failure of thermoregulation. It occurs when the body produces or absorbs more heat than it can disperse, resulting in a marked increase in core temperature. Temperatures above 40 °C can cause nerve damage, coagulation of cell proteins and death. In adults, altered consciousness, seizures and coma can occur when temperatures reach 41 °C. Unlike the febrile patient, the hyperthermic patient's thermoregulatory mechanism does not reset the hypothalamic set point. Hyperthermia can occur due to exposure to a high-temperature environment. Wearing excessive amounts of clothes, the person not being acclimatised to hot areas or poor physical fitness are just a few factors that may induce hyperthermia in a patient.

Hypothermia (<35 °C)

Hypothermia is a core temperature lower than 35 °C. This classification is typically divided into mild (<35 °C to 32 °C), moderate (<32 °C to 28 °C) and severe (<28 °C) (Brown et al., 2012). This usually occurs from prolonged exposure to a cold environment, including sudden immersion in cold water. Acute hypothermia causes peripheral vasoconstriction to shunt blood away from the colder skin to the body core to maintain body warmth and decrease heat loss. The hypothalamus stimulates shivering to increase heat production. Hypothermia also causes changes to coagulation and microcirculation, which can produce ischaemic tissue damage (McCance and Heuther, 2015). Patient presentation varies with the degree of hypothermia, which impacts on resuscitation strategies (Avellanus et al., 2012; Gordon et al., 2015). Hypothermia has a poor association with trauma outcomes (Ireland et al., 2011; Thorsen et al., 2011).

Hypothermia can affect many paramedic decisions, including rewarming, drug administration protocols and resuscitation, and impact on concurrent illnesses.

Inaccurate readings

The temperature within the ear canal and the ability of the probe to sight the tympanic membrane will influence tympanic temperature assessment. Excessive ear wax or bleeding from an injury can cover the membrane and interfere with the probe, causing a lower reading. Recent immersion in cold water can also lower readings.

Infections in an ear or lying on an ear for a period of time can raise the temperature within the ear, so that it will not necessarily be reflective of the patient's core temperature in such cases. Using another ear or allowing

Table 2.18.1 Normal infrared tympanic temperature readings for age	
Age (yrs)	**Normal tympanic temperature range**
0–2	36.4 °C to 38 °C (97.5 °F to 100.4 °F)
3–10	36.1 °C to 37.8 °C (97 °F to 100 °F)
11–65	35.9 °C to 37.6 °C (96.6 °F to 99.7 °F)
>65	35.8 °C to 37.5 °C (96.4 °F to 99.5 °F)

Source: Chamberlain et al., 1995.

time for normalisation assists with accurate assessment (Arslan et al., 2011; Gasim et al., 2013). In contrast, high ambient air temperature does not cause problems in assessing tympanic temperature (Chue et al., 2012).

If any of these problems is noted, correct it and wait for 20 minutes for the tympanic temperature to stabilise. If different readings are observed closely together, accept the highest one.

PRACTICE TIP!

For accurate infrared reading of the tympanic membrane, the ear canal must be first straightened by pulling on the outer ear. The direction of pull varies with patient age.

PRACTICE TIP!

Abnormally high readings can occur where elevated ear temperature is present, including an ear infection or lying on the ear. In either case, use the other ear or allow time for the temperature to normalise.

PRACTICE TIP!

When working in close proximity to the patient, remember that the cause of their malaise is unknown. Consider the potential cause of the fever and consider the use of P2 breathing masks and protective coverings such as Tyvec® suits if contagious illness is suspected.

TEST YOUR KNOWLEDGE QUESTIONS

1. **Why is the ear pulled during tympanic temperature assessment?**
    To align the ear canal, allowing the probe to assess the membrane.

2. **List two problems that can cause tympanic readings to be lower than actual core temperature?**
    Ears blocked with wax or blood; recent immersion in cold water.

3. **List two problems that can cause tympanic readings to be higher than normal.**
    Ear infection; lying on the ear.

4. **What three patient groups typically have higher body temperature ranges?**
    Children; females; the obese.

5. **What action is taken if a patient is found lying on an ear?**
    Assess the other ear or wait 20 minutes for temperature to stabilise.

6. **Why is tympanic membrane temperature assessment a reflection of core temperature?**
    The membrane has a common blood supply with the hypothalamus.

7. **How does older age affect body temperature?**
    Body temperature is typically lower than in people of other ages.

8. **At what temperature does severe hyperthermia exist?**
    >40 °C.

9. **At what temperature does severe hypothermia exist?**
    <28 °C.

10. **How does fever differ from hyperthermia?**
    Fever is an intentional immune response; hyperthermia is an uncontrolled elevation in body temperature.

References

Allegaert, K., Casteels, K., Van Gorp, I. and Bogaert, G., 2014. Tympanic, infrared skin, and temporal artery scan thermometers compared with rectal measurement in children: a real-life assessment. *Current Therapeutic Research*, 76, 34–38.

Arslan, G.G., Eser, I. and Khorshid, L., 2011. Analysis of the effect of lying on the ear on body temperature measurement using a tympanic thermometer. *Journal of the Pakistan Medical Association*, 61(11), 1065.

Avellanas, M.L., Ricart, A., Botella, J., Mengelle, F., Soteras, I., Veres, T. and Vidal, M., 2012. Management of severe accidental hypothermia. *Medicina Intensiva (English edition)*, 36(3), 200–212.

Barnett, B.J., Nunberg, S., Tai, J., Lesser, M.L., Fridman, V., Nichols, P., Powell, R. and Silverman, R., 2011. Oral and tympanic membrane temperatures are inaccurate to identify fever in emergency department adults. *Western Journal of Emergency Medicine*, 12(4), 505.

Batra, P. and Goyal, S., 2013. Comparison of rectal, axillary, tympanic, and temporal artery thermometry in the pediatric emergency room. *Pediatric Emergency Care*, 29(1), 63–66.

Bijur, P.E., Shah, P.D. and Esses, D., 2016. Temperature measurement in the adult emergency department: oral, tympanic membrane and temporal artery temperatures versus rectal temperature. *Emergency Medicine Journal*, emermed-2015.

Brown, D.J., Brugger, H., Boyd, J. and Paal, P., 2012. Accidental hypothermia. *New England Journal of Medicine*, 367(20), 1930–1938.

Chamberlain, J.M., Terndrup, T.E., Alexander, D.T., Silverstone, F.A., Wolf-Klein, G., O'Donnell, R. and Grandner, J., 1995. Determination of normal ear temperature with an infrared emission detection thermometer. *Annals of Emergency Medicine*, 25(1), 15–20.

Chue, A.L., Moore, R.L., Cavey, A., Ashley, E.A., Stepniewska, K., Nosten, F. and McGready, R., 2012. Comparability of tympanic and oral mercury thermometers at high ambient temperatures. *BMC Research Notes*, 5(1), 356.

Flouris, A.D. and Cheung, S.S., 2010. The validity of tympanic and exhaled breath temperatures for core temperature measurement. *Physiological Measurement*, 31(5), N35.

Gasim, G.I., Musa, I.R., Abdien, M.T. and Adam, I., 2013. Accuracy of tympanic temperature measurement using an infrared tympanic membrane thermometer. *BMC Research Notes*, 6(1), 194.

Gordon, L., Paal, P., Ellerton, J.A., Brugger, H., Peek, G.J. and Zafren, K., 2015. Delayed and intermittent CPR for severe accidental hypothermia. *Resuscitation*, 90, 46–49.

Guergova, S. and Dufour, A., 2011. Thermal sensitivity in the elderly: a review. *Ageing Research Reviews*, 10(1), 80–92.

Hasper, D., Nee, J., Schefold, J.C., Krueger, A. and Storm, C., 2011. Tympanic temperature during therapeutic hypothermia. *Emergency Medicine Journal*, 28(6), 483–485.

Höcker, J., Bein, B., Böhm, R., Steinfath, M., Scholz, J. and Horn, E.P., 2012. Correlation, accuracy, precision and practicability of perioperative measurement of sublingual temperature in comparison with tympanic membrane temperature in awake and anaesthetised patients. *European Journal of Anaesthesiology*, 29(2), 70–74.

Ireland, S., Endacott, R., Cameron, P., Fitzgerald, M. and Paul, E., 2011. The incidence and significance of accidental hypothermia in major trauma – a prospective observational study. *Resuscitation*, 82(3), 300–306.

Jefferies, S., Weatherall, M., Young, P. and Beasley, R., 2011. A systematic review of the accuracy of peripheral thermometry in estimating core temperatures among febrile critically ill patients. *Critical Care and Resuscitation*, 13(3), 194.

Levander, M.S. and Grodzinsky, E., 2017. Variation in normal ear temperature. *American Journal of the Medical Sciences*, 354(4), 370–378.

Lu, S.H., Leasure, A.R. and Dai, Y.T., 2010. A systematic review of body temperature variations in older people. *Journal of Clinical Nursing*, 19(1–2), 4–16.

Paes, B.F., Vermeulen, K., Brohet, R.M., Van der Ploeg, T. and De Winter, J.P., 2010. Accuracy of tympanic and infrared skin thermometers in children. *Archives of Disease in Childhood*, 95(12), 974–978.

Sullivan, J.E. and Farrar, H.C., 2011. Fever and antipyretic use in children. *Pediatrics*, 127(3), 580–587.

Sund-Levander, M. and Grodzinsky, E., 2013. Assessment of body temperature measurement options. *British Journal of Nursing*, 22(16), 942–950.

Terndrup, T.E. and Rajk, J., 1992. Impact of operator technique and device on infrared emission detection tympanic thermometry. *Journal of Emergency Medicine*, 10(6), 683–687.

Thorsen, K., Ringdal, K.G., Strand, K., Søreide, E., Hagemo, J. and Søreide, K., 2011. Clinical and cellular effects of hypothermia, acidosis and coagulopathy in major injury. *British Journal of Surgery*, 98(7), 894–907.

Waalen, J. and Buxbaum, J.N., 2011. Is older colder or colder older? The association of age with body temperature in 18,630 individuals. *Journals of Gerontology Series A: Biomedical Sciences and Medical Sciences*, 66(5), 487–492.

Yamakoshi, T., Matsumura, K., Rolfe, P., Tanaka, N., Yamakoshi, Y. and Takahashi, K., 2013. A novel method to detect heat illness under severe conditions by monitoring tympanic temperature. *Aviation, Space, and Environmental Medicine*, 84(7), 692–700.

Yeoh, W.K., Lee, J.K.W., Lim, H.Y., Gan, C.W., Liang, W. and Tan, K.K., 2017. Re-visiting the tympanic membrane vicinity as core body temperature measurement site. *PLoS One*, 12(4).

Zhen, C., Xia, Z., Ya Jun, Z., Long, L., Jian, S., Gui Ju, C. and Long, L., 2015. Accuracy of infrared tympanic thermometry used in the diagnosis of fever in children: a systematic review and meta-analysis. *Clinical Pediatrics*, 54(2), 114–126.

Bibliography

Craft, J., Gordon, C., Huether, S.E., McCance, K.L. and Brashers, V.L., 2015. *Understanding pathophysiology (ANZ adaptation)*. Sydney: Elsevier.

McCance, K.L. and Huether, S.E., 2015. *Pathophysiology: the biologic basis for disease in adults and children*. Sydney: Elsevier.

2.19 | Blood glucose recording

Joelene Gott

Chapter objectives

At the end of this chapter the reader will be able to:

1. Describe the rationale for assessing blood glucose levels
2. Demonstrate assessing blood glucose level
3. Accurately report on the findings

Resources required for this assessment

- Standardised patient or mannequin
- Fake blood samples created with varying glucose levels
- Glucometer
- Test strips
- Lancets
- Disposable gloves
- Antiseptic swabs
- Cotton balls/gauze
- Adhesive dressing
- Sharps container
- Clinical waste bag
- Hand decontamination agent
- Method of documenting the results

Skill matrix

This assessment requires:

- Infection control (CS 1.3)
- Communication (CS 1.5)
- Consent (CS 1.9)

This assessment is a component of:

- Patient assessment (Chapter 2)

Introduction

The measurement of blood glucose levels is an important component of the paramedic's assessment and management of patients who are either critically injured or ill or have a minor illness.

Blood glucose levels quantify the amount of glucose in the blood and are regulated by insulin and glucagon. Levels can be tested in several different ways. Point of care glucometry using capillary blood from the patient's finger is the paramedic method. It is a quick, easy and quantitative assessment enabling the determination of hypoglycaemia and hyperglycaemia. This chapter discusses effective and accurate blood glucose assessment.

Anatomy and physiology

Blood glucose levels need to be maintained by the body in a narrow range, which is allowed by hormones including glucagon and insulin. The pancreas plays the central role secreting both of these hormones to ultimately determine the patient's blood glucose levels (McCance and Heuther, 2015).

Glucagon and insulin are secreted through cells called islets of Langerhans. These islets have three different types of cells that secrete hormones. Two discussed here are the alpha cells, which secrete glucagon, and the beta cells, which secrete insulin.

Insulin secretion is activated by an increase in blood glucose levels, typically following eating. It reduces in response to lowering glucose levels. Insulin facilitates glucose uptake into cells, including glycogenesis in the liver (McCance and Heuther, 2015). Glucagon acts in the liver by increasing blood glucose through the stimulation of glycogenolysis and glucogenolysis. Glucagon levels are increased when glucose levels lower and sympathetic stimulation occurs, and they are inhibited when high glucose levels occur (McCance and Heuther, 2015; Unger and Cherrington, 2012).

Glucose is not the only sugar obtained from food and found in the blood. However, it is the main trigger for the insulin system, so it is the sugar that is most commonly referred to.

Clinical rationale

After eating, arterial blood glucose is significantly higher than that found in the capillaries until insulin redistributes it, returning levels to normal. Between meals, blood sugar is maintained by glucagon release so it remains relatively steady. The level of glucose in the arteries is slightly greater than that in the capillaries and greater again than in venous blood, with glucose being removed at the cellular level. Capillary blood readings can be up to 20% higher than venous readings (Lunt et al., 2010). The variations remain steady (Yang et al., 2012), though the unreliability of capillary readings has been noted during shock (Juneja et al., 2011). Higher than normal readings occur where there is low haematocrit (Ramljak et al., 2013).

Glucometer devices (Fig. 2.19.1a and b) are calibrated to rely on small sample volumes from capillary sources (Freckmann et al., 2012; Freckmann et al., 2014). This necessitates using a finger-prick method. Do not squeeze the finger to produce the sample, as this can cause incorrect readings. The potential for false low readings from insufficient blood availability is also reduced by modern test strips that will not test until the sufficient minimum sample is available (Lunt et al., 2010).

Blood sugar testing using a glucometer essentially involves drawing a drop of blood from a finger, typically on the side, near to the tip (less painful), using a lancet (Fig. 2.19.2). These are commonly spring loaded for ease and effectiveness. A test strip, inserted ready for use into the glucometer, is placed against the drop until enough is absorbed into it (Fig. 2.19.3). After a predetermined time, the result appears on the glucometer in either of the units mmol/L or mg/dL. The values provided for each unit will be vastly different, so be familiar with which is in use and the corresponding scales for interpretation.

Diabetics are predisposed to peripheral vascular problems, including infections. Before the finger is

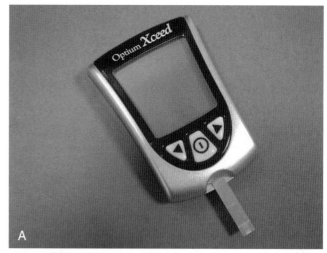
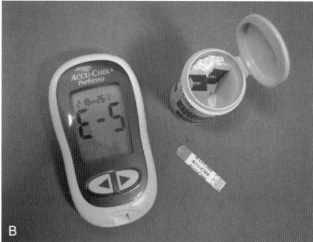

Figure 2.19.1a and b Glucometer devices with test strips

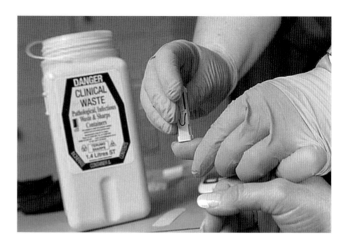

Figure 2.19.2 Using a lancet to obtain a blood droplet

pricked it should be cleaned with an antiseptic swab and allowed to dry. This is also critical for minimising the potential for reading errors. Any sugar from eating that contaminates the patient's skin can adversely affect the readings (Ginsberg, 2009). Sites other than fingers are not used, since the blood level available can vary slightly. Some patients prefer a rotation of fingers or using the sides rather than the tips, which can bother them later. Diabetics are further predisposed to peripheral neurology

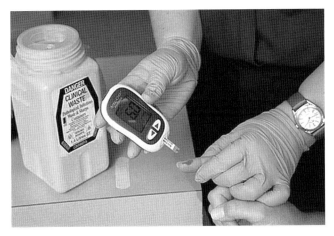

Figure 2.19.3 Using the glucometer

alterations from microcirculation disease. Using the finger ends can therefore impact on their sense of touch.

Venous blood use

Portable blood glucose measurement devices are designed to utilise capillary blood. Where intravenous cannulation simultaneously occurs, it can be tempting to make use of this blood to avoid further discomfort to the patient. In such cases, venous blood samples can provide slightly higher readings (0.3 mmol/L variance) than capillary blood (Adnan et al., 2017; Boyd et al., 2005; Yaraghi et al., 2015). The routine use of venous blood for glucometer analysis should be discouraged. However, where the patient's peripheral skin cannot be reliably cleaned, venous blood may be a suitable alternative for assessment (Yaraghi et al., 2015).

Clinical skill assessment process

The following section outlines the clinical skill assessment tools that should be used to determine a student's ability to demonstrate the safe and accurate collection and interpretation of blood glucose.
1. Clinical Skill Work Instruction
2. Formative Clinical Skill Assessment (F-CSAT)
3. Performance Improvement Plan (PIP)
4. Summative Clinical Skill Assessment (S-CSAT)
(5. Direct Observation of Procedural Skills (DOPS) – see Chapter 1.1)

Clinical Skill Work Instruction

Equipment and resources: Standardised patient or mannequin; fake blood samples created with varying glucose levels; glucometer; test strips; lancets; disposable gloves; antiseptic swabs; cotton balls/gauze; adhesive dressing; sharps container; clinical waste bag; hand decontamination agent; method of documenting results

Associated Clinical Skills: Infection control; Communication; Consent

Blood glucose recording

Activity	Critical Action	Rationale
Prepare equipment	Gather required equipment.	In readiness for use.
Prepare patient	Identify rationale for performing test. Provide clear explanation. Gain consent.	Informs patient. Failing to do so may 'startle' or 'scare' the patient and damage rapport. Be wary of response in patients experiencing altered consciousness.
Personal protection	Don appropriate PPE.	Prevents spread of communicable disease by following universal precautions.
Prepare test site	Select finger site for assessment. Vary site each time. Wipe area with antiseptic swab. Allow >30 seconds to dry.	Rotating the fingers used helps minimise scarring. Cleans fingers of any residue that may impact reading and reduces infection risk.

Blood glucose recording continued

Activity	Critical Action	Rationale
Prepare glucometer	Maintain instrument in a hygienic condition. Turn on glucometer. Unwrap test strip, ensuring no contact with either end. Insert device strip end into glucometer. Leave in place until reading is complete. Confirm device is ready.	Touching the test strip ends could cause contamination and affect result. Most devices have an indicator that says they are now ready for use. If delay occurs, device can turn off, requiring a new test strip insertion.
Draw blood droplet	Prepare lancet for use. This may involve twist removal of a cap, varying with product. Place needle discharge against test site. Discharge lancet. Allow blood droplet to appear without squeezing finger.	Lancets vary but all produce a superficial drop of capillary blood. Squeezing finger to assist corrupts the result.
Lancet disposal	Discard test lancet into sharps container.	Some lancets do not leave a needle exposed. Safe disposal is always prudent.
Apply glucometer	Touch distal end of test strip to the blood droplet. Allow blood to diffuse onto test strip. When a sufficient area of the test strip is covered the glucometer will automatically commence analysis. Hold device and wait. Read result when ready.	Test strips are designed to allow blood to creep onto them, rather than drip, until sufficient amount is applied. The operator need not do any more.
Dress test site	Cover test site with adhesive dressing. Wipe with sterile gauze first if necessary. Discard all waste into an infectious bag.	To remove blood and avoid infection.
Report	Document measurement and actions taken, and provide handover.	Accurate record kept and continuity of patient care.

Formative Clinical Skill Assessment (F-CSAT)

Equipment and resources: Standardised patient or mannequin; fake blood samples created with varying glucose levels; glucometer; test strips; lancets; disposable gloves; antiseptic swabs; cotton balls/gauze; adhesive dressing; sharps container; clinical waste bag; hand decontamination agent; method of documenting results

Associated Clinical Skills: Infection control; Communication; Consent

Staff/Student being assessed: _____

Blood glucose recording

Activity	Critical Action	Performance				
Prepares equipment	Gathers required equipment.	0	1	2	3	4
Prepares patient	Identifies rationale for performing test. Provides clear explanation. Gains consent.	0	1	2	3	4
Personal protection	Dons appropriate PPE.	0	1	2	3	4
Prepares test site	Selects finger site for assessment. Varies site each time. Wipes site with antiseptic swab and allows to dry.	0	1	2	3	4

Blood glucose recording continued

Activity	Critical Action	Performance				
Prepares glucometer	Maintains instrument in hygienic condition. Turns on glucometer and inserts test strip correctly into glucometer, confirms readiness and leaves in place.	0	1	2	3	4
Draws blood droplet	Correctly prepares lancet for use. Places against test site and discharges to produce blood. Does not squeeze finger.	0	1	2	3	4
Lancet disposal	Discards lancet safely.	0	1	2	3	4
Applies glucometer	Applies test strip correctly, waits for analysis and observes reading.	0	1	2	3	4
Dresses test site	Cleans and dresses test site. Discards waste.	0	1	2	3	4
Reports	Documents measurement and actions taken, and provides handover.	0	1	2	3	4

Standard Achieved: (please circle one)

Competent (C)   Not Yet Competent* (NYC)

Staff/Student Name: _____

Assessor (please print name)**:** _____

Signed (Assessor)**:** _____

Date of Assessment: _____

Comments:

*If Not Yet Competent (NYC) a PIP needs to be completed and a repeat of the F-CSAT

Formative Clinical Skill Assessment (F-CSAT) Key

Skill level	Standard of procedure	Quality of performance	Outcome	Level of assistance required
4 Safe for unsupervised practice	Safe Accurate Behaviour is appropriate to context	Confident Accurate Expedient	Achieved intended outcome	No supporting cues* required
3 Requires supervision	Safe Accurate Behaviour is appropriate to context	Confident Accurate Takes longer than required	Achieved intended outcome	Requires occasional supportive cues*
2 Requires assistance	Safe Accurate Behaviour generally appropriate to context	Lacks certainty	Would not have achieved outcome without support	Requires frequent verbal and occasional physical directives in addition to supportive cues*

Skill level	Standard of procedure	Quality of performance	Outcome	Level of assistance required
1 Requires direction	Safe only with guidance Not completely accurate	Unskilled Inefficient	Would not have achieved outcome without support	Requires continuous verbal and frequent physical directive cues*
0 Unsafe	Unsafe Unable to demonstrate behaviour Lack of insight into behaviour appropriate to context	Unskilled	Would not have achieved outcome	Requires continuous verbal and continuous physical directive cues*

*Refers to physical directives or verbal supportive cues

Performance Improvement Plan (PIP)

Please document the agreed education plan and completion timelines for areas assessed as less than 4.

This plan should be presented to assessor prior to commencement of summative assessment.

Where was supervisor support required?	Student summary of deficit. (Why was there a problem?)	Improvement Plan	Completed (Y/N)

Staff/Student Name: _____

Staff/Student Signature: _____

Educator Name: _____

Educator Signature: _____

Summative Clinical Skill Assessment (S-CSAT)

Equipment and resources: Standardised patient or mannequin; fake blood samples created with varying glucose levels; glucometer; test strips; lancets; disposable gloves; antiseptic swabs; cotton balls/gauze; adhesive dressing; sharps container; clinical waste bag; hand decontamination agent; method of documenting results

Associated Clinical Skills: Infection control; Communication; Consent

Staff/Student being assessed: _____

- Completed Formative Clinical Skill Assessment (F-CSAT):   YES   NO

- Completed Performance Improvement Plan (PIP):   YES   NO   N/A

Blood glucose recording

Activity	Critical Action	Achieved Without Direction	
Prepares equipment	Gathers required equipment.	NO	YES
Prepares patient	Identifies rationale for performing test. Provides clear explanation. Gains consent.	NO	YES
Infection control	Maintains instrument in a hygienic condition. Maintains universal precautions. Dons appropriate PPE.	NO	YES
Prepares test site	Selects finger site for assessment. Varies site each time. Wipes site with antiseptic swab and allows to dry.	NO	YES
Prepares glucometer	Maintains instrument in hygienic condition. Turns on glucometer and inserts test strip correctly into glucometer, confirms readiness and leaves in place.	NO	YES
Draws blood droplet	Correctly prepares lancet for use. Places against test site and discharges to produce blood. Does not squeeze finger.	NO	YES
Lancet disposal	Discards lancet safely.	NO	YES
Applies glucometer	Applies test strip correctly, waits for analysis and observes reading.	NO	YES
Dresses test site	Cleans and dresses test site. Discards waste.	NO	YES
Reports	Documents measurement and actions taken. Provides handover.	NO	YES

Standard Achieved: (please circle one)

Competent (C)   Not Yet Competent* (NYC)

Staff/Student Name: _____

Assessor (please print name): _____

Signed (Assessor): _____

Date of Assessment: _____

Comments:

*If Not Yet Competent (NYC) a PIP needs to be completed and a repeat of the F-CSAT

Clinical findings

Blood glucose level readings can be used for day-to-day monitoring by patients to guide ongoing therapy or monitor trends. In emergencies, single values can be used to assess for critical illness and prompt emergency intervention. The levels observed will be normal, too low or too high.

Normal values (4–7 mmol/L)

Normal blood glucose reading is considered to be between 4 mmol/L and 7 mmol/L (72–126 mg/dL) (American Diabetes Association, 2014), though this can rise to near 8 mmol/L soon after eating. Fasting for >8 hours can provide less variable results (Emerging Risk Factors Collaboration, 2010), but this is not suited to emergency analysis.

Hypoglycaemia (<4 mmol/L)

A patient is considered hypoglycaemic when their blood glucose levels fall below 4 mmol/L (72 mg/dL). Observable hypoglycaemia effects become more pronounced and significant as the level gets lower. Severe hypoglycaemia can be said to occur when blood sugar level drops below 2.8 mmol/L and the help of another person is required to correct it (Bonds et al., 2010; Seaquist et al., 2013). However, the value is somewhat arbitrary, as other studies refer to severe hypoglycaemia occurring at <2.2 mmol/L (Finfer et al., 2013). Patients can become symptomatic at different levels.

Hypoglycaemia can be precipitated, usually in diabetic patients, by a number of exogenous factors such as medications, alcohol or exercise. Tumours of the pancreas or inherited (endogenous) disorders can also cause hypoglycaemia. It can also be caused by functional problems such as liver disease or hyperalimentation, or simply occur spontaneously for reasons that are unclear (McCance and Huether, 2015).

Hypoglycaemia can cause a range of problems, including seizures, loss of consciousness, coma, neurological injury and even death; and it can occur in type 1 or type 2 diabetes (Bonds et al., 2010; Seaquist et al., 2013). Assessing blood sugar level is an important assessment of any change in a patient's consciousness, allowing rapid remedy where hypoglycaemia is the cause. It is an important way of excluding signs that can mimic stroke. Remedies include oral carbohydrate, intravenous glucose or SC/IM glucagon.

Hypotension leads to reduced perfusion and increased glucose utilisation. This can cause peripheral blood sugar readings to be lower than they actually are (Kotwal and Pandit, 2012).

Hyperglycaemia (>7 mmol/L)

A patient is considered hyperglycaemic when their blood glucose levels rise above 7 mmol/L. Severe hyperglycaemia is defined as levels above 11.1 mmol/L (200 mg/dL) (American Diabetes Association, 2014; Seino et al., 2010).

While diabetes is the most common cause of hyperglycaemia, there are other conditions that can cause it too, including pancreatitis, pancreatic cancer, Cushing's syndrome, unusual hormone-secreting tumours, some medications and infections/illnesses (Stöppler, n.d.).

Diabetes can be divided into four types (American Diabetes Association, 2015; Seino et al., 2010):

1. Type 1, where autoimmune destruction of the beta cells causes insufficient insulin
2. Type 2, the most common, which develops progressively and is typically due to resistance to the actions of insulin
3. Gestational diabetes that develops during pregnancy
4. Diabetes caused by a range of other problems, including drugs or being chemically induced.

The natural tendency in any of these conditions is for blood sugar levels to steadily rise with the reduced availability or effectiveness of insulin. This can commonly occur over days, offering an opportunity for intervention before it becomes too problematic. Regular monitoring of blood glucose assists with this.

Emergency presentations arise when severe hyperglycaemia goes unchecked, with thirst, dehydration and, in some cases, substantial metabolic acidosis ensuing. Blood sugar assessment can also assist in the recognition of such emergency presentations. If severe hyperglycaemia is left unchecked, the patient may present as critically unwell and become a medical emergency. Their blood sugar levels may become so high that readings may be in the 20s or register on devices as simply 'Hi'. Some devices also measure ketones, which are produced when fat is metabolised instead of sugar. Readings above 1.6–3.0 mmol/L indicate a risk of diabetic ketone acidosis (DKA).

PRACTICE TIP!

Before beginning the assessment, ensure all equipment is ready and the patient's consent is obtained. If the test strip is inserted too early, the glucometer can turn off after a period of time.

PRACTICE TIP!

Blood sugar levels are not required to be tested on every patient. However, they are a very important part of the assessment of any patient who shows symptoms/signs of blood sugar abnormality, including thirst, dehydration, increased urination or a change in consciousness or behaviour.

TEST YOUR KNOWLEDGE QUESTIONS

1. **What is a normal blood glucose level range?**
   4–7 mmol/L

2. **What is hypoglycaemia?**
   Lower than normal blood sugar levels <4 mmol/L.

3. **What does fasting do to blood sugar levels?**
   The levels stabilise without being influenced by rises caused by recent eating.

4. **What is hyperglycaemia?**
   Higher than normal blood sugar levels: >7 mmol/L.

5. **How should test strips be handled?**
   Without touching either end to avoid contamination.

6. **Why is it important to test finger blood?**
   The levels can vary at other body sites and provide inconsistent results.

7. **Why is arterial or venous blood not used with a glucometer?**
   Blood sugar levels in blood either side of the capillaries will provide differing results and the devices are calibrated to measure capillary samples.

8. **Why is glucose the sugar tested for?**
   It is the main sugar trigger for the insulin response.

9. **Why is it important to wipe the patient's finger with an antiseptic swab before testing?**
   Diabetics can have compromised peripheral circulation and be prone to infection; and any residue that may impact the result is wiped off (such as food/sugar).

10. **What presentations typically indicate blood sugar testing?**
    Signs/symptoms of thirst, dehydration or increased urination, or changes in consciousness or behaviour.

References

Adnan, M., Imam, F., Shabbir, I., Ali, Z. and Rahat, T. 2017. Correlation between capillary and venous blood glucose levels in diabetic patients. *Asian Biomedicine*, 9(1), 55–59.

American Diabetes Association, 2014. Diagnosis and classification of diabetes mellitus. *Diabetes Care*, 37(Suppl 1), S81–S90.

American Diabetes Association, 2015. Standards of medical care in diabetes – 2015 abridged for primary care providers. *Clinical Diabetes*, 33(2), 97.

Bonds, D.E., Miller, M.E., Bergenstal, R.M., Buse, J.B., Byington, R.P., Cutler, J.A., Dudl, R.J., Ismail-Beigi, F., Kimel, A.R., Hoogwerf, B. and Horowitz, K.R., 2010. The association between symptomatic, severe hypoglycaemia and mortality in type 2 diabetes: retrospective epidemiological analysis of the ACCORD study. *BMJ*, 340, b4909.

Boyd, R., Leigh, B. and Stuart, P., 2005. Capillary versus venous bedside blood glucose estimations. *Emergency Medicine Journal*, 22(3), 177–179.

Emerging Risk Factors Collaboration, 2010. Diabetes mellitus, fasting blood glucose concentration, and risk of vascular disease: a collaborative meta-analysis of 102 prospective studies. *Lancet*, 375(9733), 2215–2222.

Finfer, S., Wernerman, J., Preiser, J.C., Cass, T., Desaive, T., Hovorka, R., Joseph, J.I., Kosiborod, M., Krinsley, J., Mackenzie, I. and Mesotten, D., 2013. Clinical review: consensus recommendations on measurement of blood glucose and reporting glycemic control in critically ill adults. *Critical Care*, 17(3), 229.

Freckmann, G., Baumstark, A., Schmid, C., Pleus, S., Link, M. and Haug, C., 2014. Evaluation of 12 blood glucose monitoring systems for self-testing: system accuracy and measurement reproducibility. *Diabetes Technology & Therapeutics*, 16(2), 113–122.

Freckmann, G., Schmid, C., Baumstark, A., Pleus, S., Link, M. and Haug, C., 2012. System accuracy evaluation of 43 blood glucose monitoring systems for self-monitoring of blood glucose according to DIN EN ISO 15197. *Journal of Diabetes Science and Technology*, 6(5), 1060–1075.

Ginsberg, B.H., 2009. Factors affecting blood glucose monitoring: sources of errors in measurement. *Journal of Diabetes Science and Technology*, 3(4), 903–913.

Juneja, D., Pandey, R. and Singh, O., 2011. Comparison between arterial and capillary blood glucose monitoring in patients with shock. *European Journal of Internal Medicine*, 22(3), 241–244.

Kotwal, N. and Pandit, A., 2012. Variability of capillary blood glucose monitoring measured on home glucose monitoring devices. *Indian Journal of Endocrinology and Metabolism*, 16(Suppl 2), S248.

Lunt, H., Florkowski, C., Bignall, M. and Budgen, C., 2010. Capillary glucose meter accuracy and sources of error in the ambulatory setting. *New Zealand Medical Journal*, 123(1310), 74–85.

Ramljak, S., Lock, J.P., Schipper, C., Musholt, P.B., Forst, T., Lyon, M. and Pfützner, A., 2013. Hematocrit interference of blood glucose meters for patient self-measurement. *Journal of Diabetes Science and Technology*, 7(1), 179–189.

Seaquist, E.R., Anderson, J., Childs, B., Cryer, P., Dagogo-Jack, S., Fish, L., Heller, S.R., Rodriguez, H., Rosenzweig, J. and Vigersky, R., 2013. Hypoglycemia and diabetes: a report of a workgroup of the American Diabetes Association and the Endocrine Society. *Journal of Clinical Endocrinology & Metabolism*, 98(5), 1845–1859.

Seino, Y., Nanjo, K., Tajima, N., Kadowaki, T., Kashiwagi, A., Araki, E., Ito, C., Inagaki, N., Iwamoto, Y., Kasuga, M. and Hanafusa, T., 2010. Report of the committee on the classification and diagnostic criteria of diabetes mellitus. *Journal of Diabetes Investigation*, 1(5), 212–228.

Stöppler, M.C., n.d. 10 high blood sugar symptoms, dangers, causes, and treatment. Retrieved from: https://www.medicinenet.com/hyperglycemia/article.htm

Unger, R.H. and Cherrington, A.D., 2012. Glucagonocentric restructuring of diabetes: a pathophysiologic and therapeutic makeover. *Journal of Clinical Investigation*, 122(1), 4.

Yang, C., Chang, C. and Lin, J., 2012. A comparison between venous and finger-prick blood sampling on values of blood glucose. *International Proceedings of Chemical, Biological and Environmental Engineering*, 39, 206–210.

Yaraghi, A., Mood, N.E. and Dolatabadi, L.K., 2015. Comparison of capillary and venous blood glucose levels using glucometer and laboratory blood glucose level in poisoned patients being in coma. *Advanced Biomedical Research*, 4.

Bibliography

Craft, J., Gordon, C., Huether, S.E., McCance, K.L. and Brashers, V.L., 2015. *Understanding pathophysiology (ANZ adaptation)*. Sydney: Elsevier.

McCance, K.L. and Huether, S.E., 2015. *Pathophysiology: the biologic basis for disease in adults and children*. Sydney: Elsevier.

Chapter objectives

At the end of this chapter the reader will be able to:

1. Describe the rationale for using Aseptic Non Touch Technique (ANTT®)
2. Incorporate ANTT® into paramedic practice

Resources required for this assessment

- Standardised patient or mannequin
- Dressing kit
- Hand decontamination agent – alcohol-based hand rub (ABHR)
- Surface sanitisation wipes
- Personal protective equipment (PPE)/disposable gloves
- Clinical waste bag
- Method of documenting the results
- Items relevant to the task performed

Skill matrix

This assessment requires:

- Infection control (CS 1.3)
- Communication (CS 1.5)
- Consent (CS 1.6)

This assessment is a component of:

- Patient assessment (Chapter 2)

Introduction

Aseptic Non Touch Technique (ANTT®) is a standard aseptic technique that is used to reduce the rates of healthcare-associated infections. It aims to prevent pathogens being introduced in sufficient quantity to cause infection to susceptible sites by hands or by surfaces and equipment (NHMRC, 2010). ANTT® uses a safety approach that considers how much the patient is at risk from the healthcare worker, the technical challenge of the procedure, and the practice environment (Rowley and Clare, 2011b). In other words, ANTT® considers both the technical difficulty of procedures and the paramedic's ability to decide if procedures can be performed without touching key parts or key sites directly (NHMRC, 2010). Key parts are the critical parts of the procedure equipment that, if contaminated, are most likely to cause infection; key sites are open wounds and access sites for medical devices (Rowley and Clare, 2011b).

The ANTT® framework is based on six principles (Table 2.20.1). It has several important components and requires the paramedic to identify the risk of contamination and to choose the correct field and technique to avoid the spread of pathogens. Infective precautions are then selected to counter the risks identified; for example, the use of sterile or non-sterile gloves to maintain asepsis or freedom from infectious (pathogenic) material (NHMRC, 2010). Although the principles of aseptic technique remain constant for all procedures, the level of practice will change depending upon a standard risk assessment that considers hand hygiene, gloving, aseptic field, aseptic technique and sequencing.

ANTT® is discussed in this chapter.

Table 2.20.1 The principles of the ANTT® framework grouped by clinical practice and organisational management

Principle	Clinical practice details
Principle 1	The aim of ANTT® for invasive and clinical procedures is always asepsis.
Principle 2	Asepsis is achieved by protecting key parts and key sites from microorganism transfer from the healthcare worker and the immediate environment.
Principle 3	ANTT® needs to be efficient as well as safe. Surgical ANTT® is used for complicated procedures and Standard ANTT® for uncomplicated procedures.
Principle 4	Choice of Surgical or Standard ANTT® is based on an ANTT® risk assessment, according to the technical difficulty of protecting key part and key site asepsis. This principle relies on four safeguards. *Safeguard 1: Basic infective precautions* Precautions include hand cleaning and environmental controls, which significantly reduce the risk of contaminating key parts and key sites. *Safeguard 2: Identification of key parts & key sites* Key parts are the critical parts of the procedure equipment that, if contaminated, are most likely to cause infection. Key sites are open wounds and medical device access sites. *Safeguard 3: Non-touch technique* Non-touch technique is a critical skill that protects key parts and key sites from the healthcare worker and the procedure environment; it is used in both Surgical and Standard ANTT®. *Safeguard 4: Aseptic field management* ANTT® is a critical skill that protects key parts and key sites from the healthcare workers and the procedure environment; Surgical and Standard ANTT® require different aseptic field management.
	Organisational management details
Principle 5	Aseptic practice should be standardised.
Principle 6	Safe aseptic technique relies on effective training of healthcare workers and on environments and equipment that are fit for purpose.

Source: *Adapted from Association for Safe Aseptic Practice, 2016.*

Anatomy and physiology

Before the 1980s, common pathogens such as rotavirus, *Campylobacter*, *Legionella*, *Escherichia coli* (*E. coli*) O157 and norovirus were largely unheard of by the general public (Bloomfield et al., 2007). Furthermore, pathogens such as MRSA, VRE and *Clostridium difficile* were considered 'nosocomial infections' acquired in hospitals. Today, these pathogens are considered a major public health and financial concern for healthcare settings across the world, and are now regarded as being healthcare-associated infections (HAIs) (Bloomfield et al., 2007; Nimmo et al., 2006; ACSQHC, 2014).

In Australia, it has been estimated that there are up to 200,000 HAI cases in acute healthcare settings each year, making HAIs the most serious adverse event faced by patients during their engagement within the Australian health system (NHMRC, 2010; ACSQHC, 2014). As many as 10% of patients admitted into New Zealand hospitals can acquire infection while there, potentially doubling the length of their hospital stay (Burns et al., 2010; Read and Bhally, 2015).

Acquiring an HAI is a complicated interaction between risk factors, pathogenic microorganisms and their modes of transmission, and susceptible hosts. This interaction is called 'the chain of infection' (NHMRC, 2010). The risk factors that are important predictors of an individual's outcome after exposure to an infectious agent include immune status, age, comorbidities, severity of illness, surgery or indwelling devices, interinstitutional transfers, prolonged hospitalisation, exposure to invasive devices, and antimicrobial drugs (NHMRC, 2010; Safdar and Maki, 2002). A demographic trend towards an aging population also means that the proportion of the population in the community who are more vulnerable to HAIs is increasing. Coupled with this trend is a move towards shorter hospital stays and increased care in the community, which should raise awareness of the care of 'at-risk' groups in their home and protection from HAIs.

Clinical rationale

The aim of ANTT® for clinical practice is asepsis for all invasive clinical procedures, despite their complexity (Rowley and Clare, 2011b). The term 'asepsis' refers to the absence of pathogenic microorganisms and has replaced the terms 'sterile technique' and 'clean technique'. Sterile technique required the complete absence of microorganisms, which is not possible to achieve in typical healthcare settings due to the prevalence of microorganisms in the air. The term 'clean technique' has been discouraged as it was considered too ambiguous.

ANTT® is achieved using aseptic fields to ensure asepsis of key parts and key sites within the immediate procedural environment. The method also improves aseptic practice through standardisation of practice and efficient technique. ANTT® has assisted in the rationalisation of equipment choices and explicit sequencing act to 'prescribe out' variable practices (Rowley and Clare, 2011a).

Clinical skill assessment process

The following section outlines the clinical skill assessment tools that should be used to determine a student's ability to demonstrate the safe and accurate use of ANTT®.

1. Clinical Skill Work Instruction
2. Formative Clinical Skill Assessment (F-CSAT)
3. Performance Improvement Plan (PIP)
4. Summative Clinical Skill Assessment (S-CSAT)
(5. Direct Observation of Procedural Skills (DOPS) – see Chapter 1.1)

Clinical Skill Work Instruction

Equipment and resources: Patient or mannequin; dressing kit; hand decontamination agent; surface sanitisation wipes; PPE/gloves; clinical waste bag; method of documenting results; items relevant to task performed

Associated Clinical Skills: Infection control; Communication; Consent

Using ANTT®

Activity	Critical Action	Rationale
Perform hand hygiene	If the hands are soiled, use soap and water or detergent wipe and dry with a towel. If the hands are not soiled, use ABHR.	Removing soiling and pathogens from hands before contact with a patient or clinical environment reduces the transmission of HAIs.
Prepare patient	Gain informed patient consent. Use gloves where appropriate, such as when removing a bloodstained dressing or blood/bodily fluids (BBF). After preparing the patient, remove gloves and perform hand hygiene (ABHR).	Patients must be informed before they give consent for a procedure. To decrease risk of contact with BBF. Reduces pathogens on hands after contact with patient.
Prepare work area	Ensure ambulance work surfaces wiped clean with surface sanitisation wipes. For other uncontrolled prehospital surfaces, cover with clean linen (e.g. pillowcase/towel) or protective work sheet (e.g. bluey).	Work area may be contaminated.
Assemble equipment	Identify and gather equipment for procedure, such as dressing kits, disposable medication trays and disposable tourniquets.	To avoid need to move away from sterile field once commenced to get further equipment.
Prepare field	Perform hand hygiene (ABHR) and prepare a sterile field for the protection of key parts and key sites. Open procedure pack using corners. Make a sterile field.	This uses a sterile dressing as a typical example of preparation.
Prepare procedural equipment	After preparing the field, open procedural equipment packaging in a way that maintains asepsis and drop the required sterile equipment into the appropriate place on sterile field.	Sterile field and external potentially contaminated spaces must be kept strictly separated.
Prepare to perform procedure	If wearing gloves, remove them and perform hand hygiene (ABHR). Don required PPE. Apply new gloves if there is a risk of BBF contamination and use eye protection and masks as required. Use sterile gloves with procedures such as intraosseous needle insertion or if the hands are entering semi-critical body areas, such as the vagina during procedures to assist birthing.	Must clean hands again before they enter sterile field.
Perform procedure	Ensure all key parts/components are protected: • sterile items are used once and disposed into waste bag • only sterile items contact a key site • sterile items do not come into contact with non-sterile items.	Maintain strict separation of sterile and non-sterile fields.

Activity	Critical Action	Rationale
Post procedure	Remove gloves and dispose into clinical waste bag. Perform hand hygiene (ABHR). Clean work surface after use with a sanitising wipe if applicable, and perform hand hygiene (ABHR).	Remain vigilant against infection source transmission.
Report	Document procedure in notes, including compliance issues with ANTT®.	Accurate record kept and continuity of patient care.

Source: Adapted from NHMRC, 2010.

Formative Clinical Skill Assessment (F-CSAT)

Equipment and resources: Patient or mannequin; dressing kit; hand decontamination agent; surface sanitisation wipes; PPE/gloves; clinical waste bag, method of documenting results; items relevant to task performed

Associated Clinical Skills: Infection control; Communication; Consent

Staff/Student being assessed: _____

Using ANTT®

Activity	Critical Action	Performance				
Performs hand hygiene	Uses appropriate technique for hand hygiene.	0	1	2	3	4
Prepares patient	Gains patient consent. Prepares key site on the patient. Uses appropriate PPE to maintain safety. Removes gloves if worn and performs hand hygiene (ABHR).	0	1	2	3	4
Prepares work area	Cleans and prepares work surfaces. Performs hand hygiene (ABHR).	0	1	2	3	4
Assembles equipment	Assembles required equipment for the procedure.	0	1	2	3	4
Prepares field	Prepares sterile field.					
Prepares procedural equipment	Prepares equipment within the field.	0	1	2	3	4
Prepares to perform procedure	Performs hand hygiene (ABHR). Uses appropriate PPE.	0	1	2	3	4
Performs procedure	Ensures all key parts/components are protected.	0	1	2	3	4
Post procedure	Removes gloves and performs hand hygiene (ABHR). Cleans work surface after use while wearing appropriate PPE. Performs hand hygiene (ABHR).	0	1	2	3	4
Reports	Documents procedure in notes, including compliance issues with ANTT®.	0	1	2	3	4

Source: Adapted from NHMRC, 2010.

Standard Achieved: (please circle one)

Competent (C)   Not Yet Competent* (NYC)

Staff/Student Name: _____

Assessor (please print name)**:** _____

Signed (Assessor)**:** _____

Date of Assessment: _____

Comments:

*If Not Yet Competent (NYC) a PIP needs to be completed and a repeat of the F-CSAT

Formative Clinical Skill Assessment (F-CSAT) Key

Skill level	Standard of procedure	Quality of performance	Outcome	Level of assistance required
4 Safe for unsupervised practice	Safe Accurate Behaviour is appropriate to context	Confident Accurate Expedient	Achieved intended outcome	No supporting cues* required
3 Requires supervision	Safe Accurate Behaviour is appropriate to context	Confident Accurate Takes longer than required	Achieved intended outcome	Requires occasional supportive cues*
2 Requires assistance	Safe Accurate Behaviour generally appropriate to context	Lacks certainty	Would not have achieved outcome without support	Requires frequent verbal and occasional physical directives in addition to supportive cues*
1 Requires direction	Safe only with guidance Not completely accurate	Unskilled Inefficient	Would not have achieved outcome without support	Requires continuous verbal and frequent physical directive cues*
0 Unsafe	Unsafe Unable to demonstrate behaviour Lack of insight into behaviour appropriate to context	Unskilled	Would not have achieved outcome	Requires continuous verbal and continuous physical directive cues*

*Refers to physical directives or verbal supportive cues

Performance Improvement Plan (PIP)

Please document the agreed education plan and completion timelines for areas assessed as less than 4.

This plan should be presented to assessor prior to commencement of summative assessment.

Where was supervisor support required?	Student summary of deficit. (Why was there a problem?)	Improvement Plan	Completed (Y/N)

Staff/Student Name: _____

Staff/Student Signature: _____

Educator Name: _____

Educator Signature: _____

Summative Clinical Skill Assessment (S-CSAT)

Equipment and resources: Patient or mannequin; dressing kit; hand decontamination agent; surface sanitisation wipes; PPE/gloves; clinical waste bag; method of documenting results; items relevant to task performed

Associated Clinical Skills: Infection control; Communication; Consent

Staff/Student being assessed: _____

- Completed Formative Clinical Skill Assessment (F-CSAT):   **YES**   **NO**
- Completed Performance Improvement Plan (PIP):   **YES**   **NO**   **N/A**

Using ANTT®		Achieved Without Direction	
Activity	**Critical Action**		
Performs hand hygiene	Uses appropriate technique for hand hygiene.	NO	YES
Prepares patient	Gains consent from patient. Prepares key site on the patient. Uses appropriate PPE to maintain safety. Removes gloves if worn and performs hand hygiene (ABHR).	NO	YES
Prepares work area	Cleans and prepares work surfaces. Performs hand hygiene (ABHR).	NO	YES
Assembles equipment	Assembles required equipment for the procedure.	NO	YES
Prepares field	Prepares sterile field.	NO	YES

Using ANTT® continued

Activity	Critical Action	Achieved Without Direction	
Prepares procedural equipment	Prepares equipment within the field.	NO	YES
Prepares to perform procedure	Performs hand hygiene (ABHR). Use appropriate PPE.	NO	YES
Performs procedure	Ensures all key parts/components are protected.	NO	YES
Post procedure	Removes gloves and performs hand hygiene (ABHR). Cleans work surface after use while wearing appropriate PPE. Performs hand hygiene (ABHR).	NO	YES
Reports	Documents procedure in notes, including compliance issues with ANTT®.	NO	YES

Source: *Adapted from NHMRC, 2010.*

Standard Achieved: (please circle one)

Competent (C)   Not Yet Competent* (NYC)

Staff/Student Name: _____

Assessor (please print name)**:** _____

Signed (Assessor)**:** _____

Date of Assessment: _____

Comments:

*If Not Yet Competent (NYC) a PIP needs to be completed and a repeat of the F-CSAT

Clinical findings

The procedure should be monitored for breaches of ANTT® and these breaches reported in the patient care record and mentioned at handover.

Factors that affect the quality of ANTT®

ANTT® is reliant on appropriate hand hygiene, the use of gloves, aseptic fields, a non-touch technique, environmental hygiene and control, sequencing and clinical governance. Each of these factors is a specific skill, the individual and combined importance of which should not be overlooked.

- Hand hygiene is the single most important measure to prevent the transmission of infection in healthcare settings.
- Before performing an aseptic procedure, paramedics need to minimise environmental risks to the procedure.
- During the aseptic procedure, aseptic fields must be maintained.
- During all procedures, key parts and key sites need to be identified and protected.
- Key parts that are contaminated must be made aseptic before use.
- A non-touch technique will protect a key part or key site from contamination.
- While the principles of aseptic technique remain the same, more complex procedures require more infection prevention measures.

Frequent handwashing

Regular and repeated use of alcohol-based handwashing methods will not necessarily dry the skin – in fact, they may be less problematic than standard soap and water due to the emollients contained within the sanitising products. If skin irritation does occur, consider using a moisturising product to help counter the irritation or an alternative hand cleaning product if your skin is sensitive.

PRACTICE TIP!

Perform hand hygiene when indicated. The urgency of the procedure or a dislike of repetitive handwashing can undermine the need for vigilance.

PRACTICE TIP!

Before beginning an aseptic procedure, think through the steps to plan the sequence and ensure the infection prevention measures match the complexity of the procedure.

PRACTICE TIP!

Minimise environmental risks to the aseptic procedure. Paramedics usually work in the environment of others where infection risk must be considered ever present.

PRACTICE TIP!

ANTT® is reliant on hand hygiene, glove use, aseptic fields, environmental hygiene and control, sequencing and clinical governance. To counter the uncontrolled nature of the paramedic work environment, ambulance services typically require wearing gloves as a minimum during patient contact. This is not typical of other medical professionals, who may use gloves only when there is a risk of contact with blood/bodily fluids.

PRACTICE TIP!

Identify key parts and key sites and use a non-touch technique to protect them during aseptic procedures.

TEST YOUR KNOWLEDGE QUESTIONS

1. **What is the aim of ANTT®?**
The aim of ANTT® for invasive and clinical procedures is always asepsis (Association for Safe Aseptic Practice, 2016). ANTT is a framework for aseptic practice: the principles are intended for use in a range of settings from the operating theatre to the community.

2. **List and describe the steps in the ANTT® procedure.**
Perform hand hygiene; prepare patient; prepare the work area; assemble the equipment; prepare the fields; prepare procedural equipment; prepare to perform procedure; perform procedure; post procedure; record (see Clinical Skill Work Instruction).

3. **Define the terms 'key site' and 'key part'.**
Key sites are open wounds and access sites for medical devices; key parts are the critical parts of the procedure equipment that, if contaminated, are most likely to cause infection (Rowley and Clare, 2011b).

4. **Describe measures that may require environmental control prior to or during invasive procedures to maintain asepsis.**
Prior to aseptic procedures, healthcare workers must ensure that there are no avoidable nearby environmental risk factors, such as significant draughts, pets, people using toilets or commodes. Paramedics also need to prepare the immediate environment to decrease contamination as far as practicable.

5. **Why is it important to gain patient consent?**
Consent is enshrined in providing legal, ethical and moral healthcare.

6. **What is the most serious adverse event faced by patients during their Australian health system engagement?**
Hospital-associated infection.

7. **What risk factors are important predictors of an individual's outcomes after infectious agent exposure?**
Immune status; age; comorbidities; severity of illness; surgery; indwelling devices; interinstitutional transfers; prolonged hospitalisation; exposure to invasive devices; antimicrobial drugs.

8. **Why is all equipment gathered before any procedure commencement?**
To avoid the need to move away from the sterile field to get further equipment once the procedure is underway.

9. **Why is sterile equipment dropped into a sterile field?**
It must not be touched until contaminated gloves have been removed and sterile gloves donned.

10. **Why are work surfaces sanitised after procedures?**
To remove any infectious source that may be transmitted to the next person.

References

ACSQHC (Australian Commission on Safety and Quality in Health Care), 2014. *NSQHS Standards in 2013: transforming the safety and quality of health care*. Sydney: ACSQHC.

Association for Safe Aseptic Practice, 2016. *ANTT clinical practice framework. ANTT® Aseptic Non Touch Technique*. Retrieved from: http://www.antt.org/ANTT_Site/theory.html

Bloomfield, S.F., Aiello, A.E., Cookson, B., O'Boyle, C., Larson, E.L. and Arbor, A., 2007. The effectiveness of hand hygiene procedures in reducing the risks of infections in home and community settings including handwashing and alcohol-based hand sanitizers. *American Journal of Infection Control*, 35(10S1), S27–S64.

Burns, A., Bowers, L., Pak, N., Wignall, J. and Roberts, S., 2010. The excess cost associated with healthcare associated bloodstream infections at Auckland City Hospital. *New Zealand Medical Journal*, 123, 17–24.

NHMRC (National Health and Medical Research Council), 2010. *Australian guidelines for the prevention and control of infection in healthcare*. Canberra: Australian Government.

Nimmo, G.R., Coombs, G.W., Pearson, J.C., O'Brien, F.G., Christiansen, K.J., Turnidge, J.D., Gosbell, I.B., Collignon, P. and

McLaws, M.L, 2006. Methicillin-resistant Staphylococcus aureus in the Australian community: an evolving epidemic. *Medical Journal of Australia*, 184, 384–388.

Read, K. and Bhally, H., 2015. 'Real-time' burden of community and healthcare-related infections in medical and rehabilitation patients in a public hospital in Auckland, New Zealand. *New Zealand Medical Journal*, 128(1426), 69.

Rowley, S. and Clare, S., 2011a. Aseptic Non Touch Technique (ANTT): reducing healthcare associated infections (HCAI) by standardising aseptic technique with ANTT across large clinical workforces. *American Journal of Infection Control*, 39(5), E90.

Rowley, S. and Clare, S., 2011b. ANTT: a standard approach to aseptic technique. *Nursing Times*, 107(36), 12–14.

Safdar, N. and Maki, D.G., 2002. The commonality of risk factors for nosocomial colonization and infection with antimicrobial-resistant staphylococcus aureus, enterococcus, gram-negative bacilli, clostridium difficile, and candida. *Annals of Internal Medicine*, 136(11), 834–844.

Chapter 3

Airway and Ventilation

Chapter objectives

At the end of this chapter the reader will be able to:

1. Identify signs of choking from foreign body airway obstruction (FBAO)
2. Demonstrate effective methods of manual FBAO expulsion

Resources required for this assessment

- Standardised patient or mannequin
- Hand decontamination agent
- Disposable gloves
- Method of documenting results

Skill matrix

This assessment requires:

- Infection control (CS 1.3)
- Communication (CS 1.5)
- Consent (CS 1.6)
- Patient assessment skills (Chapter 2, CS 2.1, 2.2, 2.6, 2.8, 2.10)
- Foreign body removal/suctioning (CS 3.7)
- Chest compressions (CS 6.1)

This assessment is a component of:

- Airway and ventilation (Chapter 3)

Introduction

The proximity of the oesophageal opening and the glottis in the distal pharynx predisposes the possibility of foreign body airway obstruction. While protective airway reflexes naturally clear potential choking problems and maintain airway patency, life-threatening airway obstruction can occur if they fail. Prompt management is therefore required to correct this, to avoid a fatal outcome (Igarashi et al., 2017). This chapter discusses foreign body airway obstruction (FBAO) management in the choking patient.

Anatomy and physiology

During swallowing, food moves towards the pharynx as the tongue contracts against the oral hard palate and the nasopharynx. Oropharyngeal muscles contract, moving food downwards, and the epiglottis moves posteriorly against the glottis, preventing tracheal entry (Nikolić and Živković, 2013).

Foreign bodies (FB) can become trapped between the oropharynx and bronchi, causing obstruction. Some objects can push downwards on the epiglottis, forcing it to occlude the glottis. Others can push into the glottis itself, pushing the epiglottis forwards. Small objects can pass through the larynx into the bronchi (Iino and O'Donnell, 2010; Nikolić and Živković, 2013). Rapid fatal outcomes are commonly associated with laryngeal obstruction (Abdullat et al., 2015).

The upper airway has several protective reflexes to keep foreign bodies out or to expel any that cause problems. The cough reflex involves inspiration then forced exhalation against a closed glottis to vigorously expel the lung air when the glottis opens. Involuntary coughing is stimulated by laryngeal and respiratory tract receptors and governed by the brainstem (Widdicombe, 1995).

Clinical rationale

Deterioration following FBAO will likely be rapid, so recognition and prompt, effective management are critical. Signs of FBAO can initially be confused with those of seizure and syncope (Perkins et al., 2015).

Acute FBAO has three stages: object entry, obstruction by the object and inability to expel it (Nikolić and Živković, 2013). Once in place, the FB can cause partial or complete obstruction (Salih et al., 2016). Mild obstruction allows speaking, coughing and breathing, even if with difficulty. Severe obstruction effectively prevents any of these from being possible (Perkins et al., 2015). Cyanosis may be evident, accompanied by the almost universal throat-clutching sign (Grover et al., 2011; Pavitt, Nevett et al., 2017; Salih et al., 2016).

Food is the most common foreign body that causes obstruction (Sidell et al., 2013). Choking occurs most often during mealtimes, particularly later in the day when meat is more likely to be eaten (Coffey et al., 2014; Pavitt, Nevett et al., 2017). Peanuts are common causes of FBAO in children (Abdullat et al., 2015; Grover et al., 2011), though so are metal and plastic objects (Nikolić and Živković, 2013), coins and small toys (CIVPP, 2010). While inanimate objects remain inert in the airway, food material can cause inflammation or absorb water and swell (Salih et al., 2016).

Those at particular risk of choking include the very young and the very old (Coffey et al., 2014; Perkins et al., 2015). Neuromuscular disease and congenital and acquired brain injury can impair swallowing and airway reflexes, predisposing the person to FBAO (CIVPP, 2010; Coffey et al., 2014; Perkins et al., 2015). There is also an association between intoxication and FBAO (Coffey et al., 2014; Pavitt, Nevett et al., 2017; Perkins et al., 2015).

It is more common for FBAO to be fatal in adults when accompanied by other risk factor(s) (Coffey et al., 2014). FBAO can occur from vomitus aspiration following loss of consciousness and airway reflexes.

Children

Small children are most commonly associated with choking (Grover et al., 2011; Sidell et al., 2013), so much so that it is nicknamed 'crèche coronary' (Nikolić and Živković, 2013) and is a major cause of sudden death (CIVPP, 2010; Srivastava, 2010).

Eating requires coordination between swallowing, breathing and, in infants, sucking. These activities are not natural together, as they combine reflex and learned activities. Furthermore, infants' teeth are less developed for chewing. The reflex tendency to place objects in the mouth then suck rather than chew predisposes infants to FBAO (Abdullat et al., 2015; Salih et al., 2016).

The child airway is particularly vulnerable, given its smaller diameter than that of adults. Small obstructions cause a severe reduction in airflow. The child has cough/gag/swallow reflexes, but the force generated during coughing is less effective than in an adult. Small children can bite food but are less able to chew and grind it. They are also easily distracted and likely to try to eat while engaged in other, playful activities (CIVPP, 2010).

When sudden onset of breathing difficulty and coughing occurs in a previously healthy child, FBAO must be considered as a possible cause (Salih et al., 2016).

Management

If the patient is able, encourage them to cough. This is the most effective method of clearing a mild obstruction and differentiating between mild and severe FBAO (Perkins et al., 2015).

If the obstruction is severe and the patient unable to cough but still conscious, alternate a series of back blows and chest thrusts.

Back blows

Sharp blows between the scapulae, also called back slaps, can help remove FBAO (Blain et al., 2010; Perkins et al., 2015). To administer, stand beside or behind the patient and strike using the heel of one hand, directed inwards and slightly upwards, with sufficient force to produce a cough (Fig. 3.1.1a).

To stop movement away from the force, lean the patient forwards, braced against a table or chair or supported with one arm wrapped around their chest, while applying the blows. Deliver up to five blows, assessing each time for obstruction removal. If this method proves ineffective, attempt chest thrusts.

Lay smaller children head down across a knee, lap or arm (Maconochie et al., 2015) (Fig. 3.1.1b).

Back blows can produce less alveolar pressure change than abdominal thrusts (Pavitt, Swanton et al., 2017).

Chest thrusts

Chest thrusts can produce greater intrathoracic pressures than abdominal thrusts (Pavitt, Swanton et al., 2017). Wrap the arms around the patient with one fist placed on the mid-sternum, the other hand grasping over it. Compress the arms sharply, pulling the sternum directly inwards (Fig. 3.1.2a). Repeat in salvos of five as needed.

Alternatively, inward compressive force can be applied to the mid-sternum using the heel of one hand, with the patient leant against a firm surface such as a wall or a firm chair or braced by wrapping an arm behind them (Fig. 3.1.2b).

Position smaller children/infants supine and head down. Identify the location for performing cardiopulmonary chest compressions (CPR). Deliver five sharp compressions at a slower rate than CPR (Fig. 3.1.3) (Maconochie et al., 2015).

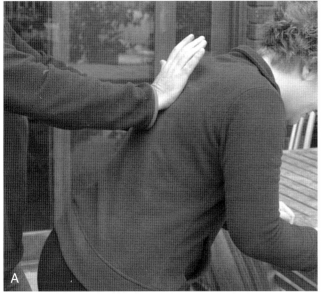

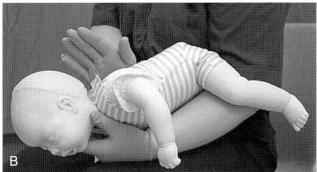

Figure 3.1.1 Performing back blows
(a) Adult. (b) Infant/small child.

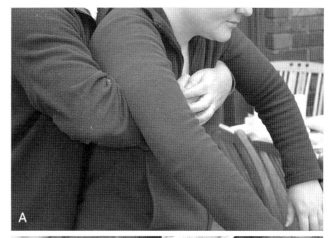

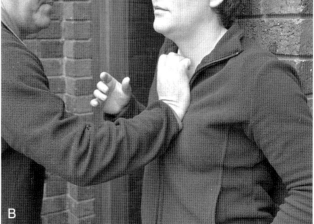

Figure 3.1.2 Performing chest thrusts
(a) From behind. (b) From the front.

Abdominal thrusts

Abdominal thrusts are an alternative to chest thrusts.

European and American resuscitation favours alternating back blows and abdominal thrusts for removing FBAO in adults (Maconochie et al., 2015; Perkins et al., 2015). The Australian and New Zealand resuscitation councils do not support abdominal thrusts, given the increased risk of internal injury (ARC, 2016). This risk can be lessened by applying inward instead of upward force, without reducing the effectiveness of the procedure. This also makes the procedure easier for smaller people to perform (Pavitt, Swanton et al., 2017).

The effectiveness of abdominal thrusts on obese patients is likely reduced (Pavitt, Swanton et al., 2017). Abdominal thrusts are not supported for use in infants and small children (Maconochie et al., 2015).

Chest compressions

Chest compressions provide similar expulsive force to chest thrusts. They improve outcomes where FBAO results in unconsciousness and collapse (Kinoshita et al., 2015). Where back blows and chest thrusts fail to dislodge the severe FBAO, the patient will likely lose consciousness quickly. Lower them to the floor in a supine position and commence CPR chest compressions (see Chapter 6.1).

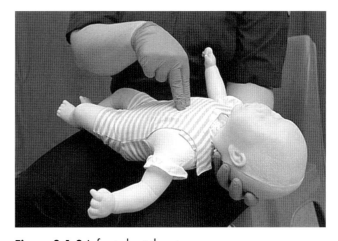

Figure 3.1.3 Infant chest thrusts

Compressions can dislodge the obstruction. Manual airway techniques will be required to remove the FBAO from the pharynx once unconsciousness occurs, including laryngoscopy, suctioning and Magill's forceps (see Chapters 3.6 and 3.7).

Clinical skill assessment process

The following section outlines the clinical skill assessment tools that should be used to determine a student's ability to demonstrate effective management of choking.

1. Clinical Skill Work Instruction
2. Formative Clinical Skill Assessment (F-CSAT)
3. Performance Improvement Plan (PIP)
4. Summative Clinical Skill Assessment (S-CSAT)
(5. Direct Observation of Procedural Skills (DOPS) – see Chapter 1.1)

Clinical Skill Work Instruction

Equipment and resources: Standardised patient or mannequin; hand decontamination agent; disposable gloves; method of documenting results

Associated Clinical Skills: Infection control; Communication; Consent; Patient assessment skills; Foreign body removal/suctioning; Chest compressions

Choking

Activity	Critical Action	Rationale
Personal protection	Don PPE gloves/mask/eyewear.	For infection control.
Assess patient	Consider coughing, throat clutching, breathing/speaking difficulty, cyanosis. Assess patient consciousness. If unconscious, commence chest compressions and proceed immediately to CS 3.7 (Foreign body removal/suctioning).	Determine if patient has FBAO. Patient coughing and the application of back blows and chest thrusts are suitable only for conscious patients.
Initial response	Encourage patient to cough if able. Manage as severe FBAO if unable. Monitor continuously until FBAO cleared or patient deteriorates.	Most effective removal option.

Severe FBAO

Activity	Critical Action	Rationale
Back blows (slaps)	Position patient standing/sitting leaning forwards. For small children, position child prone, head down across knee/lap.	Assist FBAO propulsion.
	Brace patient using one arm wrapped around their chest or leaning against chair/table.	To prevent propelling forwards.
	Strike sharply inwards and upwards with heel of hand between scapulae. Repeat up to five blows until FBAO clears.	Provide sufficient force to produce cough effect.
Chest thrusts	If FBAO still present, brace patient using one arm wrapped around their upper back or leaning against a wall. For small children, position supine, head down across knee/lap.	As counter to thrust force.
	Place heel of hand mid-sternum. Press inwards sharply as if performing CPR. Repeat up to five thrusts or until FBAO clears.	Provide sufficient force to produce cough effect.
Alternative chest thrust method	Stand behind patient with them leaning forwards. Wrap arms around patient's chest placing one fist mid-sternum. Place other hand over top of first.	In position for thrust application.
	Pull arms sharply directly inwards, applying force mid-sternum for up to five thrusts or until FBAO clears.	Provide sufficient force to produce cough effect.

Choking continued

Activity	Critical Action	Rationale
Continued therapy	Continue alternating back blow and chest thrust salvos while patient is conscious. If FBAO clears, treat accordingly. Consider transport to emergency facility. If patient has lost consciousness, commence CPR. Remove FBAO using manual airway techniques (Chapter 3.7).	Continue strategy until effective or respond according to changes in condition.
Report	Document/hand over details of FBAO, obstruction/clearance time, method(s) used.	Accurate record keeping and continuity of care.

Source: *Adapted from ARC, 2016.*

Formative Clinical Skill Assessment (F-CSAT)

Equipment and resources: Standardised patient or mannequin; hand decontamination agent; disposable gloves; method of documenting results

Associated Clinical Skills: Infection control; Communication; Consent; Patient assessment skills; Foreign body removal/suctioning; Chest compressions

Staff/Student being assessed: _____

Choking

Activity	Critical Action	Performance				
Personal protection	Dons PPE.	0	1	2	3	4
Assesses patient	Considers signs of choking. Assesses patient consciousness. If unconscious, commences chest compressions and proceeds immediately to CS 3.7 (Foreign body removal/suctioning).	0	1	2	3	4
Initial response	Encourages patient to cough. Continues to monitor. Manages as severe FBAO if appropriate.	0	1	2	3	4
Severe FBAO						
Back blows	Positions patient standing/sitting leaning forwards, or, if a small child, prone across knee/lap. Braces patient. Delivers up to five back blows correctly. Monitors effectiveness.	0	1	2	3	4
Chest thrusts	If FBAO still present, braces patient for chest thrusts or, if a small child, supine across knee/lap. Delivers up to five chest thrusts to mid-sternum correctly. Monitors effectiveness.	0	1	2	3	4
Alternative chest thrust method	Stands behind patient with them leaning forwards. Wraps arms around patient's chest, placing one fist mid-sternum and other hand on top. Pulls arms sharply inwards up to five times correctly. Monitors effectiveness.	0	1	2	3	4

Choking continued

Activity	Critical Action	Performance				
Continued therapy	Alternates back blows and chest thrusts while patient is conscious. If FBAO clears, treats accordingly. If patient has lost consciousness, commences CPR. Removes FBAO using manual airway techniques.	0	1	2	3	4
Reports	Documents/hands over correctly.	0	1	2	3	4

Source: *Adapted from ARC, 2016.*

Standard Achieved: (please circle one)

Competent (C) Not Yet Competent* (NYC)

Staff/Student Name: _____

Assessor (please print name): _____

Signed (Assessor): _____

Date of Assessment: _____

Comments:

*If Not Yet Competent (NYC) a PIP needs to be completed and a repeat of the F-CSAT

Formative Clinical Skill Assessment (F-CSAT) Key

Skill level	Standard of procedure	Quality of performance	Outcome	Level of assistance required
4 Safe for unsupervised practice	Safe Accurate Behaviour is appropriate to context	Confident Accurate Expedient	Achieved intended outcome	No supporting cues* required
3 Requires supervision	Safe Accurate Behaviour is appropriate to context	Confident Accurate Takes longer than required	Achieved intended outcome	Requires occasional supportive cues*
2 Requires assistance	Safe Accurate Behaviour generally appropriate to context	Lacks certainty	Would not have achieved outcome without support	Requires frequent verbal and occasional physical directives in addition to supportive cues*
1 Requires direction	Safe only with guidance Not completely accurate	Unskilled Inefficient	Would not have achieved outcome without support	Requires continuous verbal and frequent physical directive cues*
0 Unsafe	Unsafe Unable to demonstrate behaviour Lack of insight into behaviour appropriate to context	Unskilled	Would not have achieved outcome	Requires continuous verbal and continuous physical directive cues*

*Refers to physical directives or verbal supportive cues

Performance Improvement Plan (PIP)

Please document the agreed education plan and completion timelines for areas assessed as less than 4.

This plan should be presented to assessor prior to commencement of summative assessment.

Where was supervisor support required?	Student summary of deficit. (Why was there a problem?)	Improvement Plan	Completed (Y/N)

Staff/Student Name: _____

Staff/Student Signature: _____

Educator Name: _____

Educator Signature: _____

Summative Clinical Skill Assessment (S-CSAT)

Equipment and resources: Standardised patient or mannequin; hand decontamination agent; disposable gloves; method of documenting results

Associated Clinical Skills: Infection control; Communication; Consent; Patient assessment skills; Foreign body removal/suctioning; Chest compressions

Staff/Student being assessed: _____

- Completed Formative Clinical Skill Assessment (F-CSAT):   **YES**   **NO**

- Completed Performance Improvement Plan (PIP):   **YES**   **NO**   **N/A**

Choking		Achieved Without Direction	
Activity	**Critical Action**		
Personal protection	Dons PPE.	NO	YES
Assesses patient	Considers signs of choking. Assesses patient consciousness. If unconscious, commences chest compressions and proceeds immediately to CS 3.7 (Foreign body removal/suctioning).	NO	YES
Initial response	Encourages patient to cough. Continues to monitor. Manages as severe FBAO if appropriate.	NO	YES

Choking continued

Activity	Critical Action	Achieved Without Direction	
Severe FBAO			
Back blows	Positions patient standing/sitting leaning forwards or, if a small child, prone across knee/lap. Braces patient. Delivers up to five back blows correctly. Monitors effectiveness.	NO	YES
Chest thrusts	If FBAO still present, braces patient for chest thrusts or, if a small child, supine across knee/lap. Delivers up to five chest thrusts to mid-sternum correctly. Monitors effectiveness.	NO	YES
Alternative chest thrust method	Stands behind patient with them leaning forwards. Wraps arms around patient's chest, placing one fist mid-sternum and other hand on top. Pulls arms sharply inwards up to five times correctly. Monitors effectiveness.	NO	YES
Continued therapy	Alternates back blows and chest thrusts while patient is conscious. If FBAO clears, treats accordingly. If patient has lost consciousness, commences CPR. Removes FBAO using manual airway techniques.	NO	YES
Reports	Documents/hands over correctly.	NO	YES

Source: *Adapted from ARC, 2016.*

Standard Achieved: (please circle one)

Competent (C)   Not Yet Competent* (NYC)

Staff/Student Name: _____

Assessor (please print name)**:** _____

Signed (Assessor)**:** _____

Date of Assessment: _____

Comments: _____

*If Not Yet Competent (NYC) a PIP needs to be completed and a repeat of the F-CSAT

Clinical findings

Post-FBAO complications

The short-term complications of cyanosis, oxygen desaturation and tachycardia/bradycardia can resolve with the removal of the obstruction. However, the effects of prolonged hypoxia may not resolve so readily.

FBAO can cause pharynx/larynx injury or oedema/inflammation, hoarseness or haemoptysis (Salih et al., 2016).

Aspirated foreign bodies beyond the glottis most commonly position in the right main bronchus (Grover et al., 2011; Sidell et al., 2013). Subsequent lung pathology can vary from hyperinflation, obstructive emphysema or pneumothorax accompanied by unilateral wheezing (Grover et al., 2011; Salih et al., 2016), requiring bronchoscopic removal of the FB (Grover et al., 2011; Svrivastava, 2010).

FBAO can cause significant negative intrathoracic pressure during inspiration against a closed/obstructed glottis, leading to the formation of pulmonary oedema (Bhattacharya et al., 2016; Fremont et al., 2007; Lemyze and Mallatt, 2014; Senussi et al., 2015; Toukan et al., 2016).

However, most FBAO will clear without complications. Where cough, difficulty swallowing or breathing or throat discomfort persists, or if chest/abdominal thrusts were performed, medical follow-up is advisable (Perkins et al., 2015).

PRACTICE TIP!

Always encourage coughing first. If it is apparent the patient cannot do so, move immediately to back blows and chest thrusts.

PRACTICE TIP!

For severe FBAO, the patient will likely lose consciousness quickly. As soon as this happens, lower the patient to the floor and commence CPR chest compressions. This helps expel the FBAO until invasive airway procedures can be applied to remove it.

TEST YOUR KNOWLEDGE QUESTIONS

1. **What are the usual signs of choking?**
   Coughing; difficulty speaking and breathing; cyanosis; throat clutching.

2. **What are the signs of severe FBAO?**
   An inability to cough, speak or breathe; collapse.

3. **Who is at particular risk of FBAO?**
   The very young and very old; people with neuromuscular diseases and brain injuries; the intoxicated.

4. **What is the most effective method of FBAO clearance?**
   Coughing, if the patient is able.

5. **How many back blows or chest thrusts are provided in one salvo?**
   Up to five, but stop if the FBAO is expelled.

6. **When managing the small child with FBAO, what position is advantageous?**
   Across the knee/lap, with the head inclined downwards.

7. **Why are chest thrusts favoured over abdominal thrusts in Australia?**
   They are at least as effective and less injurious.

8. **What action is taken if the patient loses consciousness?**
   Lower them to the floor in a supine position and continue chest thrusts as for CPR.

9. **What other option is there for FBAO removal in the unconscious patient?**
   Manual airway skills including laryngoscopy, suctioning and Magill's forceps.

10. **When is medical investigation necessary post FBAO?**
    Where cough, difficulty swallowing or throat discomfort persists or if chest/abdominal thrusts were performed.

References

Abdullat, E.M., Ader-Rahman, H.A., Al Ali, R. and Hudaib, A.A., 2015. Choking among infants and young children. *Jordan Journal of Biological Sciences*, 147(3380), 1–5.

ARC (Australian Resuscitation Council), 2016. The ARC guidelines. Retrieved from: https://resus.org.au/guidelines

Bhattacharya, M., Kallet, R.H., Ware, L.B. and Matthay, M.A., 2016. Negative-pressure pulmonary edema. *Chest*, 150(4), 927–933.

Blain, H., Bonnafous, M., Grovalet, N., Jonquet, O. and David, M., 2010. The table maneuver: a procedure used with success in four cases of unconscious choking older subjects. *American Journal of Medicine*, 123(12), 1150–e7.

CIVPP (Committee on Injury, Violence, and Poison Prevention), 2010. Prevention of choking among children. *Pediatrics*, 125(3), 601–607.

Coffey, A., Pasquale-Styles, M.A. and Gill, J.R., 2014. Fatalities due to choking: internal occlusion of airway. *Academic Forensic Pathology*, 4(1), 94–99.

Fremont, R.D., Kallet, R.H., Matthay, M.A. and Ware, L.B., 2007. Postobstructive pulmonary edema: a case for hydrostatic mechanisms. *Chest*, 131(6), 1742–1746.

Grover, S., Bansal, A. and Singhi, S.C., 2011. Airway foreign body aspiration. *Indian Journal of Pediatrics*, 78(11), 1401–1403.

Igarashi, Y., Yokobori, S., Yoshino, Y., Masuno, T., Miyauchi, M. and Yokota, H., 2017. Prehospital removal improves neurological outcomes in elderly patient with foreign body airway obstruction. *American Journal of Emergency Medicine*, 35(10), 1396–1399.

Kinoshita, K., Azuhata, T., Kawano, D. and Kawahara, Y., 2015. Relationships between pre-hospital characteristics and outcome in victims of foreign body airway obstruction during meals. *Resuscitation*, 88, 63–67.

Lemyze, M. and Mallat, J., 2014. Understanding negative pressure pulmonary edema. *Intensive Care Medicine*, 40(8), 1140–1143.

Iino, M. and O'Donnell, C., 2010. Postmortem computed tomography findings of upper airway obstruction by food. *Journal of Forensic Sciences*, 55(5), 1251–1258.

Maconochie, I.K., Bingham, R., Eich, C., López-Herce, J., Rodríguez-Núnez, A., Rajka, T., Van de Voorde, P., Zideman, D.A., Biarent, D., Monsieurs, K.G. and Nolan, J.P., 2015. European Resuscitation Council guidelines for resuscitation 2015, section 6: Paediatric life support. *Resuscitation*, 95, 223–248.

Nikolić, S. and Živković, V., 2013. Choking on a grape: an unusual type of upper airway obstruction. *Forensic Science, Medicine, and Pathology*, 9(3), 452–453.

Pavitt, M.J., Nevett, J., Swanton, L.L., Hind, M.D., Polkey, M.I., Green, M. and Hopkinson, N.S., 2017. London ambulance source data on choking incidence for the calendar year 2016: an observational study. *BMJ Open Respiratory Research*, 4(1), e000215.

Pavitt, M.J., Swanton, L.L., Hind, M., Apps, M., Polkey, M.I., Green, M. and Hopkinson, N.S., 2017. Choking on a foreign body: a physiological study of the effectiveness of abdominal thrust manoeuvres to increase thoracic pressure. *Thorax*, 72(6), 576–578.

Perkins, G.D., Handley, A.J., Koster, R.W., Castrén, M., Smyth, M.A., Olasveengen, T., Monsieurs, K.G., Raffay, V., Gräsner, J.T., Wenzel, V. and Ristagno, G., 2015. European Resuscitation Council guidelines for resuscitation 2015, section 2: Adult basic life support and automated external defibrillation. *Resuscitation*, 95, 81–99.

Salih, A.M., Alfaki, M. and Alam-Elhuda, D.M., 2016. Airway foreign bodies: A critical review for a common pediatric emergency. *World Journal of Emergency Medicine*, 7(1), p. 5.

Senussi, M.H., Surath, H. and Mireles-Cabodevila, E., 2015. Shortness of breath after a choking incident. *JAMA*, 313(7), 721–722.

Sidell, D.R., Kim, I.A., Coker, T.R., Moreno, C. and Shapiro, N.L., 2013. Food choking hazards in children. *International Journal of Pediatric Otorhinolaryngology*, 77(12), 1940–1946.

Srivastava, G., 2010. Airway foreign bodies in children. *Clinical Pediatric Emergency Medicine*, 11(2), 67–72.

Toukan, Y., Gur, M. and Bentur, L., 2016. Negative pressure pulmonary edema following choking on a cookie. *Pediatric Pulmonology*, 51(7).

Widdicombe, J.G., 1995. Neurophysiology of the cough reflex. *European Respiratory Journal*, 8(7), 1193–1202.

Head positioning

John Cowell

Chapter objectives

At the end of this chapter the reader will be able to:

1. Describe the rationale for the importance of head positioning
2. Demonstrate the methods of head tilt/chin lift, neutral anatomical and sniffing head positioning
3. Accurately report on assessment findings for head positioning

Resources required for this assessment

- Standardised patient or mannequin with movement range for head positions
- Towel/pillow/padding
- Disposable gloves
- Method of documenting the results

Skill matrix

This assessment requires:

- Infection control (CS 1.3)
- Communication (CS 1.5)
- Consent (CS 1.6)
- Patient assessment skills (Chapter 2, CS 2.1, 2.2, 2.6, 2.8, 2.10)

This assessment is a component of:

- Airway and ventilation (Chapter 3)

Introduction

Airway procedures begin with basic head positioning. The range of head movement includes flexion through to extension and lateral rotation. Airway airflow can be improved or compromised by position, making basic manoeuvres important. This chapter discusses the different options for head positioning, including their advantages and indications.

Anatomy and physiology

The upper airway extends from the mouth and nose, through the oral and nasal cavities and the pharynx, to the larynx. The large tongue and epiglottis are attached at the base of the mouth and jaw. The pharynx is divided into three regions: nasopharynx, oropharynx and hypopharynx (Gurani et al., 2016).

From a sagittal view, the airway is initially posteriorly directed, curving around the tongue and epiglottis into the pharynx until directed inferiorly at the hypoglottis. The larynx is slightly anterior, with the oesophagus posterior to it. This curved anatomy forms a natural obstruction to viewing the glottis from the mouth (Greenland et al., 2010).

There are seven cervical vertebra, with the top two – C1 (atlas) and C2 (axis) – supporting the skull and allowing its mobility. The atlanto-occipital joint can be described as being at a 90° angle with the atlas facing superiorly and the occiput seated perpendicular to it. A series of anterior and posterior ligaments maintains stability during extension and flexion (Austin et al., 2014). The cervical spine has curves anteriorly (lordosis), changing to a posterior thoracic curve (kyphosis).

The occiput and the thoracic kyphosis vary in which protrudes posteriorly the most. Small children have a

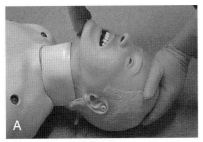

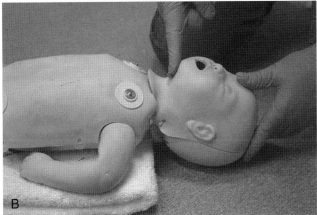

Figure 3.2.1 Head tilt
(a) Adult. (b) Infant.

relatively larger head and smaller chest diameter, so the occiput is more posterior. In adults, the kyphosis is more prominent, with the spine/shoulders posterior.

Clinical rationale

Conscious patients choose their own posture for comfort or to alleviate pain or breathing difficulty, while the paramedic can choose the patient's position if their consciousness is altered. Even if no active choice is made, the patient must be positioned in some manner. Purposeful positioning helps optimise airway care.

A supine position is common for patients, particularly for airway procedures, and it is essential during the management of cardiac arrest. There are several options for head placement when the patient is supine, including the head tilt/chin lift, neutral anatomical and sniffing positions. How these are performed can vary with the patient's age and relative head-to-body proportion.

Head tilt/chin lift

Head tilt is supine positioning with the occiput and shoulders on the same plane and the atlanto-occipital angle extended beyond 90° (Fig. 3.2.1a). In adults, one reason for this is that the occiput continues until it reaches the shoulder plane. Head flexion predisposes the adult to upper airway collapse, so head tilt during the initial rescue prevents this (Paal et al., 2007) and lifts the tongue from the glottis (Soar et al., 2015). The face angles slightly superiorly. Excessive head tilt can precipitate tracheal airway obstruction (Reber, 2016).

To perform this manoeuvre, place the palm of one hand on the patient's forehead and push downwards. Simultaneously, the chin lift is added by pressing the fingers upwards beneath the bony chin, avoiding nearby soft tissue. Moving the tongue anteriorly maximises the diameter of the pharynx. Chin lift is most effective if the mouth is closed, so a clear nasal airway is needed. It is therefore best avoided in small children, as they are nasal breathers (Reber, 2016).

For small children and newborns, the natural flexion caused by the occiput must be corrected. The desired extension angle between the head and neck is about 120° (Cruz, 2014; Gutala et al., 2014). This head tilt creates a void beneath the shoulders that must be filled with padding (Fig. 3.2.1b). It can provide ear to clavicle alignment (Chua et al., 2012; Maconochie et al., 2015).

Neutral anatomical position

As the head moves from chin to chest flexion to head tilted extension, somewhere midway it passes a point of neither flexion nor extension. This is the neutral anatomical position; the exact position of the head varies not only with age but with individuals. The head and neck are neutrally aligned when the external auditory meatus is in line with the middle of the clavicle parallel to the plane the patient is lying on.

This position can be achieved in adults by gently lifting the head and placing padding between the occiput and the surface (Fig. 3.2.2a). The head must typically be elevated by 2–5 cm to achieve neutral alignment.

For small children, neutral alignment requires the shoulders, rather than the head, to be raised with padding (Fig. 3.2.2b). This is particularly so for newborns (Chua et al., 2012; Wilton et al., 2015). Slight head extension in small children improves glottic view and airway patency (Bhalala et al., 2016; El-Orbany et al., 2011; Holm-Knudsen and Rasmussen, 2009; Tripathi et al., 2016).

Older children (about 8–12 years) lie somewhere in between these two positions (Fig. 3.2.2c). This is the only age at which neutral alignment is achieved naturally, without any alteration.

Sniffing position

Optimal alignment (angle reduction) of the mouth-pharynx-glottis is achieved in the 'sniffing position' (Fig. 3.2.3a and b). This involves forming a 35° lower cervical neck flexion combined with 15° head extension at the atlanto-occipital and atlanto-axial joints. The external auditory meatus is raised so it can be seen on the same plane as the sternal angle. The face angles perpendicular to the plane on which the patient is lying, assisted by gentle pressure on the forehead (Akhtar et al., 2017; Austin et al., 2014; El-Orbany et al., 2011; Greenland et al., 2010; Reber, 2016).

This position provides the best view of the vocal cords during laryngoscopy and intubation (Frerk et al., 2015;

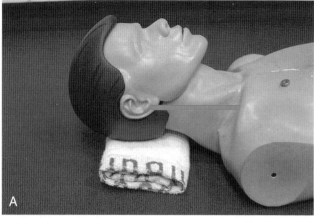

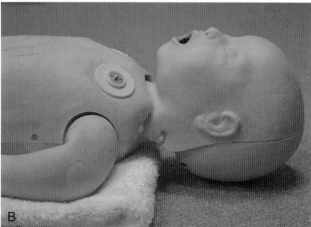

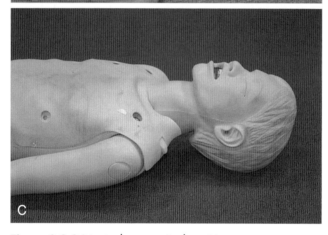

Figure 3.2.2 Neutral anatomical position
(a) Adult. (b) Infant. (c) Older child.

Myatra et al., 2016). Airway volume is increased and resistance minimised in the sniffing position, making it ideal for bag/valve/mask ventilation (Wei et al., 2017). However, it is undesirable for use in patients with a spinal injury (Myatra et al., 2016).

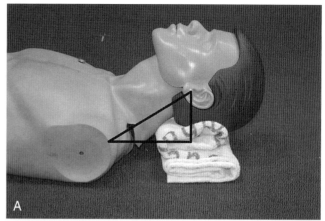

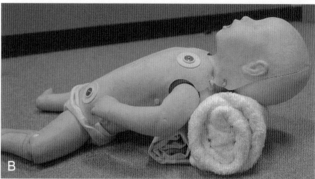

Figure 3.2.3 Sniffing position
(a) Adult. (b) Infant.

In adults, the sniffing position is achieved by placing 7–9 cm of padding beneath the occiput. For small children, to accommodate the relatively larger occiput, padding is placed beneath the neck (not shoulders) to create the desired neck flexion. It is unclear from the available evidence whether this is superior to the neutral position in this age group (Chua et al., 2012).

Clinical skill assessment process

The following section outlines the clinical skill assessment tools that should be used to determine a student's ability to demonstrate effective patient head positioning when the patient is supine.
1. Clinical Skill Work Instruction
2. Formative Clinical Skill Assessment (F-CSAT)
3. Performance Improvement Plan (PIP)
4. Summative Clinical Skill Assessment (S-CSAT)
(5. Direct Observation of Procedural Skills (DOPS) – see Chapter 1.1)

Clinical Skill Work Instruction

Equipment and resources: Standardised patient or mannequin with movement range for head positions; towel/pillow/padding; disposable gloves; method of documenting results

Associated Clinical Skills: Infection control; Communication; Consent; Patient assessment skills

Head positioning

Activity	Critical Action	Rationale
Personal protection	Don PPE as required.	For infection control.
Prepare patient	Assess for suspected spinal injury.	Excludes head tilt and sniffing positions.
	Place patient supine with head returned midline.	Aligns the head and body.
	Determine head position required.	Varies with need and injuries.
	Position paramedic beside patient's head.	Best position for head movements.
Head tilt/chin lift	Place palm of one hand on patient's forehead and push downwards. Maintain for stability.	To provide impetus for head tilt.
	Simultaneously place the first two fingers just beneath patient's chin. Push anteriorly and superiorly to lift chin. The mouth should partly close in doing so.	Chin lift pulls tongue away from pharynx and adds to impetus for head tilt.
	Ensure patient's neck is extended at an approximately 120° angle to the atlanto-occipital joint. For small children, ensure adequate shoulder padding to support body and avoid hyperextension.	Maximises pharyngeal diameter.
Neutral anatomical position	Gently lift head until external auditory meatus is on the same plane as the mid-clavicle, parallel to the body plane with the head facing anteriorly. For small children, lift the body instead.	Removes flexion and extension from the cervical spine.
	Place sufficient padding (usually 2–5 cm) beneath the occiput (adults) or shoulders (small children) to maintain position.	To maintain in position.
	Visually verify correct alignment. Adjust padding if necessary.	Add or remove padding as needed.
Sniffing position	Gently lift head until there is 35° flexion at the lower neck. Tilt the head 15° until facing anteriorly. The external auditory meatus is on the same plane as the sternum angle parallel to the body plane.	To create artificial neck angles to optimise mouth-pharynx-glottic alignment for advanced airway procedures.
	Place sufficient padding beneath the occiput (adults) or neck arch (small children) to maintain. Apply forehead pressure if necessary to ensure anterior facial alignment.	To support in correct position.
	Visually verify correct alignment. Adjust padding if necessary.	
Report	Accurately document/hand over findings.	Accurate record kept and patient care continuity.

Formative Clinical Skill Assessment (F-CSAT)

Equipment and resources: Standardised patient or mannequin with movement range for head positions; towel/pillow/padding; disposable gloves; method of documenting results

Associated Clinical Skills: Infection control; Communication; Consent; Patient assessment skills

Staff/Student being assessed: _____

Head positioning

Activity	Critical Action	Participant Performance				
Personal protection	Dons PPE as required.	0	1	2	3	4
Prepares patient	Assesses for suspected spinal injury.	0	1	2	3	4
	Places patient supine with head returned midline.	0	1	2	3	4
	Determines head position required.	0	1	2	3	4
	Positions beside patient's head.	0	1	2	3	4
Head tilt/chin lift	Places palm of one hand on patient's forehead and pushes firmly downwards.	0	1	2	3	4
	Simultaneously places first two fingers just beneath patient's chin. Pushes anteriorly and superiorly to lift chin.	0	1	2	3	4
	Ensures patient's neck is extended at an approximately 120° angle to the atlanto-occipital joint. For small children, ensures adequate shoulder padding to support body.	0	1	2	3	4
Neutral anatomical position	Gently lifts head until external auditory meatus is on the same plane as mid-clavicle, parallel to the body plane with head facing anteriorly. For small children, lifts the body instead.	0	1	2	3	4
	Places sufficient padding (usually 2–5 cm) beneath the occiput (adults) or shoulders (small children) to maintain position.	0	1	2	3	4
	Visually verifies correct alignment. Adjusts padding if necessary.	0	1	2	3	4
Sniffing position	Gently lifts head until there is 35° flexion at the lower neck. Tilts the head 15° until facing anteriorly. The external auditory meatus is on the same plane as the sternum angle parallel to the body plane.	0	1	2	3	4
	Places sufficient padding beneath the occiput (adults) or neck arch (small children) to maintain position.	0	1	2	3	4
	Visually verifies correct alignment. Adjusts padding if necessary.	0	1	2	3	4
Reports	Accurately documents/hands over findings.	0	1	2	3	4

Standard Achieved: (please circle one)

Competent (C)   Not Yet Competent* (NYC)

Staff/Student Name: _____

Assessor (please print name): _____

Signed (Assessor): _____

Date of Assessment: _____

Comments:

*If Not Yet Competent (NYC) a PIP needs to be completed and a repeat of the F-CSAT

Formative Clinical Skill Assessment (F-CSAT) Key

Skill level	Standard of procedure	Quality of performance	Outcome	Level of assistance required
4 Safe for unsupervised practice	Safe Accurate Behaviour is appropriate to context	Confident Accurate Expedient	Achieved intended outcome	No supporting cues* required
3 Requires supervision	Safe Accurate Behaviour is appropriate to context	Confident Accurate Takes longer than required	Achieved intended outcome	Requires occasional supportive cues*
2 Requires assistance	Safe Accurate Behaviour generally appropriate to context	Lacks certainty	Would not have achieved outcome without support	Requires frequent verbal and occasional physical directives in addition to supportive cues*
1 Requires direction	Safe only with guidance Not completely accurate	Unskilled Inefficient	Would not have achieved outcome without support	Requires continuous verbal and frequent physical directive cues*
0 Unsafe	Unsafe Unable to demonstrate behaviour Lack of insight into behaviour appropriate to context	Unskilled	Would not have achieved outcome	Requires continuous verbal and continuous physical directive cues*

*Refers to physical directives or verbal supportive cues

Performance Improvement Plan (PIP)

Please document the agreed education plan and completion timelines for areas assessed as less than 4.

This plan should be presented to assessor prior to commencement of summative assessment.

Where was supervisor support required?	Student summary of deficit. (Why was there a problem?)	Improvement Plan	Completed (Y/N)

Staff/Student Name: _____

Staff/Student Signature: _____

Educator Name: _____

Educator Signature: _____

Summative Clinical Skill Assessment (S-CSAT)

Equipment and resources: Standardised patient or mannequin with movement range for head positions; towel/pillow/padding; disposable gloves; method of documenting results

Associated Clinical Skills: Infection control; Communication; Consent; Patient assessment skills

Staff/Student being assessed: _____

• Completed Formative Clinical Skill Assessment (F-CSAT):   **YES   NO**

• Completed Performance Improvement Plan (PIP):   **YES   NO   N/A**

Head positioning			
Activity	**Critical Action**	**Achieved Without Direction**	
Personal protection	Dons PPE as required.	NO	YES
Prepares patient	Assesses for suspected spinal injury.	NO	YES
	Places patient supine with head returned midline.	NO	YES
	Determines head position required.	NO	YES
	Positions beside patient's head.	NO	YES

		Achieved Without Direction	
Activity	**Critical Action**		
Head tilt/chin lift	Places palm of one hand on patient's forehead and pushes firmly downwards.	NO	YES
	Simultaneously places the first two fingers just beneath patient's chin. Pushes anteriorly and superiorly to lift chin.	NO	YES
	Ensures patient's neck is extended at an approximately 120° angle to the atlanto-occipital joint. For small children, ensures adequate shoulder padding to support body.	NO	YES
Neutral anatomical position	Gently lifts head until external auditory meatus is on the same plane as mid-clavicle, parallel to the body plane with head facing anteriorly. For small children, lifts the body instead.	NO	YES
	Places sufficient padding (usually 2–5 cm) beneath the occiput (adults) or shoulders (small children) to maintain position.	NO	YES
	Visually verifies correct alignment. Adjusts padding if necessary.	NO	YES
Sniffing position	Gently lifts head until there is 35° flexion at the lower neck. Tilts the head 15° until facing anteriorly. The external auditory meatus is on the same plane as the sternum angle parallel to the body plane.	NO	YES
	Places sufficient padding beneath the occiput (adults) or neck arch (small children) to maintain position.	NO	YES
	Visually verifies correct alignment. Adjusts padding if necessary.	NO	YES
Reports	Accurately documents/hands over findings.	NO	YES

Standard Achieved: (please circle one)

Competent (C)   Not Yet Competent* (NYC)

Staff/Student Name: _____

Assessor (please print name): _____

Signed (Assessor): _____

Date of Assessment: _____

Comments:

*If Not Yet Competent (NYC) a PIP needs to be completed and a repeat of the F-CSAT

Clinical findings

Obese patients

The sniffing position may not prove sufficient for laryngoscopy in obese patients, as their increased chest diameter may impede neck flexion. To achieve the correct angle, 'ramping' can be used. This is done either by stacking padding beneath the shoulders and head or by raising the upper back of the bed/trolley to place the patient's entire back into a semi-upright posture of approximately 25°. Alignment of the external auditory meatus with the sternum remains the goal (Frerk et al., 2015; Troop, 2016; Reber, 2016). There is debate regarding the effectiveness of this position, with some suggestion that it may actually worsen glottis view and not assist oxygenation (Rahiman and Keane, 2018; Semler et al., 2017).

Reduced neck movement

Neck movement is not always possible. Ankylosing spondylitis and kyphosis can cause excessive posterior curve of the thoracic spine, forcing the head forwards and reducing neck movement. The head may have to be managed in the position in which it is found, and should not be forcibly moved. This increases the difficulty of some procedures, particularly advanced airway procedures where mouth opening and access to the trachea and front of the neck are all reduced (Ali et al., 2012; Hariharasudhan et al., 2016; Kang et al., 2013; Ma et al., 2016; Saricicek et al., 2014; Woodward and Kam, 2009).

Spinal injury

Neutral position is preferred for suspected neck trauma management (Farag, 2016; Jung, 2015). Flexion can stretch the spinal cord while extension decreases its length and vertebral space. Neither options are favourable for spinal injuries, making sniffing and head tilt positions unsuitable (Austin et al., 2014; Jose et al., 2016; Jung, 2015; Prasarn et al., 2014).

PRACTICE TIP!

Head position can be critical, including during advanced airway procedures. Attention to this basic method could prove the difference between success and difficulty or failure.

PRACTICE TIP!

Basic head position cannot be ignored – all patients must be postured somehow. Decide whether a specific position will add benefit or carries risk.

PRACTICE TIP!

All patients are anatomically different. Placement in the correct position requires visual inspection and adjustment where necessary for anatomical alignment.

PRACTICE TIP!

Airway procedures should always be managed as high risk for exposure to body fluid and infection. Protective eyewear and respiratory masks should be worn as appropriate.

TEST YOUR KNOWLEDGE QUESTIONS

1. **What three positions are suitable for supine patients?**
Head tilt/chin lift; neutral anatomical; sniffing.

2. **Define the neutral anatomical head position.**
Where the external auditory meatus is on the same plane as the mid-clavicle.

3. **How does the neutral anatomical head position differ from the sniffing position?**
In the sniffing position, the neck is flexed at 35° and extended 15° again at the head to raise the external auditory meatus to the plane of the sternum angle.

4. **Which is the preferred head position for patients with a spinal injury?**
Supine in neutral anatomical position.

5. **How is the neutral anatomical position achieved in the adult?**
Lift the head to the correct plane, then support with 2–5 cm padding beneath the occiput.

6. **How is the neutral anatomical position achieved in the small child?**
Lift the shoulders to the correct plane and place 2–5 cm padding beneath the shoulders.

7. **How is the sniffing position achieved in the adult?**
Place 7–9 cm padding beneath the patient's occiput and light pressure on the forehead to maintain anterior facial alignment.

8. **How is the sniffing position achieved in the child?**
Padding is placed beneath the neck arch to create flexion, then the face is tilted until it is in anterior view alignment.

9. **How might positioning of the obese patient vary from that of other patients?**
It may be necessary to raise the head and upper body by 25° using padding or bed angle, to add to the sniffing position.

10. **What is the main advantage of the sniffing position?**
It best improves the mouth-pharynx-glottis view, which is useful during intubation.

References

Akhtar, M., Ali, Z., Hassan, N., Mehdi, S., Wani, G.M. and Mir, A.H., 2017. A randomized study comparing the sniffing position with simple head extension for glottis visualization and difficulty in intubation during direct laryngoscopy. *Anesthesia, Essays and Researches*, 11(3), 762.

Ali, Q.E., Amir, S.H., Siddiqui, O.A., Nadeem, A. and Azhar, A.Z., 2012. Airtraq® optical laryngoscope for tracheal intubation in patients with severe ankylosing spondylitis: a report of two cases. *Indian Journal of Anaesthesia*, 56(2), 165.

Austin, N., Krishnamoorthy, V. and Dagal, A., 2014. Airway management in cervical spine injury. *International Journal of Critical Illness and Injury Science*, 4(1), 50.

Bhalala, U.S., Hemani, M., Shah, M., Kim, B., Gu, B., Cruz, A., Arunachalam, P., Tian, E., Yu, C., Punnoose, J. and Chen, S., 2016. Defining optimal head-tilt position of resuscitation in neonates and young infants using magnetic resonance imaging data. *PLOS ONE*, 11(3), e0151789.

Chua, C., Schmölzer, G.M. and Davis, P.G., 2012. Airway manoeuvres to achieve upper airway patency during mask ventilation in newborn infants – an historical perspective. *Resuscitation*, 83(4), 411–416.

Cruz, A., 2014. Defining head-tilt position of resuscitation. In *2014 AAP National Conference and Exhibition*, American Academy of Pediatrics.

El-Orbany, M., Woehlck, H. and Salem, M.R., 2011. Head and neck position for direct laryngoscopy. *Anesthesia & Analgesia*, 113(1), 103–109.

Farag, E., 2016. Airway management for cervical spine surgery. *Best Practice & Research Clinical Anaesthesiology*, 30(1), 13–25.

Frerk, C., Mitchell, V.S., McNarry, A.F., Mendonca, C., Bhagrath, R., Patel, A., O'Sullivan, E.P., Woodall, N.M. and Ahmad, I., 2015. Difficult Airway Society 2015 guidelines for management of unanticipated difficult intubation in adults. *British Journal of Anaesthesia*, 115(6), 827–848.

Greenland, K.B., Edwards, M.J., Hutton, N.J., Challis, V.J., Irwin, M.G. and Sleigh, J.W., 2010. Changes in airway configuration with different head and neck positions using magnetic resonance imaging of normal airways: a new concept with possible clinical applications. *British Journal of Anaesthesia*, 105(5), 683–690.

Gurani, S.F., Di Carlo, G., Cattaneo, P.M., Thorn, J.J. and Pinholt, E.M., 2016. Effect of head and tongue posture on the pharyngeal airway dimensions and morphology in three-dimensional imaging: a systematic review. *Journal of Oral & Maxillofacial Research*, 7(1).

Gutala, D., Hemani, M., Chen, S., Kitchen, G., Allen, R., Acharya, S., Bosemani, T. and Bhalala, U., 2014. Defining head-tilt position of resuscitation. *Critical Care Medicine*, 42(12), 12.

Hariharasudhan, B., Mane, R.S., Gogate, V.A. and Dhorigol, M.G., 2016. Successful management of difficult airway: a case series. *Journal of the Scientific Society*, 43(3), 151.

Holm-Knudsen, R.J. and Rasmussen, L.S., 2009. Paediatric airway management: basic aspects. *Acta Anaesthesiologica Scandinavica*, 53(1), 1–9.

Jose, A., Nagori, S.A., Agarwal, B., Bhutia, O. and Roychoudhury, A., 2016. Management of maxillofacial trauma in emergency: an update of challenges and controversies. *Journal of Emergencies, Trauma, and Shock*, 9(2), 73.

Jung, J.Y., 2015. Airway management of patients with traumatic brain injury/C-spine injury. *Korean Journal of Anesthesiology*, 68(3), 213–219.

Kang, J.M., Lee, K.W., Kim, D.O. and Yi, J.W., 2013. Airway management of an ankylosing spondylitis patient with severe temporomandibular joint ankylosis and impossible mouth opening. *Korean Journal of Anesthesiology*, 64(1), 84–86.

Ma, L.L., Yu, X.R., Zhu, B., Huang, Y.G., Shen, J.X. and Zhang, J.G., 2016. Difficult airway for patients undergoing spine surgeries. *Chinese Medical Journal*, 129(6), 749.

Maconochie, I.K., Bingham, R., Eich, C., López-Herce, J., Rodríguez-Núñez, A., Rajka, T., Van de Voorde, P., Zideman, D.A., Biarent, D., Monsieurs, K.G. and Nolan, J.P., 2015. European Resuscitation Council guidelines for resuscitation 2015, section 6: Paediatric life support. *Resuscitation*, 95, 223–248.

Myatra, S.N., Shah, A., Kundra, P., Patwa, A., Ramkumar, V., Divatia, J.V., Raveendra, U.S., Shetty, S.R., Ahmed, S.M., Doctor, J.R. and Pawar, D.K., 2016. All India Difficult Airway Association 2016 guidelines for the management of unanticipated difficult tracheal intubation in adults. *Indian Journal of Anaesthesia*, 60(12), 885.

Paal, P., Goedecke, A.V., Brugger, H., Niederklapfer, T., Lindner, K.H. and Wenzel, V., 2007. Head position for opening the upper airway. *Anaesthesia*, 62(3), 227–230.

Prasarn, M.L., Horodyski, M., Scott, N.E., Konopka, G., Conrad, B. and Rechtine, G.R., 2014. Motion generated in the unstable upper cervical spine during head tilt–chin lift and jaw thrust maneuvers. *Spine Journal*, 14(4), 609–614.

Rahiman, S.N. and Keane, M., 2018. Ramped position: what the 'neck'! *Chest*, 153(2), 567–568.

Reber, A., 2016. Airway characteristics and safe management of spontaneously breathing patients: risks of sedation and analgesia and changes in wakefulness. *International Journal of Clinical Medicine*, 7(11), 726–735.

Saricicek, V., Mizrak, A., Gul, R., Goksu, S. and Cesur, M., 2014. GlideScope video laryngoscopy use tracheal intubation in patients with ankylosing spondylitis: a series of four cases and literature review. *Journal of Clinical Monitoring and Computing*, 28(2), 169–172.

Semler, M.W., Janz, D.R., Russell, D.W., Casey, J.D., Lentz, R.J., Zouk, A.N., Santanilla, J.I., Khan, Y.A., Joffe, A.M., Stigler, W.S. and Rice, T.W., 2017. A multicenter, randomized trial of ramped position vs sniffing position during endotracheal intubation of critically ill adults. *Chest*, 152(4), 712–722.

Soar, J., Nolan, J.P., Böttiger, B.W., Perkins, G.D., Lott, C., Carli, P., Pellis, T., Sandroni, C., Skrifvars, M.B., Smith, G.B. and Sunde, K., 2015. European Resuscitation Council guidelines for resuscitation 2015, section 3: Adult advanced life support. *Resuscitation*, 95, 100–147.

Tripathi, S.S., Pal, J.K., Singh, R.R., Awasthi, S. and Mishra, S.P., 2016. Airway management of trauma patient of paediatric age group. *International Journal of Life-Sciences Scientific Research*, 2(6), 644–650.

Troop, C., 2016. The difficult airway and or obesity and the importance of positioning. *British Journal of Anaesthesia*, 117(5), 674–674.

Wei, W., Huang, S.W., Chen, L.H., Qi, Y., Qiu, Y.M. and Li, S.T., 2017. Airflow behavior changes in upper airway caused by different head and neck positions: comparison by computational fluid dynamics. *Journal of Biomechanics*, 52, 89–94.

Wilton, N., Lee, C. and Doyle, E., 2015. Developmental anatomy of the airway. *Anaesthesia & Intensive Care Medicine*, 16(12), 611–615.

Woodward, L.J. and Kam, P.C.A., 2009. Ankylosing spondylitis: recent developments and anaesthetic implications. *Anaesthesia*, 64(5), 540–548.

3.3 | Jaw thrust
John Cowell

Chapter objectives

At the end of this chapter the reader will be able to:

1. Describe the rationale for jaw thrust application
2. Demonstrate the method of jaw thrust application

Resources required for this assessment

- Standardised patient or mannequin allowing jaw and head movement
- Disposable gloves, eyewear, mask
- Method of documenting the results

Skill matrix

This assessment requires:
- Infection control (CS 1.3)
- Communication (CS 1.5)
- Consent (CS 1.6)
- Patient assessment skills (Chapter 2, CS 2.1, 2.2, 2.6, 2.8, 2.10)
- Head positioning (CS 3.2)

This assessment is a component of:
- Airway and ventilation (Chapter 3)

Introduction

Maintenance of airway patency can involve one or more methods, ranging from simple manipulations through to advanced procedures. The option(s) selected must adequately address the underlying obstruction. The value of simple physical options should not be underestimated. One of the most effective of such options is jaw thrust. This chapter discusses the application of jaw thrust for providing airway care.

Anatomy and physiology

The tongue is a large (intrinsic) muscle attached to the skull and hyoid bone by four extrinsic muscles on either side. Most significantly, the tongue is attached to the floor of the mouth and mandible. Movement of the lower jaw also moves the tongue.

At the base of the tongue are the vallecula and the epiglottis within the oropharynx. Superior to the epiglottis are the soft palate, uvula and nasopharynx.

During swallowing, the soft palate contacts with and closes the nasopharynx. The tongue base pulls posteriorly and the pharynx shortens. The hyoid and larynx are pulled upwards under the base of the tongue, covered by the epiglottis, and the vocal cords close to seal the glottis.

Clinical rationale

Lying supine poses a risk to the upper airway if the patient loses consciousness and airway reflexes. Loss of tongue control allows the tongue to fall backward and obstruct the nasopharynx, oropharynx and hypoglottis. This may be indicated by upper airway snoring or ineffective ventilation.

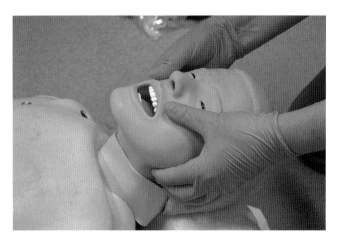

Figure 3.3.1 Positioning the fingers for jaw thrust

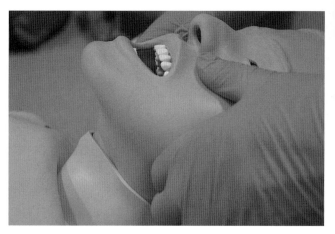

Figure 3.3.2 Applying jaw thrust

Moving the jaw anteriorly moves the mouth floor forwards, countering the natural obstructive tongue position when supine. This is known as jaw thrust. It increases pharyngeal dimension and improves ventilation (Albrecht and Schoettker, 2010; Aoyama et al., 2000; Chua et al., 2012; Gurani et al., 2016; Han et al., 2013; Isono, 2008; Uzun et al., 2005; Wittels, 2018). It can also be helpful in improving glottis view if maintained during intubation (Aoyama et al., 2000; Corda et al., 2012; Han et al., 2013; Patil et al., 2016).

Jaw thrust is effective in managing the paediatric airway (Bingham and Proctor, 2008; Harless et al., 2014; Maconochie et al., 2015; von Ungern-Sternberg et al., 2005) where the tongue and epiglottis is relatively larger, more problematic and less easily displaced (Holm-Knudsen and Rasmussen, 2009). It is more effective than chin lift (Reber, 2016).

The combination of head tilt, jaw thrust and mouth opening is referred to as 'triple airway manoeuvre' (Isono, 2008; Joffe et al., 2010).

Application

The ideal position from which to apply jaw thrust is superior to the patient's head, facing towards them. Place a hand on either side of the face, with a thumb on each cheekbone and the fingers beneath the jaw angle (see Fig. 3.3.1). Firmly pull the jaw anteriorly and slightly superiorly while simultaneously pushing down with the thumbs on the cheekbone until the lower teeth are in front of the upper jaw (Fig. 3.3.2). Increased force can be applied if the palms are placed on the cheeks rather than just the thumbs. If necessary, the thumbs can then be used to open the mouth (Soar et al., 2015).

No specific patient head position is required first before jaw thrust is applied. The neutral anatomical or sniffing

positions can be combined for optimal benefit (Chua et al., 2012). Positioning the patient semi-upright at 20–25° can reduce the gravity effect on the tongue and particularly at the soft palate level, improving the effectiveness of jaw thrust (Chang et al., 2015; Isono, 2008; Weingart and Levitan, 2012).

Jaw thrust can be performed with one hand during positive pressure ventilation by pressing the mask downwards while using the fingers from the same hand to pull the jaw upwards (see Chapter 3.11). Alternatively, use two hands to push the mask into the face while the fingers simultaneously pull the jaw angles upwards. While the two-handed method is more effective, it has the disadvantage of requiring a second person if any other airway or ventilation procedure is required (Joffe et al., 2010).

Maintaining jaw thrust is physically demanding on the hands, so it will be necessary to change paramedics if it is required for prolonged periods. Jaw thrust can be used in conjunction with oropharyngeal or nasopharyngeal airway devices (see Chapters 3.4 and 3.5). This method does not do anything to protect against gastric aspiration or insufflation.

Clinical skill assessment process

The following section outlines the clinical skill assessment tools that should be used to determine a student's ability to demonstrate the effective application of jaw thrust.
1. Clinical Skill Work Instruction
2. Formative Clinical Skill Assessment (F-CSAT)
3. Performance Improvement Plan (PIP)
4. Summative Clinical Skill Assessment (S-CSAT)
(5. Direct Observation of Procedural Skills (DOPS) – see Chapter 1.1)

Clinical Skill Work Instruction

Equipment and resources: Standardised patient or mannequin allowing jaw and head movement; disposable gloves, eyewear and mask; method of documenting results

Associated Clinical Skills: Infection control; Communication; Consent; Patient assessment skills; Head positioning

Jaw thrust

Activity	Critical Action	Rationale
Personal protection	Don PPE as required.	For infection control.
Prepare patient	Assess for suspected spinal injury.	Excludes head tilt and sniffing positions.
	Place patient supine with head returned midline. Choose head tilt, neutral anatomical or sniffing position, as desired.	Head and body aligned.
	Position paramedic superior to patient's head, looking inferiorly to them.	Best position for this manoeuvre.
Apply jaw thrust	Place hands either side of patient's face. If patient is on the floor or low surface, it may be more effective if paramedic rests elbows against surface.	In preparation for correct placement.
	Press one thumb against either cheekbone.	Ready for downward pressure.
	With each hand, place two or three fingers beneath angle of the jaw on each side of face.	Ready for upward pressure.
	Firmly press down thumbs into the cheekbones while simultaneously pulling jaw anteriorly and superiorly. Avoid causing lateral movement.	Correct application. Minimal cervical spine impact.
	Visually inspect jaw and lower teeth relocation forwards relative to upper teeth.	To assess movement effectiveness.
Reassess	Assess breathing and airway patency for effectiveness.	To assess outcome.
Report	Accurately document/hand over findings, including therapeutic benefit or adverse reaction.	Accurate record kept and patient care continuity.

Formative Clinical Skill Assessment (F-CSAT)

Equipment and resources: Standardised patient or mannequin allowing jaw and head movement; disposable gloves, eyewear and mask; method of documenting results

Associated Clinical Skills: Infection control; Communication; Consent; Patient assessment skills; Head positioning

Staff/Student being assessed: _____

Jaw thrust

Activity	Critical Action	Participant Performance				
Personal protection	Dons appropriate PPE, including protective gloves and eyewear.	0	1	2	3	4
Prepares patient	Assesses for suspected spinal injury.	0	1	2	3	4
	Places patient supine with head returned midline. Places head in desired position.	0	1	2	3	4
	Adopts a position superior to patient's head, looking inferiorly to them.	0	1	2	3	4
Applies jaw thrust	Places hands either side of patient's face.	0	1	2	3	4
	Presses one thumb against either cheekbone.	0	1	2	3	4
	With each hand, places two or three fingers beneath angle of the jaw on each side of face.	0	1	2	3	4
	Firmly presses down thumbs into the cheekbones while simultaneously pulling jaw anteriorly and superiorly. Avoids causing lateral movement.	0	1	2	3	4
	Visually inspects jaw and lower teeth relocation forwards relative to upper teeth.	0	1	2	3	4
Reassesses	Assesses breathing and airway patency for effectiveness.	0	1	2	3	4
Reports	Accurately documents/hands over findings, including therapeutic benefit or adverse reaction.	0	1	2	3	4

Standard Achieved: (please circle one)

Competent (C)   Not Yet Competent* (NYC)

Staff/Student Name: _____

Assessor (please print name): _____

Signed (Assessor): _____

Date of Assessment: _____

Comments:

*If Not Yet Competent (NYC) a PIP needs to be completed and a repeat of the F-CSAT

Formative Clinical Skill Assessment (F-CSAT) Key

Skill level	Standard of procedure	Quality of performance	Outcome	Level of assistance required
4 Safe for unsupervised practice	Safe Accurate Behaviour is appropriate to context	Confident Accurate Expedient	Achieved intended outcome	No supporting cues* required
3 Requires supervision	Safe Accurate Behaviour is appropriate to context	Confident Accurate Takes longer than required	Achieved intended outcome	Requires occasional supportive cues*
2 Requires assistance	Safe Accurate Behaviour generally appropriate to context	Lacks certainty	Would not have achieved outcome without support	Requires frequent verbal and occasional physical directives in addition to supportive cues*
1 Requires direction	Safe only with guidance Not completely accurate	Unskilled Inefficient	Would not have achieved outcome without support	Requires continuous verbal and frequent physical directive cues*
0 Unsafe	Unsafe Unable to demonstrate behaviour Lack of insight into behaviour appropriate to context	Unskilled	Would not have achieved outcome	Requires continuous verbal and continuous physical directive cues*

*Refers to physical directives or verbal supportive cues

Performance Improvement Plan (PIP)

Please document the agreed education plan and completion timelines for areas assessed as less than 4.

This plan should be presented to assessor prior to commencement of summative assessment.

Where was supervisor support required?	Student summary of deficit. (Why was there a problem?)	Improvement Plan	Completed (Y/N)

Staff/Student Name: _____

Staff/Student Signature: _____

Educator Name: _____
Educator Signature: _____

Summative Clinical Skill Assessment (S-CSAT)

Equipment and resources: Standardised patient or mannequin allowing jaw and head movement; disposable gloves, eyewear and mask; method of documenting results

Associated Clinical Skills: Infection control; Communication; Consent; Patient assessment skills; Head positioning

Staff/Student being assessed: _____

- Completed Formative Clinical Skill Assessment (F-CSAT):   **YES**   **NO**
- Completed Performance Improvement Plan (PIP):   **YES**   **NO**   **N/A**

Jaw thrust

Activity	Critical Action	Achieved Without Direction	
Prepares operator	Dons appropriate PPE, including protective gloves and eyewear.	NO	YES
Prepares patient	Assesses for suspected spinal injury.	NO	YES
	Places patient supine with head returned midline. Places head in desired position.	NO	YES
	Adopts a position superior to patient's head, looking inferiorly to them.	NO	YES
Applies jaw thrust	Places hands either side of patient's face.	NO	YES
	Presses one thumb against either cheekbone.	NO	YES
	With each hand, places two or three fingers beneath angle of the jaw on each side of face.	NO	YES
	Firmly presses down thumbs into the cheekbones while simultaneously pulling jaw anteriorly and superiorly. Avoids causing lateral movement.		
	Visually inspects jaw and lower teeth relocation forwards relative to upper teeth.	NO	YES
Reassesses	Assesses breathing and airway patency for effectiveness.	NO	YES
Reports	Accurately documents/hands over findings, including therapeutic benefit or adverse reaction.	NO	YES

Standard Achieved: (please circle one)

Competent (C)   Not Yet Competent* (NYC)

Staff/Student Name: _____

Assessor (please print name)**:** _____

Signed (Assessor)**:** _____

Date of Assessment: _____

Comments:

*If Not Yet Competent (NYC) a PIP needs to be completed and a repeat of the F-CSAT

Clinical findings

Spinal injury

Jaw thrust alone was previously preferred as an alternative to head tilt/chin lift where spinal injury is suspected, given its reduced movement of the cervical spine (Crosby, 2006; Prasarn et al., 2014; Reber, 2016). This recommendation has recently been revised, and first-aiders are now recommended to use the head tilt/chin lift in early resuscitation, regardless of any suspected spinal injury (Perkins et al., 2015). The modified jaw thrust method (without head tilt) remains valid where the head is restricted to the neutral anatomical position (Koo et al., 2014) and can be applied where there are spinal injury concerns.

Facial/mandibular trauma

Injury to the mandible and face can compromise the airway, particularly if there is posterior displacement. There is no absolute contraindication of jaw thrust in the presence of facial/mandibular injury, although its effectiveness will be uncertain. It may offer benefit or, conversely, be too difficult to apply (Jose et al., 2016). Attempt jaw thrust only where the manoeuvre is necessary.

PRACTICE TIP!

It is possible for a single paramedic to apply jaw thrust and assisted ventilation simultaneously (see Chapter 3.11). If there is doubt about the effectiveness of doing so, two paramedics must be allocated, with one holding the mask and applying jaw thrust while the second ventilates.

PRACTICE TIP!

Jaw thrust is an airway procedure that requires close proximity to the patient. As with all such methods, personal protection, including gloves, eyewear and respiratory mask, should be worn.

PRACTICE TIP!

Jaw thrust can require strong force applied by the fingers and thumbs. For increased force, consider using the palm instead of the thumbs. Also consider alternating paramedics to avoid finger cramping.

TEST YOUR KNOWLEDGE QUESTIONS

1. **What are the two physical movements required to perform jaw thrust?**
   Pushing down on the cheek while pulling jaw angles anteriorly and superiorly.

2. **How can the effectiveness of jaw thrust be evaluated?**
   Visualising anterior jaw displacement until the lower teeth are in front of the upper jaw.

3. **For which concurrent injury can jaw thrust be used to support the neutral anatomical position?**
   Suspected spinal injury.

4. **What airway obstruction can jaw thrust assist with?**
   Pharyngeal obstruction caused by the tongue/epiglottis collapsing posteriorly when the patient is supine.

5. **What impact does jaw thrust have during an intubation attempt?**
   It can improve the view of the glottis.

6. **How can jaw thrust cause tongue movement?**
   The tongue is attached to the mouth floor and to the jaw. Movement of the jaw moves the tongue with it.

7. **How can jaw thrust be applied during assisted ventilation?**
   Either by one paramedic using one hand to hold the mask and jaw or by two paramedics, one holding the mask and jaw and the other ventilating.

8. **What head position is required before jaw thrust can be applied?**
   Any position, including head tilt, neutral anatomical and sniffing.

9. **What benefit is offered by posturing the patient upright at 20–25°?**
   It can reduce the gravity effect on the tongue and particularly at the soft palate level, improving the effectiveness of jaw thrust.

10. **What is the impact of facial injury when considering whether to apply jaw thrust?**
    Injury to the mandible and face can compromise the airways and cause posterior displacement. The effectiveness of jaw thrust will be uncertain: it may be too difficult to apply or might prove beneficial.

References

Albrecht, E. and Schoettker, P., 2010. The jaw-thrust maneuver. *New England Journal of Medicine*, 363(21), e32.

Aoyama, K., Takenaka, I., Nagaoka, E. and Kadoya, T., 2000. Jaw thrust maneuver for endotracheal intubation using a fiberoptic stylet. *Anesthesia & Analgesia*, 90(6), 1457–1458.

Bingham, R.M. and Proctor, L.T., 2008. Airway management. *Pediatric Clinics of North America*, 55(4), 873–886.

Chang, J.E., Min, S.W., Kim, C.S., Kwon, Y.S. and Hwang, J.Y., 2015. Effects of the jaw-thrust manoeuvre in the semi-sitting position on securing a clear airway during fibreoptic intubation. *Anaesthesia*, 70(8), 933–938.

Chua, C., Schmölzer, G.M. and Davis, P.G., 2012. Airway manoeuvres to achieve upper airway patency during mask ventilation in newborn infants – an historical perspective. *Resuscitation*, 83(4), 411–416.

Crosby, E.T., 2006. Airway management in adults after cervical spine trauma. *Anesthesiology*, 104(6), 1293–1318.

Corda, D.M., Riutort, K.T., Leone, A.J., Qureshi, M.K., Heckman, M.G. and Brull, S.J., 2012. Effect of jaw thrust and cricoid pressure maneuvers on glottic visualization during GlideScope videolaryngoscopy. *Journal of Anesthesia*, 26(3), 362–368.

Gurani, S.F., Di Carlo, G., Cattaneo, P.M., Thorn, J.J. and Pinholt, E.M., 2016. Effect of head and tongue posture on the pharyngeal airway dimensions and morphology in three-dimensional imaging: a systematic review. *Journal of Oral & Maxillofacial Research*, 7(1).

Han, S.H., Oh, A.Y., Jung, C.W., Park, S.J., Kim, J.H. and Nahm, F.S., 2013. The effect of the jaw-thrust manoeuvre on the ability to advance a tracheal tube over a bronchoscope during oral fibreoptic intubation. *Anaesthesia*, 68(5), 472–477.

Harless, J., Ramaiah, R. and Bhananker, S.M., 2014. Pediatric airway management. *International Journal of Critical Illness and Injury Science*, 4(1), 65.

Holm-Knudsen, R.J. and Rasmussen, L.S., 2009. Paediatric airway management: basic aspects. *Acta Anaesthesiologica Scandinavica*, 53(1), 1–9.

Isono, S., 2008. One hand, two hands, or no hands for maximizing airway maneuvers?. *Anesthesiology*, 109(4), 576–577.

Joffe, A.M., Hetzel, S. and Liew, E.C., 2010. A two-handed jaw-thrust technique is superior to the one-handed 'EC-clamp' technique for mask ventilation in the apneic unconscious person. *Anesthesiology*, 113(4), 873–879.

Jose, A., Nagori, S.A., Agarwal, B., Bhutia, O. and Roychoudhury, A., 2016. Management of maxillofacial trauma in emergency: an update of challenges and controversies. *Journal of Emergencies, Trauma, and Shock*, 9(2), 73.

Koo, S.K., Lee, H.J., Kim, Y.J., Kim, Y.J. and Jung, S.H., 2014. Change of obstruction site by modified jaw thrust maneuver in obstructive sleep apnea patients. *Sleep Medicine Research*, 5(2), 49–53.

Maconochie, I.K., Bingham, R., Eich, C., López-Herce, J., Rodríguez-Núnez, A., Rajka, T., Van de Voorde, P., Zideman, D.A., Biarent, D., Monsieurs, K.G. and Nolan, J.P., 2015. European Resuscitation Council guidelines for resuscitation 2015, section 6: Paediatric life support. *Resuscitation*, 95, 223–248.

Patil, M.C., Sanikop, C.S. and Dhorigol, M.G., 2016. Effect of cricoids pressure and jaw thrust maneuvers on glottis visualization during C-MAC videolaryngoscopy. *International Journal of Recent Scientific Research*, 7(2).

Perkins, G.D., Travers, A.H., Berg, R.A., Castren, M., Considine, J., Escalante, R., Gazmuri, R.J., Koster, R.W., Lim, S.H., Nation, K.J. and Olasveengen, T.M., 2015. Part 3: Adult basic life support and automated external defibrillation: 2015 international consensus on cardiopulmonary resuscitation and emergency cardiovascular care science with treatment recommendations. *Resuscitation*, 95, e43–e69.

Prasarn, M.L., Horodyski, M., Scott, N.E., Konopka, G., Conrad, B. and Rechtine, G.R., 2014. Motion generated in the unstable upper cervical spine during head tilt–chin lift and jaw thrust maneuvers. *Spine Journal*, 14(4), 609–614.

Reber, A., 2016. Airway characteristics and safe management of spontaneously breathing patients: risks of sedation and analgesia and changes in wakefulness. *International Journal of Clinical Medicine*, 7(11), 726.

Soar, J., Nolan, J.P., Böttiger, B.W., Perkins, G.D., Lott, C., Carli, P., Pellis, T., Sandroni, C., Skrifvars, M.B., Smith, G.B. and Sunde, K., 2015. European Resuscitation Council guidelines for resuscitation 2015, section 3: Adult advanced life support. *Resuscitation*, 95, 100–147.

Uzun, L., Ugur, M.B., Altunkaya, H., Ozer, Y., Ozkocak, I. and Demirel, C.B., 2005. Effectiveness of the jaw-thrust maneuver in opening the airway: a flexible fiberoptic endoscopic study. *ORL*, 67(1), 39–44.

von Ungern-Sternberg, B.S., Erb, T.O., Reber, A. and Frei, F.J., 2005. Opening the upper airway – airway maneuvers in pediatric anesthesia. *Pediatric Anesthesia*, 15(3), 181–189.

Weingart, S.D. and Levitan, R.M., 2012. Preoxygenation and prevention of desaturation during emergency airway management. *Annals of Emergency Medicine*, 59(3), 165–175.

Wittels, K.A., 2018. Basic airway management in adults. Retrieved from: https://www.uptodate.com

3.4 | Oropharyngeal airway

Gavin Smith

Chapter objectives

At the end of this chapter the reader will be able to:

1. Describe the rationale for oropharyngeal airway (OPA) insertion
2. Demonstrate effective and safe placement of an OPA
3. Accurately report on the performance of OPA placement

Resources required for this assessment

- Airway mannequin suitable for OPA insertion
- OPA device in range of sizes
- Disposable gloves, protective eyewear, respiratory mask
- Method of documenting the results

Skill matrix

This assessment requires:

- Infection control (CS 1.3)
- Consent (CS 1.6)
- Patient assessment skills (Chapter 2, CS 2.1, 2.2, 2.6, 2.8, 2.10)
- Airway and ventilation skills (Chapter 3, CS 3.2, 3.3, 3.6, 3.7)

This assessment is a component of:

- Airway and ventilation (Chapter 3)

Introduction

In any unconscious patient there is risk of physical upper airway obstruction through poor anatomical positioning. There are numerous strategies and adjuncts to respond to this. This chapter discusses the oropharyngeal airway (OPA).

Anatomy and physiology

The oral cavity and oropharynx are the upper airway structures that commence at the lips and continue inwards past the base of the tongue, soft palate and pharynx. The oral cavity is mostly rigid, as is the larynx at the distal end of the upper airway. The pharynx in between them is largely smooth muscle that can collapse whenever muscle tone is lost. This contributes to sleep apnoea and is worsened by obesity (Isono, 2012; Ma et al., 2016).

The cartilaginous epiglottis is at the base of the tongue, designed to flap back over the glottis during swallowing when the larynx rises towards it. There are several airway reflexes within and around the larynx, including cough, gag and swallow.

Tongue and pharynx muscle tone and airway reflexes deteriorate and eventually fail with loss of consciousness.

Clinical rationale

An OPA, or Guedel airway, is an orally invasive semi-flexible silicon implement used to secure the tongue anteriorly. This helps prevent airway obstruction caused by poor positioning of the epiglottis and collapsing soft airway muscles in the pharynx (Pozner et al., 2015; Soar et al., 2015). This is particularly helpful when the patient must be left supine, such as during the management of cardiac arrest.

The requirement for OPA insertion is the loss of airway reflexes, particularly accompanying altered consciousness. The primary action of the device is to support a physical passage that enables unhindered airflow through the upper airway to the glottis.

Although OPA insertion does not have to be aseptic, it should be performed as cleanly as possible to avoid unnecessary exposure of the patient to contaminants.

Patient positioning

Some patients must be positioned supine. Given that many training devices are designed for a supine posture, this is the most likely position for practising the skill. In such cases, the head can be placed in any position, preferably neutral anatomical and sniffing (see Chapter 3.2) where some longitudinal traction is placed on the soft airway, helping to hold it open.

Insertion is possible in any position, including the lateral position where gravity can assist or in cases of patient entrapment, such as motor vehicle rescue, where difficult patient posture can be imposed.

Airway preparation

Foreign material must be physically removed from the mouth and oropharynx, either manually or by mechanical suction, before insertion of the OPA (see Chapter 3.7). This includes vomitus and saliva, foreign bodies and any damaged tissue (such as teeth) resulting from trauma.

As the OPA device is not designed to prevent aspiration of foreign objects into the lower airways, ongoing airway clearance can require an alternative option such as supraglottic airway or intubation.

Device measurement

To select the appropriate size of device, it must be individually measured against the patient's anatomy using one of two variations. The OPA can be placed with one end against the angle of the jaw and the other reaching the central incisor on that side (Fig. 3.4.1a) (Kim et al., 2016). Alternatively, the OPA can be placed with one end against the tragus and the other reaching the corner of the mouth on that side (Fig. 3.4.1b).

Inserting an OPA that is too large risks damaging the posterior soft pharyngeal tissue. If too small a device is used, it may fail to achieve airway patency by failing to either displace the tongue forwards or support the soft airway. OPA devices come in a range of sizes, typically colour-coded and with their length measured in millimetres.

Insertion method

Once the patient is positioned correctly and foreign material has been cleared, the oropharynx can be held open further using jaw thrust (see Chapter 3.3).

Remove the selected size of device from its packaging. While it does not absolutely require lubrication, water or even the patient's own saliva can be used if this is deemed beneficial.

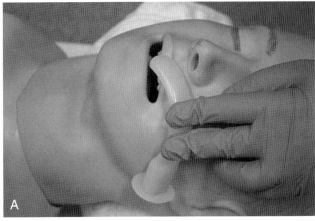
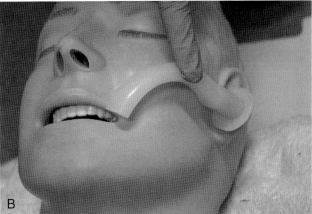

Figure 3.4.1 Measuring the OPA for size
(a) OPA with one end against the angle of the jaw and the other reaching the central incisor. (b) OPA with one end against the tragus and the other reaching the corner of the mouth.

Insertion of the OPA in an adult is accomplished by holding the device by the flanged end, with the curve in opposition to that of the oral cavity. It is then inserted slowly and carefully into the mouth to approximately half its length, and then gently rotated 180° prior to inserting the remainder of the device.

Provided the correct size is available, OPA devices can also be inserted into child patients. Instead of inserting the OPA inverted, as with adults, the same contour as the tongue is followed to avoid any injury to the softer hard palate. This is also necessary given the child's relatively larger tongue. If necessary, depress the tongue with a spatula or laryngoscope first.

Ideally, jaw thrust should be maintained throughout and following insertion. This may require two operators. To be confident of oropharyngeal placement, apply jaw thrust just prior to final placement of the OPA by pulling anteriorly on the jaw angles with both hands and completing the OPA insertion using the free thumbs (Fig. 3.4.2).

Once the device is completely inserted, the flanged end should rest against the patient's lips, with no pinching (Fig. 3.4.3).

Respiratory assessment can now be performed, with emphasis on the air passage. The size, number of attempts

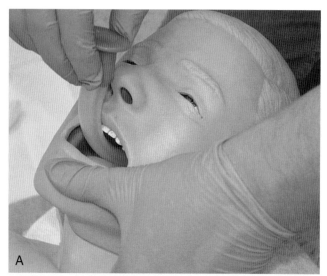

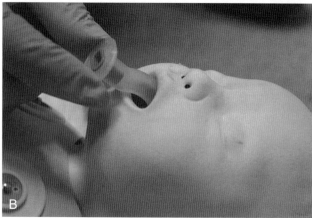

Figure 3.4.2 OPA insertion
(a) Adult. (b). Child.

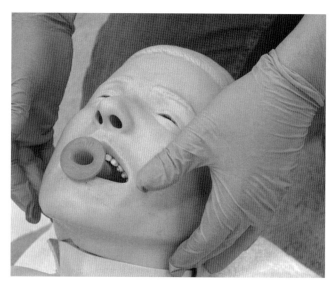

Figure 3.4.3 A correctly inserted OPA

required for success and insertion time are noted in the patient care record.

Clinical skill assessment process

The following section outlines the clinical skill assessment tools that should be used to determine a student's ability to demonstrate safe and accurate placement of the oropharyngeal airway.
1. Clinical Skill Work Instruction
2. Formative Clinical Skill Assessment (F-CSAT)
3. Performance Improvement Plan (PIP)
4. Summative Clinical Skill Assessment (S-CSAT)
(5. Direct Observation of Procedural Skills (DOPS) – see Chapter 1.1)

Clinical Skill Work Instruction

Equipment and resources: Airway mannequin suitable for OPA insertion; OPA device in range of sizes; disposable gloves, eyewear and mask; method of documenting results

Associated Clinical Skills: Infection control; Consent; Patient assessment skills; Airway and ventilation skills

Oropharyngeal airway

Activity	Critical Action	Rationale
Personal protection	Don PPE as required.	All airway procedures are considered high infection risk.
Assess indications	Assess patient consciousness, airway reflexes and respiratory status. Consider OPA contraindications/precautions.	Ensure appropriate use.
Prepare equipment	Lay out OPA and other airway resuscitation equipment on a clean surface.	Other airway devices might also be required.

Oropharyngeal airway continued

Activity	Critical Action	Rationale
Prepare patient	Place patient supine, with head in neutral anatomical or sniffing position (preferred) or allowing effective paramedic access to head and face (if unable to move patient).	Appropriate position assists airway patency and insertion.
	Ensure adequate FBAO clearance has been performed before insertion. (If there is copious vomitus, consider definitive airway management.) Provide simultaneous jaw thrust if support personnel are available.	OPA does not address any FBAO present. Displacing the jaw and tongue forwards improves access by the OPA device.
Measure OPA size	Measure appropriate size OPA using chosen method (one of two).	It is important to select the correct size.
Insert OPA	Hold the OPA by the flanged end.	In readiness for insertion.
	Lubricate the selected OPA (with water, patient saliva) if necessary.	To ease insertion.
	Adult: Insert distal end into patient's mouth, inverting curve in opposition to oral cavity. Child: Insert directly without inversion.	To avoid pushing the adult's tongue inwards. To avoid damaging the child's palate.
	Slide the OPA forwards approximately halfway into the mouth between the hard palate and tongue.	To avoid the tongue.
	Rotate the device 180° (adults only), then continue insertion until flange sits against lips without being pinched against teeth. Apply jaw thrust to ensure OPA seats in oropharynx.	To position correctly in oropharynx.
Reassess	Ensure no airway reflex is triggered by placement and that respiratory status is effective. Remove if airway reflexes are present.	To ensure OPA effectiveness. Gag reflex may result in vomiting.
Report	Accurately document/hand over time of insertion, OPA size, and any relevant information regarding placement or insertion.	Accurate record kept and continuity of patient care.

Formative Clinical Skill Assessment (F-CSAT)

Equipment and resources: Airway mannequin suitable for OPA insertion; OPA device in range of sizes; disposable gloves, eyewear and mask; method of documenting results

Associated Clinical Skills: Infection control; Consent; Patient assessment skills; Airway and ventilation skills

Staff/Student being assessed: _____

Oropharyngeal airway

Activity	Critical Action	Participant Performance				
Personal protection	Dons PPE as required.	0	1	2	3	4
Assesses indications	Assesses patient consciousness, airway reflexes and respiratory status. Considers OPA contraindications/precautions.	0	1	2	3	4
Prepares equipment	Lays out OPA and other airway resuscitation equipment on a clean surface.	0	1	2	3	4

Oropharyngeal airway continued

Activity	Critical Action	Participant Performance				
Prepares patient	Places patient supine, with head in neutral anatomical or sniffing position, or allows effective paramedic access to head and face.	0	1	2	3	4
	Provides adequate FBAO clearance prior to insertion. Provides simultaneous jaw thrust if support personnel are available.	0	1	2	3	4
Measures OPA size	Measures appropriate size of OPA using chosen method.	0	1	2	3	4
Inserts OPA	Holds the OPA by the flanged end.	0	1	2	3	4
	Lubricates the selected OPA (water, patient saliva) if necessary.	0	1	2	3	4
	Adult: Inserts distal end into patient's mouth, inverting curve in opposition to oral cavity. Children: Inserts into mouth without inversion.	0	1	2	3	4
	Slides OPA forwards approximately halfway into the mouth between the hard palate and tongue.	0	1	2	3	4
	Rotates the device 180° (adults only), then continues insertion until flange sits against lips without being pinched against teeth. Applies jaw thrust to ensure OPA seats in oropharynx.	0	1	2	3	4
Reassesses	Ensures no airway reflex is triggered by placement and that respiratory status is effective. Removes if gag reflex is present.	0	1	2	3	4
Reports	Accurately documents/hands over time of insertion, OPA size, and any relevant information regarding placement or insertion.	0	1	2	3	4

Standard Achieved: (please circle one)

Competent (C)   Not Yet Competent* (NYC)

Staff/Student Name: _____

Assessor (please print name)**:** _____

Signed (Assessor)**:** _____

Date of Assessment: _____

Comments:

*If Not Yet Competent (NYC) a PIP needs to be completed and a repeat of the F-CSAT

Formative Clinical Skills Assessment (F-CSAT) Key

Skill level	Standard of procedure	Quality of performance	Outcome	Level of assistance required
4 Safe for unsupervised practice	Safe Accurate Behaviour is appropriate to context	Confident Accurate Expedient	Achieved intended outcome	No supporting cues* required
3 Requires supervision	Safe Accurate Behaviour is appropriate to context	Confident Accurate Takes longer than required	Achieved intended outcome	Requires occasional supportive cues*
2 Requires assistance	Safe Accurate Behaviour generally appropriate to context	Lacks certainty	Would not have achieved outcome without support	Requires frequent verbal and occasional physical directives in addition to supportive cues*
1 Requires direction	Safe only with guidance Not completely accurate	Unskilled Inefficient	Would not have achieved outcome without support	Requires continuous verbal and frequent physical directive cues*
0 Unsafe	Unsafe Unable to demonstrate behaviour Lack of insight into behaviour appropriate to context	Unskilled	Would not have achieved outcome	Requires continuous verbal and continuous physical directive cues*

*Refers to physical directives or verbal supportive cues

Performance Improvement Plan (PIP)

Please document the agreed education plan and completion timelines for areas assessed as less than 4.

This plan should be presented to assessor prior to commencement of summative assessment.

Where was supervisor support required?	Student summary of deficit. (Why was there a problem?)	Improvement Plan	Completed (Y/N)

Staff/Student Name: _____

Staff/Student Signature: _____

Educator Name: _____

Educator Signature: _____

Summative Clinical Skill Assessment (S-CSAT)

Equipment and resources: Airway mannequin suitable for OPA insertion; OPA device in range of sizes; disposable gloves, eyewear and mask; method of documenting results

Associated Clinical Skills: Infection control; Consent; Patient assessment skills; Airway and ventilation skills

Staff/Student being assessed: _____

- Completed Formative Clinical Skill Assessment (F-CSAT): **YES** **NO**
- Completed Performance Improvement Plan (PIP): **YES** **NO** **N/A**

Oropharyngeal airway

Activity	Critical Action	Achieved Without Direction	
Personal protection	Dons PPE as required.	NO	YES
Assesses indications	Assesses patient consciousness, airway reflexes and respiratory status. Considers OPA contraindications/precautions.	NO	YES
Prepares equipment	Lays out OPA and other airway resuscitation equipment on a clean surface.	NO	YES
Prepares patient	Places patient supine, with head in neutral anatomical or sniffing position, or allows effective paramedic access to head and face.	NO	YES
	Provides adequate FBAO clearance prior to insertion. Provides simultaneous jaw thrust if support personnel are available.	NO	YES
Measures OPA size	Measures appropriate size OPA using chosen method.	NO	YES
Inserts OPA	Holds the OPA by the flanged end.	NO	YES
	Lubricates the selected OPA (water, patient saliva) if necessary.	NO	YES
	Adult: Inserts distal end into patient's mouth, inverting curve in opposition to oral cavity. Children: Inserts into mouth without inversion.	NO	YES
	Slides OPA forwards approximately halfway into the mouth between the hard palate and tongue.	NO	YES
	Rotates the device 180° (adults only) then continues insertion until flange sits against lips without being pinched against teeth. Applies jaw thrust to ensure OPA seats in oropharynx.	NO	YES
Reassesses	Ensures no airway reflex is triggered by placement and that respiratory status is effective. Removes if gag reflex is present.	NO	YES
Reports	Accurately documents/hands over time of insertion, OPA size, and any relevant information regarding placement or insertion.	NO	YES

Standard Achieved: (please circle one)

Competent (C)   Not Yet Competent* (NYC)

Staff/Student Name: _____

Assessor (please print name): _____

Signed (Assessor): _____

Date of Assessment: _____

Comments:

*If Not Yet Competent (NYC) a PIP needs to be completed and a repeat of the F-CSAT

Clinical findings

Airway reflexes

Following insertion, airway reflexes can sometimes be stimulated unexpectedly, creating a risk of vomiting or passive regurgitation. Unwanted gagging is also associated with stimulating the vagus nerve and triggering a rise in intracranial pressure. Remove the device where this happens and consider an alternative option. In some cases, uncontrolled teeth clenching/trismus may preclude insertion, also forcing the consideration of alternatives.

The patient should be observed continually for the return of gag reflex signs. If these are noted, the OPA should be removed immediately. Additionally, if the device slowly ejects from the mouth, it is too large and should be removed and replaced with a smaller one.

Aspiration

Even without airway reflexes, the OPA does nothing to prevent passive regurgitation of gastric content or subsequent entry into the trachea. Where this is of concern, such as when administering positive pressure ventilation, more substantial airway protection will be necessary.

Injury

Careless or rough OPA insertion can result in localised tissue damage, leading to bleeding and oedema. Do not force against any obstruction, including clenched teeth.

Although trauma to the mandible and maxilla are not contraindications, care should be taken to prevent exacerbation of existing injury during and post insertion. In patients with difficult airway access or facial trauma, a laryngoscope may be used to visualise the passage over the tongue.

Other uses

Since the OPA sits in the posterior oropharynx, a narrow, flexible suction catheter can be inserted into it, passed along its length until beyond the distal tip and used to provide oropharyngeal suctioning. This should be measured against the OPA length to identify when the tip will enter the oropharynx. Similarly, a duodenal tube can be passed down the length of the OPA to facilitate gastric emptying. In this case, the OPA will not be able to be subsequently removed while the duodenal tube remains in situ.

The OPA can also be inserted for use as a bite block when protecting an intubated patient from the return of any airway reflexes.

PRACTICE TIP!

The OPA has a specific and limited purpose. Monitor the patient continuously and reconsider requirements following any change in condition.

PRACTICE TIP!

The insertion of an OPA suggests a critically unwell patient requiring immediate intervention, multiple therapies and urgent transport. The allocation of a paramedic to continuously monitor the patient's airways must remain a priority.

PRACTICE TIP!

To ensure the OPA tip seats correctly in the oropharynx, measure the device first and apply jaw thrust, particularly at the point of final placement.

TEST YOUR KNOWLEDGE QUESTIONS

1. **What are the two ways to measure an OPA device?**
From the angle of the jaw to the incisor on that side; from the tragus to the corner of the mouth on that side.

2. **Why is the OPA inserted with the tip initially facing into the roof of the mouth?**
To avoid pushing the tongue posteriorly.

3. **Why is the OPA inserted curving downwards in children?**
To avoid injuring the undeveloped hard palate.

4. **Which patient head position is chosen when inserting an OPA?**
Essentially any position can be used, though supine in a neutral anatomical or sniffing position is common.

5. **What does the OPA offer protection against?**
Epiglottis collapse against the glottis and collapse of the soft palate airway.

6. **What airway problems does the OPA not assist with?**
Obstruction by foreign body material, including vomitus.

7. **What should be done if the patient shows signs of airway reflexes returning?**
Remove the OPA device.

8. **What physical action helps ensure the OPA seats correctly in the oropharynx?**
Jaw thrust, particularly just at the point of seating.

9. **Where should the flanged OPA end seat if it is placed correctly?**
Gently against the lips, without compressing them.

10. **Why is it important to monitor the patient post OPA insertion?**
Airway reflexes might return, causing gagging or vomiting.

References

Isono, S., 2012. Obesity and obstructive sleep apnoea: mechanisms for increased collapsibility of the passive pharyngeal airway. *Respirology*, 17(1), 32–42.

Kim, H.J., Kim, S.H., Min, N.H. and Park, W.K., 2016. Determination of the appropriate sizes of oropharyngeal airways in adults: correlation with external facial measurements: a randomised crossover study. *European Journal of Anaesthesiology*, 33(12), 936–942.

Ma, M.A., Kumar, R., Macey, P.M., Yan-Go, F.L. and Harper, R.M., 2016. Epiglottis cross-sectional area and oropharyngeal airway length in male and female obstructive sleep apnea patients. *Nature and Science of Sleep*, 8, 297.

Pozner, C.N., Walls, R.M., Page, R.L. and Grayzel, J., 2015. Advanced cardiac life support (ACLS) in adults. Retrieved from: https://www.uptodate.com

Soar, J., Nolan, J.P., Böttiger, B.W., Perkins, G.D., Lott, C., Carli, P., Pellis, T., Sandroni, C., Skrifvars, M.B., Smith, G.B. and Sunde, K., 2015. European Resuscitation Council guidelines for resuscitation 2015, section 3: Adult advanced life support. *Resuscitation*, 95, 100–147.

Bibliography

Craft, J., Gordon, C., Huether, S.E., McCance, K.L. and Brashers, V.L., 2015. *Understanding pathophysiology (ANZ adaptation)*. Sydney: Elsevier.

McCance, K.L. and Huether, S.E., 2015. *Pathophysiology: the biologic basis for disease in adults and children*. Sydney: Elsevier.

Chapter objectives

At the end of this chapter the reader will be able to:

1. Describe the rationale for nasopharyngeal airway (NPA) insertion
2. Demonstrate effective and safe placement of an NPA
3. Accurately report on the performance of NPA placement

Resources required for this assessment

- Airway mannequin suitable for NPA insertion
- NPA device in range of sizes
- Disposable gloves, protective eyewear, respiratory mask
- Water-based gel lubricant
- Method of documenting the results

Skill matrix

This assessment requires:

- Infection control (CS 1.3)
- Patient assessment skills (Chapter 2, CS 2.1, 2.2, 2.6, 2.8, 2.10)
- Airway and ventilation skills (Chapter 3, CS 3.2, 3.3, 3.6, 3.7)

This assessment is a component of:

- Airway and ventilation (Chapter 3)

Introduction

The risk of physical upper airway obstruction through poor anatomical positioning increases with loss of consciousness. This can be mitigated with basic positioning that is supported by minimally invasive devices suited to that purpose. This chapter discusses one such device, the nasopharyngeal airway (NPA).

Anatomy and physiology

The nose has two nostril openings that remain divided through the nasal cavity by the septum before uniting in the posterior nasopharynx. The roof of the nasal cavity is the skull base, and its base the roof of the mouth. The lining of the nasal cavity is soft and highly vascular tissue that allows air warmth and humidification. The airway continues inferiorly past the uvula to the oropharynx.

Like the oral cavity, the nasal cavity is relatively rigid, as is the distal larynx. The soft nasopharynx and oropharynx is comprised of smooth muscle that can collapse whenever muscle tone is lost (Isono, 2012; Ma et al., 2016).

At the distal upper airway are the tongue base and epiglottis. The latter covers the glottis during swallowing when the larynx rises towards it. Backwards movement of the tongue into the pharynx can press the uvula anteriorly, occluding the nasopharynx as well as the oropharynx. Airway reflexes within and around the larynx include cough, gag and swallow. Reflexes and muscle control deteriorate and eventually fail as consciousness diminishes and is lost.

Clinical rationale

A nasopharyngeal airway device (NPA), sometimes called a nasal trumpet, is a nasally invasive physical implement constructed of latex-free polyvinylchloride that is used to provide physical patency of the distal nasopharynx. It is different from the oropharyngeal airway (OPA) in that it is much softer and narrower and is inserted via a nostril, which provides one of its major advantages: it can be used where trismus or strong jaw tone preclude oral entry.

The NPA helps prevent posterior tongue and uvula displacement in the nasopharynx, preventing upper airway obstruction by invading the posterior nasopharynx (Pozner et al., 2015; Soar et al., 2015; Stoneham, 1993).

While the requirement for insertion of the OPA and NPA is loss of airway reflexes, there is notably less stimulation of the gag reflex by NPA placement, since a correctly sized and placed NPA sits just above the epiglottis (Kumar et al., 2015; Stoneham, 1993; Roberts et al., 2005). This makes it useful where airway reflexes remain present and make an OPA intolerable.

Although NPA insertion does not have to be aseptic, it should be performed as cleanly as possible to avoid unnecessary patient exposure to contaminants.

Patient positioning

Patients will commonly be positioned supine, ideally using either a neutral anatomical or sniffing head position (see Chapter 3.2). However, insertion is possible using the lateral position or, in cases of patient entrapment, such as during road trauma, any posture that is initially imposed during rescue.

Airway preparation

The physical removal of foreign material from the nasal cavity and oropharynx is essential prior to insertion (see Chapter 3.7). This includes vomitus, blood and saliva, as well as any damaged tissue (such as teeth) resulting from trauma.

Where ongoing airway clearance is required, the NPA may not be the right option, and an alternative such as supraglottic airway or intubation may be preferred.

Device measurement

There are two sizes to consider when using the NPA:
• internal diameter
• device length.
The NPA size is described according to the internal diameter measurement in millimetres. Longer devices are also wider. NPA length is the significant measurement when selecting the size of the device (Roberts et al., 2005).

The appropriate size of NPA must be selected for the device to position correctly in the nasopharynx. This is anatomically measured by holding one end of the NPA against the tragus and the other end to the nostril on that side (Fig. 3.5.1). Alternatively, one end can be held at the angle of the mandible and the other to the same nostril (Bailie et al., 2008; Stoneham, 1993).

An NPA that is too large can reach and injure the nasal and soft posterior pharyngeal tissue. The diameter of the NPA should pass through the nostril without causing blanching to the skin. If it is too long, the distal tip can

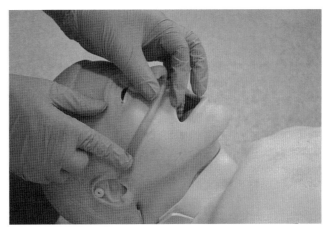

Figure 3.5.1 Measuring the NPA for size

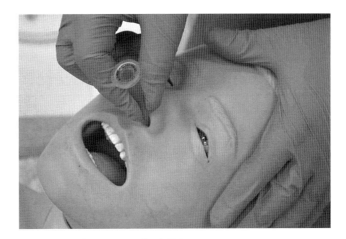

Figure 3.5.2 Inserting the NPA

become occluded if in the vallecular or misplaced into the oesophagus, or even cause laryngospasm. Conversely, a device that is too small will not position in the nasopharynx to support collapsed soft tissue or displace the tongue (Stoneham, 1993).

Insertion method

Lubrication of the NPA is necessary before insertion. Apply water-based lubricant along the sides of the NPA near the tip.

Inspect the patient's nose for injury, deformity or abnormal tissue that might predispose them to difficulty or bleeding.

Insertion is accomplished by holding the flanged end and placing the bevelled tip into the nostril. The right nostril is described as larger and straighter, and so is often preferred (Sanuki et al., 2010; Smith and Reid, 2001). The temptation at this point can be to point the NPA upwards in line with the contour of the outer nose. This is incorrect. Place one finger on the tip of the nose and gently tilt it superiorly to open the view of the nostril. Place the bevel inside the nostril facing the septum (Fig. 3.5.2). Once inside, direct the NPA posteriorly with no upward inclination. Continue pushing it forwards, following the base of the nasal cavity, until the correct insertion depth is achieved, usually with the flange resting just outside the nostril. The flange ensures the device cannot be too deeply inserted.

Apply jaw thrust throughout the insertion (see Chapter 3.3) if possible. This may require a second paramedic to temporarily assist. To be confident of the correct pharyngeal placement, ensure jaw thrust is being performed just prior to the final placement of the NPA by pulling anteriorly on the jaw angles with both hands and completing the NPA insertion using the free thumbs (Fig. 3.5.3a and b). Jaw thrust may have to be maintained since it remains possible for tongue displacement to occlude the pharynx even with the NPA in place (Stoneham, 1993).

The patient should be observed for any sign of airway reflex, including gag.

Reassess the patient's respiratory status, with an emphasis on air passage. The size, number of attempts required for success, any difficulties and time of insertion should be noted in the patient care record.

Clinical skill assessment process

The following section outlines the clinical skill assessment tools that should be used to determine a student's ability to demonstrate safe and accurate insertion of nasopharyngeal airway.

1. Clinical Skill Work Instruction
2. Formative Clinical Skill Assessment (F-CSAT)
3. Performance Improvement Plan (PIP)
4. Summative Clinical Skill Assessment (S-CSAT)
(5. Direct Observation of Procedural Skills (DOPS) – see Chapter 1.1)

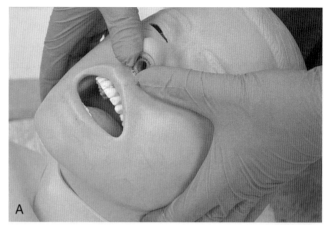

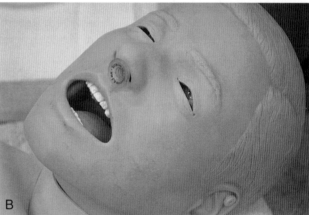

Figure 3.5.3 Completing the NPA insertion
(a) Using the free thumbs. (b) Final NPA seating.

Clinical Skill Work Instruction

Equipment and resources: Airway mannequin suitable for NPA insertion; NPA device in range of sizes; gloves, eyewear and mask; water-based gel lubricant; method of documenting results

Associated Clinical Skills: Infection control; Patient assessment skills; Airway and ventilation skills

Nasopharyngeal airway		
Activity	**Critical Action**	**Rationale**
Personal protection	Don PPE as required.	All airway procedures are considered high infection risk.
Assess indications	Assess patient consciousness, airway reflexes and respiratory status. Consider NPA contraindications/precautions.	Ensure appropriate use.
Prepare equipment	Lay out NPA and other airway resuscitation equipment on a clean surface.	Other airway devices may also be required.

Nasopharyngeal airway continued

Activity	Critical Action	Rationale
Prepare patient	Place patient supine, with head in neutral anatomical or sniffing position (preferred) or allowing effective paramedic access to head and face (if unable to move patient).	Appropriate position assists airway patency and insertion.
	Ensure adequate airway clearance has been performed prior to insertion. (If there is copious vomitus, consider definitive airway management.) Provide jaw thrust if support personnel are available.	NPA does not address any FBAO present. Displacing the jaw and tongue forwards improves access by the NPA device.
Measure NPA size	Measure appropriate size NPA using chosen method (one of two).	Correct size is important.
Insert NPA	Hold the NPA by the flanged end.	In readiness for insertion.
	Lubricate NPA with water-based gel.	To ease insertion.
	Lift tip of nose superiorly to expose nostrils. Insert distal end into one nostril with bevel facing septum and curve facing downwards.	To ease access into nose without snagging.
	Gently twist as NPA slides inwards along base of nasal cavity, directed posteriorly.	To free bevel from any resistance and avoid injury.
	Apply jaw thrust to ensure NPA seats in nasopharynx.	To position correctly in nasopharynx.
Reassess	Ensure no airway reflex is triggered by placement and that respiratory status is effective.	To ensure NPA effectiveness.
Report	Document time of insertion, NPA size, and any relevant information regarding placement or insertion.	Accurate record kept and continuity of patient care.

Formative Clinical Skill Assessment (F-CSAT)

Equipment and resources: Airway mannequin suitable for NPA insertion; NPA device in range of sizes; gloves, eyewear and mask; water-based gel lubricant; method of documenting results

Associated Clinical Skills: Infection control; Patient assessment skills; Airway and ventilation skills

Staff/Student being assessed: _____

Nasopharyngeal airway

Activity	Critical Action	Participant Performance				
Personal protection	Dons PPE as required.	0	1	2	3	4
Assesses indications	Assesses patient consciousness, airway reflexes and respiratory status. Considers NPA contraindications/precautions.	0	1	2	3	4
Prepares equipment	Lays out NPA and other airway resuscitation equipment on a clean surface.	0	1	2	3	4

Nasopharyngeal airway continued

Activity	Critical Action	Participant Performance				
Prepares patient	Places patient supine, with head in neutral anatomical or sniffing position, or allows effective paramedic access to head and face.	0	1	2	3	4
	Provides adequate airway clearance prior to insertion. Provides jaw thrust if support personnel are available.	0	1	2	3	4
Measures NPA size	Measures appropriate size NPA using chosen method.	0	1	2	3	4
Inserts NPA	Holds the NPA by the flanged end.	0	1	2	3	4
	Lubricates NPA with water-based gel.	0	1	2	3	4
	Lifts tip of nose superiorly to expose nostrils. Inserts distal end into one nostril with bevel facing septum and curve facing downwards.	0	1	2	3	4
	Gently twists as NPA slides inwards along base of nasal cavity, directed posteriorly.	0	1	2	3	4
	Applies jaw thrust to ensure NPA seats in nasopharynx.	0	1	2	3	4
Reassesses	Ensures no airway reflex is triggered by placement and that respiratory status is effective.	0	1	2	3	4
Reports	Accurately documents/hands over time of insertion, NPA size, and any relevant information regarding placement or insertion.	0	1	2	3	4

Standard Achieved: (please circle one)

Competent (C)   Not Yet Competent* (NYC)

Staff/Student Name: _____

Assessor (please print name): _____

Signed (Assessor): _____

Date of Assessment: _____

Comments:

*If Not Yet Competent (NYC) a PIP needs to be completed and a repeat of the F-CSAT

Formative Clinical Skill Assessment (F-CSAT) Key

Skill level	Standard of procedure	Quality of performance	Outcome	Level of assistance required
4 Safe for unsupervised practice	Safe Accurate Behaviour is appropriate to context	Confident Accurate Expedient	Achieved intended outcome	No supporting cues* required
3 Requires supervision	Safe Accurate Behaviour is appropriate to context	Confident Accurate Takes longer than required	Achieved intended outcome	Requires occasional supportive cues*

Skill level	Standard of procedure	Quality of performance	Outcome	Level of assistance required
2 Requires assistance	Safe Accurate Behaviour generally appropriate to context	Lacks certainty	Would not have achieved outcome without support	Requires frequent verbal and occasional physical directives in addition to supportive cues*
1 Requires direction	Safe only with guidance Not completely accurate	Unskilled Inefficient	Would not have achieved outcome without support	Requires continuous verbal and frequent physical directive cues*
0 Unsafe	Unsafe Unable to demonstrate behaviour Lack of insight into behaviour appropriate to context	Unskilled	Would not have achieved outcome	Requires continuous verbal and continuous physical directive cues*

*Refers to physical directives or verbal supportive cues

Performance Improvement Plan (PIP)

Please document the agreed education plan and completion timelines for areas assessed as less than 4.

This plan should be presented to assessor prior to commencement of summative assessment.

Where was supervisor support required?	Student summary of deficit. (Why was there a problem?)	Improvement Plan	Completed (Y/N)

Staff/Student Name: _____

Staff/Student Signature: _____

Educator Name: _____

Educator Signature: _____

Summative Clinical Skill Assessment (S-CSAT)

Equipment and resources: Airway mannequin suitable for NPA insertion; NPA device in range of sizes; gloves, eyewear and mask; water-based gel lubricant; method of documenting results

Associated Clinical Skills: Infection control; Patient assessment skills; Airway and ventilation skills

Staff/Student being assessed: _____

- Completed Formative Clinical Skill Assessment (F-CSAT): **YES**   **NO**

- Completed Performance Improvement Plan (PIP): **YES**   **NO**   **N/A**

Nasopharyngeal airway

Activity	Critical Action	Achieved Without Direction	
Personal protection	Dons PPE as required.	NO	YES
Assesses indications	Assesses patient consciousness, airway reflexes and respiratory status. Considers NPA contraindications/precautions.	NO	YES
Prepares equipment	Lays out NPA and other airway resuscitation equipment on a clean surface.	NO	YES
Prepares patient	Places patient supine, with head in neutral anatomical or sniffing position, or allows effective paramedic access to head and face.	NO	YES
	Provides adequate airway clearance prior to insertion. Provides jaw thrust if support personnel are available.	NO	YES
Measures NPA size	Measures appropriate size NPA using chosen method.	NO	YES
Inserts NPA	Holds the NPA by the flanged end.	NO	YES
	Lubricates NPA with water-based gel.	NO	YES
	Lifts tip of nose superiorly to expose nostrils. Inserts distal end into one nostril with bevel facing septum and curve facing downwards.	NO	YES
	Gently twists as NPA slides inwards along base of nasal cavity, directed posteriorly.	NO	YES
	Applies jaw thrust to ensure NPA seats in nasopharynx.	NO	YES
Reassesses	Ensures no airway reflex is triggered by placement and that respiratory status is effective.	NO	YES
Reports	Accurately documents/hands over time of insertion, NPA size, and any relevant information regarding placement or insertion.	NO	YES

Standard Achieved: (please circle one)

Competent (C)   Not Yet Competent* (NYC)

Staff/Student Name: _____

Assessor (please print name): _____

Signed (Assessor): _____

Date of Assessment: _____

Comments:

*If Not Yet Competent (NYC) a PIP needs to be completed and a repeat of the F-CSAT

Clinical findings

Resistance

If resistance is encountered during insertion, gently rotate the NPA to allow the bevel to manoeuvre around the obstruction. The NPA is soft and so cannot be forced. If the resistance cannot be overcome, attempt insertion into the other nostril (Roberts et al., 2005).

Airway remains non-patent

Where the NPA fails to provide effective airway patency, assess for obstruction (including kinking or compression) by passing a suitably sized suction catheter through its length. The alternative could be the NPA being too short and occluded by the tongue, in which case consider inserting a longer device.

Cough/gag reflex stimulated

The NPA is intended to sit just above where airway reflexes can be initiated, and so it is less likely to stimulate unwanted or problematic airway reflexes than an OPA. If reflex responses are observed, withdraw the NPA 1–2 cm and reassess its effectiveness. Consider inserting a more appropriate size if the NPA selected is too large.

Soft tissue injury

The nasal cavity mucosa is soft and highly vascular. It can be easily torn during the insertion of an NPA, causing bleeding. Correct diameter selection and gentle insertion can minimise this risk (Roberts et al., 2005).

Cardiovascular effects

NPA insertion can cause a transient but not alarming rise in blood pressure during insertion, which usually settles within minutes (Tong and Smith, 2004). Persistent gagging can cause an unwanted rise in intracranial pressure (Roberts et al., 2005).

Facial injury

Maxillofacial trauma complications include maxilla and mandible fracture, displaced and loose teeth and a bleeding and blood-filled pharynx (Barak et al., 2015; Jain et al., 2016). NPA insertion may not be possible with facial trauma. Conversely, the attempt at insertion can cause further injury and bleeding (Barak et al., 2015; Krausz et al., 2015; Schade et al., 2000; Swanson et al., 2016). Use of an NPA should therefore be avoided where there is significant facial trauma.

Basal skull fracture

A limited number of examples of incorrectly positioned NPAs, intruding into anterior brain through basal skull fractures, have been reported (Martin et al., 2004; Schade et al., 2000; Swanson et al., 2016), making this arguably the most significant complication of the procedure. It can also expose cerebrospinal fluid to contamination. Wherever possible, if basal skull fracture is suspected, avoid inserting an NPA (Krausz et al., 2015; Barak et al., 2015).

However, airway patency remains a priority at all times. Where trismus presents no alternative for airway management and patency is threatened, careful NPA insertion may offer a last, temporary solution. Lifting the nostrils and inserting the NPA away from the nasal cavity roof and along its floor minimises the risk (Roberts et al., 2005).

Aspiration

The NPA does nothing to prevent passive regurgitation of gastric content or its subsequent entry into the trachea. Where this is of concern, such as when administering positive pressure ventilation, more substantial airway protection is necessary.

Children

Children have a relatively larger tongue, epiglottis and tonsils and shorter mandible, predisposing them to upper airway obstruction (Harless et al., 2014). They are also principally nasal breathers. Where the correct size is available, NPA devices can be used in paediatric emergencies (Harless et al., 2014; Russo and Becke, 2015; Tripathi et al., 2016; Shoukry and Sharaf, 2018).

PRACTICE TIP!

During patient preparation, assess the nostrils for injury or deformity and identify the larger of the two as the preferred insertion point.

PRACTICE TIP!

Epistaxis will complicate airway management. Approach all insertion attempts with care, particularly patients on anticoagulant medication.

PRACTICE TIP!

NPA insertion should be considered in any patient where risk of mechanical upper airway obstruction is caused by posture and decreased conscious state. The procedure may offer an advantage where residual gag reflex or trismus are present.

TEST YOUR KNOWLEDGE QUESTIONS

1. **What are the two ways to measure an NPA device?**
   From the angle of the jaw to the nostril on that side; from the tragus to the nostril on that side.

2. **What action can help open the nostril before insertion?**
   Touching the nose tip and pushing it superiorly.

3. **What is the direction of NPA insertion?**
   Directly posteriorly into the nostril along the nasal cavity floor.

4. **Which head position is chosen when inserting an NPA?**
   Essentially any position can be used, though supine in a neutral anatomical or sniffing position is common.

5. **What should be done if there is resistance during insertion?**
   Gently rotate the device to free the bevel; remove it and attempt in the other nostril.

6. **List two injuries that can preclude NPA insertion.**
   Severe facial/nasal trauma; suspected basal skull fracture.

7. **What are two advantages of the NPA?**
   It can be inserted where there is trismus; it is less likely to stimulate airway reflexes.

8. **What physical action helps ensure the NPA seats correctly in the oropharynx?**
   Jaw thrust, particularly just at the point of seating.

9. **Where should the flanged NPA end seat if it is placed correctly?**
   Gently against the outer nostril.

10. **Why is it important to monitor the patient post NPA insertion?**
    Though less likely than with an OPA, airway reflexes might return, causing gagging or vomiting.

References

Bailie, R.K., Mannion, D., Russell, J., Hone, S., O'Hare, B., 2008. *Is APLS right? A pilot study to assess the best anatomical measurement for estimation of appropriate length of a nasopharyngeal airway.* Paper presented at the Association of Anaesthetists of Great Britain and Ireland, May, London.

Barak, M., Bahouth, H., Leiser, Y. and Abu El-Naaj, I., 2015. Airway management of the patient with maxillofacial trauma: review of the literature and suggested clinical approach. *BioMed Research International*, doi: https://doi.org/10.1155/2015/724032.

Harless, J., Ramaiah, R. and Bhananker, S.M., 2014. Pediatric airway management. *International Journal of Critical Illness and Injury Science*, 4(1), 65.

Isono, S., 2012. Obesity and obstructive sleep apnoea: mechanisms for increased collapsibility of the passive pharyngeal airway. *Respirology*, 17(1), 32–42.

Jain, U., McCunn, M., Smith, C.E. and Pittet, J.F., 2016. Management of the traumatized airway. *Anesthesiology*, 124(1), 199–206.

Krausz, A.A., Krausz, M.M. and Picetti, E., 2015. Maxillofacial and neck trauma: a damage control approach. *World Journal of Emergency Surgery*, 10(1), 31.

Kumar, A.R., Guilleminault, C., Certal, V., Li, D., Capasso, R. and Camacho, M., 2015. Nasopharyngeal airway stenting devices for obstructive sleep apnoea: a systematic review and meta-analysis. *Journal of Laryngology & Otology*, 129(1), 2–10.

Ma, M.A., Kumar, R., Macey, P.M., Yan-Go, F.L. and Harper, R.M., 2016. Epiglottis cross-sectional area and oropharyngeal airway length in male and female obstructive sleep apnea patients. *Nature and Science of Sleep*, 8, 297.

Martin, J.E., Mehta, R., Aarabi, B., Ecklund, J.E., Martin, A.H. and Ling, G.S., 2004. Intracranial insertion of a nasopharyngeal airway in a patient with craniofacial trauma. *Military Medicine*, 169(6), 496–497.

Pozner, C.N., Walls, R.M., Page, R.L. and Grayzel, J., 2015. *Advanced cardiac life support (ACLS) in adults.* Retrieved from: https://www.uptodate.com

Roberts, K., Whalley, H. and Bleetman, H., 2005. The nasopharyngeal airway: dispelling the myths and establishing the facts, *Emergency Medical Journal*, 22, 394–396.

Russo, S.G. and Becke, K., 2015. Expected difficult airway in children. *Current Opinion in Anesthesiology*, 28(3), 321–326.

Sanuki, T., Hirokane, M. and Kotani, J., 2010. Epistaxis during nasotracheal intubation: a comparison of nostril sides. *Journal of Oral and Maxillofacial Surgery*, 68(3), 618–621.

Schade, K., Borzotta, A. and Michaels, A., 2000. Intracranial malposition of nasopharyngeal airway. *Journal of Trauma and Acute Care Surgery*, 49(5), 967–968.

Shoukry, A.A. and Sharaf, A.G.S., 2018. Nasopharyngeal airway versus laryngeal mask airway during diagnostic flexible fiber-optic bronchoscope in children. *Open Anesthesiology Journal*, 12(1).

Smith, J.E. and Reid, A.P., 2001. Identifying the more patent nostril before nasotracheal intubation. *Anaesthesia*, 56(3), 258–262.

Soar, J., Nolan, J.P., Böttiger, B.W., Perkins, G.D., Lott, C., Carli, P., Pellis, T., Sandroni, C., Skrifvars, M.B., Smith, G.B. and Sunde, K., 2015. European Resuscitation Council guidelines for resuscitation 2015, section 3: Adult advanced life support. *Resuscitation*, 95, 100–147.

Stoneham, M.D., 1993. The nasopharyngeal airway. *Anaesthesia*, 48(7), 575–580.

Swanson, K.I., Nickele, C.M. and Kuo, J.S., 2016. Iatrogenic intracranial placement of nasopharyngeal airway after trauma. *British Journal of Neurosurgery*, 30(4), 448–449.

Tong, J.L. and Smith, J.E., 2004. Cardiovascular changes following insertion of oropharyngeal and nasopharyngeal airways. *British Journal of Anaesthesia*, 93(3), 339–342.

Tripathi, S.S., Pal, J.K., Singh, R.R., Awasthi, S. and Mishra, S.P., 2016. Airway management of trauma patient of paediatric age group. *International Journal of Life-Sciences Scientific Research*, 2(6), 644–650.

Bibliography

Craft, J., Gordon, C., Huether, S.E., McCance, K.L. and Brashers, V.L., 2015. *Understanding pathophysiology (ANZ adaptation).* Sydney: Elsevier.

McCance, K.L. and Huether, S.E., 2015. *Pathophysiology: the biologic basis for disease in adults and children.* Sydney: Elsevier.

Chapter objectives

At the end of this chapter the reader will be able to:

1. Identify occasions when laryngoscopy can be performed
2. Demonstrate safe and effective laryngoscopy
3. Identify and resolve common difficulties during laryngoscopy

Resources required for this assessment

- Airway mannequin
- Laryngoscope and blade
- Gloves, respiratory mask, eyewear
- Suction equipment
- Towel/pillow
- Method of documenting the results

Skill matrix

This assessment requires:

- Infection control (CS 1.3)
- Communication (CS 1.5)
- Consent (CS 1.6)
- Patient assessment skills (Chapter 2, CS 2.1, 2.2, 2.6, 2.8, 2.10)
- Airway and ventilation skills (Chapter 3, CS 3.2, 3.3, 3.7)

This assessment is a component of:

- Airway and ventilation (Chapter 3)

Introduction

Laryngoscopy is a foundation airway management skill, allowing laryngopharynx view in the unconscious patient. A laryngoscope comprises a handle and blade with a light source that is inserted via the oropharynx to displace the tongue and gain laryngeal view (Mireles-Cabodevila and Siddiqui, 2014; Sanders et al., 2007).

Many techniques and tools have been developed to assist this occasionally difficult skill. An understanding of airway anatomy and patient positioning, and a familiarity with the equipment and technique selected, are required for effective laryngoscopy (Frerk et al., 2015; Mireles-Cabodevila and Siddiqui, 2014; Levitan, 2007). This chapter discusses these essential elements.

Anatomy and physiology

The upper airway is comprised of the oro- (mouth), naso- (nose) and laryngo- (or hypo) pharynx. While the nose, mouth and upper throat may be examined in the conscious patient, the laryngopharynx remains largely obscured by the tongue and the presence of protective gag reflexes (Beachey, 2012) (Fig. 3.6.1a).

The larynx sits anteriorly to the laryngopharynx. It is comprised of the epiglottis, thyroid, cricoid and several smaller cartilages, muscles and ligaments (including vocal cords; Figure 3.6.1b) connecting the upper airway to the trachea. Its primary function is to protect the lungs from the aspiration of food or oral secretions (Beachey, 2012; Klinger and Infosino, 2018).

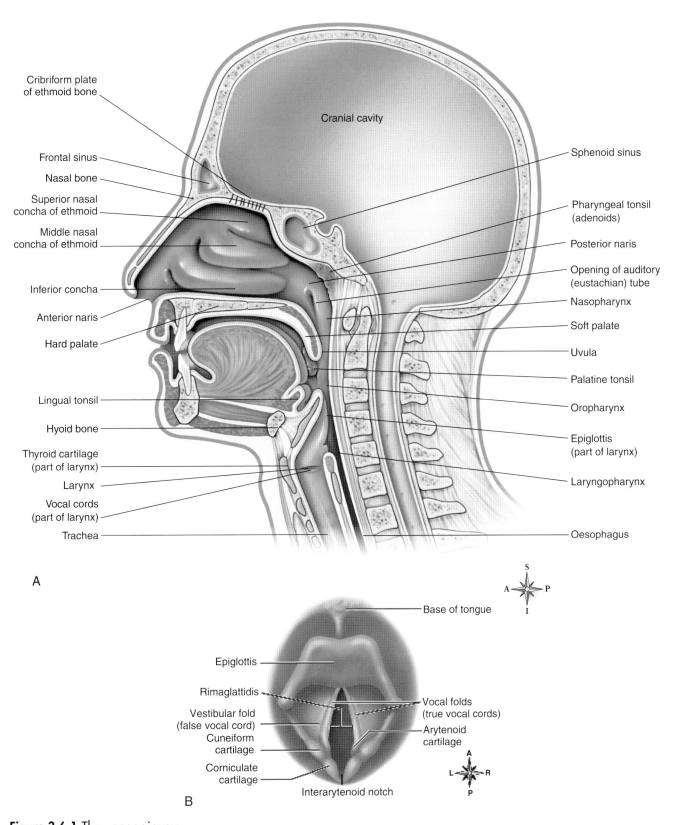

Figure 3.6.1 The upper airway

(a) Anatomy of the upper airway; sagittal section of the head and neck. The nasal septum has been removed, exposing the right lateral wall of the nasal cavity so that the nasal conchae can be seen. Note also the divisions of the pharynx and the position of the tonsils. (b) Superior view of the vocal cords and epiglottis.

Source: *Patton, K.T. and Thibodeau, G.A., 2020,* Structure & function of the body, *16th edn (Chapter 15, Figure 15-4), Elsevier.*

During swallowing, the epiglottis, a semi-rigid flap connected to the base of the tongue at the vallecular groove, approximates to the glottic opening of the thyroid cartilage, preventing food entering the trachea (Beachey, 2012).

Posteriorly, the laryngopharynx is continuous with the oesophagus.

Branches of the glossopharyngeal and vagal cranial nerves innervate the posterior pharynx and larynx. These mediate swallowing and protective gag reflexes (Beachey, 2012; Klinger and Infosino, 2018).

Stimulation of the larynx causes reflex catecholamine release, leading to tachycardia and hypertension, but it may also cause vagal-mediated bradycardia and hypotension, especially in children (Brown and Walls, 2014; Donoghue and Walls, 2008; Rothrock, 2008). Intracranial pressure (ICP) elevates, though the exact mechanism is poorly understood. Laryngoscopy should be avoided in traumatic or non-traumatic brain injury patients unless they are paralysed, to avoid increasing ICP (Brown and Walls, 2014; Kenneally et al., 2015).

Larynx stimulation can cause laryngospasm, closing the glottic opening and compromising ventilation (Sanders et al., 2007; Roman, 2004). This is generally self-limiting but may persist, causing hypoxia. It is more commonly problematic in paediatrics (Kenneally et al., 2015, Roman, 2004).

The tongue, foreign bodies, blood, secretions or vomitus may obstruct the laryngopharynx of the unconscious patient (Kenneally et al., 2015; Roman, 2004; Sanders et al., 2007). Passive regurgitation secondary to oesophageal sphincter relaxation may occur without external vomiting signs (Beachey, 2012; Kenneally et al., 2015).

Clinical rationale

Laryngoscopy by direct visualisation (or video laryngoscope) is a fundamental skill in securing the upper airway by endotracheal intubation (Levitan, 2007; Mireles-Cabodevila and Siddiqui, 2014).

Direct laryngoscopy uses a guttered blade that is inserted in the right side of the mouth to displace the tongue to the left and out of view (Klinger and Infosino, 2018; Mireles-Cabodevila and Siddiqui, 2014; Sanders et al., 2007). By advancing down the tongue, the epiglottis is located (Danzl and Vissers, 2004; Sanders et al., 2007). Identification of the epiglottis is fundamental to visualising the glottis and successful laryngoscopy. Advancing down the midline may assist if identifying the epiglottis is difficult.

If using a curved blade laryngoscope (e.g. Macintosh), place the tip in the vallecular groove at the junction of the tongue and the epiglottis (Fig. 3.6.2a) (Danzl and Vissers, 2004; Kenneally et al., 2015; Mireles-Cabodevila and Siddiqui, 2014). This process should utilise minimal force to avoid damage to soft pharyngeal mucosa, tongue, teeth and vocal cords (Mireles-Cabodevila and Siddiqui, 2014).

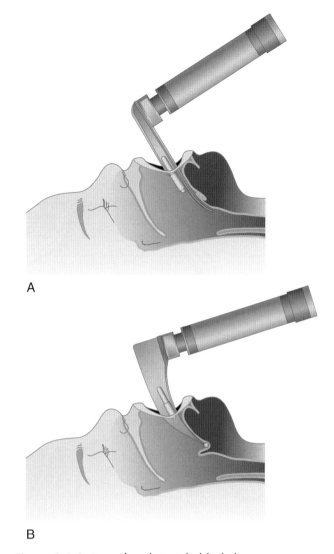

A

B

Figure 3.6.2 Curved and straight blade laryngoscopy (tip placement)

(a) Correct position and exposure of glottic opening with a curved laryngoscope blade. (b) Correct position and exposure of glottic opening with a straight laryngoscope blade.

Source: Jill, B., Steven, R., John, B., Lance, B., 2008, Pediatric emergency medicine *(Figure 4-3)*, Elsevier.

Once the blade tip is seated in the vallecular, the laryngoscope is moved up and away, in line with the handle, to distract the mandible (Danzl and Vissers, 2004; Mireles-Cabodevila and Siddiqui, 2014). This tips the epiglottis anteriorly, exposing the posterior notch of the glottis. Rotation or 'levering' of the laryngoscope may fracture incisors and does not improve visualisation (Kenneally et al., 2015; Klinger and Infosino, 2018).

Straight (e.g. Millar) blade laryngoscopy (Fig. 3.6.2b) lifts the epiglottis directly against the tongue to expose the glottis (Donoghue and Walls, 2008; Mireles-Cabodevila and Siddiqui, 2014; Sanders et al., 2007). It is a useful technique in neonates and small infants due to their relatively large epiglottis (Padlipsky and Gausche-Hill, 2008, Rubin and Sadovnikoff, 2004). Straight blade laryngoscopy increases the risk of larynx stimulation, which may increase sympathetic or vagal tone, laryngospasm and ICP (Rothrock, 2008).

Indirect or video laryngoscopes use a blade with a distal end camera providing glottis view without necessarily aligning the oral, pharyngeal and tracheal axes. The image is displayed on a monitor on the laryngoscope or beside the patient, effectively allowing the paramedic to 'see around the corner' (Klinger and Infosino, 2018).

The blade of the video laryngoscope is inserted down the midline, as the tongue is unlikely to obstruct the camera view on the distal blade (Brown and Walls, 2014).

Many video laryngoscopes use standard Macintosh- or Millar-style blades to allow direct laryngoscopy using familiar techniques as well as indirect laryngoscopy. The monitor display can be used for instructional purposes (Brown and Walls, 2014; Klinger and Infosino, 2018).

Hyper-angulated video blades enhance glottic view in the patient with anterior laryngeal anatomy, minimising the need for flexion and extension of the head and neck (Klinger and Infosino, 2018).

Paramedics should be able to use both curved- (more common) and straight-blade direct and video techniques to manage a wide range of anatomically varied airways (Sanders et al., 2007).

Airway assessment

Before commencing laryngoscopy, an assessment of the patient's airway is undertaken. Although no assessment is both sensitive and specific for difficult laryngoscopy, studies suggest the increased likelihood of problematic airways being identified beforehand (Apfelbaum et al., 2013; Yentis, 2002).

Although it is rarely available to paramedics, a history of previous difficult intubation is considered predictive (Apfelbaum et al., 2013). Dietary history is useful to determine potential for aspiration in non-fasted patients, though this should be assumed in prehospital patients (Kenneally et al., 2015).

Assess facial and airway anatomy. Facial hair increases difficulty in bag/mask ventilation, an important adjunct to laryngoscopy (Danzl and Vissers, 2004). Small mouths, difficulty opening the mouth, prominent (or loose) teeth and recessed jaw make laryngoscope insertion and epiglottis identification difficult (Apfelbaum et al., 2013; Danzl and Vissers, 2004; Kenneally et al., 2015).

Assess mouth opening (vertically between incisors), hyomental distance (hyoid bone to the posterior edge of the front of the jaw) or alternately thyromental distance (measured from top of the more prominent thyroid cartilage or Adam's apple). Less than 3 fingers in any may predict difficult laryngoscopy (Apfelbaum et al., 2013; Kenneally et al., 2015; Klinger and Infosino, 2018; Yu et al., 2015). Mouth opening to assess tongue base to mouth roof (Mallampati scoring) is questionable in emergency or prehospital settings (Kenneally et al., 2015; Levitan et al., 2004; Yu et al., 2015).

Assess for facial, throat and neck trauma, which may impact on laryngoscopy. Swelling caused by upper airway

infection, burns or anaphylaxis may occlude the larynx (Beachey, 2012; Boudewyns et al., 2010; Padlipsky and Gausche-Hill, 2008). Laryngoscopy in young patients with croup or epiglottitis may precipitate laryngospasm and cardiac arrest, and so should be limited to paediatric specialists, preferably in controlled hospital environments (Boudewyns et al., 2010; Rubin and Sadovnikoff, 2004).

Airway visualisation may be difficult in patients with short necks or decreased neck movement range due to age, degenerative disease or spinal trauma immobilisation (Apfelbaum et al., 2013; Kenneally et al., 2015; Rubin and Sadovnikoff, 2004). An inability to adequately elevate the head decreases glottic view and may require alternative

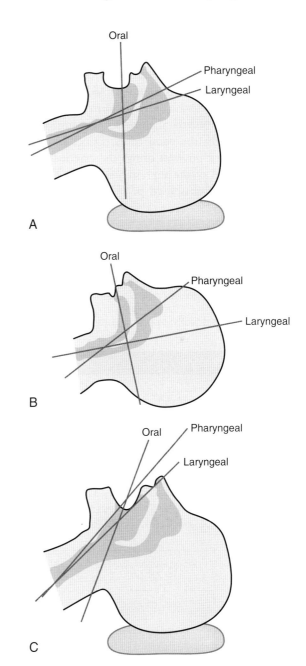

Figure 3.6.3 Airway axes

(a) The three axes with the head in the 'sniffing' position. (b) The three axes of the airway with the head in a neutral position. (c) The three axes after extending the head.

Source: *Peate, I., 2019, Learning to care: the nursing associate (Chaper 19, Figure 19.5), Elsevier.*

positioning or techniques (Danzl and Vissers, 2004; Klinger and Infosino, 2018).

Obese, large-breasted or pregnant patients provide challenges to laryngoscope blade insertion and an increased risk of aspiration and desaturation (Kenneally et al., 2015; Weingart and Levitan, 2012). Using a short-handled laryngoscope or inserting the blade with the handle rotated 90° to the right, then rotating back into alignment, may make it easier to place the blade in the mouth (Kenneally et al., 2015; Mireles-Cabodevila and Siddiqui, 2014).

Positioning

To gain a direct view of the glottis, the oral, pharyngeal and laryngeal axes need to be aligned (Klinger and Infosino, 2018). This occurs in the 'sniffing' position (Fig. 3.6.3a) but not in the neutral anatomical position (Fig. 3.6.3b) (see Chapter 3.2). To achieve an optimal view, cervical manipulation is required to align the axes.

Using blankets to elevate the head horizontally can bring these axes into improved alignment, allowing a greater opportunity to sight the vocal cords (Danzl and Vissers, 2004). The optimal position brings the external auditory meatus to the level of the suprasternal notch (El-Orbany et al., 2011). The neck should be minimally extended to ensure the face is horizontal (facing the roof; see Fig. 3.6.3c) (El-Orbany et al., 2011; Greenland et al., 2010; Levitan et al., 2003). In obese patients, multiple blankets may be required to achieve sufficient elevation of the shoulders and then the head to achieve the 'face to roof' position (Collins et al., 2004; El-Orbany et al., 2011).

Head elevation above the stomach decreases atelectasis, improves ventilation/perfusion ratios and decreases passive regurgitation and aspiration risk (Klinger and Infosino, 2018; Levitan et al., 2003; Myatt and Haire, 2010; Rao et al., 2008; Weingart and Levitan, 2012). Elevating the stretcher head achieves similar results (Rao et al., 2008; Reddy et al., 2016).

Clinical skill assessment process

The following section outlines the clinical skill assessment tools that should be used to determine a student's ability to demonstrate safe and accurate laryngoscopy.
1. Clinical Skill Work Instruction
2. Formative Clinical Skill Assessment (F-CSAT)
3. Performance Improvement Plan (PIP)
4. Summative Clinical Skill Assessment (S-CSAT)
(5. Direct Observation of Procedural Skills (DOPS) – see Chapter 1.1)

Clinical Skill Work Instruction

Equipment and resources: Airway mannequin; laryngoscope and blades; gloves, respiratory mask and eyewear; suction equipment; towel/pillow; method of documenting results

Associated Clinical Skills: Infection control; Consent; Patient assessment skills; Airway and ventilation skills

Laryngoscopy

Activity	Critical Action	Rationale
Personal protection	Don gloves, respiratory mask, eyewear.	Infection risk management – high-risk procedure.
Prepare equipment	Select blade and attach to laryngoscope. Verify light is functioning. Ensure suction/Magill's/other airway devices as required are available.	Laryngoscope must be functional with appropriate bright light.
Airway assessment	Check facial hair, mouth opening, integrity of teeth, thyromental distance, neck length and mobility.	Improved awareness and anticipation of expected difficulties.
Prepare patient	Position ear to sternal notch, face parallel to roof.	Aligns oral, pharyngeal and laryngeal axes to improve view.
Pre-oxygenate	Ventilate/oxygenate as appropriate.	Create/improve oxygen reserve.
Insert laryngoscope	Open mouth with right hand. Holding laryngoscope in left hand, insert blade in right side of mouth. Rotate to right if required.	Failure to adequately open mouth prevents laryngoscopy.
Advance blade	Advance blade down right side of tongue until epiglottis is sighted. Place blade tip in vallecular groove (may use ELM to improve vallecular access).	Allows glottis to be located and exposed.

Laryngoscopy continued

Activity	Critical Action	Rationale
Glottis view	Distract mandible forwards to expose glottis. Suction if required, using right hand.	Tilts epiglottis anteriorly, exposing glottis.
Vocalise finding	Communicate grade view achieved.	Team awareness of critical airway finding.
Perform adjunct procedure	Clear airway/intubate/insert gastric tube.	As indicated.
Report	Document/hand over airway view, difficulties and adjuncts used.	Accurate record kept and continuity of patient care.

Formative Clinical Skill Assessment (F-CSAT)

Equipment and resources: Airway mannequin; laryngoscope and blades; gloves, respiratory mask and eyewear; suction equipment; towel/pillow; method of documenting results

Associated Clinical Skills: Infection control; Consent; Patient assessment skills; Airway and ventilation skills

Staff/Student being assessed: _____

Laryngoscopy

Activity	Critical Action	Participant Performance				
Personal protection	Dons gloves, respiratory mask, eyewear.	0	1	2	3	4
Prepares equipment	Selects blade and attaches to laryngoscope. Verifies light is functioning. Ensures suction/Magill's/other airway devices as required are available.	0	1	2	3	4
Airway assessment	Checks facial hair, mouth opening, integrity of teeth, thyromental distance, neck length and mobility.	0	1	2	3	4
Prepares patient	Positions ear to sternal notch, face parallel to roof.	0	1	2	3	4
Pre-oxygenates	Ventilates/oxygenates as appropriate.	0	1	2	3	4
Inserts laryngoscope	Opens mouth with right hand. Holding laryngoscope in left hand, inserts blade in right side of mouth.	0	1	2	3	4
Advances blade	Advances blade down right side of tongue until epiglottis is sighted. Places tip of blade in vallecular groove.	0	1	2	3	4
Glottis view	Distracts mandible forwards to expose glottis. Suctions if required.	0	1	2	3	4
Vocalises finding	Communicates grade view achieved.	0	1	2	3	4
Performs adjunct procedure	Clears airway clearance/intubates/inserts gastric tube.	0	1	2	3	4
Reports	Documents/hands over airway view, difficulties and adjuncts used.	0	1	2	3	4

Standard Achieved: (please circle one)

Competent (C)   Not Yet Competent* (NYC)

Staff/Student Name: _____

Assessor (please print name): _____

Signed (Assessor): _____

Date of Assessment: _____

Comments:

*If Not Yet Competent (NYC) a PIP needs to be completed and a repeat of the F-CSAT

Formative Clinical Skill Assessment (F-CSAT) Key

Skill level	Standard of procedure	Quality of performance	Outcome	Level of assistance required
4 Safe for unsupervised practice	Safe Accurate Behaviour is appropriate to context	Confident Accurate Expedient	Achieved intended outcome	No supporting cues* required
3 Requires supervision	Safe Accurate Behaviour is appropriate to context	Confident Accurate Takes longer than required	Achieved intended outcome	Requires occasional supportive cues*
2 Requires assistance	Safe Accurate Behaviour generally appropriate to context	Lacks certainty	Would not have achieved outcome without support	Requires frequent verbal and occasional physical directives in addition to supportive cues*
1 Requires direction	Safe only with guidance Not completely accurate	Unskilled Inefficient	Would not have achieved outcome without support	Requires continuous verbal and frequent physical directive cues*
0 Unsafe	Unsafe Unable to demonstrate behaviour Lack of insight into behaviour appropriate to context	Unskilled	Would not have achieved outcome	Requires continuous verbal and continuous physical directive cues*

*Refers to physical directives or verbal supportive cues

Performance Improvement Plan (PIP)

Please document the agreed education plan and completion timelines for areas assessed as less than 4.

This plan should be presented to assessor prior to commencement of summative assessment.

Where was supervisor support required?	Student summary of deficit. (Why was there a problem?)	Improvement Plan	Completed (Y/N)

Staff/Student Name: _____

Staff/Student Signature: _____

Educator Name: _____

Educator Signature: _____

Summative Clinical Skill Assessment (S-CSAT)

Equipment and resources: Airway mannequin; laryngoscope and blades; gloves, respiratory mask and eyewear; suction equipment; towel/pillow; method of documenting results

Associated Clinical Skills: Infection control; Consent; Patient assessment skills; Airway and ventilation skills

Staff/Student being assessed: _____

- Completed Formative Clinical Skill Assessment (F-CSAT): **YES**   **NO**
- Completed Performance Improvement Plan (PIP): **YES**   **NO**   **N/A**

Laryngoscopy

Activity	Critical Action	Achieved Without Direction	
Personal protection	Dons gloves, respiratory mask, eyewear.	NO	YES
Prepares equipment	Selects blade and attaches to laryngoscope. Verifies light is functioning. Ensures suction/Magill's/other airway devices as required are available.	NO	YES
Airway assessment	Checks facial hair, mouth opening, integrity of teeth, thyromental distance, neck length and mobility.	NO	YES
Prepares patient	Positions ear to sternal notch, face parallel to roof.	NO	YES
Pre-oxygenates	Ventilates/oxygenates as appropriate.	NO	YES
Inserts laryngoscope	Opens mouth with right hand. Holding laryngoscope in left hand, inserts blade in right side of mouth.	NO	YES
Advances blade	Advances blade down right side of tongue until epiglottis is sighted. Places tip of blade in vallecular groove.	NO	YES

Laryngoscopy continued

Activity	Critical Action	Achieved Without Direction	
Glottis view	Distracts mandible forwards to expose glottis. Suctions if required.	NO	YES
Vocalises finding	Communicates grade view achieved.	NO	YES
Performs adjunct procedure	Clears airway/intubates/inserts gastric tube.	NO	YES
Reports	Documents/hands over airway view, difficulties and adjuncts used.	NO	YES

Standard Achieved: (please circle one)

Competent (C)   Not Yet Competent* (NYC)

Staff/Student Name: _____

Assessor (please print name): _____

Signed (Assessor): _____

Date of Assessment: _____

Comments:

*If Not Yet Competent (NYC) a PIP needs to be completed and a repeat of the F-CSAT

Clinical findings

Airway view

Glottic view in laryngoscopy is commonly recorded using Cormack-Lehane grades (Fig. 3.6.4) and, more recently, the modified Cormack-Lehane (Brown and Walls, 2014; Yentis and Lee, 1998). Full glottis view is described as Grade 1. Grade 2a views the posterior cartilages and part vocal cords. Grade 2b views posterior cartilages only; Grade 2b makes up approximately 20% of Cormack-Lehane Grade 2 views. Grade 3 views the epiglottis only and Grade 4 indicates the epiglottis is not visible (Brown and Walls, 2014).

Grade 2b, 3 and 4 views are associated with increased difficulty in intubation. Understanding the manipulations that may improve grade view is important to successful laryngoscopy.

Video laryngoscopy

Video laryngoscopy can improve laryngeal view and intubation success in logistically difficult settings

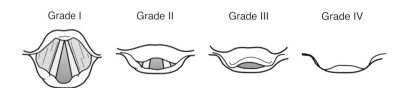

Grade I   Grade II   Grade III   Grade IV

Figure 3.6.4 Cormack-Lehane grades 1–4

The Cormack-Lehane system for grading laryngoscopic view at intubation. Difficulty of direct laryngoscopy correlates with the best view of the glottis, as defined by the Cormack-Lehane scale. With this scale, a Grade 1 view connotes a full view of the entire glottic aperture, Grade 2 represents a partial glottic view, Grade 3 represents visualisation of the epiglottis only and Grade 4 represents an inability to visualise even the epiglottis.

Source: Robbins, K.T., Flint, P.W., Lesperance, M.M., Lund, V.J., Francis, H.W., Thomas, J.R. and Haughey, B.H., 2021, Cummings otolaryngology: head and neck surgery, 7th edn (Chapter 5, Figure 5.2), Elsevier.

(Boehringer et al., 2015; Natt et al., 2016). It may also decrease complications in an emergency setting (Hinkelbein et al., 2015).

Video laryngoscopy, particularly with hyper-angulated blades, may assist with Grade 3/4 views arising from decreased mouth opening or neck range motion, or from immobilisation of the cervical spine (Brown and Walls, 2014; Klinger and Infosino, 2018; Smereka et al., 2017). However, it may be less useful in soiled airways due to blurring of the screen image (Mihara et al., 2015). Airway suctioning before inserting the video laryngoscope can minimise this issue (Law et al., 2013).

Video laryngoscopy has a clear role in training for direct laryngoscopy, facilitating the observation, real-time instruction and intervention of experienced clinicians (Brown and Walls, 2014, Natt et al., 2016). Novices have demonstrated improved success rates and learning curves when using video laryngoscopy (Hinkelbein et al., 2015).

Failure to visualise landmarks

Foreign body

Foreign bodies, vomit, excess secretions or blood can obstruct the view of the glottis and should be cleared. Bodily fluids and inadequate positioning are common reasons for inferior views in laryngoscopy (Prekker et al., 2014). Magill's forceps should be available for removing solid objects (Chapter 3.7). Laryngopharynx visualisation facilitates the targeted suction and removal of impacted foreign bodies (Kenneally et al., 2015; Mireles-Cabodevila and Siddiqui, 2014; Sanders et al., 2007).

Incorrect blade position

If the glottis view is inadequate despite adequate head positioning, reconsider laryngoscope placement in the vallecular. Minor changes in tip placement and the force applied can significantly alter glottis view (Levitan et al., 2003). Consider a longer blade if you are unable to reach the vallecular (Law et al., 2013).

Laryngeal manipulation

External laryngeal manipulation (ELM), or bimanual laryngoscopy, using the right hand to press down and moving the larynx posteriorly, improve vallecular access and glottic view (Law et al., 2013; Levitan et al., 2006; Levitan et al., 2002; Schmitt and Mang, 2002). An assistant may provide ELM, with their hand guided by the laryngoscopist (Hwang et al., 2013).

Inadequate head position

If inadequate view persists despite optimised blade placement and ELM, increasing the head lift above 'ear to sternal notch' may improve glottis view (Law et al., 2013; Levitan et al., 2003; Schmitt and Mang, 2002). An assistant can help elevate the head to an optimal position (Schmitt and Mang, 2002) (see Chapter 3.2).

Obstructive epiglottis

Occasionally, a large/floppy epiglottis causes a Grade 3 view. Changing to a straight (Miller) blade may improve view where specific anatomic finding suggests benefit (Law et al., 2013).

Inability to insert laryngoscope blade

The 'scissor' technique can be used to open the mouth by applying opposing forces with the thumb and index or third finger. An assistant can distract the right corner of the mouth laterally, increasing access to the oropharynx. Avoid pinching the lips between the laryngoscope and teeth (Klinger and Infosino, 2018; Sanders et al., 2007).

Mechanical obstructions to opening the jaw (such as partial dislocation or surgical fusion) generally prevent continuation with laryngoscopy (Law et al., 2013). Trismus or intact gag requires the use of sedation/muscle relaxant prior to laryngoscopy and intubation.

PRACTICE TIP!

A common error is to place a pillow behind the patient's head, flexing the head/neck rather than elevating it. This makes inserting the laryngoscope and sighting the glottis more difficult (El-Orbany et al., 2011; Roman, 2004). Ensure the face is positioned horizontally for effective access to the mouth and glottis.

PRACTICE TIP!

Commence laryngoscopy with a rigid suction catheter in the right hand. As the laryngoscope is advanced slowly through the oropharynx, suction pooled fluids as required. This decreases soiling of the laryngoscope light source.
The sucker can be used to dab the posterior pharynx, aiding identification of the epiglottis (see suctioning methods, including SALAD, in Chapter 3.7).

PRACTICE TIP!

ELM should be distinguished from Backward/ Upward/Rightward/Pressure (BURP) applied by an assistant. By applying ELM themselves, the paramedic can immediately gauge the effectiveness of the manoeuvre and adjust accordingly. An assistant can then maintain the position, freeing the paramedic's right hand for other interventions.

PRACTICE TIP!

During practice, the airway mannequin should tend to slide away if laryngoscope force is applied correctly. If the mannequin slides towards the operator, the laryngoscope force is likely being applied rotationally, risking damage to the teeth and not improving the view.

PRACTICE TIP!

The airway paramedic should communicate their findings during laryngoscopy, allowing assistants to anticipate and prepare adjuncts or manoeuvres to assist.

PRACTICE TIP!

Airway secretions increase infection transmission. Airway procedures require appropriate PPE (respiratory face mask and goggles/face shield).

TEST YOUR KNOWLEDGE QUESTIONS

1. **What are the indications for laryngoscopy?**
    Airway inspection; removal of foreign body obstruction; suctioning; intubation.

2. **What complications may occur secondary to laryngoscopy?**
    Hypoxia from prolonged attempts or laryngospasm; trauma to the soft tissue, dental or vocal cord; vagal tone, leading to bradycardia and hypotension; increased intracranial pressure.

3. **When should laryngoscopy be avoided?**
    In conscious patients with an intact gag reflex and patients with upper airway inflammatory disease (e.g. croup, epiglottitis).

4. **What adjuncts are essential to laryngoscopy?**
    Head positioning; functioning suction; Magill's forceps; alternate laryngoscope; blades; artificial airways.

5. **What patient position is optimal during laryngoscopy?**
    The sniffing position. Ramping using blankets under the shoulders may help in obese patients. Upper body elevation using stretcher head inclination may assist and improve respiratory function.

6. **If breast tissue makes laryngoscope placement in the mouth difficult, what alternatives can be used?**
    Use a short handle if available; insert the blade 90° to the right then rotate it back to normal; remove the blade, place it the mouth and then reattach the handle.

7. **If encountering persistent, uncontrolled regurgitation, what steps may assist?**
    Lateral position if the patient is vomiting or there is massive soiling. If the patient is not vomiting, cricoid pressure performed by an assistant may prevent ongoing passive regurgitation, allowing suction to clear the airway.

    Suctioning methods, including SALAD.

8. **If you are unable to identify the epiglottis, what steps should you take?**
    Dab the posterior pharynx wall with the suction catheter, suctioning excess fluids/secretion films. If the epiglottis still cannot be identified, move the blade to the midline and advance slowly until it is located.

9. **If the attempts to lift the epiglottis fail, what steps may be taken?**
    Ensure the laryngoscope is adequately advanced in the vallecular. Apply ELM to move the larynx posteriorly, optimising the view. If a Grade 3 view persists, lift the head into an increasingly elevated position.

10. **If you are unable to view the glottis despite optimisation, what options are available?**
    Video laryngoscopy with hyper-angulated blade improves glottis viewing in an unsoiled airway. A straight blade laryngoscope may allow the epiglottis to be lifted directly.

References

Apfelbaum, J.L., Hagberg, C.A., Caplan, R.A., Blitt, C.D., Connis, R.T., Nickinovich, D.G., Benumof, J.L., Berry, F.A., Bode, R.H., Cheney, F.W., Guidry, O.F. and Ovassapian A., 2013. Practice guidelines for management of the difficult airway: an updated report by the American Society of Anesthesiologists Task Force on Management of the Difficult Airway. *Anesthesiology*, 118(2), 251–270.

Beachey, W., 2012. *Respiratory care anatomy and physiology: foundations for clinical practice*, 3rd edn. St Louis: Mosby.

Boehringer, B., Choate, M., Hurwitz, S., Tilney, P.V. and Judge, T., 2015. Impact of video laryngoscopy on advanced airway management by critical care transport paramedics and nurses using the cmac pocket monitor. *BioMed Research International*. Retrieved from: https://www.hindawi.com/journals/bmri/2015/821302

Boudewyns, A., Claes, J. and van de Heyning, P., 2010. Clinical practice: an approach to stridor in infants and children. *European Journal of Pediatrics*, 169(2): 135–141, 2010.

Brown, C.A. and Walls, R.M., 2014. Airway. In Marx, J.A., Hockberger, R.S. and Walls, R.M. (eds), *Rosen's emergency medicine – concepts in clinical practice*, 8th edn. Philidelphia: Elsevier, pp. 3–22.

Collins, J.S., Lemmens, H.J., Brodsky, J.B., Brock-Utne, J.G. and Levitan, R.M., 2004. Laryngoscopy and morbid obesity: a comparison of the 'sniff' and 'ramped' positions. *Obesity Surgery*, 14(9), 1171–1175.

Danzl, D.F. and Vissers, R.J., 2004. Tracheal intubation and mechanical ventilation. In Tintinalli, J.E., Kelen, G.D. and Stapczynski, J.S. (eds), *Emergency medicine – a comprehensive study guide*, 6th edn. New York: McGraw-Hill, pp. 108–119.

Donoghue, A.J. and Walls, R.M., 2008. Intubation, rescue devices, and airway adjuncts. In Baren, J.M., Rothrock, S.G., Brennan, J.A., Brown, L. and Goldman, R.D. (eds), *Pediatric emergency medicine*, Philadelphia: Elsevier, pp. 37–49.

El-Orbany, M., Woehlck, H. and Salem, M.R., 2011. Head and neck position for direct laryngoscopy. *Anesthesia & Analgesia*, 113(1), 103–109.

Frerk, C., Mitchell, V.S., McNarry, A.F., Mendonca, C., Bhagrath, R., Patel, A., O'Sullivan, E.P., Woodall, N.M. and Ahmad, I., 2015. Difficult Airway Society Intubation Guidelines Working Group: Difficult Airway Society 2015 guidelines for management of unanticipated difficult intubation in adults. *British Journal of Anaesthesia*, 115(6), 827–848.

Greenland, K.B., Edwards, M.J., Hutton, N.J., Challis, V.J., Irwin M.G. and Sleigh J.W., 2010. Changes in airway configuration with different head and neck positions using magnetic resonance imaging of normal airways: a new concept with possible clinical applications. *British Journal of Anaesthesia*, 105(5), 683–690.

Hinkelbein, J., Cirillo, F., de Robertis, E. and Spelten, O., 2015. Update on video laryngoscopy in the emergency environment: the most important publications of the last 12 months. *Trends in Anaesthesia and Critical Care*, 5(6), 188–194.

Hwang, J., Park, S., Huh, J., Kim, J., Kim, K., Oh, A. and Han S., 2013. Optimal external laryngeal manipulation: modified bimanual laryngoscopy. *American Journal of Emergency Medicine*, 31(1), 32–36.

Kenneally, J., Marshall, T. and Jarvie, I., 2015. *MICA paramedic rapid sequence intubation*, 5th edn. Melbourne: Ambulance Victoria.

Klinger, K. and Infosino, A., 2018. Airway management. In Pardo, M.C. and Miller R.D. (eds), *Basics of anesthesia*, 7th edn. Philadelphia: Elsevier, pp. 239–272.

Law, J.A., Broemling, N., Cooper, R., Drolet, P., Duggan, L.V., Griesdale, D.E., Hung, O.R., Jones, P.M., Kovacs, G., Massey, S., Morris, I.R., Mullen, T., Murphy, M.F., Preston, R., Naik, V.N., Scott, J., Stacey, S., Turkstra, T.P. and Wong, D.T., 2013. Canadian Airway Focus Group: the difficult airway with recommendations for management, part 1: Difficult tracheal intubation encountered in an unconscious/induced patient. *Canadian Journal of Anesthesia*, 60(11), 1089–1118.

Levitan, R.M., 2007. The mystique of direct laryngoscopy. *Respiratory Care*, 52(1), 21–23.

Levitan, R.M., Everett, W.W. and Ochroch, E.A., 2004. Limitations of difficult airway prediction in the emergency department. *Annals of Emergency Medicine*, 44, 307–313.

Levitan, R.M., Kinkle, W.C., Levin, W.J. and Everett, W.W., 2006. Laryngeal view during laryngoscopy: a randomized trial comparing cricoid pressure, backward-upward-rightward pressure, and bimanual laryngoscopy. *Annals of Emergency Medicine*, 47(6), 548–555.

Levitan, R.M., Mechem, C.C., Ochroch, E.A., Shofer, F.S. and Hollander, J.E., 2003. Head-elevated laryngoscopy position: improving laryngeal exposure during laryngoscopy by increasing head elevation. *Annals of Emergency Medicine*, 41(3), 322–330.

Levitan, R.M., Mickler, T. and Hollander, J.E., 2002. Bimanual laryngoscopy: a videographic study of external laryngeal manipulation by novice intubators. *Annals of Emergency Medicine*, 40(1), 30–37.

Mihara, R., Komasawa, N., Matsunami, S. and Minami, T., 2015. Comparison of direct and indirect laryngoscopes in vomitus and hematemesis settings: a randomized simulation trial. *BioMed Research International*, doi:10.1155/2015/806243.

Mireles-Cabodevila, E. and Siddiqui, M.F., 2014. Airway management and emergency resuscitation equipment. In Volsko, T.A., Chatburn, R.L. and El-Khatib, M.F. (eds), *Equipment for respiratory care*. Burlington: Jones & Bartlett, pp. 97–149.

Myatt, J. and Haire, K., 2010. Airway management in obese patients. *Current Anaesthesia & Critical Care*, 21, 9–15.

Natt, B.S., Malo, J., Hypes, C.D., Sakles, J.C. and Mosier, J.M., 2016. Strategies to improve first attempt success at intubation in critically ill patients. *British Journal of Anaesthesia*, 117(1), i60–i68.

Padlipsky, P.S. and Gausche-Hill, M., 2008. Respiratory distress and respiratory failure. In Baren, J.M., Rothrock, S.G., Brennan, J.A., Brown, L. and Goldman, R.D. (eds), *Pediatric emergency medicine*. Philadelphia: Elsevier, pp. 13–27.

Prekker, M.E., Kwok, H., Shin, J., Carlbom, D., Grabinski, A. and Rea, T., 2014. The process of prehospital airway management: challenges and solutions during paramedic endotracheal intubation. *Critical Care Medicine*, 42(6), 1372–1378.

Rao, S.L., Kunselman, A.R., Schuler, H.G. and DesHarnais, S., 2008. Laryngoscopy and tracheal intubation in the head-elevated position in obese patients: a randomized, controlled, equivalence trial. *Anesthesia & Analgesia*, 107(6), 1912–1918.

Reddy, R.M., Adke, M., Patil, P., Kosheleva, I. and Ridley, S., 2016. Comparison of glottic views and intubation times in the supine and 25 degree back-up positions. *BMC Anesthesiology*, 16(1), 113.

Roman, M.A., 2004. Noninvasive airway management. In Tintinalli, J.E., Kelen, G.D. and Stapczynski, J.S. (eds), *Emergency medicine: a comprehensive study guide*, 6th edn. New York: McGraw-Hill, pp. 102–108.

Rothrock, S.G., 2008. Rapid sequence intubation. In Baren, J.M., Rothrock, S.G., Brennan, J.A., Brown, L. and Goldman, R.D. (eds), *Pediatric emergency medicine*. Philadelphia: Elsevier, pp. 28–36.

Rubin, M. and Sadovnikoff, N., 2004. Pediatric airway management. In Tintinalli, J.E., Kelen, G.D. and Stapczynski, J.S. (eds), *Emergency medicine: a comprehensive study guide*, 6th edn. New York: McGraw-Hill, pp. 88–94.

Sanders, M., McKenna, K.D., Lewis, L.M. and Quick, G., 2007. *Mosby's paramedic textbook*. St Louis: Mosby.

Schmitt, H.J. and Mang, H., 2002. Head and neck elevation beyond the sniffing position improves laryngeal view in cases of difficult direct laryngoscopy. *Journal of Clinical Anesthesia*,14(5), 335–338.

Smereka, J., Ladny, J.R., Naylor, A., Ruetzler, K. and Szarpak, L., 2017. C-MAC compared with direct laryngoscopy for intubation in patients with cervical spine immobilization: a manikin trial. *American Journal of Emergency Medicine*, 35(8), 1142–1146.

Weingart, S.D. and Levitan, R.M., 2012. Preoxygenation and prevention of desaturation during emergency airway management. *Annals of Emergency Medicine*, 59(3), 165–175.

Yentis, S.M., 2002. Predicting difficult intubation – worthwhile exercise or pointless ritual? *Anaesthesia*, 57(2), 105–109.

Yentis, S.M. and Lee, D.J., 1998. Evaluation of an improved scoring system for the grading of direct laryngoscopy. *Anaesthesia*, 53(11), 1041–1044.

Yu, T., Wang, B., Jin, X.J., Wu, H., He, J.J., Yao, W.D. and Li, Y.H., 2015. Predicting difficult airways: 3-3-2 rule or 3-3 rule? *Irish Journal of Medical Science*, 184(3), 677–683.

3.7 Foreign body removal/suctioning

Dianne Inglis

Chapter objectives

At the end of this chapter the reader will be able to:

1. Describe the types of foreign body airway obstruction (FBAO)
2. Demonstrate removing solid and liquid FBAO
3. Accurately report findings

Resources required for this assessment

- Airway mannequin
- Suction device with tubing/Yankauer sucker
- Magill's forceps
- Laryngoscope
- Disposable gloves, eyewear, respiratory mask
- Hand decontamination agent
- Clinical waste bag
- Method of documenting the results

Skill matrix

This assessment requires:

- Infection control (CS 1.3)
- Communication (CS 1.5)
- Consent (CS 1.6)
- Patient assessment skills (Chapter 2, CS 2.1, 2.2, 2.6, 2.7, 2.8, 2.10)
- Airway and ventilation skills (Chapter 3, CS 3.1, 3.2, 3.6)

This assessment is a component of:

- Airway and ventilation (Chapter 3)

Introduction

The initial measures for removing a foreign body airway obstruction (FBAO) involve creating an expulsive force to propel the object from the glottis, which is the most common site of upper airway obstruction (see Chapter 3.1). Where this is not achievable, respiratory failure quickly follows, along with loss of consciousness and airway reflexes. This necessitates direct FBAO removal, including with Magill's forceps for solid objects and suction for liquid/friable foreign bodies. This chapter discusses these methods.

Anatomy and physiology

The airway is divisible into upper and lower levels. Upper FBAO most commonly occurs just above the glottis in the hypopharynx, within the glottis itself or just distal to the glottis, where the airway diameter reduces considerably. Typically, upper FBAO compromises all or at least partial airway patency. However, this upper location also allows the possibility of visualisation and manual removal.

Clinical rationale

Children are at greatest risk of FBAO, due to their tendency to insert objects into their mouths and noses. The most commonly inserted objects are coins, buttons and food items, including nuts (Baral et al., 2010; Gupta and Gupta, 2010; Ishii and Yonekura, 2016; Oncel et al., 2017; Passàli et al., 2010). The risk of FBAO increases with age in adults over 50 years old (Hewlett et al., 2017); it is also associated with neurological changes, including stroke, dysphagia or altered consciousness.

The initial presentation of choking includes coughing, difficulty breathing and sometimes stridor (see Chapter 3.1). Wheezing may be heard if a smaller obstruction reaches the lower airway. This can be problematic where the initial presentation does not immediately suggest FBAO, leading to misdiagnosis (Hewlett et al., 2017).

Suspicion is key to diagnosis: FBAO must be considered from the outset in the event of a sudden such presentation in a smaller child (Gupta and Gupta, 2010; Passàli et al., 2010; Srivastava, 2010). Identifying the patient's activities immediately prior to onset, including eating or playing with objects, assists with diagnosis. FBAO can also occur in trauma, particularly from dislodged teeth (Hewlett et al., 2017).

If the patient's condition deteriorates following initial attempts at FBAO expulsion, manual removal becomes necessary. This should be accompanied by continued chest compression to expel the FBAO (see Chapter 3.1).

When the foreign body is trapped in the supraglottic or glottic region, forceps can be used to retrieve solid, graspable objects (Oncel et al., 2017). However, forceps should not be used to remove soft and friable objects, as this could cause fragmentation that is harder to remove or enters deeper into the airway. Take care to not push the obstruction further into the airway (Hewlett et al., 2017). Where possible, quick visualisation of a similar object to the foreign body, or at least gaining a description of its size and shape, can be helpful to identify any potential difficulties that might be encountered during the removal process.

Magill's forceps

Magill's forceps have multiple uses, including assisting the passage of endotracheal or duodenal tubes into position, and have a critical role in solid FBAO removal. The forceps have two circular handles, like scissors, with two long arms tipped with rounded, ridged ends for grasping. The arms can be manipulated open and closed as required. There are adult and smaller child sizes.

FBAO removal is performed under laryngoscopy, which allows a direct view of the glottis/object. Accompanying the left-handed laryngoscope, Magill's forceps are for right-hand use. The thumb and ring finger fit into the circular handles, with the index finger running along the arms for tip guidance (Fig. 3.7.1).

Placing the patient's head into the sniffing position optimises laryngoscopic view (see Chapter 3.2). Insert the closed Magill's tips into the mouth and direct them along the laryngoscope blade towards the object in view. Suction can be used if liquid obscures the view. When the forceps tips are within 1–2 cm of the object, open them, and surround and grasp the object. Gently withdraw the object straight from the mouth.

After removing the object, sweep left and right with the laryngoscope to ensure that there is no further obstructing material. Visualise to confirm the glottis is clear. Remove the laryngoscope and immediately provide assisted ventilation or oxygenation to support spontaneous breathing.

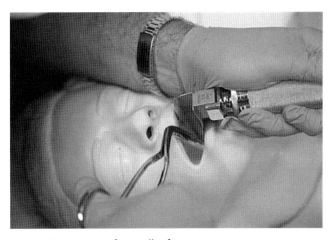

Figure 3.7.1 Use of Magill's forceps

Upper airway suctioning

An FBAO does not have to be solid to void airway patency. Liquid or semi-liquid sources include regurgitated gastric content and material entering the mouth during drinking, drowning or retained secretions. Fluid can accumulate in the upper and lower airway of unconscious or sedated patients. This is the most common prehospital obstruction, so suction should be made available whenever laryngoscopy occurs (Prekker et al., 2014).

The presentation of liquid or semi-liquid FBAO may differ from that of solid FBAO. There may be little or no warning of the presence of regurgitated gastric content, which is particularly problematic for supine patients with reduced airway reflexes. The event may not have been precipitated by choking, playing with an object or eating. Instead of the stridor or wheezing audible with a solid obstruction, gurgling or a moist-sounding cough may be heard. The patient may have an increasing respiratory rate and decreasing pulse oximetry.

There are multiple indications for airway suction, both routine and emergency, with and without other airway adjuncts in situ. This discussion focuses on oral clearance in FBAO.

Airway suctioning removes not only liquid but also air from the upper and lower airway, potentially leading to hypoxia. The longer the duration of suction, the greater the possibility of this complication. Suctioning attempts should therefore ideally be <10 seconds.

Suction vacuum is around 80–120 mmHg for adults and 60–80 mmHg for children. Excessive suction can remove air from the airway too quickly or cause soft tissue/mucous membrane injury.

Preparation

Suctioning should be clean but not necessarily sterile. Direct oropharynx suctioning usually requires a solid, wider Yankauer sucker inserted into the mouth (never the nose). Since this can stimulate airway reflexes if they are present, this option should only be used when reflexes are compromised or absent. If there is an oro/nasopharyngeal airway in situ, remove it to allow full oral access.

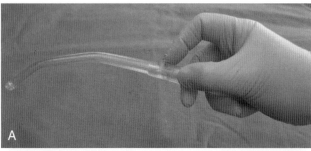
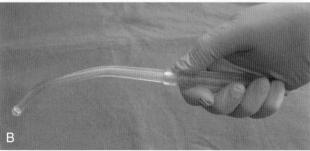

Figure 3.7.2 Yankauer sucker grip
(a) With finger over the hole. (b) With thumb over the hole.

The Yankauer sucker has a distal hole for fluid entry; larger particles cannot be withdrawn through this. The tip is a bulbous shape to reduce the potential for soft tissue injury. Midway along the shaft is a second, top hole. When this hole is uncovered, air is preferentially withdrawn through it, reducing suction at the tip and air removal. Once the sucker is in position, placing a finger or thumb over the hole diverts suction to the tip. The grip/hold on the Yankauer sucker varies with the digit used (Fig. 3.7.2a and b), so experiment to determine which offers you best control of the device.

Although a rigid Yankauer sucker can be reused, do be mindful that it will be soiled, so placing it on surfaces contaminates clean or sterile items and poses an infection risk. A suitable receptacle for isolating the soiled sucker is therefore essential. If this is not available, discard and replace the used item.

Position the patient, if appropriate, in the sniffing position (see Chapter 3.2). Attach the sucker to suction hose that is long enough to allow its effective use. Dip the sucker into a small container of water to test function. This same water can be used periodically during suctioning to unclog thick fluid and ensure continued effective suction. A replacement sucker must be at hand, along with a clinical waste bag so that the used item can be discarded immediately.

Visualise the hypopharynx/glottis under laryngoscopy (see Chapter 3.6). Insert the Yankauer sucker along the laryngoscope blade, progressing gently until the tip reaches the fluid obstruction. Cover the Yankauer top hole and visualise the fluid being removed. Visualise left and right of the glottis to ensure the airway is clear. Uncover the top hole again, withdraw the sucker and discard or place it into a suitable receptacle.

Check the patient immediately after suctioning to evaluate the effectiveness of the procedure, including for evidence of fluid removal. Suctioned liquid should be collected in a suitable receptacle so that the amount removed can be examined. However, even if large amounts of liquid have been removed, this does not guarantee that there is no further gastric content or fragmented material in the airway. Provide rapid re-oxygenation and consider further airway options as necessary.

Clinical skill assessment process

The following section outlines the clinical skill assessment tools that should be used to determine a student's ability to demonstrate effective upper airway foreign body removal in an unconscious patient.

1. Clinical Skill Work Instruction
2. Formative Clinical Skill Assessment (F-CSAT)
3. Performance Improvement Plan (PIP)
4. Summative Clinical Skill Assessment (S-CSAT)
(5. Direct Observation of Procedural Skills (DOPS) – see Chapter 1.1)

Clinical Skill Work Instruction

Equipment and resources: Airway mannequin; suction device with tubing/Yankauer sucker; laryngoscope; Magill's forceps; laryngoscope; disposable gloves, eyewear and mask; clinical waste bag; method of documenting results

Associated Clinical Skills: Infection control; Communication; Consent; Patient assessment skills; Airway and ventilation skills

Foreign body removal/suctioning

Activity	Critical Action	Rationale
PPE	Don appropriate PPE: eyewear, respiratory mask, gloves.	Airway procedures are high infection risk.
Patient assessment	Establish likelihood of FBAO: • history • respiratory effort, breathing sounds, pulse oximetry, air entry.	To support need for clearance.

Foreign body removal/suctioning continued

Activity	Critical Action	Rationale
Prepare patient	Position head in sniffing position.	Optimises glottis view.
Prepare equipment	Lay out Magill's forceps. Attach Yankauer sucker to suction tubing. Ensure all suction system components attached, including collection bottle. If available, fill a cup/container with water. Test suction function by dipping tip into water and occluding top hole.	To ensure suction is effective before use. Water allows suction testing and hose clearance during use.
Perform laryngoscopy	Insert laryngoscope until tip is located in vallecular. Identify glottis or FBAO.	To visualise FBAO.

Solid FBAO: Magill's forceps removal

Insert forceps	Grasp Magill's forceps in right hand, with thumb and ring finger in the circular handles and index finger along forceps length. Insert forceps along laryngoscope blade until 1–2 cm from FBAO. Open forceps tips. Grasp object.	In preparation for solid object removal. Opening only when ready to grasp the object reduces the risk of tissue injury.
Remove FBAO	Withdraw FBAO back along blade length. Discard object into waste bag. Sweep laryngoscope tip left and right to confirm pharynx is clear and glottis visible. Attempt should take <10 seconds. Repeat procedure if further obstruction exists. Place forceps into separate waste bag for later cleaning.	To allow effective removal without injuring soft tissue and identify any further FBAO.

Liquid FBAO: Airway suctioning

Insert sucker	Grasp Yankauer sucker in right hand. Depending on preference, hold device so either thumb or index finger can cover top hole. Progress the sucker inwards along length of laryngoscope blade until it reaches the fluid.	Ability to manoeuvre sucker and control suction application is essential. To delay suctioning in order to minimise tissue injury and hypoxia.
Apply suction	When sucker tip is in position, cover top hole to commence suction. Sweep laryngoscope tip left and right, with sucker tip following, until pharynx is clear and glottis visible. Attempt should take <10 seconds.	To ensure fluid removal from entire hypopharynx.
Withdraw sucker	Either discard and replace used sucker or place it into clean, isolated container. If further suction is necessary, repeat process. If fluid occludes suction hose, dip sucker tip into clean water briefly, under suction, to clear it.	Used sucker can contaminate anything it contacts. Thick fluid can clog the sucker; this can be cleared with water.
Re-oxygenate	Provide oxygenation/assisted ventilation as necessary.	To counter hypoxia.
Assess effectiveness	Visualise airway clarity before exiting. Reassess earlier FBAO signs for improvement.	To ensure entire FBAO cleared.
Report	Document/hand over FBAO nature, removal method and patient condition.	Accurate record keeping and care continuity.

Formative Clinical Skill Assessment (F-CSAT)

Equipment and resources: Airway mannequin; suction device with tubing/Yankauer sucker; laryngoscope; Magill's forceps; laryngoscope; disposable gloves, eyewear and mask; clinical waste bag; method of documenting results

Associated Clinical Skills: Infection control; Communication; Consent; Patient assessment skills; Airway and ventilation skills

Staff/Student being assessed: _____

Foreign body removal/suctioning

Activity	Critical Action	Performance				
PPE	Dons appropriate PPE.	0	1	2	3	4
Patient assessment	Establishes likelihood of FBAO: • history • patient presentation.	0	1	2	3	4
Prepares patient	Positions head in sniffing position.	0	1	2	3	4
Prepares equipment	Lays out Magill's forceps. Attaches Yankauer sucker to tubing, then to suction device. Tests suction.	0	1	2	3	4
Performs laryngoscopy	Inserts laryngoscope. Identifies glottis or FBAO.	0	1	2	3	4

Solid FBAO: Magill's forceps removal

Inserts forceps	Grasps forceps correctly. Inserts tips along laryngoscope until 1–2 cm from FBAO. Opens tips, grasps object.	0	1	2	3	4
Removes FBAO	Withdraws FBAO along blade. Discards object correctly. Sweeps pharynx to ensure clarity. Repeats procedure if necessary. Sets aside forceps correctly for cleaning.	0	1	2	3	4

Liquid FBAO: Airway suctioning

Inserts sucker	Grasps Yankauer sucker in right hand. Holds device, allowing top hole to be covered. Inserts sucker along laryngoscope correctly.	0	1	2	3	4
Applies suction	Covers top hole with tip in position to suction. Sights pharynx after suctioning to confirm clarity.	0	1	2	3	4
Withdraws sucker	Discards sucker or places it in clean receptacle for further use. Repeats as necessary. Uses water to clear suction occlusion.	0	1	2	3	4
Re-oxygenates	Provides oxygenation/assisted ventilation as necessary.	0	1	2	3	4
Assesses effectiveness	Visualises airway clarity. Reassesses for improvement.	0	1	2	3	4
Reports	Documents/hands over FBAO nature, removal method and patient condition.	0	1	2	3	4

Standard Achieved: (please circle one)

Competent (C)   Not Yet Competent* (NYC)

Staff/Student Name: _____

Assessor (please print name): _____

Signed (Assessor): _____

Date of Assessment: _____

Comments:

*If Not Yet Competent (NYC) a PIP needs to be completed and a repeat of the F-CSAT

Formative Clinical Skill Assessment (F-CSAT) Key

Skill level	Standard of procedure	Quality of performance	Outcome	Level of assistance required
4 Safe for unsupervised practice	Safe Accurate Behaviour is appropriate to context	Confident Accurate Expedient	Achieved intended outcome	No supporting cues* required
3 Requires supervision	Safe Accurate Behaviour is appropriate to context	Confident Accurate Takes longer than required	Achieved intended outcome	Requires occasional supportive cues*
2 Requires assistance	Safe Accurate Behaviour generally appropriate to context	Lacks certainty	Would not have achieved outcome without support	Requires frequent verbal and occasional physical directives in addition to supportive cues*
1 Requires direction	Safe only with guidance Not completely accurate	Unskilled Inefficient	Would not have achieved outcome without support	Requires continuous verbal and frequent physical directive cues*
0 Unsafe	Unsafe Unable to demonstrate behaviour Lack of insight into behaviour appropriate to context	Unskilled	Would not have achieved outcome	Requires continuous verbal and continuous physical directive cues*

*Refers to physical directives or verbal supportive cues

Performance Improvement Plan (PIP)

Please document the agreed education plan and completion timelines for areas assessed as less than 4.

This plan should be presented to assessor prior to commencement of summative assessment.

Where was supervisor support required?	Student summary of deficit. (Why was there a problem?)	Improvement Plan	Completed (Y/N)

Staff/Student Name: _____

Staff/Student Signature: _____

Educator Name: _____

Educator Signature: _____

Summative Clinical Skill Assessment (S-CSAT)

Equipment and resources: Airway mannequin; suction device with tubing/Yankauer sucker; laryngoscope; Magill's forceps; laryngoscope; disposable gloves, eyewear and mask; clinical waste bag; method of documenting results

Associated Clinical Skills: Infection control; Communication; Consent; Patient assessment skills; Airway and ventilation skills

Staff/Student being assessed: _____

- Completed Formative Clinical Skill Assessment (F-CSAT): **YES   NO**

- Completed Performance Improvement Plan (PIP): **YES   NO   N/A**

Foreign body removal/suctioning

Activity	Critical Action	Achieved Without Direction	
PPE	Dons appropriate PPE.	NO	YES
Patient assessment	Establishes likelihood of FBAO: • history • patient presentation.	NO	YES
Prepares patient	Positions head in sniffing position.	NO	YES
Prepares equipment	Lays out Magill's forceps. Attaches Yankauer sucker to tubing, then to suction device. Tests suction.	NO	YES
Performs laryngoscopy	Inserts laryngoscope. Identifies glottis or FBAO.	NO	YES

Activity	Critical Action	Achieved Without Direction	
Foreign body removal/suctioning continued			
Solid FBAO: Magill's forceps removal			
Inserts forceps	Grasps forceps correctly. Inserts forceps along laryngoscope until 1–2 cm from FBAO. Opens tips, grasps object.	NO	YES
Removes FBAO	Withdraws FBAO along blade. Discards object correctly. Sweeps pharynx to ensure clarity. Repeats procedure if necessary. Sets aside forceps correctly for cleaning.	NO	YES
Liquid FBAO: Airway suctioning			
Inserts sucker	Grasps Yankauer sucker in right hand. Holds device, allowing top hole to be covered. Inserts sucker along laryngoscope correctly.	NO	YES
Applies suction	Covers top hole with tip in position to suction. Visualises pharynx after suctioning to confirm clarity.	NO	YES
Withdraws sucker	Discards sucker or places in clean receptacle for further use. Repeats as necessary. Uses water to clear suction occlusion.	NO	YES
Re-oxygenates	Provides oxygenation/assisted ventilation as necessary.	NO	YES
Assesses effectiveness	Visualises airway clarity. Reassesses for improvement.	NO	YES
Reports	Documents/hands over FBAO nature, removal method and patient condition.	NO	YES

Standard Achieved: (please circle one)

Competent (C)   Not Yet Competent* (NYC)

Staff/Student Name: _____

Assessor (please print name): _____

Signed (Assessor): _____

Date of Assessment: _____

Comments:

*If Not Yet Competent (NYC) a PIP needs to be completed and a repeat of the F-CSAT

Clinical findings

Oesophageal obstruction

Many foreign bodies lodge in the oesophagus, usually at the laryngeal level, where they can cause distress and require removal. Although they are rarely life threatening, they can be problematic if the object is large enough to compress the trachea and cause respiratory difficulty or is sharp and able to penetrate the oesophagus (Baral et al., 2010; Gupta and Gupta, 2010). Button-sized batteries are particularly problematic because of their corrosive nature (Ishii and Yonekura, 2016; Oncel et al., 2017; Srivastava, 2010).

Suctioning during intubation

Suction assisted laryngoscopic airway decontamination (SALAD) is a technique for managing ongoing regurgitation that is unresponsive to cricoid pressure, where intubation is envisaged. As the laryngoscope blade is inserted the sucker follows the tip, clearing liquid and preventing the laryngoscope light from being soiled. Once the tip is in the vallecular, the Yankauer sucker can be left in the proximal oesophagus in the left of the mouth, pinned by the laryngoscope itself. This allows continued suctioning of any gastric content that might appear during the intubation attempt. To achieve this, the top sucker hole must be covered with tape first (DuCanto et al., 2017).

Lower airway suctioning and Y-suction catheters

Softer, narrower and more flexible Y-suction catheters can be selected as an alternative for suctioning. They are attached to the suction tubing and the hole is covered by a finger during use, in a similar fashion to when using the Yankauer sucker. These devices offer less guidance control than the Yankauer sucker and are typically chosen for suctioning other airway devices, including endotracheal tubes, through supraglottic airway device gastric ports or tracheostomy tubes. Their smaller size and flexibility also allows insertion into the nasal cavity and paediatric airways.

Lower airway suctioning through an endotracheal or tracheostomy tube requires a narrower and flexible Y-suction catheter. Differing diameter options are available, depending on the tube diameter. To determine the insertion length, the catheter can be compared against an equivalent endotracheal/tracheostomy tube and the correct point marked. Catheter protrusion from an endotracheal tube can contact the carina at the bronchial bifurcation, causing vagal stimulation and bradycardia. If contact is felt, withdraw the catheter 1–2 cm to minimise soft tissue injury and avoid stimulation. Always use a new catheter from sterile packaging, insert it once only and then discard it immediately into an infectious waste bag. Never suction the lower airway with a soiled or used catheter.

For conscious patients, suction can be unpleasant due to hypoxia or carina contact. Warning must be given and consent obtained prior to elective procedures. Avoid hypoxia with pre-oxygenation and short suction durations of <10 seconds. Apply suction once the catheter is inserted to the desired position, and also during withdrawal of the catheter from within the endotracheal/tracheostomy tube. If the suction attempt must be repeated, re-oxygenate the patient first.

FBAO removal failure

Where an FBAO cannot be removed, and therefore spontaneous patient respiration or assisted ventilation cannot occur, an alternative airway route must be found. Surgical airway must be established immediately (see Chapter 3.10) (Hewlett et al., 2017). The eventual removal of the object may need to be done in hospital, such as by bronchoscopy.

PRACTICE TIP!

Prior inspection and testing of, and familiarity with, equipment are critical before encountering any emergency. Briefly test suction immediately before use, to be certain/confident it is functioning properly.

PRACTICE TIP!

FBAO requires urgent intervention to avoid irreversible hypoxia occurring. Attention to universal precautions comes first, but airway intervention should not be otherwise delayed.

PRACTICE TIP!

The FBAO may not be exclusively solid or liquid. Both forms may be encountered together and solid objects may fragment. Be prepared to use forceps or suction, or even to alternate them, to gain clearance.

PRACTICE TIP!

Airway procedures create a risk of infection through sputum, exhalation and exposure to gastric content. Gloves, protective eyewear and respiratory masks must therefore be worn, including by assistants.

TEST YOUR KNOWLEDGE QUESTIONS

1. **What is the major complication of FBAO removal?**
   Hypoxia from a prolonged procedure and air removal from the airway.

2. **How might the presentation of solid FBAO differ from that of liquid?**
   Liquid may appear passively during loss of consciousness; solid may be preceded by choking, coughing or breathing difficulty.

3. **Why are airway procedures high risk?**
   They create exposure to sputum, patient breath and gastric content.

4. **What groups are at a greater risk of FBAO?**
   Adults over 50 years of age; small children; people with neurological changes, including stroke, difficulty swallowing and altered consciousness.

5. **Which hand is used to hold the forceps or suction catheter during use and why?**
   The right hand; both are performed under laryngoscopy, which is a left-handed method.

6. **At what moment is suction applied and why?**
   When the sucker tip is within contact of the fluid; to avoid soft tissue injury and minimise air removal during the procedure.

7. **What is the ideal duration of any attempt at removing an FBAO?**
   <10 seconds.

8. **What is the method of clearing a suction catheter if it becomes occluded during use?**
   Dip the suction tip briefly into water with the suction active.

9. **If a Yankauer sucker is to be reused, what precaution must be included?**
   Place the sucker into a suitable container where it cannot contaminate anything else.

10. **What must be done immediately following FBAO removal?**
    Sight the hypopharynx/glottis to verify airway clarity, and reassess the patient for improvement.

References

Baral, B.K., Joshi, R.R., Bhattarai, B.K. and Sewal, R.B., 2010. Removal of coin from upper esophageal tract in children with Magill's forceps under propofol sedation. *Nepal Medical College Journal*, 12(1), 38–41.

DuCanto, J., Serrano, K.D. and Thompson, R.J., 2017. Novel airway training tool that simulates vomiting: suction-assisted laryngoscopy assisted decontamination (SALAD) system. *Western Journal of Emergency Medicine*, 18(1), 117.

Gupta, K. and Gupta, P.K., 2010. Laryngoscopic removal of unusual metallic foreign body of the subglottic region of the larynx. *Anesthesia, Essays and Researches*, 4(2), 106.

Hewlett, J.C., Rickman, O.B., Lentz, R.J., Prakash, U.B. and Maldonado, F., 2017. Foreign body aspiration in adult airways: therapeutic approach. *Journal of Thoracic Disease*, 9(9), 3398.

Ishii, T. and Yonekura, T., 2016. Foreign body extraction. In Taguchi, T., Iwanaka, T. and Okamatsu, T. (eds), *Operative general surgery in neonates and infants*. Tokyo: Springer, pp. 31–35.

Oncel, M., Sunam, G.S., Elsurer, C. and Yildiran, H., 2017. Use of Magill forceps to remove foreign bodies in children. *Surgery Journal*, 3(2), e91.

Passàli, D., Lauriello, M., Bellussi, L., Passali, G.C., Passali, F.M. and Gregori, D., 2010. Foreign body inhalation in children: an update. *Acta Otorhinolaryngologica Italica*, 30(1), 27.

Prekker, M.E., Kwok, H., Shin, J., Carlbom, D., Grabinski, A. and Rea, T., 2014. The process of prehospital airway management: challenges and solutions during paramedic endotracheal intubation. *Critical Care Medicine*, 42(6), 1372–1378.

Srivastava, G., 2010. Foreign bodies in the oropharynx, gastrointestinal tract, ear, and nose. *Clinical Pediatric Emergency Medicine*, 11(2), 81–94.

Bibliography

Curtis, K. and Ramsden, C., 2015. *Emergency and trauma care for nurses and paramedics*. Philadelphia: Elsevier.

Johnson, M., Boyd, L., Grantham, H.J. and Eastwood, K., 2014. *Paramedic principles and practice ANZ*. Sydney: Harcourt.

McCance, K.L. and Huether, S.E., 2015. *Pathophysiology: the biologic basis for disease in adults and children*. Sydney: Elsevier.

3.8 | Laryngeal mask airway

Nick Holden and Gavin Smith

Chapter objectives

At the end of this chapter the reader will be able to:

1. Describe the rationale for laryngeal mask airway (LMA) insertion
2. Demonstrate effective and safe insertion of an LMA
3. Accurately report on the performance of LMA insertion

Resources required for this assessment

- Airway mannequin suitable for LMA insertion
- Various sized LMA/i-gel® devices
- 50/60 mL syringe if using inflatable cuff LMA
- Disposable gloves, protective eyewear, respiratory mask
- Water-based gel lubricant
- Method of documenting the results

Skill matrix

This assessment requires:

- Infection control (CS 1.3)
- Patient assessment skills (Chapter 2, CS 2.1, 2.2, 2.6, 2.8, 2.10)
- Airway and ventilation skills (Chapter 3, CS 3.2, 3.3, 3.6, 3.7, 3.11)

This assessment is a component of:

- Airway and ventilation (Chapter 3)

Introduction

Airway patency has a simple definition: it is where airflow moves freely between atmosphere and alveoli without obstruction. There are multiple potential obstructions to this air movement, including anatomical obstructions by upper airway structures and the regurgitation of gastric content. The risk of these increases with compromised patient positioning and loss of consciousness. Some airway obstructions can be mitigated using a supraglottic airway device, including the laryngeal mask airway (LMA), which is discussed in this chapter. Inflatable and non-inflatable mask or cuff (i.e. i-gel®) devices are discussed for use in emergency indications. The term 'LMA' refers to both options unless otherwise specified.

Anatomy and physiology

The upper airway can be divided into three distinct segments: the rigid oral and nasal cavities, the soft pharynx and the rigid larynx.

The pharynx is comprised largely of smooth muscle that can collapse as muscle tone is lost (Isono, 2012; Ma et al., 2016). This creates difficulties during sleep, but can be life threatening when consciousness is lost.

The pharynx and larynx contain protective airway reflexes, including cough, gag and swallow. Mechanically, the epiglottis at the base of the tongue can cause glottis obstruction if muscle tone is lost.

The oesophagus opens immediately posterior to the laryngopharynx. Upper and lower oesophageal sphincters prevent regurgitation and air entry into the stomach (Boeckxstaens, 2005; Singh and Hamdy, 2005). Loss of consciousness impairs sphincter function, allowing both of these complications to occur. The risk of pulmonary aspiration also increases with age and severity of illness (Lee et al., 2014); aspiration can lead to both foreign body airway obstruction and pulmonary injury from acidic gastric content (Hu et al., 2015). Insufflation occurs during positive pressure ventilation.

Clinical rationale

Supraglottic airway devices include a broad range of options for supporting upper airway patency in patients presenting with loss of consciousness and cough or gag airway reflexes. The most common devices include varieties of LMA. All sit invasively above the glottis, secure the oesophagus and allow pulmonary ventilation through them (Almeida et al., 2016; Cook and Kelly, 2015; Moser et al., 2017). Their deep pharyngeal positioning necessitates their use only where airway reflexes are absent.

The LMA is less invasive than endotracheal intubation and it is a quicker, more easily inserted alternative in emergencies (Benger et al., 2016; Soar et al., 2015). A cuffed distal end sits over the hypoglottis, creating a seal. Its tip invades the upper oesophagus, isolating the gastric content beyond and avoiding gastric insufflation during ventilation (Venugopal et al., 2016). Unlike intubation, the vocal cords are avoided. The mask joins to a stem that exits the mouth and allows attachment to standard bag/valve/mask (BVM) resuscitators (Moser et al., 2017).

Subsequent (second-generation) LMA versions have been refined. A wider, hardened stem prevents biting and occlusion if the airway reflexes inadvertently return. In some devices, a gastric port runs from the proximal end, through the stem to the distal tip, allowing insertion of a duodenal tube into the stomach (Cook and Kelly, 2015;

Moser et al., 2017; Timmermann et al., 2015; Park et al., 2015; Pournajafian et al., 2015).

The LMA has proven effective in a range of circumstances, including routine, emergency and prolonged use, airway rescue during unsuccessful intubation, as a portal for intubation, and in a variety of positions, including in prone and obese patients (Cook and Kelly, 2015; Moser et al., 2017; Timmermann et al., 2015).

Inflatable cuff/mask devices

Many LMA devices have a distal cuff that requires correct inflation before use (Fig. 3.8.1). There are slight variations among the wide range of options available, including shape, material, colour, angle of the distal cuff and method of evaluating the inflation pressure. Devices can vary in their method of cuff preparation for insertion, and reference to specific manufacturer instructions is therefore recommended. This discussion provides generic instruction that is suitable for most devices.

Non-inflatable cuff/mask i-gel® airway

The i-gel® airway has a soft, latex-free, thermoplastic, gel-like non-inflatable cuff that is as effective at gaining an airway seal as the inflatable cuff varieties (Acharya and Dave, 2016). It has a wide stem that serves as a bite block and to hold seated against the hypoglottis (Park et al., 2015). The solid cuff allows faster insertion and fewer steps during emergencies than inflatable-cuffed devices (Park et al., 2015; Pournajafian et al., 2015) (Fig. 3.8.2).

Patient positioning

The LMA can be inserted and used with the patient in a variety of positions, and can be effective with head flexion, extension and rotation (Mishra et al., 2015). The preferred option is supine in either a neutral anatomical or a sniffing head position (see Chapter 3.2). Changing the patient's

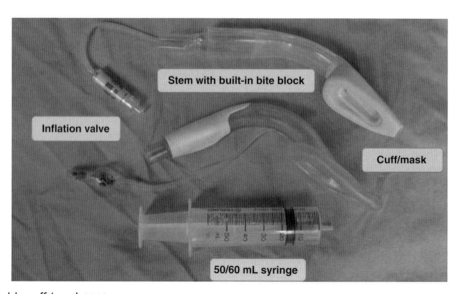

Figure 3.8.1 Inflatable cuff/mask LMA

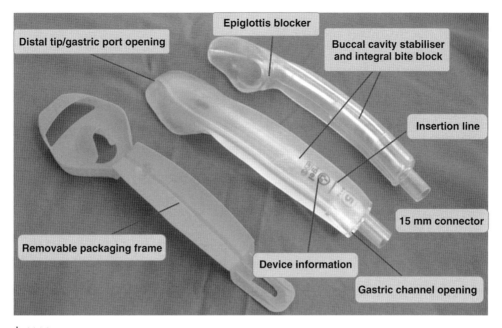

Figure 3.8.2 I-gel® LMA

head position once the device has been inserted can affect the cuff leak pressure and the ability to ventilate.

Airway preparation

While the LMA can be effective at preventing gastric aspiration, it cannot remove material that is already in the airway. Before insertion, remove foreign material from the oropharynx (see Chapter 3.7), including vomitus, blood and saliva.

Device measurement

As with all airway devices, the appropriate size of LMA must first be selected. The selection of size is based on the patient's body weight and varies with the brand. This information is printed on the LMA packaging and on the device stem.

As an example, i-gel® adult sizes are:
Size 3: 30–60 kg body weight
Size 4: 50–90 kg body weight
Size 5: >90 kg body weight

There is scope for overlap between sizes. If insertion or gaining an effective seal is difficult with one size, consider changing up or down as appropriate. Selecting a size that is smaller than required is a common error (Suibhne et al., 2018).

Cuff inflation (if required)

Cuff inflation volumes are printed on the packaging and on the LMA stem. The i-gel® does not require cuff inflation, which is a distinct advantage during emergency use. Where an LMA has a cuff, inflate and inspect it before use.

Inflation volumes are not precise but have a maximum value that must not be exceeded. Over-inflation can cause pharyngeal mucosal injury and incorrect positioning of the LMA, allowing gastric escape and ineffective ventilation.

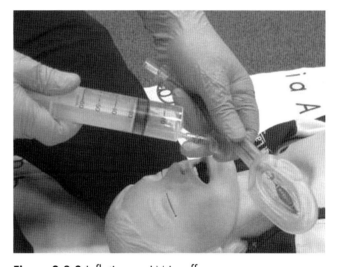

Figure 3.8.3 Inflating an LMA cuff

Cuff inflation pressure is also quoted on the packaging and device stem. This relates to the performance of the cuff itself rather than its impact on airway mucosa. Increasing the inflation pressure causes the cuff to force airway tissue to mould to it, rather than the other way around (Bick et al., 2014).

Attach an empty 50/60 mL syringe to the injection port. Gently withdraw all air from the cuff until it is fully deflated (Fig. 3.8.3). Detach the syringe. Draw up into the same syringe the maximum air volume that the specific device recommends. Inject sufficient air via the injection port into the completely deflated cuff to just form its inflated shape. This typically uses around half the air in the syringe. After insertion, if an effective seal or ventilation is not obtained and a leak can be heard, inject enough of the remaining air to correct this. Never draw up more air, as this can outwardly displace the cuff from its correct seating; instead, consider whether the LMA is

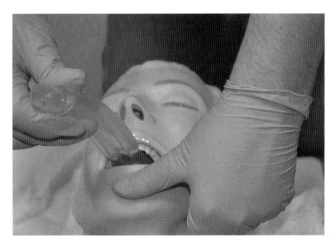

Figure 3.8.4 Inserting an LMA

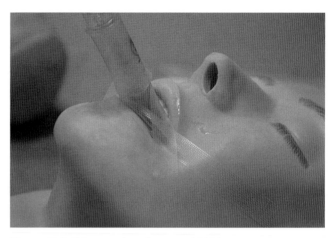

Figure 3.8.5 Inserted and secured LMA

correctly positioned or if the size is incorrect (Bick et al., 2014).

If the cuff is not seated correctly in the oesophagus and over the hypoglottis, air leakage, failure to ventilate the lungs, gastric regurgitation and pulmonary aspiration and increased sympathetic stimulation can occur (Pournajafian et al., 2015).

Insertion method

Before insertion, water-based lubricant must be applied along the back, sides and tip of the LMA mask. The LMA can then be left in its opened packaging, ready for use.

Typical insertion is blind and does not require visualisation under laryngoscopy. On insertion, the LMA tip/mask can push the tongue inwards, preventing further advancement. Open the mouth wide, using chin lift, to help avoid this (see Chapter 3.3) and also to prevent contact between the teeth and an inflatable cuff.

Holding the stem of the LMA, insert the tip into the mouth, back against the roof to avoid contact with the tongue (Fig. 3.8.4). Once past the tongue, continue gently pushing the LMA posteriorly along the palate towards the pharynx. A rotating left and right movement can be used if resistance is encountered (Nalini et al., 2016). Continue until firm resistance is felt as the tip reaches the oropharynx and oesophagus. If cricoid pressure is being applied, it must be released to allow correct placement.

If the tongue obstructs insertion, it must be splinted in place first. This can be done using a laryngoscope and then passing the LMA over it. The fingers can be used to splint the tongue or push at cuff level, being mindful of the risk of biting in patients who are not anaesthetised. Some LMA devices are inserted with the cuff deflated to reduce the likelihood of tongue contact during early insertion (Nalini et al., 2016).

Following insertion, observe for airway reflex signs, including gag, that may prompt removal of the LMA.

Once completely inserted, the proximal end sits just outside the patient's lips. The i-gel® has a marker indicating approximate lip length after insertion. Critically, the stem *must* sit midline to avoid left or right cuff displacement from the hypopharynx. This can happen when a BVM resuscitator is attached and allowed to hang to one side. The incisors sit against the integral bite block.

Secure the LMA by running adhesive tape from the patient's upper cheek, circling the stem once and then attaching the tape to the lower cheek on that side. Repeat for the other cheek (Fig. 3.8.5). Alternatively, tie a clove hitch knot around the LMA stem using endotracheal securing tape, then secure it around the patient's head/neck and tie off. LMA devices dislodge easily and require monitoring during use (Benger et al., 2016).

Reassess ventilation, particularly air passage or leakage. High airway pressures, such as during asthma, can cause the seal to leak. Document the size of device used, the number of attempts required and the time of insertion.

At a convenient time, a narrow gastric tube can be inserted into the lubricated duodenal port (if present), allowing aspiration of air and gastric content (Moser et al., 2017).

Contraindications

An LMA cannot be inserted where a patient has intact airway reflexes, trismus or too small a mouth.

Clinical skill assessment process

The following section outlines the clinical skill assessment tools that should be used to determine a student's ability to demonstrate safe and accurate insertion of a laryngeal mask airway.

1. Clinical Skill Work Instruction
2. Formative Clinical Skill Assessment (F-CSAT)
3. Performance Improvement Plan (PIP)
4. Summative Clinical Skill Assessment (S-CSAT)
(5. Direct Observation of Procedural Skills (DOPS) – see Chapter 1.1)

Clinical Skill Work Instruction

Equipment and resources: Airway mannequin suitable for LMA insertion; various sized LMA/i-gel® devices; 50/60 mL syringe if using inflatable cuff LMA; gloves, eyewear and mask; water-based gel lubricant; method of documenting results

Associated Clinical Skills: Infection control; Head positioning; Jaw thrust; Foreign body removal/suctioning; Intermittent positive pressure ventilation

Laryngeal mask airway

Activity	Critical Action	Rationale
Personal protection	Don PPE as required.	All airway procedures are considered high infection risk.
Assess indications	Assess consciousness and airway reflexes.	To ensure appropriate use.
Select device size	Choose appropriate size of LMA/i-gel® for patient's body weight. Open packaging, maintaining hygiene. If using i-gel®, remove from protective cradle.	Correct size is important for function.
Prepare equipment	Lay out LMA/i-gel® and other airway resuscitation equipment on a clean surface.	Other airway devices might also be required.
Prepare patient	Place patient supine with head in neutral anatomical or sniffing position.	Appropriate position assists airway patency and insertion.
	Ensure any foreign material is cleared from airway before inserting LMA.	The LMA/i-gel® does not address this issue.
Prepare cuff	If device used has an inflatable cuff/mask, attach empty 50/60 mL syringe to inflation cuff, depressing the valve. Withdraw all air from cuff to cause complete inward collapse. Detach syringe. Fill syringe with maximum air volume for device, as specified on product packaging. Reattach syringe to inflation cuff. Inject sufficient air slowly into cuff to just cause full reinflation. Save remaining air in syringe.	Ensures correct inflation pressure within cuff for effectiveness in use. Remaining air in syringe allows for later adjustment of cuff if necessary.
	Lubricate back, sides and tip of distal LMA/i-gel® mask with water-based gel.	To ease insertion.
Insert LMA	Perform chin lift to open mouth sufficiently wide to allow mask insertion.	To create maximum access.
	Hold stem firmly. Introduce tip into mouth. Gently direct upwards along mouth roof, away from the tongue.	To free mask from any resistance and avoid injury.
	Once clear of tongue, continue pushing posteriorly, following palate curve into pharynx. If tongue cannot be cleared or resistance is encountered, gently rotate left and right to continue progress.	The LMA follows the airway curve to its destination. The tongue is the main impediment.
	Gently apply sufficient force to seat tip of device in oesophagus until no further progress can be made.	To seat correctly in oesophagus, covering hypoglottis.
Reassess	Ensure no airway reflex is triggered by placement.	To avoid regurgitation of gastric contents.
Ventilate	Attach BVM resuscitator. Ventilate patient appropriately.	Unconscious patient may require ventilation assistance.

Laryngeal mask airway continued

Activity	Critical Action	Rationale
Adjust seal	If a leak is suspected (air escaping audible or inadequate chest expansion) in the air-filled cuff LMA, titrate in some or all of the remaining air in the syringe.	Minor cuff inflation adjustment may be necessary to effect seal. Further air administration can cause LMA displacement superiorly.
Secure LMA	Once confident of LMA placement and effectiveness, secure in place, using adhesive tape attached to face and device or cloth tape tied off. Maintain LMA midline in the mouth, with incisors on the integral bite block.	Correct placement maintains effectiveness of gastric and hypoglottic seal.
Duodenal tube	When convenient, insert appropriate size of duodenal tube through gastric port (if device has one) into stomach. This may require slight initial lubrication applied to port first. Withdraw air/gastric content using 50/60 mL catheter tip syringe.	To further reduce pulmonary aspiration risk.
Report	Document/hand over insertion time, LMA size, and any relevant information regarding placement or insertion.	Accurate record kept and continuity of patient care.

Formative Clinical Skill Assessment (F-CSAT)

Equipment and resources: Airway mannequin suitable for LMA insertion; various sized LMA/i-gel® devices; 50/60 mL syringe if using inflatable cuff LMA; gloves, eyewear and mask; water-based gel lubricant; method of documenting results

Associated Clinical Skills: Infection control; Head positioning; Jaw thrust; Foreign body removal/suctioning; Intermittent positive pressure ventilation

Staff/Student being assessed: _____

Laryngeal mask airway insertion

Activity	Critical Action	Participant Performance				
Personal protection	Dons PPE as required.	0	1	2	3	4
Assesses indications	Assesses consciousness and airway reflexes.	0	1	2	3	4
Selects device size	Chooses appropriate size of LMA/i-gel® for patient's body weight. Opens packaging, maintaining hygiene. If using i-gel®, removes from protective cradle.	0	1	2	3	4
Prepares equipment	Lays out LMA/i-gel® and other airway resuscitation equipment on a clean surface.	0	1	2	3	4
Prepares patient	Places patient supine with head in neutral anatomical or sniffing position.	0	1	2	3	4
	Clears any foreign material from airway before inserting LMA.	0	1	2	3	4

Laryngeal mask airway insertion continued

Activity	Critical Action	Participant Performance				
Prepares cuff	If device used has an inflatable cuff/mask, attaches empty 50/60 mL syringe to inflation cuff, depressing valve. Withdraws all air from cuff to cause complete inward collapse. Detaches syringe. Fills syringe with maximum air volume for device, as specified on product packaging. Reattaches syringe to inflation cuff. Injects sufficient air slowly into cuff to just cause full reinflation. Saves remaining air in syringe.	0	1	2	3	4
	Lubricates back, sides and tip of distal mask with water-based gel.	0	1	2	3	4
Inserts LMA	Performs chin lift to open mouth sufficiently wide to allow mask insertion.	0	1	2	3	4
	Holds stem firmly. Introduces tip into mouth. Gently directs upwards along mouth roof, away from the tongue.	0	1	2	3	4
	Once clear of tongue, continues pushing posteriorly, following palate curve into pharynx. If tongue cannot be cleared or resistance is encountered, gently rotates left and right to continue progress.	0	1	2	3	4
	Gently applies sufficient force to seat tip of device in oesophagus until no further progress can be made.	0	1	2	3	4
Reassesses	Ensures no airway reflex is triggered by placement.	0	1	2	3	4
Ventilates	Attaches BVM and ventilates.	0	1	2	3	4
Adjusts seal	If an air leak is suspected in the air-filled cuff LMA, titrates in some or all of the remaining air in the syringe.	0	1	2	3	4
Secures LMA	Once confident of LMA placement, secures in place in midline.	0	1	2	3	4
Duodenal tube	When convenient, inserts appropriate size of duodenal tube through gastric port and aspirates air/gastric content.	0	1	2	3	4
Reports	Accurately documents/hands over insertion time, LMA size, and any relevant information regarding placement or insertion.	0	1	2	3	4

Standard Achieved: (please circle one)

Competent (C)   Not Yet Competent* (NYC)

Staff/Student Name: _____

Assessor (please print name)**:** _____

Signed (Assessor)**:** _____

Date of Assessment: _____

Comments:

*If Not Yet Competent (NYC) a PIP needs to be completed and a repeat of the F-CSAT

Formative Clinical Skill Assessment (F-CSAT) Key

Skill level	Standard of procedure	Quality of performance	Outcome	Level of assistance required
4 Safe for unsupervised practice	Safe Accurate Behaviour is appropriate to context	Confident Accurate Expedient	Achieved intended outcome	No supporting cues* required
3 Requires supervision	Safe Accurate Behaviour is appropriate to context	Confident Accurate Takes longer than required	Achieved intended outcome	Requires occasional supportive cues*
2 Requires assistance	Safe Accurate Behaviour generally appropriate to context	Lacks certainty	Would not have achieved outcome without support	Requires frequent verbal and occasional physical directives in addition to supportive cues*
1 Requires direction	Safe only with guidance Not completely accurate	Unskilled Inefficient	Would not have achieved outcome without support	Requires continuous verbal and frequent physical directive cues*
0 Unsafe	Unsafe Unable to demonstrate behaviour Lack of insight into behaviour appropriate to context	Unskilled	Would not have achieved outcome	Requires continuous verbal and continuous physical directive cues*

*Refers to physical directives or verbal supportive cues

Performance Improvement Plan (PIP)

Please document the agreed education plan and completion timelines for areas assessed as less than 4.

This plan should be presented to assessor prior to commencement of summative assessment.

Where was supervisor support required?	Student summary of deficit. (Why was there a problem?)	Improvement Plan	Completed (Y/N)

Staff/Student Name: _____

Staff/Student Signature: _____

Educator Name: _____

Educator Signature: _____

Summative Clinical Skill Assessment (S-CSAT)

Equipment and resources: Airway mannequin suitable for LMA insertion; various sized LMA/i-gel® devices; 50/60 mL syringe if using inflatable cuff LMA; gloves, eyewear and mask; water-based gel lubricant; method of documenting results

Associated Clinical Skills: Infection control; Head positioning; Jaw thrust; Foreign body removal/suctioning; Intermittent positive pressure ventilation

Staff/Student being assessed: _____

• Completed Formative Clinical Skill Assessment (F-CSAT): **YES** **NO**

• Completed Performance Improvement Plan (PIP): **YES** **NO** **N/A**

Laryngeal mask airway insertion

Activity	Critical Action	Achieved Without Direction	
Personal protection	Dons PPE as required.	NO	YES
Assesses indications	Assesses patient consciousness and airway reflexes.	NO	YES
Selects device size	Chooses appropriate size of LMA/i-gel® for patient's body weight. Opens packaging, maintaining hygiene. If using i-gel®, removes from protective cradle.	NO	YES
Prepares equipment	Lays out LMA/i-gel® and other airway resuscitation equipment on a clean surface.	NO	YES
Prepares patient	Places patient supine with head in neutral anatomical or sniffing position.	NO	YES
	Clears any foreign material from airway before inserting LMA.	NO	YES
Prepares cuff	If device used has an inflatable cuff/mask, attaches empty 50/60 mL syringe to inflation cuff, depressing valve. Withdraws all air from cuff to cause complete inward collapse. Detaches syringe. Fills syringe with maximum air volume for device, as specified on product packaging. Reattaches syringe to inflation cuff. Injects sufficient air slowly into cuff to just cause full reinflation. Saves remaining air in syringe.	NO	YES
	Lubricates back, sides and tip of distal mask with water-based gel.	NO	YES
Inserts LMA	Performs chin lift to open mouth sufficiently wide to allow mask insertion.	NO	YES
	Holds stem firmly. Introduces tip into mouth. Gently directs upwards along mouth roof, away from the tongue.	NO	YES
	Once clear of tongue, continues pushing posteriorly, following palate curve into pharynx. If tongue cannot be cleared or resistance is encountered, gently rotates left and right to continue progress.	NO	YES
	Gently applies sufficient force to seat tip of device in oesophagus until no further progress can be made.	NO	YES
Reassesses	Ensures no airway reflex is triggered by placement.	NO	YES
Ventilates	Attaches BVM and ventilates.	NO	YES
Adjusts seal	If an air leak is suspected in the air-filled cuff LMA, titrates in some or all of the remaining air in the syringe.	NO	YES
Secures LMA	Once confident of LMA placement, secures in place in midline.	NO	YES

Laryngeal mask airway insertion continued		Achieved Without Direction	
Activity	**Critical Action**		
Duodenal tube	When convenient, inserts appropriate size of duodenal tube through gastric port and aspirates air/gastric content.	NO	YES
Reports	Accurately documents/hands over insertion time, LMA size, and any relevant information regarding placement or insertion.	NO	YES

Standard Achieved: (please circle one)

Competent (C)   Not Yet Competent* (NYC)

Staff/Student Name: _____

Assessor (please print name)**:** _____

Signed (Assessor)**:** _____

Date of Assessment: _____

Comments:

*If Not Yet Competent (NYC) a PIP needs to be completed and a repeat of the F-CSAT

Clinical findings

Return of airway reflexes

Airway reflexes may be absent on insertion but return during patient care. They may be denoted by the onset of gagging, coughing or even attempts to reach up and remove the device. LMA devices are not intended for such patients. They are typically removed when airway reflexes return and alternative options are sought.

Pharyngeal injury

Sore throat, dysphagia and minor bleeding can be noted after LMA use when consciousness returns – more so with air-inflated cuffs (Park et al., 2015) than with i-gel® use (de Montblanc et al., 2014; Moser et al., 2017; Pournajafian et al., 2015). The use of LMA reduces the incidence of upper airway injury compared to endotracheal intubation (Kishnani et al., 2016; van Esch et al., 2017). Lower cuff inflation pressure can reduce these complications (Bick et al., 2014; Venugopal et al., 2016). Injuries are more likely associated with unnecessary force or poor insertion technique.

Cardiovascular effects

Both laryngoscopy and endotracheal intubation can cause laryngeal and sympathetic stimulation, leading to tachycardia and hypertension. This can be problematic in at-risk patients, such as those with underlying cardiovascular problems or cerebrovascular disease, where elevations in intracranial pressure should be avoided.

LMA use is much less implicated than laryngoscopy and endotracheal intubation in causing these problems (Jarineshin et al., 2015; Kashani et al., 2017; Kishnani et al., 2016).

Intubation

A few LMA devices allow endotracheal intubation through them once they are in position. First verify that the specific device is intended for this use. Though the i-gel® was not, it can successfully allow this intubation to occur (Choudhary et al., 2016; Naik et al., 2016).

Children

The paediatric upper airway varies from that of adults, as children have a relatively larger tongue, epiglottis and tonsils and a shorter mandible. These predispose to upper airway obstruction (Harless et al., 2014) and intubation difficulty (Acharya and Dave, 2016).

The use of an appropriately sized LMA provides upper airway support and an alternative where intubation cannot be achieved (Keil et al., 2016; Maconochie et al., 2015). I-gel® devices are available in paediatric sizes (Acharya and Dave, 2016; Choi et al., 2014).

LMA removal

The LMA/i-gel® cannot remain in situ if airway reflexes return. If possible, suction the upper airway first, then position the patient laterally. Remove the device during coughing or exhalation and dispose of it immediately as clinical waste.

PRACTICE TIP!

The tongue poses the greatest problem during the insertion of an LMA. Using chin lift and aiming for the roof of the mouth roof are essential to avoid this issue.

PRACTICE TIP!

LMA insertion should be considered where a risk of gastric aspiration exists, including during prolonged BVM ventilation. It is expedient to insert an LMA even during cardiopulmonary resuscitation. Conversely, it is an alternative if intubation fails.

PRACTICE TIP!

Where positive pressure ventilation will be applied, such as during cardiac arrest, an LMA can be inserted quickly instead of an initial OPA/NPA.

PRACTICE TIP!

As LMA insertion is an airway procedure, it is considered high risk for infection. PPE should be used, including eyewear and a respiratory mask.

TEST YOUR KNOWLEDGE QUESTIONS

1. **How is an LMA sized for use?**
   Based on the patient's weight.

2. **What is the main impediment to LMA insertion?**
   The tongue.

3. **What mouth action assists LMA insertion?**
   Chin lift to open the mouth.

4. **Which head position is preferred when inserting an LMA?**
   Supine with the head in a neutral anatomical or sniffing position.

5. **What airway problems does LMA insertion assist with?**
   Tongue/epiglottis occlusion; soft palate collapse; gastric insufflation; oesophageal regurgitation.

6. **What contraindications preclude LMA insertion?**
   Intact airway reflexes; trismus; a mouth that is too small.

7. **Why must the LMA be maintained midline in the mouth?**
   To ensure it remains effectively seated over the hypoglottis.

8. **Where is information about LMA cuff inflation volume and pressure found?**
   On the packaging and the LMA stem.

9. **Why is there a maximum cuff air volume that must not be exceeded?**
   Excess inflation pressure can cause mucosal injury and LMA malposition.

10. **Why is the i-gel® specifically advantageous in emergency use?**
    It has a solid cuff, reducing the number of steps required for insertion.

References

Almeida, G., Costa, A.C. and Machado, H.S., 2016. Supraglottic airway devices: a review in a new era of airway management. *Journal of Anesthesia and Clinical Research*, 7, 647.

Acharya, R. and Dave, N.M., 2016. Comparison between i-gel airway and the ProSeal laryngeal mask airway in pediatric patients undergoing general anesthesia. *Pediatric Anesthesia and Critical Care Journal*, 4(2), 97–102.

Benger, J., Coates, D., Davies, S., Greenwood, R., Nolan, J., Rhys, M., Thomas, M. and Voss, S., 2016. Randomised comparison of the effectiveness of the laryngeal mask airway supreme, i-gel and current practice in the initial airway management of out of hospital cardiac arrest: a feasibility study. *British Journal of Anaesthesia*, 116(2), 262–268.

Bick, E., Bailes, I., Patel, A. and Brain, A.I.J., 2014. Fewer sore throats and a better seal: why routine manometry for laryngeal mask airways must become the standard of care. *Anaesthesia*, 69(12), 1304–1308.

Boeckxstaens, G.E., 2005. The lower oesophageal sphincter. *Neurogastroenterology & Motility*, 17(s1), 13–21.

Choi, G.J., Kang, H., Baek, C.W., Jung, Y.H., Woo, Y.C. and Cha, Y.J., 2014. A systematic review and meta-analysis of the i-gel* vs laryngeal mask airway in children. *Anaesthesia*, 69(11), 1258–1265.

Choudhary, B., Karnawat, R., Mohammed, S., Gupta, M., Srinivasan, B. and Kumar, R., 2016. Comparison of endotracheal intubation through i-gel and intubating laryngeal mask airway. *Open Anesthesiology Journal*, 10(1).

Cook, T.M. and Kelly, F.E., 2015. Time to abandon the 'vintage' laryngeal mask airway and adopt second-generation supraglottic airway devices as first choice. *British Journal of Anaesthesia*, 115(4), 497–499.

de Montblanc, J., Ruscio, L., Mazoit, J.X. and Benhamou, D., 2014. A systematic review and meta-analysis of the i-gel® vs laryngeal mask airway in adults. *Anaesthesia*, 69(10), 1151–1162.

Harless, J., Ramaiah, R. and Bhananker, S.M., 2014. Pediatric airway management. *International Journal of Critical Illness and Injury Science*, 4(1), 65.

Hu, X., Lee, J.S., Pianosi, P.T. and Ryu, J.H., 2015. Aspiration-related pulmonary syndromes. *Chest*, 147(3), 815–823.

Isono, S., 2012. Obesity and obstructive sleep apnoea: mechanisms for increased collapsibility of the passive pharyngeal airway. *Respirology*, 17(1), 32–42.

Jarineshin, H., Kashani, S., Vatankhah, M., Baghaee, A.A., Sattari, S. and Fekrat, F., 2015. Better hemodynamic profile of laryngeal mask airway insertion compared to laryngoscopy and tracheal intubation. *Iranian Red Crescent Medical Journal*, 17(8).

Kashani, S., Khosravi, F. and Jarineshin, H., 2017. Hemodynamic responses to insertion of the laryngeal mask airway versus Combitube. *Hormozgan Medical Journal*, 20.

Keil, J., Jung, P., Schiele, A., Urban, B., Parsch, A., Matsche, B., Eich, C., Becke, K., Landsleitner, B., Russo, S.G. and Bernhard, M., 2016. Interdisciplinary consensus statement on alternative airway management with supraglottic airway devices in pediatric emergency medicine: laryngeal mask is state of the art. *Anaesthesist*, 65(1), 57–66.

Kishnani, P.P., Tripathi, D.C., Trivedi, L., Shah, K., Patel, J. and Ladumor, J., 2016. Hemodynamic stress response during insertion of ProSeal laryngeal mask airway and endotracheal tube – a prospective randomized comparative study. *International Journal of Research Medicine*, 5(2), 34–38.

Lee, A., Festic, E., Park, P.K., Raghavendran, K., Dabbagh, O., Adesanya, A., Gajic, O. and Bartz, R.R., 2014. Characteristics and outcomes of patients hospitalized following pulmonary aspiration. *Chest*, 146(4), 899–907.

Ma, M.A., Kumar, R., Macey, P.M., Yan-Go, F.L. and Harper, R.M., 2016. Epiglottis cross-sectional area and oropharyngeal airway length in male and female obstructive sleep apnea patients. *Nature and Science of Sleep*, 8, 297.

Maconochie, I.K., Bingham, R., Eich, C., López-Herce, J., Rodríguez-Núnez, A., Rajka, T., Van de Voorde, P., Zideman, D.A., Biarent, D., Monsieurs, K.G. and Nolan, J.P., 2015. European Resuscitation Council guidelines for resuscitation 2015, section 6: Paediatric life support. *Resuscitation*, 95, 223–248.

Mishra, S.K., Nawaz, M., Satyapraksh, M.V.S., Parida, S., Bidkar, P.U., Hemavathy, B. and Kundra, P., 2015. Influence of head and neck position on oropharyngeal leak pressure and cuff position with the ProSeal laryngeal mask airway and the i-gel: a randomized clinical trial. *Anesthesiology Research and Practice*, doi: 10.1155/2015/705869.

Moser, B., Brimacombe, J., Sharma, B., Dutta, A. and Sood, J., 2017. Prolonged use of the laryngeal mask airway ProSeal™: a report of seven cases lasting 5–11 h. *Journal of Anesthesia and Clinical Research*, 8(717), 2.

Naik, L., Bhardwaj, N., Sen, I.M. and Sondekoppam, R.V., 2016. Intubation success through i-gel* and Intubating Laryngeal Mask Airway* using flexible silicone tubes: a randomised noninferiority trial. *Anesthesiology Research and Practice*, doi: 10.1155/2016/7318595.

Nalini, K.B., Shivakumar, S., Archana, S., Rani, D.C.S. and Mohan, C.V.R., 2016. Comparison of three insertion techniques of ProSeal laryngeal mask airway: a randomized clinical trial. *Journal of Anaesthesiology Clinical Pharmacology*, 32(4), 510.

Park, S.K., Choi, G.J., Choi, Y.S., Ahn, E.J. and Kang, H., 2015. Comparison of the i-gel and the Laryngeal Mask Airway ProSeal during general anesthesia: a systematic review and meta-analysis. *PLOS ONE*, 10(3), e0119469.

Pournajafian, A., Alimian, M., Rokhtabnak, F., Ghodraty, M. and Mojri, M., 2015. Success rate of airway devices insertion: laryngeal mask airway versus supraglottic gel device. *Anesthesiology and Pain Medicine*, 5(2).

Singh, S. and Hamdy, S., 2005. The upper oesophageal sphincter. *Neurogastroenterology & Motility*, 17(s1), 3–12.

Soar, J., Nolan, J.P., Böttiger, B.W., Perkins, G.D., Lott, C., Carli, P., Pellis, T., Sandroni, C., Skrifvars, M.B., Smith, G.B. and Sunde, K., 2015. European Resuscitation Council guidelines for resuscitation 2015, section 3: Adult advanced life support. *Resuscitation*, 95, 100–147.

Suibhne, P.M., White, D. and Riain, S.Ó., 2018. AB220. 113. An audit of adult laryngeal mask airway size selection. *Mesentery and Peritoneum*, 2(2).

Timmermann, A., Bergner, U.A. and Russo, S.G., 2015. Laryngeal mask airway indications: new frontiers for second-generation supraglottic airways. *Current Opinion in Anesthesiology*, 28(6), 717–726.

van Esch, B.F., Stegeman, I. and Smit, A.L., 2017. Comparison of laryngeal mask airway vs tracheal intubation: a systematic review on airway complications. *Journal of Clinical Anesthesia*, 36, 142–150.

Venugopal, A., Jacob, R.M. and Koshy, R.C., 2016. A randomized control study comparing the pharyngolaryngeal morbidity of laryngeal mask airway versus endotracheal tube. *Anesthesia, Essays and Researches*, 10(2), 189.

Bibliography

Craft, J., Gordon, C., Huether, S.E., McCance, K.L. and Brashers, V.L., 2015. *Understanding pathophysiology (ANZ adaptation)*. Sydney: Elsevier.

McCance, K.L. and Huether, S.E., 2015. *Pathophysiology: the biologic basis for disease in adults and children*. Sydney: Elsevier.

3.9 | Endotracheal intubation

Nick Holden

Chapter objectives

At the end of this chapter the reader will be able to:

1. Describe the rationale for performing endotracheal intubation
2. Demonstrate the successful method of endotracheal intubation
3. Identify difficulties and complications with endotracheal intubation
4. Recognise and respond to difficult airway problems that can arise

Resources required for this assessment

- Mannequin with airway and airway structures
- Endotracheal intubation equipment
- Hand decontamination agent
- Disposable gloves, respiratory mask, protective eyewear
- Clinical waste bag
- Method of documenting results

Skill matrix

This assessment requires:

- Infection control (CS 1.3)
- Consent (CS 1.6)
- Patient assessment skills (Chapter 2, CS 2.1, 2.6, 2.7, 2.8, 2.10)
- Airway and ventilation skills (Chapter 3, CS 3.2, 3.3, 3.6, 3.7, 3.11)

This assessment is a component of:

- Airway and ventilation (Chapter 3)

Introduction

Endotracheal intubation is described as the 'gold standard' for airway protection in patients who are unable to maintain a patent airway (Gregory and Mursell, 2010; Hillman et al., 2003). However, maintaining airway patency is not restricted to endotracheal intubation. Supine posturing can allow gravity to collapse the soft palate and the tongue/epiglottis to obstruct the glottis/ trachea. Lateral position, oro/nasopharyngeal airway devices and jaw thrust/chin lift can therefore assist (see Chapters 3.1.2–3.5). While supraglottic airway devices can provide gastric protection (Chapter 3.8), these are not always sufficient.

This chapter describes the skill of intubation in the adult patient with absent airway reflexes.

Anatomy and physiology

The upper airway comprises the nasal cavity and mouth, leading to the softer nasopharynx and oropharynx curving inferiorly and posteriorly. The tongue is at the base of the mouth, with the epiglottis posterior to it. Between the base of the tongue and the epiglottis is the vallecular groove. Behind the epiglottis are the glottis and the vocal cords on its left and right. Beyond are the larynx and trachea (see Chapter 3.6).

Airway patency forms the basis of many emergency resuscitation guidelines. A patent airway means an unobstructed pathway between the mouth/nose atmospheric opening and the lower alveoli where gas exchange occurs.

The upper airway provides a major role in protection against potential obstructions, employing several anatomical and reflex features. These include the glottis (and vocal cords within), which not only has a role in speech but can close when irritated to reduce the passage of foreign bodies. Nerve reflexes include sneezing, gagging, swallowing and coughing (Nishino, 2000).

Pharyngeal muscles maintain upper airway patency when the person is conscious. Airway reflexes and patency become depressed with reduced consciousness, age, anaesthesia, some drugs and some diseases, such as stroke. The pharynx is collapsible, compared to the nasal cavity and larynx/trachea on either side and, with reduced airway reflexes, is a vulnerable point.

Clinical rationale

Endotracheal intubation

Endotracheal intubation is indicated when an adequate airway cannot be maintained through less-invasive airway devices (Field et al., 2012). This can occur in acute respiratory insufficiency or cardiac arrest. Some key indications include the patient:
- with no response to painful stimuli
- with no gag or cough reflex
- who requires ongoing ventilation.

Patients with loss of airway reflexes or those being positive-pressure ventilated are at risk of passive gastric content aspiration, and all prehospital patients are considered to be unfasted.

Special note: Only experienced paramedics should attempt endotracheal tube insertion after careful assessment of any difficulties anticipated or risks. Intubation should not be attempted if difficulties are considered prohibitive, as the procedure performance itself may lead to prolonged hypoxia or deterioration of the patient's condition. It should also not be attempted where there is sufficient consciousness for airway reflexes to be present. In such cases, prior drug facilitation is necessary to both provide sufficient sedation to remove any physiological and conscious awareness that the patient may have, as well as muscle relaxation (paralysis) to remove motor (gag/cough) responses.

Equipment

The following equipment is required for safe and effective intubation:
- personal protective equipment, including respiratory mask and eyewear; airway procedures are always considered high risk for infection transmission
- stethoscope
- endotracheal tubes (ETT) in assorted sizes, usually cuffed:
  - adult male: 8.0–9.0 mm internal diameter
  - adult female: 7.0–8.0 mm internal diameter
- bougie and introducing stylet appropriately sized for endotracheal tubes
- failed intubation airway devices, including supraglottic and oro/nasopharyngeal options

- laryngoscope with size 3 and 4 Macintosh blades
- Magill's forceps
- airway lubricant
- oxygen supply
- suction unit with suction catheter
- bag/valve/mask (BVM) with end tidal CO_2 and bacterial filter attached
- 10 mL syringe and manometer
- securing device (tape or device such as the Thomas Tube Holder).

Equipment should be laid out on a clean surface on the right-hand side of the patient's head. Ensure everything is pre-gathered to cater for all unforeseen contingencies. Inspect the equipment for correct functioning. Prepare each item of equipment for use, including insertion of intubating stylet into the ETT.

Endotracheal tubes

A range of ETT are available. There are minor cosmetic differences between them, but the majority share distinct features (Fig. 3.9.1), including:
- a pilot balloon, for verifying cuff pressure
- a cuff, which holds about 10 mL of air but should be inflated with only 6–7 mL of air (20–30 cm H_2O pressure) to seal the airway and avoid excessive pressure on the trachea wall (Carhart et al., 2016)
- a Murphy's eye – a small hole across from the bevel (distal tube end) to reduce the risk of tip obstruction.

To aid correct placement of the ETT, the paramedic may use a stylet (a pliable metal device) to help guide the ETT. This is placed inside the ETT, with the tip sitting near the Murphy eye. A J-shaped bend (Fig. 3.9.2) is usually preformed for use. Alternatively, a bougie (a 70 cm long pliable plastic catheter) with a diameter of 4.6 mm (14 Fr) can be used. The bougie is placed in the trachea first and then the ETT is fed over the top. A bougie is used with tubes greater than 6 mm in diameter.

Head position

Placing the head in the sniffing position with lower cervical flexion and upper cervical extension, aligning the ear opening with sternum angle, enhances pharyngeal airway tension and decreases collapse. It also improves glottic view under laryngoscopy (see Chapters 3.2 and 3.6) (Frerk et al., 2015).

Intubation

The ETT is passed with the right hand, since laryngoscopy is a left-handed procedure. With the epiglottis and airway landmarks identified, laryngoscopy exposes the glottis to view. Either the pre-shaped introducer stylet/ETT or the bougie is introduced into the right corner of the patient's mouth (see Fig. 3.9.2). Using the J-shaped stylet or the curved bougie tip allows the clinician to direct the ETT tip towards the anteriorly located glottis.

The ETT is slowly advanced while maintaining a continuous view of the glottis. Gently approach the glottis and place the ETT tip between the cords. Advance

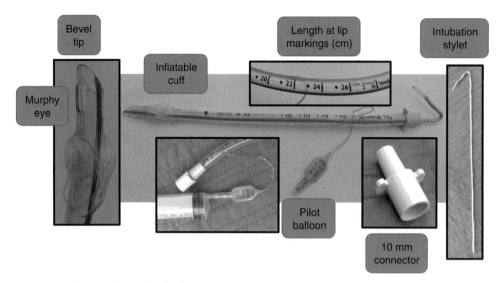

Figure 3.9.1 Components of an endotracheal tube

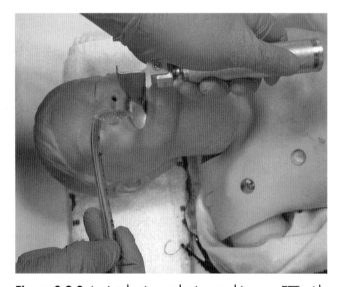

Figure 3.9.2 An intubation stylet inserted into an ETT with a J-shaped bend added

forwards, watching the entry of the tip and then the cuff. Just proximal to the cuff are black line(s) that prompt the correct depth of ETT as it passes through the glottis. However, these can vary, and so provide an initial guide only (Goel and Lim, 2003).

Where the bougie is used, it must first be positioned with the curve tip passed into the trachea. The bougie is often used where the glottis cannot be seen; if possible, observe its passage between vocal cords. Avoid pushing too far downwards due to the risk of stimulating or traumatising the carina (Frerk et al., 2015). While holding the bougie in place, pass the ETT over it until it reaches the required insertion depth (Fig. 3.9.3). An assistant may be helpful for this.

Post confirmation

Once the ETT is positioned, the paramedic must confirm that it is correctly placed in the trachea and not the oesophagus (Frerk et al., 2015). This is performed by:

- observing the ETT pass between the vocal cords
- auscultating for distinctive gastric gurgling sounds over the stomach during ventilation
- auscultating both lungs to assess for lung inflation and air movement during ventilation
- confirming chest rise and fall during ventilation
- condensation (misting) inside the ETT with each ventilation
- where available, attaching end tidal CO_2 monitoring to detect readings and waveform.

Where there is any doubt about placement, remove the ETT and return to BVM/oxygenation.

Once tracheal placement has been confirmed, assess its depth at the lips using the numerical markings along the ETT length. The ETT is typically placed approximately 2.5 cm above the sensitive carina at the bronchial bifurcation. The ETT marking at the patient's lips is the reference used (see Fig. 3.9.1). The positioning is 21–23 cm for adult males and 19–21 cm for adult females, varying with height (Roberts et al., 1995; Sitzwohl et al., 2010).

Secure the ETT in place using cloth or adhesive tying tape tied in clove hitch around the ETT stem, near the lip length position, and then passed around patient's neck, without impacting on circulation. Alternative manufactured securing devices can be used (Carlson et al., 2007).

Clinical skill assessment process

The following section outlines the clinical skill assessment tools that should be used to determine a student's ability to demonstrate safe and accurate endotracheal intubation.

1. Clinical Skill Work Instruction
2. Formative Clinical Skill Assessment (F-CSAT)
3. Performance Improvement Plan (PIP)
4. Summative Clinical Skill Assessment (S-CSAT)
(5. Direct Observation of Procedural Skills (DOPS) – see Chapter 1.1)

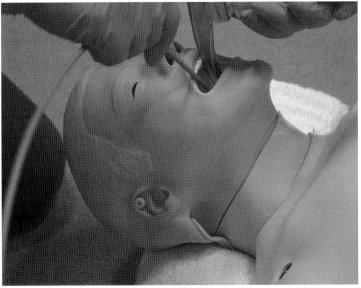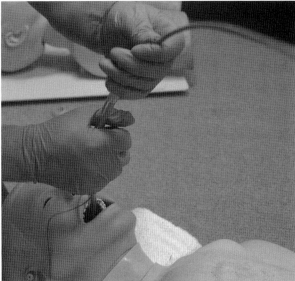

Figure 3.9.3 Inserting an ETT using a bougie

Clinical Skill Work Instruction

Equipment and resources: Airway mannequin; endotracheal intubation equipment; hand decontamination agent; disposable gloves, mask and eyewear; clinical waste bag; method of documenting results

Associated Clinical Skills: Infection control; Consent; Patient assessment skills; Airway and ventilation skills

Endotracheal intubation

Activity	Critical Action	Rationale
Prepare paramedic	Don gloves, eyewear and respiratory mask.	To provide protection from blood-borne or bodily fluids during procedure.
Prepare equipment	Lay out all equipment in preparation. Ensure operation of laryngoscope suction and tube cuff, including difficult airway devices.	Preparation ensures all available equipment needed is functional.
Prepare patient	Pre-oxygenate using BVM and positive pressure ventilation, if necessary, with high-flow oxygen for at least 3 minutes.	Intubation takes time, during which no oxygen is being supplied to the patient. Pre-oxygenation and de-nitrogenation help reduce onset of hypoxia during the procedure (Frerk et al., 2015).
	Position patient's head in the sniffing position with padding. (If spinal injury is suspected, consider using neutral anatomical position and manual in-line stabilisation.)	Appropriate positioning of the patient's head improves vocal cord view and helps achieve 'first pass intubation'.
	Assess risks for difficult intubation.	Advance warning of difficulties can allow prior consideration of solutions or avoidance.
Perform laryngoscopy	Pick up laryngoscope in left hand. Ensure blade is locked in position with the light on. Perform laryngoscopy as in Chapter 3.6. Note airway structures during insertion, particularly epiglottis.	Anatomical landmarks will assist in locating vocal cords/glottis.

Endotracheal intubation continued

Activity	Critical Action	Rationale
Visualise glottic opening	Visualise glottic opening and vocal cords and keep them in sight.	Consider view grade while visualising cords and consider difficulty and requirement for stylet and ET sizing.
Direct ETT passage	If using ETT with inner stylet, insert into right side of patient's mouth. Follow tip passage into oropharynx and pass between vocal cords until cuff and line markings move distal.	The ETT is placed just through the glottis into the trachea.
Bougie passage	Insert bougie into the right side of the mouth and through the glottis, feeling for tracheal clicks (the sound and feeling of the bougie running over the tracheal rings).	Passing the bougie through the trachea provides a guide for ETT.
Intubation over bougie	Holding bougie in place at lips, feed or have assistant 'railroad' the ETT over the bougie until at required lip length. Gentle rotation may be required during passage if the tip meets any resistance.	Visualising the procedure can aid in confirming tracheal placement. The bougie will have to be held above the ETT as it nears the lips.
Remove bougie	Hold ETT in place at lips. Withdraw bougie.	Until it is secured, the tube is easily displaced.
Inflate cuff and confirm placement	Inflate the ETT cuff. Confirm ETT placement.	Oesophageal or bronchial placement can be catastrophic.
Secure ETT	Secure the ETT with tape or Thomas device.	Securing prevents the tube inadvertently being pulled out.
Report	Accurately document/hand over the findings.	Accurate record keeping and continuity of care.

Formative Clinical Skill Assessment (F-CSAT)

Equipment and resources: Airway mannequin; endotracheal intubation equipment; hand decontamination agent; disposable gloves, mask and eyewear; clinical waste bag; method of documenting results

Associated Clinical Skills: Infection control; Consent; Patient assessment skills; Airway and ventilation skills

Staff/Student being assessed: _____

Endotracheal intubation

Activity	Critical Action	Performance				
Prepares paramedic	Dons gloves, eyewear and respiratory mask.	0	1	2	3	4
Prepares equipment	Lays out all equipment in preparation. Ensures operation of laryngoscope suction and tube cuff, including difficult airway devices.	0	1	2	3	4
Prepares patient	Pre-oxygenates with BVM/high-flow oxygen for at least 3 minutes.	0	1	2	3	4
	Positions patient's head in sniffing position with padding. (Modifies appropriately for suspected spinal injury.)	0	1	2	3	4
	Assesses risks for difficult intubation.	0	1	2	3	4
Performs laryngoscopy	Performs laryngoscopy as per procedures and notes airway structures visible.	0	1	2	3	4

Endotracheal intubation continued

Activity	Critical Action	Performance				
Visualises glottic opening	Visualises glottic opening and vocal cords, and keeps them in sight.	0	1	2	3	4
Directs ETT passage	If using ETT/stylet, inserts into right side of patient's mouth. Passes into oropharynx and places between vocal cords correctly.	0	1	2	3	4
Bougie passage	Inserts bougie into right side of the mouth and through the glottis, feeling for tracheal clicks.	0	1	2	3	4
Intubation over bougie	Holding bougie in place at lips, feeds or has assistant 'railroad' ETT over the bougie until at required lip length.	0	1	2	3	4
Removes bougie	Holds ETT in place at lips. Withdraws bougie.	0	1	2	3	4
Inflates cuff and confirms placement	Inflates ETT cuff. Confirms ETT placement.	0	1	2	3	4
Secures ETT	Secures ETT with tape or Thomas device.	0	1	2	3	4
Reports	Accurately documents/hands over the findings.	0	1	2	3	4

Standard Achieved: (please circle one)

Competent (C)   Not Yet Competent* (NYC)

Staff/Student Name: _____

Assessor (please print name)**:** _____

Signed (Assessor)**:** _____

Date of Assessment: _____

Comments:

*If Not Yet Competent (NYC) a PIP needs to be completed and a repeat of the F-CSAT

Formative Clinical Skill Assessment (F-CSAT) Key

Skill level	Standard of procedure	Quality of performance	Outcome	Level of assistance required
4 Safe for unsupervised practice	Safe Accurate Behaviour is appropriate to context	Confident Accurate Expedient	Achieved intended outcome	No supporting cues* required
3 Requires supervision	Safe Accurate Behaviour is appropriate to context	Confident Accurate Takes longer than required	Achieved intended outcome	Requires occasional supportive cues*

Skill level	Standard of procedure	Quality of performance	Outcome	Level of assistance required
2 Requires assistance	Safe Accurate Behaviour generally appropriate to context	Lacks certainty	Would not have achieved outcome without support	Requires frequent verbal and occasional physical directives in addition to supportive cues*
1 Requires direction	Safe only with guidance Not completely accurate	Unskilled Inefficient	Would not have achieved outcome without support	Requires continuous verbal and frequent physical directive cues*
0 Unsafe	Unsafe Unable to demonstrate behaviour Lack of insight into behaviour appropriate to context	Unskilled	Would not have achieved outcome	Requires continuous verbal and continuous physical directive cues*

*Refers to physical directives or verbal supportive cues

Performance Improvement Plan (PIP)

Please document the agreed education plan and completion timelines for areas assessed as less than 4.

This plan should be presented to assessor prior to commencement of summative assessment.

Where was supervisor support required?	Student summary of deficit. (Why was there a problem?)	Improvement Plan	Completed (Y/N)

Staff/Student Name: _____

Staff/Student Signature: _____

Educator Name: _____

Educator Signature: _____

Summative Clinical Skill Assessment (S-CSAT)

Equipment and resources: Airway mannequin; endotracheal intubation equipment; hand decontamination agent; disposable gloves, mask and eyewear; clinical waste bag; method of documenting results

Associated Clinical Skills: Infection control; Consent; Patient assessment skills; Airway and ventilation skills

Staff/Student being assessed: _____

- Completed Formative Clinical Skill Assessment (F-CSAT): **YES** **NO**

- Completed Performance Improvement Plan (PIP): **YES** **NO** **N/A**

Endotracheal intubation

Activity	Critical Action	Achieved Without Direction	
Prepares paramedic	Dons gloves, eyewear and respiratory mask.	NO	YES
Prepares equipment	Lays out all equipment in preparation. Ensures operation of laryngoscope suction and tube cuff, including difficult airway devices.	NO	YES
Prepares patient	Pre-oxygenates with BVM/high flow oxygen for at least 3 minutes.	NO	YES
	Positions patient's head in sniffing position with padding. (Modifies appropriately for suspected spinal injury.)	NO	YES
	Assesses risks for difficult intubation.	NO	YES
Performs laryngoscopy	Performs laryngoscopy as per procedures and notes airway structures visible.	NO	YES
Visualises glottic opening	Visualises the glottic opening and vocal cords, and keeps them in sight.	NO	YES
Directs ETT passage	If using ETT/stylet, inserts into right side of patient's mouth. Passes into oropharynx and places between vocal cords correctly.	NO	YES
Bougie passage	Inserts bougie into right side of the mouth and through the glottis, feeling for tracheal clicks.	NO	YES
Intubation over bougie	Holding bougie in place at lips, feeds or has assistant 'railroad' ETT over the bougie until at required lip length.	NO	YES
Removes bougie	Holds ETT in place at lips. Withdraws bougie.	NO	YES
Inflates cuff and confirms placement	Inflates ETT cuff. Confirms ETT placement.	NO	YES
Secures ETT	Secures ETT with tape or Thomas device.	NO	YES
Reports	Accurately documents/hands over the findings.	NO	YES

Standard Achieved: (please circle one)

Competent (C)   Not Yet Competent* (NYC)

Staff/Student: _____

Assessor (please print name): _____

Signed (Assessor): _____

Date of Assessment: _____

Comments:

*If Not Yet Competent (NYC) a PIP needs to be completed and a repeat of the F-CSAT

Clinical findings

Hypoxia

Intubation implies the temporary absence of oxygenation or ventilation. Pre-oxygenation and alveolar de-nitrogenation can prolong the period before desaturation occurs, but this is finite in emergencies. Short intubation attempts not exceeding 20 seconds are advised, with a return to oxygenation afterwards. Monitoring pulse oximetry is essential.

Soiled airway

Glottic view may be impeded by vomitus or foreign body obstruction. If necessary, remove this appropriately (see Chapter 3.7). Properly applied cricoid pressure (Sellick's manoeuvre) can be applied before and during intubation to avoid the passive escape of gastric contents (Frerk et al., 2015).

Airway reflexes present

If the patient has airway gag reflexes present, vomiting may be stimulated. This can also raise intracranial pressure, which is to be avoided in neurological emergencies. In either case, abandon the procedure and use drug-facilitated intubation.

Difficult airway assessment

Before attempting intubation, assess the patient for difficult airway predictors, including obesity, a large neck circumference, a small mouth opening, large teeth, a large tongue, decreased neck length, limited head/neck flexion or extension, a small jaw, facial trauma/oedema, high Mallampati score or decreased thyromental distance (Gaither et al., 2014; Hillman et al., 2003; Joshi et al., 2017; Riad et al., 2016; Sakles et al., 2014). Depending on the level of difficulty, either abandon the attempt or use assist methods to overcome the problem (Frerk et al., 2015).

Difficulty assist methods

If, despite optimal head position and laryngoscope technique, it is still not possible to view the glottis, assist methods may be used. Commonly, the glottis will be anatomically anteriorly positioned upwards, out of view. Pressure can be applied by the paramedic/assistant pushing downwards on the larynx to bring the vocal cords in view if possible. Alternatively, the bougie or J-curved intubating stylet can be directed upwards into the area where the glottis is estimated to be, despite being out of sight, for an attempt at blind intubation (Frerk et al., 2015).

Cannot intubate

Occasionally, intubation will not be possible despite the paramedic's best efforts. In such cases, an immediate return to BVM/oxygenation is required, using the most appropriate alternative airway method. If this cannot be achieved, surgical airway must be considered (see Chapter 3.10).

Patient movements

Whenever an intubated patient is moved, the ETT should be held with thumb and forefinger while the remaining fingers hook gently under the jaw. The patient's head must not be allowed to move, either laterally or through flexion/extension, to avoid inadvertent displacement of the ETT. Recheck its position following every move.

PRACTICE TIP!

Preparation for intubation must include the orderly layout of equipment and inspection in advance. Unpredictable requirements for devices can occur, and equipment failure can prove disastrous.

PRACTICE TIP!

Intubation is ideally performed using an airway team. One paramedic will perform the intubation and at least one other paramedic will assist to prepare, test and pass equipment. Assistance with laryngeal manipulation, bougie intubation and vital sign monitoring is important.

PRACTICE TIP!

The most qualified and experienced paramedic on scene should usually perform the intubation. A team leader is essential to ensure paramedic team performs in a timely, safe and effective manner.

PRACTICE TIP!

Prepare a tube size above and below the estimated size in case it is required. This assists by having an alternative ready for use if the first size chosen is not suitable (Jones & Bartlett Learning, 2013).

PRACTICE TIP!

Airway procedures are always considered high risk for exposure to infectious blood or bodily fluids. The use of gloves, respiratory masks and eyewear is important for the protection of all attending paramedics.

TEST YOUR KNOWLEDGE QUESTIONS

1. **What key indications for intubation exist?**
    No response to painful stimuli; absent gag/cough reflex; ongoing need for ventilation.

2. **What hazard exists with loss of airway reflex or during positive pressure ventilation?**
    The risk of passive gastric content aspiration.

3. **When should intubation not be attempted?**
    If difficulties are considered prohibitive or if there is sufficient consciousness for airway reflexes to be present.

4. **What two methods can be used to pass the ETT through the vocal cords?**
    Passing the ETT over an intubating stylet; railroading over a bougie that is already in position.

5. **What lip length is usually selected for ETT insertion depth?**
    21–23 cm for adult males, 19–21 cm for adult females.

6. **List three confirmation checks of intubation placement.**
    Visualise ETT pass between vocal cords; auscultate stomach gurgling sounds; lung ventilation; chest rise and fall; ETT misting; end tidal CO_2.

7. **What is the usual optimal head position for intubation?**
    Sniffing position with head elevated to align ear opening with sternum angle.

8. **ETT cuffs are usually filled with what air volume/pressure?**
    6-7 mL air at 20–30 cm H_2O pressure.

9. **How long should a single intubation attempt last and why?**
    No more than 20 seconds to minimise the risk of oxygen desaturation.

10. **List three features that suggest difficult airway.**
    Obesity; large neck circumference; small mouth opening; large teeth; large tongue; decreased neck length; limited head/neck flexion or extension; small jaw; facial trauma/oedema; high Mallampati score; decreased thyromental distance.

References

Carhart, E., Stuck, L.H. and Salzman, J.G., 2016. Achieving a safe endotracheal tube cuff pressure in the prehospital setting: is it time to revise the standard cuff inflation practice? *Prehospital Emergency Care*, 20(2), 273–277.

Carlson, J., Mayrose, J., Krause, R. and Jehle, D., 2007. Extubation force: tape versus endotracheal tube holders. *Annals of Emergency Medicine*, 50(6), 686–691.

Field, J., Kudenchuk, P., O'Conner, R. and VandenHoek, T., 2012. *The textbook of emergency cardiovascular care and CPR.* Philadelphia: Lippincott Willliams & Wilkins.

Frerk, C., Mitchell, V.S., McNarry, A.F., Mendonca, C., Bhagrath, R., Patel, A., O'Sullivan, E.P., Woodall, N.M. and Ahmad, I., 2015. Difficult Airway Society 2015 guidelines for management of unanticipated difficult intubation in adults. *British Journal of Anaesthesia*, 115(6), 827–848.

Gaither, J.B., Spaite, D.W., Stolz, U., Ennis, J., Mosier, J. and Sakles, J.J., 2014. Prevalence of difficult airway predictors in cases of failed prehospital endotracheal intubation. *Journal of Emergency Medicine*, 47(3), 294–300.

Goel, S. and Lim, S.L., 2003. The intubation depth marker: the confusion of the black line. *Pediatric Anesthesia*, 13(7), 579–583.

Gregory, P. and Mursell, I., 2010. *Manual of clinical paramedic procedures.* Chichester: Wiley-Blackwell.

Hillman, D.R., Platt, P.R. and Eastwood, P.R., 2003. The upper airway during anaesthesia. *British Journal of Anaesthesia*, 91(1), 31–39.

Jones & Bartlett Learning, 2013. *Endotracheal procedure.* Burlington: Jones & Bartlett Learning.

Joshi, R., Hypes, C.D., Greenberg, J., Snyder, L., Malo, J., Bloom, J.W., Chopra, H., Sakles, J.C. and Mosier, J.M., 2017. Difficult airway characteristics associated with first-attempt failure at intubation using video laryngoscopy in the intensive care unit. *Annals of the American Thoracic Society*, 14(3), 368–375.

Nishino, T., 2000. Physiological and pathophysiological implications of upper airway reflexes in humans. *Japanese Journal of Physiology*, 50(1), 3–14.

Riad, W., Vaez, M.N., Raveendran, R., Tam, A.D., Quereshy, F.A., Chung, F. and Wong, D.T., 2016. Neck circumference as a predictor of difficult intubation and difficult mask ventilation in morbidly obese patients: a prospective observational study. *European Journal of Anaesthesiology*, 33(4), 244–249.

Roberts, J.R., Spadafora, M. and Cone, D.C., 1995. Proper depth placement of oral endotracheal tubes in adults prior to radiographic confirmation. *Academic Emergency Medicine*, 2, 20–24.

Sakles, J.C., Patanwala, A.E., Mosier, J.M. and Dicken, J.M., 2014. Comparison of video laryngoscopy to direct laryngoscopy for intubation of patients with difficult airway characteristics in the emergency department. *Internal and Emergency Medicine*, 9(1), 93–98.

Sitzwohl, C., Langheinrich, A., Schober, A., Krafft, P., Sessler, D.I., Herkner, H., Gonano, C., Weinstabl, C. and Kettner, S.C., 2010. Endobronchial intubation detected by insertion depth of endotracheal tube, bilateral auscultation, or observation of chest movements: randomised trial. *BMJ*, doi: 10.1136/bmj.c5943.

Bibliography

Brunner, L.S. and Smeltzer, S.C., 2010. *Brunner & Suddarth's textbook of medical-surgical nursing.* Philadelphia: Wolters Kluwer/Lippincott Williams & Wilkins.

Hagberg, C., 2013. *Benumof and Hagberg's airway management.* Philadelphia: Elsevier.

3.10 | Surgical airway

Jeff Kenneally

Chapter objectives

At the end of this chapter the reader will be able to:

1. Describe the rationale for establishing a surgical airway
2. Demonstrate the method of surgical cricothyroidotomy
3. Identify difficulties and complications with emergency cricothyroidotomy

Resources required for this assessment

- Airway mannequin with surgical airway capability
- Scalpel and blade (size 10)
- Bougie
- 5.0/6.0 mm cuffed endotracheal tubes
- Bag/valve/mask (BVM) resuscitator
- Hand decontamination agent
- Disposable gloves, respiratory mask, protective eyewear
- Clinical waste bag
- Sharps waste container
- Method of documenting the results

Skill matrix

This assessment requires:

- Infection control (CS 1.3)
- Communication (CS 1.5)
- Consent (CS 1.6)
- Patient assessment skills (Chapter 2, CS 2.1, 2.6, 2.7, 2.8, 2.10)
- Airway and ventilation skills (Chapter 3, CS 3.2, 3.11)

This assessment is a component of:

- Airway and ventilation (Chapter 3)

Introduction

On rare occasions, the paramedic will be confronted with the feared 'cannot intubate–cannot ventilate/oxygenate' (CICV/O) situation. This may be where an intubation attempt is considered unfeasible or it may follow an unsuccessful attempt. In any case, where upper airway patency compromise is life threatening and no other alternative exists, emergency surgical or percutaneous cricothyroidotomy is the last option.

This chapter describes surgical cricothyroidotomy in the adult patient where all other attempts at airway patency and ventilation have failed.

Anatomy and physiology

The distal upper airway extends from the hypopharynx to the trachea. It is largely comprised of the larynx, made up of a number of cartilages including the epiglottis, the large thyroid and the cricoid. The thyroid is attached to the hyoid bone via the thyrohyoid membrane ligament.

The cricoid cartilage ring forms the inferior point for tracheal attachment. The cricothyroid membrane (ligament) attaches the cricoid to the thyroid cartilage with around 10 mm between (Ince and Melachuri, 2017; Myatra et al., 2016). Laterally are the cricothyroid muscles, which are used in speech.

The larynx is dividable into the supraglottis, the glottis (containing the vocal cords) about 10 mm above the cricothyroid membrane and the subglottis. The entire structure is innervated by the vagus and laryngeal nerves.

The movement of the pharynx and larynx, the closure of the epiglottis over the glottis, and the glottis itself all participate in protecting the airway against the entry of foreign bodies, through swallowing, coughing and closure of the vocal cords.

The superior and inferior laryngeal artery and vein service the larynx. These run laterally to the structure, as do the carotid artery, jugular veins and thyroid vessels. All are well clear of the anterior cricothyroid membrane.

Clinical rationale

Emergency cricothyroidotomy accesses the anterior cricothyroid membrane (Melchiors et al., 2016). Cricothyroidotomy is a temporary intervention that is frequently replaced by tracheotomy afterwards (Andersson et al., 2014; Ince and Melachuri, 2017).

If cricothyroidotomy is to be attempted, inform all paramedics about the life-threatening situation of the airway. There are multiple 'front of neck access' methods, none of which are necessarily better than any other (Asai, 2016; Frerk et al., 2015; Kristensen et al., 2015; Marshall, 2016; Mallari et al., 2016; Myatra et al., 2016).

For paramedics, who are almost always relatively inexperienced with these procedures, the surgical method is favoured over percutaneous methods due to the relative speed with which it can be performed and its significantly higher success rates (Asai, 2016; Chrisman et al., 2016; Frerk et al., 2015; Heymans et al., 2016; Kristensen et al., 2015; Pracy et al., 2016). All methods share the principle of incision through the cricothyroid membrane and insertion of a tube into the trachea through the wound.

Surgical cricothyroidotomy involves a larger incision, or forceps dissection, through the cricothyroid membrane and then passage of a bougie into the trachea, followed by an endotracheal tube over it. This uses the equipment already available without necessitating purpose-designed devices. It provides airway protection through the inflatable cuff (Kristensen et al., 2015).

Percutaneous cricothyroidotomy involves needle access. The Seldinger method, which can sometimes be difficult to perform, inserts a hollow needle through an incision in the cricothyroid membrane, feeding a guide wire through the needle. In turn, a dilator/cannula is fed over the wire to expand the opening size.. Needle insertion directly into the cricothyroid membrane is an alternative, but the diameter of the needle is typically smaller (<4 mm) and more likely to kink or occlude (Asai, 2016; Frerk et al., 2015; Kristensen et al., 2015; Marshall, 2016; Myatra et al., 2016). Following penetration of the skin, the insertion is angled slightly towards the lungs to ensure the correct direction (Ince and Melachuri, 2017). Larger sized needle kits exist but these require considerable insertion force and have a high failure rate (Ince and Melachuri, 2017).

Patients considered difficult for intubation are more likely to require emergency cricothyroidotomy (Marshall, 2016). Despite the urgency in life-threatening situations, cricothyroidotomy is frequently attempted too late (Ince and Melachuri, 2017).

Head position

It is likely that the patient will be in a sniffing position for airway intervention. For cricothyroidotomy, the optimal head position should be changed to one with neck extended, exposing the larynx. Remove pillows/padding from beneath the occiput and consider raising the shoulders a few centimetres to facilitate the procedure (Frerk et al., 2015; Ince and Melachuri, 2017; Myatra et al., 2016; Patel and Meyer, 2014).

The paramedic should be positioned at the patient's head, either superiorly or to one side. If positioned to one side, keep the dominant hand closest to the patient. A second paramedic should continue ventilation attempts throughout (Frerk et al., 2015).

Site identification

Palpation of the small insertion site can be difficult, particularly in patients with short, fat or oedematous necks or where there are neck burns or trauma (Kristensen et al., 2015). If necessary, begin with an identifiable landmark, such as the sternal notch. Moving superiorly is the hard cricoid cartilage ring (Fig. 3.10.1a). Running the fingers upwards and over its surface contacts the small cricothyroid membrane. Immediately above that, the larger larynx can be palpated with the other hand by placing a second finger and thumb either side and running the forefinger down to the cricothyroid membrane (Fig. 3.10.1b). Palpation may be more useful than visualisation (Melchiors et al., 2016).

Mark the cricothyroid membrane with a pen or marker (Ince and Melachuri, 2017; Patel and Meyer, 2014). The emergency nature of the procedure may allow minimal opportunity for site swabbing, so this can be done during early airway preparation.

Insertion method

Make a scalpel incision (typically using a size 10 blade) into the cricothyroid membrane by plunging the blade straight into the site, perpendicular to the trachea (Fig. 3.10.2). Extend the cut to the left and right to accommodate the airway catheter (Ince and Melachuri, 2017; Myatra et al., 2016). Reluctance and anxiety are common at this point (Heymans et al., 2016; Ince and Melachuri, 2017; Kristenson et al., 2015; Melchiors et al., 2016).

If the membrane cannot be located, a vertical incision down the larynx and cricoid cartilage can be cut first, allowing further (i.e. finger) penetration into the wound in search of the membrane (Frerk et al., 2015; Heymans et al., 2016; Myatra et al., 2016; Patel and Meyer, 2014). This may cause bleeding; ignore it for the moment and continue securing the airway.

Once the opening is large enough, insert the tip of the bougie into the wound, and angle it inferiorly towards the

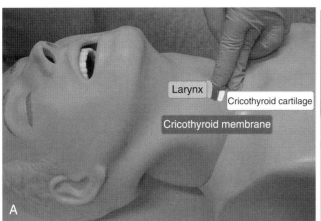
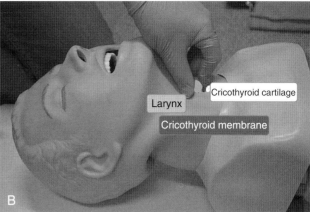

Figure 3.10.1 Palpating the cricothyroid membrane

(a) Palpate the sternal notch and move fingers superiorly to the hard cricoid cartilage ring. Continue upwards and over its surface to the cricothyroid membrane. (b) Palpate the larynx by placing a second finger and thumb on either side of it and running the forefinger down to the cricothyroid membrane.

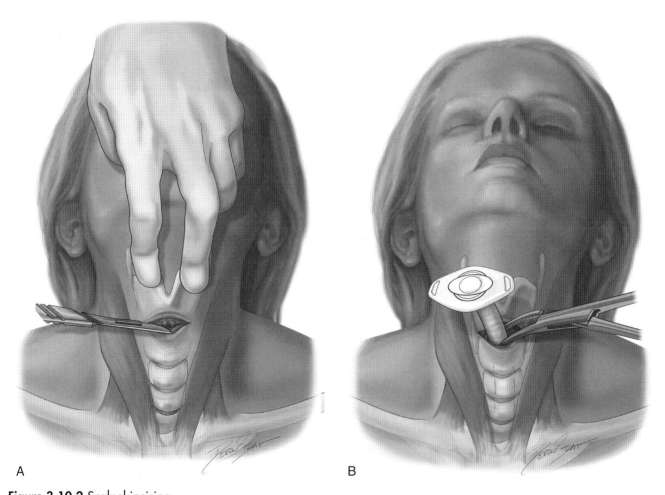

Figure 3.10.2 Scalpel incision

For an emergency surgical airway, the non-dominant hand stabilises the trachea while the other hand incises down to the trachea.

Source: *Tiwana, P.S. and Kademani, D., 2015, Atlas of oral & maxillofacial surgery (Chapter 97, Figure 97-3), Elsevier.*

lungs. Pass sufficient length to ensure tracheal placement. The bougie may contact the carina, but ideally this should be avoided. Holding the bougie in place, feed 5–6 mm internal diameter endotracheal tube over it (Melchiors et al., 2016). Continue pushing through the opening, monitoring progress, until the deflated cuff is completely within the trachea. Beware of pushing too far; this is already below the vocal cords and near the carina and bronchi. Secure the tube in place with cloth or adhesive tape.

For percutaneous options, the cricothyroidotomy needle is now inserted into the wound with the bevel facing upwards. It is then immediately directed at a downwards angle to avoid the posterior tracheal wall. Air can be aspirated via syringe as the needle is advanced to confirm tracheal placement. Insert the needle sufficiently to ensure its distal opening is within the tracheal lumen. Now feed off the cannula fully into the trachea, and withdraw the needle and discard it.

Ventilation

The standard 15 mm attachment at the proximal end of the endotracheal tube allows attachment of a bag/valve/mask (BVM) resuscitator. With the cuff inflated, sufficient air escape allows end tidal CO_2 monitoring and normal tidal volume/ventilation rates to be used (Myatra et al., 2016).

Where the needle is narrow diameter (<4 mm), jet ventilation is necessary (Asai, 2016). Jet ventilation does not require normal minute volume since the intention is oxygenation rather than ventilation (Marshall, 2016; Ince and Melachuri, 2017; Myatra et al., 2016).

Clinical skill assessment process

The following section outlines the clinical skill assessment tools that should be used to determine a student's ability to demonstrate the safe and accurate performance of surgical cricothyroidotomy.
1. Clinical Skill Work Instruction
2. Formative Clinical Skill Assessment (F-CSAT)
3. Performance Improvement Plan (PIP)
4. Summative Clinical Skill Assessment (S-CSAT)
(5. Direct Observation of Procedural Skills (DOPS) – see Chapter 1.1)

Clinical Skill Work Instruction

Equipment and resources: Airway mannequin with surgical airway capability; scalpel and blade (size 10); bougie; 5/6 mm cuffed endotracheal tube; BVM resuscitator; hand decontamination agent; disposable gloves, respiratory mask and protective eyewear; clinical waste bag; sharps waste container; method of documenting the results

Associated Clinical Skills: Infection control; Communication; Consent; Respiratory status

Surgical airway

Activity	Critical Action	Rationale
Personal protection	Don gloves, eyewear and respiratory mask.	Protection from blood/body fluids during procedure. May already be donned.
Correct indication	Identify cannot intubate–cannot ventilate situation with all other airway and ventilation options exhausted.	No alternative, as no delay is tolerable.
Prepare team	Announce to team urgency and strategy.	To ensure total focus on crisis.
	Second paramedic continues to ventilate patient throughout procedure.	Some oxygenation might still be achieved.
Prepare equipment	Lay out required equipment in preparation.	For immediate use. Likely this was done during earlier airway preparation.
Prepare patient	Position head hyperextended. Consider padding beneath shoulders to obtain correct position.	To improve cricothyroid exposure.
	Palpate/visualise insertion site. Locate cricoid cartilage and feel for cricothyroid membrane. Simultaneously grasp thyroid cartilage between thumb and middle finger of other hand and run forefinger inferiorly to locate cricothyroid membrane.	Locations meet at the cricothyroid membrane site.
	Swab and mark site with marker.	For asepsis and ready identification. This step may be performed early, in anticipation.

Surgical airway continued

Activity	Critical Action	Rationale
Perform surgical incision	Using size 10 scalpel, plunge straight into site aiming posteriorly, with the blade perpendicular to trachea. Withdraw, reverse blade direction and reinsert scalpel.	To ensure surgical incision large enough for tube insertion.
	If membrane cannot be located, cut a vertical incision down the larynx and cricoid cartilage midline first, to allow finger penetration into wound to assist search.	Allows opening of the cricoid membrane longitudinally.
	When opening is large enough, dispose of scalpel in sharps container.	Sharps safety is critical, but don't dispose of scalpel until incision is complete.
Bougie insertion	When opening is large enough, insert bougie tip into wound. Angle inferiorly towards the lungs. Pass several centimetres' length for tracheal placement.	Bougie provides guide for tube to follow.
Tube insertion	Holding bougie in place, feed 5–6 mm endotracheal tube over it. Continue pushing tube through opening until deflated cuff is completely sitting within the trachea.	Small adult ETT to fit small opening. Tip must be placed above carina/bifurcation.
Inflate cuff	Inflate tube cuff with 6–7 mL air from 10 mL syringe.	To secure airway and allow effective ventilation.
Secure tube	Using cloth tape, tie clove hitch knot around tube near lips and secure around patient's neck without compromising circulation.	To avoid tube dislodgement.
End tidal CO_2	Attach end tidal capnography. Confirm correct placement via auscultation.	For monitoring ventilation effectiveness.
Ventilate	Ventilate at 6 mL/kg, 14 per minute.	For normal ventilation.
Report	Accurately document/hand over findings.	Accurate record kept and continuity of patient care.

Source: *Adapted from Ince and Melachuri, 2017.*

Formative Clinical Skill Assessment (F-CSAT)

Equipment and resources: Airway mannequin with surgical airway capability; scalpel and blade (size 10); bougie, 5/6 mm cuffed endotracheal tube; BVM resuscitator; hand decontamination agent; disposable gloves, respiratory mask and protective eyewear; clinical waste bag; sharps waste container; method of documenting the results

Associated Clinical Skills: Infection control; Communication; Consent; Respiratory status

Staff/Student being assessed: _____

Surgical airway

Activity	Critical Action	Performance				
Personal protection	Dons gloves, eyewear and respiratory mask.	0	1	2	3	4
Verifies indication	Identifies cannot intubate–cannot ventilate situation, with all other airway and ventilation options exhausted.	0	1	2	3	4
Prepares team	Announces urgency and strategy to team.	0	1	2	3	4
	Second paramedic continues assisting patient ventilation throughout procedure.	0	1	2	3	4

Surgical airway continued

Activity	Critical Action	Performance				
Prepares equipment	Lays out equipment in preparation.	0	1	2	3	4
Prepares patient	Positions patient's head hyperextended.	0	1	2	3	4
	Palpates/visualises insertion site.	0	1	2	3	4
	Swabs and marks site with marker.	0	1	2	3	4
Performs surgical incision	Plunges scalpel straight into site, aiming posteriorly, perpendicular to trachea. Withdraws, reverses blade direction and reinserts scalpel.	0	1	2	3	4
	If membrane cannot be located, makes vertical incision down the larynx and cricoid cartilage midline to allow finger penetration into wound to assist search.	0	1	2	3	4
	When opening is large enough, disposes of scalpel in sharps container.	0	1	2	3	4
Bougie insertion	Inserts bougie tip into wound. Angles inferiorly towards the lungs. Proceeds several centimetres for tracheal placement.	0	1	2	3	4
Tube insertion	Holding bougie in place, feeds 5–6 mm of endotracheal tube over it. Continues pushing tube through opening until deflated cuff is completely sitting within the trachea.	0	1	2	3	4
Inflates cuff	Inflates tube cuff with 6–7 mL air from 10 mL syringe.	0	1	2	3	4
Secures tube	Secures tube without compromising circulation.	0	1	2	3	4
End tidal CO_2	Attaches end tidal capnography. Confirms correct placement.	0	1	2	3	4
Ventilates	Ventilates at 6 mL/kg, 14 per minute.	0	1	2	3	4
Reports	Accurately documents/hands over findings.	0	1	2	3	4

Source: *Adapted from Ince and Melachuri, 2017.*

Standard Achieved: (please circle one)

Competent (C)   Not Yet Competent* (NYC)

Staff/Student Name: _____

Assessor (please print name): _____

Signed (Assessor): _____

Date of Assessment: _____

Comments:

*If Not Yet Competent (NYC) a PIP needs to be completed and a repeat of the F-CSAT

Formative Clinical Skill Assessment (F-CSAT) Key

Skill type	Standard of procedure	Quality of performance	Outcome	Level of assistance required
4 Safe for unsupervised practice	Safe Accurate Behaviour is appropriate to context	Confident Accurate Expedient	Achieved intended outcome	No supporting cues* required
3 Requires supervision	Safe Accurate Behaviour is appropriate to context	Confident Accurate Takes longer than required	Achieved intended outcome	Requires occasional supportive cues*
2 Requires assistance	Safe Accurate Behaviour generally appropriate to context	Lacks certainty	Would not have achieved outcome without support	Requires frequent verbal and occasional physical directives in addition to supportive cues*
1 Requires direction	Safe only with guidance Not completely accurate	Unskilled Inefficient	Would not have achieved outcome without support	Requires continuous verbal and frequent physical directive cues*
0 Unsafe	Unsafe Unable to demonstrate behaviour Lack of insight into behaviour appropriate to context	Unskilled	Would not have achieved outcome	Requires continuous verbal and continuous physical directive cues*

*Refers to physical directives or verbal supportive cues

Performance Improvement Plan (PIP)

Please document the agreed education plan and completion timelines for areas assessed as less than 4.

This plan should be presented to assessor prior to commencement of summative assessment.

Where was supervisor support required?	Student summary of deficit. (Why was there a problem?)	Improvement Plan	Completed (Y/N)

Staff/Student Name: _____

Staff/Student Signature: _____

Educator Name: _____

Educator Signature: _____

Summative Clinical Skill Assessment (S-CSAT)

Equipment and resources: Airway mannequin with surgical airway capability; scalpel and blade (size 10); bougie, 5/6 mm cuffed endotracheal tube; BVM resuscitator; hand decontamination agent; disposable gloves, respiratory mask and protective eyewear; clinical waste bag; sharps waste container; method of documenting the results

Associated Clinical Skills: Infection control; Communication; Consent; Respiratory status

Staff/Student being assessed: _____

- Completed Formative Clinical Skill Assessment (F-CSAT):   **YES**   **NO**
- Completed Performance Improvement Plan (PIP):   **YES**   **NO**   **N/A**

Surgical airway

Activity	Critical Action	Achieved Without Direction	
Personal protection	Dons gloves, eyewear and respiratory mask.	NO	YES
Verifies indication	Identifies cannot intubate–cannot ventilate situation, with all other airway and ventilation options exhausted.	NO	YES
Prepares team	Announces urgency and strategy to team.	NO	YES
	Second paramedic continues assisting patient ventilation throughout procedure.	NO	YES
Prepares equipment	Lays out all equipment in preparation.	NO	YES
Prepares patient	Positions patient's head hyperextended.	NO	YES
	Palpates/visualises insertion site.	NO	YES
	Swabs and marks site with marker.	NO	YES
Performs surgical incision	Plunges scalpel straight into site, aiming posteriorly, perpendicular to trachea. Withdraws, reverses blade direction and reinserts scalpel.	NO	YES
	If membrane cannot be located, makes vertical incision down the larynx and cricoid cartilage midline to allow finger penetration into wound to assist search.	NO	YES
	When opening is large enough, disposes of scalpel in sharps container.	NO	YES
Bougie insertion	Inserts bougie tip into wound. Angles inferiorly towards the lungs. Proceeds several centimetres' length to allow tracheal placement.	NO	YES
Tube insertion	Holding bougie in place, feeds 5–6 mm endotracheal tube over it. Continues pushing tube through opening until deflated cuff is completely sitting within the trachea.	NO	YES
Inflates cuff	Inflates tube cuff with 6–7 mL air from 10 mL syringe. Confirms correct placement.	NO	YES
Secures tube	Secures tube without compromising circulation.	NO	YES
End tidal CO_2	Attaches end tidal capnography.	NO	YES
Ventilates	Ventilates at 6 mL/kg, 14 per minute.	NO	YES
Reports	Accurately documents/hands over the findings.	NO	YES

Source: *Adapted from Ince and Melachuri, 2017.*

Standard Achieved: (please circle one)

Competent (C)   Not Yet Competent* (NYC)

Staff/Student Name: _____

Assessor (please print name)**:** _____

Signed (Assessor)**:** _____

Date of Assessment: _____

Comments:

*If Not Yet Competent (NYC) a PIP needs to be completed and a repeat of the F-CSAT

Clinical findings

Contraindications

Cricothyroidotomy is the ultimate airway-saving method. It is not appropriate where effective airway patency can be obtained with an alternative option. It is also not appropriate where there is major front of neck trauma that allows no prospect of success.

The child patient (<10 years of age) requires a much smaller needle/catheter device. The risk of trauma and permanent larynx injury is greater in children (Patel and Meyer, 2014). The limited cricothyroid space further precludes the surgical method described in this chapter (Melchiors et al., 2016).

Difficult patients

Developing oedema or neck injury, including burns, progressively obscures landmarks and the insertion site.

The cricothyroidotomy insertion site is similarly more difficult to locate in obese patients, who are already difficult to intubate (Howes et al., 2015; Kristensen et al., 2015; Melchiors et al., 2016).

> **PRACTICE TIP!**
>
> Advanced airway management (intubation) should have the cricoid membrane marked and the neck area swabbed clean as routine preparation to assist readiness if airway difficulty arises.

> **PRACTICE TIP!**
>
> This skill will be rarely, if ever, performed. When it is, it must be performed precisely and when under great duress. The only effective method of reliably achieving this is to maintain regular simulated practice.

Complications

Bleeding from the surgical site can complicate cricothyroidotomy, though it is not usually profuse as the correct site location is sufficiently clear of major blood vessels. Damage to the larynx from incision or insertion is possible, particularly subglottic stenosis scarring. If insertion is unsuccessful, the catheter can be forced into the surrounding neck tissue instead, causing injury and failed airway (Patel and Meyer, 2014).

Needle cricothyroidotomy can be problematic where complete upper airway obstruction is present. In such cases, only minimal air escape is possible through the needle itself. This predisposes to gas retention and pulmonary barotrauma (Patel and Meyer, 2014), which can be exacerbated by jet ventilation (Asai, 2016; Ince and Melachuri, 2017; Myatra et al., 2016). Posterior tracheal wall injury is possible with a needle approach (Asai, 2016).

> **PRACTICE TIP!**
>
> The decision to perform a cricothyroidotomy must be made quickly and resolutely. Delays could prove fatal (Myatra et al., 2016).

> **PRACTICE TIP!**
>
> The cricothyroidotomy must be performed in minimal time, with little warning and likely without previous experience, other than training. The stress of the situation will be significant.

> **PRACTICE TIP!**
>
> Airway procedures are always considered high risk for exposure to infectious blood and body fluids. Gloves, respiratory masks and eyewear are important for protection.

TEST YOUR KNOWLEDGE QUESTIONS

1. **What are the criteria for emergency cricothyroidotomy?**
   Unable to intubate or ventilate and there is no other airway alternative.

2. **What is the difference between surgical and percutaneous cricothyroidotomy?**
   Percutaneous uses needle entry into the trachea; surgical uses large incision.

3. **Why is the anterior cricothyroid membrane chosen for surgical airway?**
   The site is easier to locate, less fatty and away from muscular and vascular structures.

4. **Why is surgical favoured over percutaneous cricothyroidotomy?**
   For paramedics, who almost always have relative inexperience with any surgical airway procedures, the surgical method is comparatively faster to perform, with significantly higher success rates than needle methods.

5. **What head position is preferred for cricothyroidotomy?**
   Neck extended, possibly with padding under the shoulders.

6. **Where is the paramedic positioned to perform cricothyroidotomy?**
   At the patient's head, either superiorly or to one side; if to one side, the side that allows the dominant hand to be closest to the patient.

7. **What else should occur during the procedure?**
   A second paramedic should continue ventilation attempts.

8. **What size endotracheal tube is suitable for use?**
   5.0–6.0 mm internal diameter.

9. **In which patients will the cricothyroid membrane be difficult to identify?**
   Patients with short, fat or oedematous necks or where there are neck burns or trauma.

10. **What can be done if the cricoid membrane cannot be located?**
    A vertical incision down the larynx and cricoid cartilage can be cut first, allowing further penetration into the wound in search of the membrane.

References

Andersson, M.L., Møller, A.M. and Pace, N.L., 2014. *Emergency cricothyroidotomy for airway management.* Online: The Cochrane Library.

Asai, T., 2016. Surgical cricothyrotomy, rather than percutaneous cricothyrotomy, in 'cannot intubate, cannot oxygenate' situation. *Anesthesiology*, 125(2), 269–271.

Chrisman, L., King, W., Wimble, K., Cartwright, S., Mohammed, K.B. and Patel, B., 2016. Surgicric 2: A comparative bench study with two established emergency cricothyroidotomy techniques in a porcine model. *British Journal of Anaesthesia*, 117(2), 236–242.

Frerk, C., Mitchell, V.S., McNarry, A.F., Mendonca, C., Bhagrath, R., Patel, A., O'Sullivan, E.P., Woodall, N.M. and Ahmad, I., 2015. Difficult Airway Society 2015 guidelines for management of unanticipated difficult intubation in adults. *British Journal of Anaesthesia*, 115(6), 827–848.

Heymans, F., Feigl, G., Graber, S., Courvoisier, D.S., Weber, K.M. and Dulguerov, P., 2016. Emergency cricothyrotomy performed by surgical airway–naive medical personnel: a randomized crossover study in cadavers comparing three commonly used techniques. *Anesthesiology*, 125(2), 295–303.

Howes, T.E., Lobo, C.A., Kelly, F.E. and Cook, T.M., 2015. Rescuing the obese or burned airway: are conventional training manikins adequate? A simulation study. *British Journal of Anaesthesia*, 114(1), 136–142.

Ince, M. and Melachuri, V.K., 2017. Emergency front of neck access. *Indian Journal of Respiratory Care*, 6(2), 793.

Kristensen, M.S., Teoh, W.H.L. and Baker, P.A., 2015. Percutaneous emergency airway access; prevention, preparation, technique and training. *British Journal of Anaesthesia* 114(3), 357–361.

Marshall, S.D., 2016. Evidence is important: safety considerations for emergency catheter cricothyroidotomy. *Academic Emergency Medicine*, 23(9), 1074–1076.

Mallari, C.A., Ross, E.E. and Vieux, E.E., 2016. Emergency airway: cricothyroidotomy. In Taylor, D.A., Sherry, S.P. and Sing, R.F. (eds), *Interventional Critical Care.* Cham: Springer, pp. 59–65.

Melchiors, J., Todsen, T., Konge, L., Charabi, B. and von Buchwald, C., 2016. Cricothyroidotomy – the emergency surgical airway. *Head Neck*, 38(7), 1129–1131.

Myatra, S.N., Ahmed, S.M., Kundra, P., Garg, R., Ramkumar, V., Patwa, A., Shah, A., Raveendra, U.S., Shetty, S.R., Doctor, J.R. and Pawar, D.K., 2016. The All India Difficult Airway Association 2016 guidelines for tracheal intubation in the intensive care unit. *Indian Journal of Anaesthesia*, 60(12), 922.

Patel, S.A. and Meyer, T.K., 2014. Surgical airway. *International Journal of Critical Illness and Injury Science*, 4(1), 71.

Pracy, J.P., Brennan, L., Cook, T.M., Hartle, A.J., Marks, R.J., McGrath, B.A., Narula, A. and Patel, A., 2016. Surgical intervention during a Can't Intubate Can't Oxygenate (CICO) event: emergency Front-of-Neck Airway (FONA)? *British Journal of Anaesthesia*, 117(4), 426–428.

3.11 | Intermittent positive pressure ventilation

Jeff Kenneally

Chapter objectives

At the end of this chapter the reader will be able to:

1. Describe physiological differences between spontaneous respiration and intermittent positive pressure ventilation (IPPV)
2. Describe the component parts of a bag/valve/mask (BVM) ventilation device
3. Demonstrate the method of using BVM to provide IPPV and oxygenation
4. Recognise and rectify difficulties and adverse effects of IPPV

Resources required for this assessment

- Simulated patient capable of ventilation
- Airway devices
- BVM ventilator
- Oxygen source
- Protective gloves, mask, eyewear
- Method of documenting results

Skill matrix

This assessment requires:

- Infection control (CS 1.3)
- Communication (CS 1.5)
- Consent (CS 1.6)
- Patient assessment skills (Chapter 2, CS 2.1, 2.6, 2.7, 2.8, 2.10)
- Airway and ventilation skills (Chapter 3, CS 3.2, 3.3, 3.4, 3.5, 3.6, 3.7)

This assessment is a component of:

- Airway and ventilation (Chapter 3)

Introduction

Intermittent positive pressure ventilation (IPPV) is an essential skill for all medical emergency responders when managing inadequately breathing patients. To be effective it must be performed correctly, as discussed in this chapter.

Anatomy and physiology

The airway extends from the mouth/nose, through the trachea and the bronchi until the terminal bronchioles. These are dead space since they convey air without providing alveoli gas exchange. Normal adult lung volume at rest (tidal volume) is typically 500 mL, with dead space being one-third of this (Joffe et al., 2010).

The regulation of oxygen delivery and/or carbon dioxide removal can be achieved by varying either ventilation rate or tidal volume (Joffe et al., 2010).

$$\text{Ventilation rate} \times \text{Tidal volume} = \text{Minute volume}$$

Lung (alveoli) volumes can expand during physical exertion or illness several times more greater than resting tidal volume. There is a maximum expansion before barotrauma occurs (Joffe et al., 2010). Chest wall connective tissue provides elastic resistance to expansion and expiratory recoil.

Normal breathing has a positive effect on circulation. Chest expansion lowers alveoli and intrathoracic pressure. Right ventricle venous return increases, as does pulmonary vasculature capacity, absorbing this increased blood flow as the alveoli fill. With expiration, intrathoracic pressure rises again, decreasing venous return and pulmonary vasculature volume.

Clinical rationale

A patent airway is necessary before IPPV (see Chapter 3.1). Correct obstructions and provide jaw thrust concurrently (Henline et al., 2014; Joffe et al., 2010; Parry and Higginson, 2016).

The patient should ideally be placed in the neutral anatomical or sniffing position (see Chapter 3.2) (Henline et al., 2014; Weingart and Levitan, 2012), although lateral posture is also suitable. Tilting the upper body to 20° can reduce posterior atelectasis, particularly for obese patients (Weingart and Levitan, 2012).

Paramedic-assisted methods of lung ventilation most commonly employ the use of a bag/valve/mask (BVM) device. There are two broad BVM methods to consider: IPPV or oxygenation for spontaneously breathing patients (Weingart and Levitan, 2012).

Using the BVM to provide IPPV

IPPV physically pushes air into the lungs using a BVM device to counter a slow or absent breathing rate and/or insufficient tidal volume. The ventilation rate is typically within the normal respiratory rate range for the patient's age, with a few exceptions that will be discussed later.

Adjusting either tidal volume or the ventilation rate changes minute volume. Increasing the rate adds to minute volume but also to dead space. Some of the increased air movement does not contribute to actual gas exchange.

In contrast, increased tidal volume adds to minute volume only. If tidal volume decreases until it is equal to or less than dead space, no alveolar gas exchange occurs.

IPPV aims to provide sufficient alveolar ventilation to maintain effective oxygenation and carbon dioxide removal. A volume of 6–7 mL/kg provides qualities that protect the lungs by avoiding continued overdistension, reducing pulmonary endothelium injury and inflammatory responses while still achieving effective ventilation (Guest, 2000; Hsu et al., 2016; Khoury et al., 2015; Lipes et al., 2012; Liu et al., 2016; Weingart and Levitan, 2012).

Using the BVM to provide oxygenation

The BVM can be used for oxygenation of the spontaneously breathing patient where other options prove insufficient. Increasing the fraction of inspired oxygen displaces alveolar nitrogen. The increased oxygen reserve makes this oxygenation method useful preceding advanced airway procedures such as endotracheal intubation (Weingart and Levitan, 2012). It also has a therapeutic benefit in managing decompression illness or carbon monoxide poisoning.

Oxygenation requires adequate spontaneous respiration to ensure carbon dioxide removal.

BVM use

BVM devices come in newborn, child and adult sizes (Fig. 3.11.1).

Masks range from newborn to larger adult sizes (Fig. 3.11.2). All fit over the mouth and nose. Smaller options can be circular, while larger ones can be triangular with the narrow end fitting above the nose, the rounder end across the chin. It is better to use a slightly larger size mask than one that is too small (Bauman et al., 2010; Otten et al., 2014).

Some masks have air-filled cushions, others a silicone structure. Some can adjust the volume of air in the cushion, allowing face contouring. Do not fill it to more

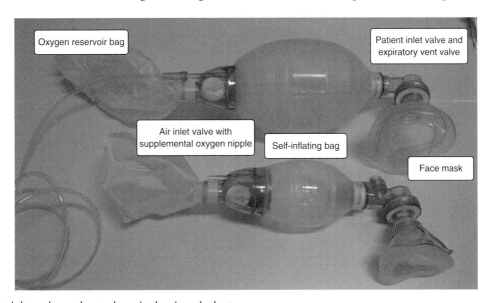

Figure 3.11.1 Adult and paediatric bag/valve/mask devices

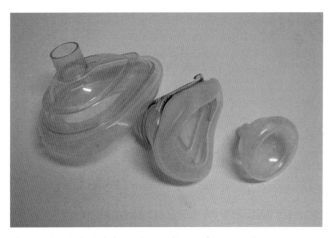

Figure 3.11.2 Adult and paediatric face masks

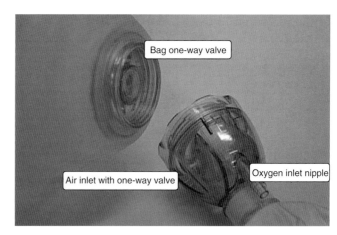

Figure 3.11.4 Air/oxygen inlet valve and reservoir bag

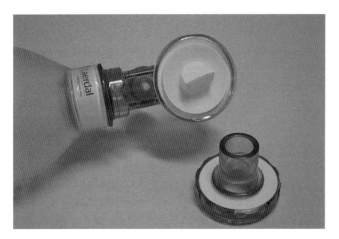

Figure 3.11.3 Valve structure

than 80% of capacity (Bauman et al., 2010; Otten et al., 2014).

Masks attach to the L-shaped valve structure, allowing 360° rotation during use (Fig. 3.11.3). Within the valve a rubber diaphragm directs airflow (Khoury et al., 2014). Airflow from the bag towards the mask opens the valve, allowing entry in one of two ways. The first is to manually squeeze the bag and push air through (Weingart and Levitan, 2012). The second is during spontaneous inspiration, which reduces pressure within the mask, drawing air towards the patient. The inlet valve must open to ensure adequate oxygenation. Small tidal volumes that occur in patients with respiratory failure may not be sufficient to achieve this (Weingart and Levitan, 2012).

Exhaled air must escape to the atmosphere and not be rebreathed. The inlet valve only allows airflow from the bag to the patient. It is surrounded by a second rubber ring that vents expired air.

Excessive inflation pressure risks barotrauma and stomach inflation. Some devices have a blow-off valve that limits ventilation pressure by releasing at about 35 cm/H_2O.

Positive expiratory end pressure (PEEP) valves can be fitted to some BVM devices where pressure support is indicated.

The valve structure attaches to the self-inflating bag, which reinflates following each ventilation. Adult recoil bags are typically 1600 mL, paediatric 500 mL and newborn 240 mL (Siegler et al., 2016). The force of the bag compression varies the volume delivered.

At the distal end, another one-way valve allows fresh gas to entrain following each ventilation. To increase the fraction of inspired oxygen, the device includes an oxygen inlet nipple and reservoir bag (Fig. 3.11.4).

Reservoir bags do not recoil. They fill from supplemental oxygen; the available gas volume varies with the supply flow rate and BVM use. Larger minute volumes require a larger flow rate. For pre-oxygenation, flow rates of about 15 L/min can usually achieve 95% oxygen delivery.

For IPPV or oxygenation, ensure the mask seal is sufficient to open the inspiratory valve, prevent the mask from leaking and ensure exhaled air is vented. An effective seal is achieved by placing the mask in position against the face and pressing posteriorly, using the EC/C3 grip. Alternatively, place the mask on one side of the face and then roll it to the other side (Bauman et al., 2010; Grant et al., 2016; Otten et al., 2014).

The EC/C3 grip involves placing the thumb and forefinger across the top of the mask in a C shape (Fig. 3.11.5a and b) and then pushing posteriorly creating the seal. This also pushes the tongue posteriorly, causing tongue obstruction. To counter this, the remaining fingers run along the jawline/angle, pulling it anteriorly into the mask (jaw thrust). These three fingers have an E-shaped appearance, hence the name 'EC' or 'C3' (Otten et al., 2014; Parry and Higginson, 2016).

Applying jaw thrust and seal maintenance can be challenging using one hand. If this is unachievable, use two hands to provide bilateral jaw thrust while simultaneously maintaining the seal (Grant et al., 2016; Joffe et al., 2010; Otten et al., 2014) (Fig. 3.11.6). This demands a second paramedic to ventilate. The lifesaving nature of this procedure means that other tasks are less important. If it takes two paramedics to perform it correctly, then so be it.

The delicate soft tissue under the jaw of the small child or newborn is easily injured, so take care to handle it gently and avoid pressing fingers into the flesh.

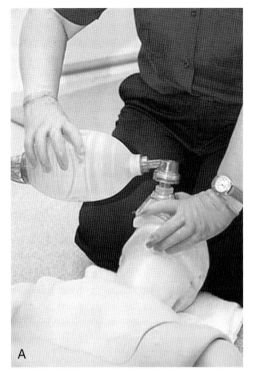

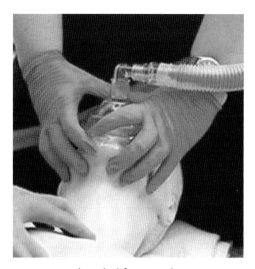

Figure 3.11.6 Two-handed face mask grip

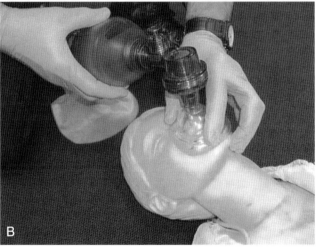

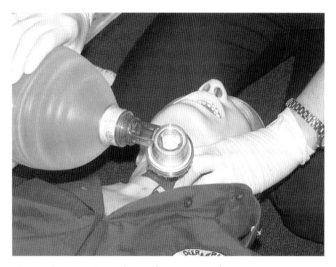

Figure 3.11.7 Cricothyroidotomy ventilation

Figure 3.11.5 EC (or C3) grip
(a) Adult. (b) Child.

Tidal volume is around one-third of total bag volume; use only one hand for compression. Using two hands or placing the BVM on a surface and pushing on it can overventilate the patient (Hsu et al., 2016; Liu et al., 2016; Seigler et al., 2016).

The BVM resuscitator can be attached to advanced airway options, including endotracheal tubes, supraglottic devices and cricothyroidotomy tubes with standard connections (Fig. 3.11.7). Take care to not dislodge airway devices during such use.

Tidal volume delivery with a BVM must be estimated. Watch for suitable chest rise and fall in order to assess the volume, supported by observations of improvements in skin colour, pulse oximetry and, where available, end tidal capnography.

Bag compression is typically performed using a low pressure, slow squeeze approach. Compression should not be applied rapidly or sharply, but instead gently over 1–2 seconds (Seigler et al., 2016).

Expiration takes longer than inspiration due to its passive nature. Allow three to four times as long as inspiration, supported by observing chest relaxation.

Clinical skill assessment process

The following section outlines the clinical skill assessment tools that should be used to determine a student's ability to demonstrate safe and accurate IPP ventilation.
1. Clinical Skill Work Instruction
2. Formative Clinical Skill Assessment (F-CSAT)
3. Performance Improvement Plan (PIP)
4. Summative Clinical Skill Assessment (S-CSAT)
(5. Direct Observation of Procedural Skills (DOPS) – see Chapter 1.1)

Clinical Skill Work Instruction

Equipment and resources: Mannequin for ventilating; airway devices; BVM resuscitator; oxygen source; protective gloves, mask and eyewear; method of documenting results

Associated Clinical Skills: Infection control; Communication; Consent; Patient assessment skills; Airway and ventilation skills

Intermittent positive pressure ventilation

Activity	Critical Action	Rationale
Prepare paramedic	Don PPE, including eyewear, respiratory mask and gloves.	Airway procedures are high risk for infection transmission.
	Kneel superiorly to patient's head, facing towards their feet.	Allows for position of mask and visualisation of chest rise and fall.
Position patient	Place patient's head in required anatomical position.	Position may vary with circumstances and presentation.
Patient airway	Remove mechanical/foreign body obstructions as required.	Prior airway patency is essential.
Prepare equipment	Ensure BVM resuscitator is assembled for use. Test function by occluding patient ventilation valve to assess resistance. The bag should not be able to be compressed. Release valve and compress bag. Air should flow freely and the bag fully reinflate immediately after.	Device must deliver IPPV and reinflate.
	Select and attach correct size of mask. Inflate air cushion to 80% of maximum if adjustable.	Ensure adequate patient fit; 80% allows for malleability of mask to achieve seal.
	Attach supplemental oxygen therapy to BVM nipple at appropriate flow rate if indicated.	The BVM device will inflate lungs with air only.
Apply mask seal	Place mask on face over mouth and nose. Press posteriorly with the thumb and forefinger to gain seal. Alternatively, place the mask on one side of the face and roll onto the other side to gain seal.	An effective seal is essential to ensure air flows in and out of the lungs effectively.
Apply jaw thrust	Place the fifth finger at jaw angle, the third finger at the point of the jaw and the fourth finger under the jaw in between. Pull the jaw anteriorly into mask to provide jaw thrust.	To remove tongue obstruction.
Ventilate patient	With one hand holding the mask and jaw, hold the middle of the self-inflating bag with other hand. Compress bag with one hand, watching for sufficient chest rise/fall.	One-handed use avoids lung over-inflation. Chest rise and fall indicates effective air entry.
	If unable to maintain seal and ventilation, adjust grip and mask position. Attempt again.	Corrects air escape and inadequate ventilation.
	If still unable to maintain seal and ventilation, change to a two-handed grip method, with a second paramedic compressing the bag.	Corrects seal issues and applies bilateral jaw thrust.
	Provide ventilation rate and tidal volume as appropriate for patient's presentation.	Ensures care is appropriate for patient's size and age.
Report	Accurately document/hand over findings, including ventilation rate and tidal volume provided.	Accurate record kept and continuity of patient care.

Formative Clinical Skill Assessment (F-CSAT)

Equipment and resources: Mannequin for ventilating; airway devices; BVM resuscitator; oxygen source; protective gloves, mask and eyewear; method of documenting results

Associated Clinical Skills: Infection control; Communication, Consent; Patient assessment skills; Airway and ventilation skills

Staff/Student being assessed: _____

Intermittent positive pressure ventilation

Activity	Critical Action	Participant Performance				
Prepares paramedic	Dons PPE.	0	1	2	3	4
	Kneels superiorly to patient's head, facing towards their feet.	0	1	2	3	4
Positions patient	Places patient's head in required anatomical position.	0	1	2	3	4
Patent airway	Removes mechanical/foreign body obstructions as required.	0	1	2	3	4
Prepares equipment	Ensures BVM resuscitator is assembled. Tests function.	0	1	2	3	4
	Selects and attaches correct size of mask. Adjusts air cushion if necessary.	0	1	2	3	4
	Attaches supplemental oxygen therapy to BVM nipple at appropriate flow rate if indicated.	0	1	2	3	4
Applies mask seal	Places mask on face over patient's mouth and nose. Presses posteriorly with thumb and forefinger and gains seal.	0	1	2	3	4
Applies jaw thrust	Places fifth finger at the jaw angle, third finger at the point of the jaw and fourth finger under the jaw in between. Pulls jaw anteriorly into mask.	0	1	2	3	4
Ventilates patient	With one hand holding mask and jaw, holds and compresses self-inflating bag with one hand, watching for sufficient chest rise and fall.	0	1	2	3	4
	If seal and ventilation are ineffective, adjusts grip and mask position and attempts again.	0	1	2	3	4
	If seal and ventilation are still ineffective, changes to two-handed grip method, with second paramedic compressing bag.	0	1	2	3	4
	Provides ventilation at rate and tidal volume appropriate for patient's presentation.	0	1	2	3	4
Reports	Accurately documents/hands over findings, including ventilation rate and tidal volume provided.	0	1	2	3	4

Standard Achieved: (please circle one)

Competent (C)   Not Yet Competent* (NYC)

Staff/Student Name: _____

Assessor (please print name): _____

Signed (Assessor): _____

Date of Assessment: _____

Comments:

*If Not Yet Competent (NYC) a PIP needs to be completed and a repeat of the F-CSAT

Formative Clinical Skill Assessment (F-CSAT) Key

Skill level	Standard of procedure	Quality of performance	Outcome	Level of assistance required
4 Safe for unsupervised practice	Safe Accurate Behaviour is appropriate to context	Confident Accurate Expedient	Achieved intended outcome	No supporting cues* required
3 Requires supervision	Safe Accurate Behaviour is appropriate to context	Confident Accurate Takes longer than required	Achieved intended outcome	Requires occasional supportive cues*
2 Requires assistance	Safe Accurate Behaviour generally appropriate to context	Lacks certainty	Would not have achieved outcome without support	Requires frequent verbal and occasional physical directives in addition to supportive cues*
1 Requires direction	Safe only with guidance Not completely accurate	Unskilled Inefficient	Would not have achieved outcome without support	Requires continuous verbal and frequent physical directive cues*
0 Unsafe	Unsafe Unable to demonstrate behaviour Lack of insight into behaviour appropriate to context	Unskilled	Would not have achieved outcome	Requires continuous verbal and continuous physical directive cues*

*Refers to physical directives or verbal supportive cues

Performance Improvement Plan (PIP)

Please document the agreed education plan and completion timelines for areas assessed as less than 4.

This plan should be presented to assessor prior to commencement of summative assessment.

Where was supervisor support required?	Student summary of deficit. (Why was there a problem?)	Improvement Plan	Completed (Y/N)

Staff/Student Name: _____

Staff/Student Signature: _____

Educator Name: _____

Educator Signature: _____

Summative Clinical Skill Assessment (S-CSAT)

Equipment and resources: Mannequin for ventilating; airway devices; BVM resuscitator; oxygen source; protective gloves, mask and eyewear; method of documenting results

Associated Clinical Skills: Infection control; Communication; Consent; Patient assessment skills; Airway and ventilation skills

Staff/Student being assessed: _____

• Completed Formative Clinical Skill Assessment (F-CSAT): **YES   NO**

• Completed Performance Improvement Plan (PIP): **YES   NO   N/A**

Intermittent positive pressure ventilation

Activity	Critical Action	Achieved Without Direction	
Prepares paramedic	Dons PPE.	NO	YES
	Kneels superiorly to patient's head, facing towards their feet.	NO	YES
Positions patient	Places patient's head in required anatomical position.	NO	YES
Patent airway	Removes mechanical/foreign body obstructions as required.	NO	YES
Prepares equipment	Ensures BVM resuscitator is assembled for use. Tests function.	NO	YES
	Selects and attaches correct size of mask. Adjusts air cushion if necessary.	NO	YES
	Attaches supplemental oxygen therapy to BVM nipple at appropriate flow rate if indicated.	NO	YES
Applies mask seal	Places mask on face over patient's mouth and nose. Presses posteriorly with thumb and forefinger and gains seal.	NO	YES
Applies jaw thrust	Places fifth finger at the jaw angle, third finger at the point of the jaw and fourth finger under the jaw in between. Pulls jaw anteriorly into mask.	NO	YES
Ventilates patient	With one hand holding mask and jaw, holds and compresses self-inflating bag with one hand, watching for sufficient chest rise and fall.	NO	YES
	If seal and ventilation are ineffective, adjusts grip and mask position and attempts again.	NO	YES
	If seal and ventilation are still ineffective, changes to two-handed grip method, with second paramedic compressing bag.	NO	YES
	Provides ventilation at rate and tidal volume appropriate for patient's presentation.	NO	YES
Reports	Accurately documents/hands over findings, including ventilation rate and tidal volume provided.	NO	YES

Standard Achieved: (please circle one)

Competent (C)   Not Yet Competent* (NYC)

Staff/Student Name: _____

Assessor (please print name)**:** _____

Signed (Assessor)**:** _____

Date of Assessment: _____

Comments:

*If Not Yet Competent (NYC) a PIP needs to be completed and a repeat of the F-CSAT

Clinical findings

Failure to secure effective seal

Failure to achieve a seal renders the use of a BVM ineffective. Even when using two hands, other variables can interfere with the seal. For example, the mask size may be incorrect. Adjust the air cushions where possible, or choose either a larger or smaller mask size as needed (Weingart and Levitan, 2012).

The removal of dentures alters the facial structure, so leave them in place if possible. If they have been removed, consider reinserting them back into position in the mouth. Also consider moving the mask slightly superiorly on the face to seek sufficient facial structure to secure the seal.

Facial hair and beards can also impact the seal. Consider sticking occlusive tape or rubbing water-based lubricant onto the hair to improve the mask's contact.

Compromised perfusion

IPPV has the opposite effect on intrathoracic pressure to that of spontaneous breathing. It increases intrathoracic pressure, and decreases venous return and pulmonary vascular filling as the alveoli fill (Henlin et al., 2014; Khoury et al., 2014; Kreit, 2014; Mesquida et al., 2012). Cardiac output reduces.

This is problematic when the right ventricular preload is vulnerable, including where there is depleted vascular volume, vasodilation from sepsis or reduced cardiac output from arrhythmia, ventricular failure or cardiac arrest.

Where IPPV compromises circulation, consider reducing the ventilation rate or tidal volume while addressing perfusion. A notable example is during cardiopulmonary resuscitation (Nagao et al., 2012) using slower ventilation rates.

Matching ventilation to problem

Failure to provide adequate alveolar ventilation leads to hypoxia, anaerobic metabolism, hypercapnoea and respiratory acidosis.

Overventilating through excessive rate or volume leads to hypocapnea and respiratory alkalosis. Controlled hyperventilation is occasionally used to cause hypocapnea in order to manage raised intracranial pressure.

Respiratory alkalosis, by hyperventilating, can offset metabolic ketoacidosis or reduce toxic activity from tricyclic acid medication overdose.

Barotrauma

Pulmonary barotrauma can be caused by excessive pressure, alveoli overdistention or the expose of weakened lung tissue to IPPV (Lipes et al., 2012). Defining excessive pressure is difficult, as it is not measurable nor equal throughout the airways and alveoli.

Barotrauma is relatively uncommon, its likelihood being minimised by correct ventilation volume, pressure and rate.

Gastric inflation

Loss of consciousness decreases oesophageal sphincter tones. Lung inflation pressure is usually less than required for stomach inflation. Stomach insufflation can happen when ventilation pressure exceeds 20 cm/H_2O in adults or 15 cm/H_2O in children (Grant et al., 2016; Henlin et al., 2014; Khoury et al., 2014; Lagarde et al., 2010; Nagao et al., 2012; Steigler et al., 2016), causing a risk of gastric aspiration.

An inflated stomach can reduce diaphragm movement and lung expansion, particularly in smaller children. Paediatric size BVM minimises the risk of this occurring.

Airway resistance

Expiratory airflow resistance, such as bronchospasm, requires higher ventilation pressures. Prolonged expiratory phase requires longer than normal expiratory time.

Ventilate using higher pressure or a slow compression time for chest expansion and a slower than normal rate to allow air escape. The rate may be as slow as 5 per minute in adult patients.

PRACTICE TIP!

Effective IPPV requires a patent airway, including head position, supportive airway devices and jaw thrust.

PRACTICE TIP!

IPPV requires an effective face mask seal. A correctly sized mask, cushion inflation, patient dentures and overcoming difficulties with facial hair all help to achieve this. Where an effective seal cannot be achieved, it is essential to use two rescuers.

PRACTICE TIP!

IPPV is a lifesaving skill. Ineffective performance must be recognised and rectified immediately. Monitor its effectiveness for suitable rise and fall of the patient's chest, improvements in skin colour and pulse oximetry readings.

PRACTICE TIP!

Airway procedures are high risk for infection transmission. Don gloves, eyewear and respiratory masks during IPPV.

TEST YOUR KNOWLEDGE QUESTIONS

1. **What patient position is possible during IPPV?**
   Supine, lateral or even sitting are acceptable.

2. **Which three factors are considered when establishing effective minute volume?**
   Ventilation rate; tidal volume; dead space.

3. **What is the most favourable patient position when performing IPPV?**
   Supine in a neutral anatomical or sniffing position and with the upper body tilted to 20°.

4. **What is the effect of insufficient minute volume?**
   Hypoxia from insufficient oxygen delivery and hypercapnoea from insufficient carbon dioxide removal, leading to respiratory acidosis.

5. **What are the complications of excessive ventilation?**
   Excessive carbon dioxide removal, causing respiratory alkalosis; raised intrathoracic pressure, decreasing venous return and cardiac output; barotrauma; stomach inflation, leading to diaphragmatic embarrassment and regurgitation.

6. **Which is most effective for increasing minute volume: increased rate or tidal volume?**
   Increased rate alone increases minute volume and dead space. Increased tidal volume alone increases only alveolar ventilation, so this is more effective.

7. **Why is an effective facial seal important during IPPV?**
   Without a seal, ventilated air escapes without ventilating the lungs. During oxygenation, the inlet valve will not operate to ensure oxygen/air is delivered and exhaled gas is vented from the mask.

8. **What strategies can improve facial seal?**
   Adjust the mask position; change the cushion air pressure; reinsert the patient's dentures; use tape or gel to manipulate facial hair.

9. **How does ventilation of the patient with bronchospasm differ from that of most other patients?**
   To allow for airway resistance and slower expiration, a slow rate is used, with higher pressure for effective tidal volume.

10. **Must the reservoir bag be attached to the BVM device?**
    Only to increase inspiratory oxygen fraction. The device delivers ambient air without the bag attached.

References

Bauman, E.B., Joffe, A.M., Lenz, L., DeVries, S.A., Hetzel, S. and Seider, S.P., 2010. An evaluation of bag-valve-mask ventilation using an ergonomically designed facemask among novice users: a simulation-based pilot study. *Resuscitation*, 81(9), 1161–1165.

Guest, W., 2000. Ventilation with lower tidal volumes as compared with traditional tidal volumes for acute lung injury and the acute respiratory distress syndrome. *New England Journal of Medicine*, 342, 1301–1308.

Grant, S., Khan, F., Keijzers, G., Shirran, M. and Marneros, L., 2016. Ventilator-assisted preoxygenation: protocol for combining non-invasive ventilation and apnoeic oxygenation using a portable ventilator. *Emergency Medicine Australasia*, 28(1), 67–72.

Henlin, T., Michalek, P., Tyll, T., Hinds, J.D. and Dobias, M., 2014. Oxygenation, ventilation, and airway management in out-of-hospital cardiac arrest: a review. *BioMed Research International*, doi: 10.1155/2014/376871.

Hsu, L., Anderson, R.J., Joshua, J., Tyagi, S., Beitler, J.R. and Ghafouri, T.B., 2016. Lower tidal volume is associated with favorable neurologic outcome following out-of-hospital cardiac arrest. In *C49. Respiratory failure: clinical and translational aspects of vili and lung protective MV*. American Thoracic Society, May, pp. A5239–A5239.

Joffe, A.M., Hetzel, S. and Liew, E.C., 2010. A two-handed jaw-thrust technique is superior to the one-handed 'EC-clamp' technique for mask ventilation in the apneic unconscious person. *Anesthesiology*, 113(4), 873–879.

Khoury, A., de Luca, A., Sall, F.S., Pazart, L. and Capellier, G., 2015. Performance of manual ventilation: how to define its efficiency in bench studies? A review of the literature. *Anaesthesia*, 70(8), 985–992.

Khoury, A., Hugonnot, S., Cossus, J., de Luca, A., Desmettre, T., Sall, F.S. and Capellier, G., 2014. From mouth-to-mouth to bag-valve-mask ventilation: evolution and characteristics of actual devices – a review of the literature. *BioMed Research International*, 27.

Kreit, J.W., 2014. Systolic blood pressure variation during mechanical ventilation. *Annals of the American Thoracic Society*, 11(3), 462–465.

Lagarde, S., Semjen, F., Nouette-Gaulain, K., Masson, F., Bordes, M., Meymat, Y. and Cros, A.M., 2010. Facemask pressure-controlled ventilation in children: what is the pressure limit? *Anesthesia & Analgesia*, 110(6), 1676–1679.

Lipes, J., Bojmehrani, A. and Lellouche, F., 2012. Low tidal volume ventilation in patients without acute respiratory distress syndrome: a paradigm shift in mechanical ventilation. *Critical Care Research and Practice*, doi:10.1155/2012/416862.

Liu, Y., Lou, J.S., Mi, W.D., Yuan, W.X., Fu, Q., Wang, M. and Qu, J., 2016. Pulse pressure variation shows a direct linear correlation with tidal volume in anesthetized healthy patients. *BMC Anesthesiology*, 16(1), 75.

Mesquida, J., Kim, H.K. and Pinsky, M.R., 2012. Effect of tidal volume, intrathoracic pressure, and cardiac contractility on variations in pulse pressure, stroke volume, and intrathoracic blood volume. In Pinsky, M.R., Brochard, L., Mancebo, J. and Hedenstierna, G. (eds), *Applied physiology in intensive care medicine*. Berlin Heidelberg: Springer, pp. 255–262.

Nagao, T., Kinoshita, K., Sakurai, A., Yamaguchi, J., Furukawa, M., Utagawa, A., Moriya, T., Azuhata, T. and Tanjoh, K., 2012. Effects of bag-mask versus advanced airway ventilation for patients undergoing prolonged cardiopulmonary resuscitation in pre-hospital setting. *Journal of Emergency Medicine*, 42(2), 162–170.

Otten, D., Liao, M.M., Wolken, R., Douglas, I.S., Mishra, R., Kao, A., Barrett, W., Drasler, E., Byyny, R.L. and Haukoos, J.S., 2014. Comparison of bag-valve-mask hand-sealing techniques in a simulated model. *Annals of Emergency Medicine*, 63(1), 6–12.

Parry, A. and Higginson, R., 2016. How to use a self-inflating bag and face mask. *Nursing Standard*, 30(19), 36–38.

Siegler, J., Kroll, M., Wojcik, S. and Moy, H.P., 2016. Can EMS providers provide appropriate tidal volumes in a simulated adult-sized patient with a pediatric-sized bag-valve-mask? *Prehospital Emergency Care*, 28, 1–5.

Weingart, S.D. and Levitan, R.M., 2012. Preoxygenation and prevention of desaturation during emergency airway management. *Annals of Emergency Medicine*, 59(3), 165–175.

Bibliography

Craft, J., Gordon, C., Huether, S.E., McCance, K.L. and Brashers, V.L., 2015. *Understanding pathophysiology (ANZ adaptation)*. Sydney: Elsevier.

McCance, K.L. and Huether, S.E., 2015. *Pathophysiology: the biologic basis for disease in adults and children*. Sydney: Elsevier.

Chapter 4
Medication Administration

4.1 | Administering oral medications

Amanda Hlushak

Chapter objectives

At the end of this chapter the reader will be able to:

1. Identify when a patient may require oral medication
2. Identify the different oral medication forms
3. Demonstrate safe delivery of oral medications

Resources required for this assessment

- Simulated patient/mannequin
- Sample oral medications of various forms: tablet, liquid, spray
- Hand decontamination agent
- Disposable gloves
- Clinical waste bag
- Method of documenting the results

Skill matrix

This assessment requires:

- Infection control (CS 1.3)
- Communication (CS 1.5)
- Consent (CS 1.6)

This assessment is a component of:

- Medication administration (Chapter 4)

Introduction

The delivery of medication depends on the patient's presentation. While some medications are delivered via a parenteral route, the paramedic should consider all routes of administration, including oral (enteral). Oral medications may be swallowed, delivered sublingually or buccally.

In general terms, enteral administration is the most common method of medication delivery. It is typically safe and usually the most economical route. However, absorption can be slow and unreliable, with frequent variations in gastrointestinal tract absorption caused by food, emotion, physical activity or previously absorbed drugs. This makes enteral administration less ideal in many emergency situations.

This chapter will discuss instances and methods of administering oral medication.

Anatomy and physiology

During enteral ingestion, medication is generally absorbed from one or more of four body areas: oral cavity, stomach, small intestine, or colon/rectum.

Oral cavity absorption

The oral cavity has a thin lining that has a rich blood supply and a slightly acidic pH. Many enteral medications are not absorbed in the mouth because they contain a protective coating or are quickly swallowed. However, some medications dissolve rapidly when encountering salivary secretions, including those intended for sublingual and buccal administration; for example, glyceryl trinitrate and ondansetron. Sublingual (under the tongue) and buccal (placed in the cheek) administration allows medication to be absorbed up to 10 times faster than by the oral route, through direct membrane absorption into the systemic circulation. Sublingual uptake is faster than buccal (Narang and Sharma, 2011).

Medications absorbed sublingually enter the systemic circulation without entering the portal system and so bypass the liver. The liver is responsible for first-pass metabolism, which in turn reduces the efficacy of the remaining circulating drug. Without this first-pass effect, sublingual medication absorption is fast and rapid, with the effects of the medication appearing as soon as a few minutes after dissolution.

Stomach absorption

The stomach is not a very effective site for absorption. Despite having a rich blood supply, the low pH, thick layer of protective mucus and relatively small surface area reduce the opportunity for absorption (Ensign et al., 2012). However, the amount of time the medication remains in the stomach affects absorption in the small intestine. The longer it takes for food to empty from the stomach (gastric emptying), the longer it takes for the drug to be effective and the greater the risk of acid-labile drugs being destroyed. That is why some medications are required to be taken on an empty stomach. Conversely, some drugs can cause gastric irritation and should be taken with food to minimise the risk of this occurring.

Small intestine absorption

The small intestine is highly vascular, with a significantly larger and more permeable absorption area than the stomach. This is the primary absorption site for orally administered drugs. Since the small intestine has a pH close to neutral, the extent of ionisation is influenced by the acid-base combination of the drug ingested. Lipophilic medications are readily absorbed as they can pass through cell membranes. Ionised hydrophilic medications, particularly those that have a smaller molecular size, pass between cells.

If a patient has increased motility from diarrhoea or other drugs, absorption may be decreased because of reduced exposure time in the small intestine. This may lead to the medication having an ineffective therapeutic effect.

Colon and rectum absorption

Drug uptake from the colon is much less than from the small intestine, as the latter lacks villi and so has a reduced surface area. Slower uptake and transit time in the colon allows the opportunity to metabolise the remaining medication (Philip and Philip, 2010). The rectum, the last part of the large intestine, is small but very vascular. The superior rectal veins drain into the portal vein and allow first-pass metabolism of the drug that is taken up. The lower rectal veins drain into the inferior vena cava, bypassing the liver. As much as 50% of medication taken up in the rectum avoids first-pass metabolism, and more if it is rectally administered, making the rectum an effective drug route (Lakshmi Prasanna et al., 2012). The corollary is that most of the drug is already absorbed before this point if it is administered orally. The presence of faeces can impact on the uptake time of medication in the rectum. Rectal administration is generally used for unconscious patients who are unable to swallow, or when severe vomiting is present.

Clinical rationale

In a conscious acute and non-acute patient requiring medication administration, the oral route is a safe and effective method of administration. The paramedic must remember that the absorption of medication may be affected by several factors that can change its efficacy, including medication solubility, gastric emptying, vomiting, the food eaten, emotion and physical activity.

For sublingual or buccal administration, medications must be left where they are placed, without any attempt to chew or swallow them.

Medications intended for oral uptake should not always be considered acceptable for crushing and delivery via nasogastric/gastric tube, so this should be verified beforehand (Elliott and Liu, 2010).

Solid and liquid oral medication comes in various forms:

- capsules (medication within either a hard or soft shell, intended for swallowing)
- time-release capsules
- lozenges (intended to dissolve slowly in the mouth)
- tablet (doses of medication in solid form – can also be administered other than orally, e.g. via the rectum)
- pills (small, round, swallowable tablets)
- caplets (smooth, oval, swallowable tablets)
- oral (mouth) disintegrating tablets (ODTs)
- elixirs (medicinal liquids)
- emulsions
- suspensions
- syrups
- sprays.

Before administering any medication, at least nine factors must be first verified for patient safety. The first are the traditional five rights:

1. Right patient (where there is more than one person being treated)
2. Right medication (double check and confirm the packaging, including the expiry date; also check allergies/sensitivities)
3. Right route
4. Right time (the interval of administration or in line with eating if required)
5. Right dose (in some cases, a tablet may need to be broken along scored lines if other than a full dose is required; this must happen before offering it to the patient and confirmed during checking)

To this can be added:

6. Right documentation (always applicable in emergencies or otherwise; includes documentation during handover)
7. Right action (the medication matches the condition it is intended to treat)

8. Right form (some medications come in multiple route options)
9. Right response (reassess for effect) (Elliott and Liu, 2010)

Handing over medication

Ideally, medication should be handled only when wearing clean gloves. Asepsis is not typically necessary for oral medication. Remove the medication from its normal packaging, place it into a disposable receptacle and hand it to the patient. This is hygienic, aesthetically more pleasant and ensures the patient receives only the required medication.

Where such a receptacle is not available, the patient can be allowed to remove the medication directly from the palm of the paramedic's upturned hand, provided clean gloves are worn.

Avoid placing the medication directly into the patient's mouth. This not only distributes patient body fluid but it risks the paramedic being bitten and can be distasteful to some patients.

If any medication is scored and broken for the administration of smaller doses, discard any part of it that is not given to the patient. Do not return any medication back into its storage bottle.

Contraindications to oral drug administration

Due to the risk of aspiration, oral drug administration may be unsafe for patients who have difficulty swallowing, including due to suspected or post stroke and for those with altered consciousness or who are fed via enteric means.

Clinical skill assessment process

The following section outlines the clinical skill assessment tools that should be used to determine a student's ability to demonstrate safe and accurate oral medication administration.

1. Clinical Skill Work Instruction
2. Formative Clinical Skill Assessment (F-CSAT)
3. Performance Improvement Plan (PIP)
4. Summative Clinical Skill Assessment (S-CSAT)
(5. Direct Observation of Procedural Skills (DOPS): see Chapter 1.1)

Clinical Skill Work Instruction

Equipment and resources: Simulated patient/mannequin; sample oral medications of various forms: tablet, liquid, spray; hand decontamination agent; disposable gloves; clinical waste bag; method of documenting the results

Associated Clinical Skills: Infection control; Communication; Consent

Administering oral medications

Activity	Critical Action	Rationale
Prepare paramedic	Wash and clean hands. Wear protective gloves as required.	To prevent infection transmission.
Confirm patient	Check the correct patient has been identified for the medication/indication.	Ensures patient should receive the medication.
Confirm medication	Check correct medication is chosen as indicated/prescribed and in the correct form for the chosen route.	Ensures correct medication is administered.
Conform dose	Check dose is appropriate for indication/prescription.	Ensures medication matches necessary route and dose.
Confirm right time	Check frequency required and relationship to food ingestion. Check correct time for administration as indicated/prescribed.	Ensures medication is to be administered at right time and interval.
Medication presentation	Withdraw medication from bottle/container and place into clean container for presentation to patient. Break scored tablets as required for smaller doses if indicated.	To ensure only the required tablet is provided to the patient.
Patient preparation	Inform patient of medication they are to receive, including potential effects. Ensure consent.	Informed consent is essential, including any warnings/advice.

Administering oral medications continued

Activity	Critical Action	Rationale
Instruct administration method	Provide specific instruction as to how to take the medication, particularly if they are to swallow or otherwise.	Instruction ensures medication is taken correctly.
Confirm allergies/ sensitivities	Reconfirm patient has no allergies or previous sensitivities to medication.	To avoid adverse reaction.
Oral delivery	Ideally have the patient sit upright. Hand medication to them and observe placing medication in their own mouth. Provide enough water to allow drug to be swallowed if appropriate.	A dry mouth can make it difficult to swallow.
Sublingual/ buccal delivery	Offer medication to patient as for oral delivery, ensuring this time that the patient places medication against either inner cheek for buccal or under one side of the tongue for sublingual. Ensure patient does not swallow and leaves medication in place.	Swallowing renders medication ineffective.
Report	Document dose, delivery, time and effects of the drug. Monitor the patient for adverse effects. Hand over, including therapeutic benefit/adverse reaction.	For continuity of care and to avoid risk of inadvertent readministering. Adverse reactions identified and managed, and accurate record maintained.

Source: *Adapted from Elliott and Liu, 2010.*

Formative Clinical Skill Assessment (F-CSAT)

Equipment and resources: Simulated patient/mannequin; sample oral medications of various forms: tablet, liquid, spray; hand decontamination agent; disposable gloves; clinical waste bag; method of documenting the results

Associated Clinical Skills: Infection control; Communication; Consent

Staff/Student being assessed: _____

Administering oral medications

Activity	Critical Action	Performance				
Prepares paramedic	Washes hands and dons protective gloves.	0	1	2	3	4
Confirms patient	Checks correct patient for medication/indication.	0	1	2	3	4
Confirms medication	Checks correct medication and in correct form for chosen route.	0	1	2	3	4
Confirms dose	Checks appropriate dose for indication/prescription.	0	1	2	3	4
Confirms right time	Checks correct time for administration.	0	1	2	3	4
Medication presentation	Withdraws medication and places into clean container for presentation. Breaks scored tablet if required.	0	1	2	3	4
Patient preparation	Informs patient about medication. Ensures consent.	0	1	2	3	4
Instructs administration method	Provides specific instruction to taking medication.	0	1	2	3	4
Confirms allergies/ sensitivities	Reconfirms patient has no allergies/sensitivities.	0	1	2	3	4

Administering oral medications continued

Activity	Critical Action	Performance				
Oral delivery	Ideally, sits patient upright. Hands patient medication and observes them place it in their mouth.	0	1	2	3	4
Sublingual/buccal delivery	Ensures patient places medication correctly for buccal or sublingual delivery, without swallowing.	0	1	2	3	4
Reports	Documents/hands over dose, delivery, time, effects of the drug.	0	1	2	3	4

Source: Adapted from Elliott and Liu, 2010.

Standard Achieved: (please circle one)

Competent (C)   Not Yet Competent* (NYC)

Staff/Student Name: _____

Assessor (please print name): _____

Signed (Assessor): _____

Date of Assessment: _____

Comments:

*If Not Yet Competent (NYC) a PIP needs to be completed and a repeat of the F-CSAT

Formative Clinical Skill Assessment (F-CSAT) Key

Skill level	Standard of procedure	Quality of performance	Outcome	Level of assistance required
4 Safe for unsupervised practice	Safe Accurate Behaviour is appropriate to context	Confident Accurate Expedient	Achieved intended outcome	No supporting cues* required
3 Requires supervision	Safe Accurate Behaviour is appropriate to context	Confident Accurate Takes longer than required	Achieved intended outcome	Requires occasional supportive cues*
2 Requires assistance	Safe Accurate Behaviour generally appropriate to context	Lacks certainty	Would not have achieved outcome without support	Requires frequent verbal and occasional physical directives in addition to supportive cues*
1 Requires direction	Safe only with guidance Not completely accurate	Unskilled Inefficient	Would not have achieved outcome without support	Requires continuous verbal and frequent physical directive cues*
0 Unsafe	Unsafe Unable to demonstrate behaviour Lack of insight into behaviour appropriate to context	Unskilled	Would not have achieved outcome	Requires continuous verbal and continuous physical directive cues*

*Refers to physical directives or verbal supportive cues

Performance Improvement Plan (PIP)

Please document the agreed education plan and completion timelines for areas assessed as less than 4.

This plan should be presented to assessor prior to commencement of summative assessment.

Where was supervisor support required?	Student summary of deficit. (Why was there a problem?)	Improvement Plan	Completed (Y/N)

Staff/Student Name: _____

Staff/Student Signature: _____

Educator Name: _____

Educator Signature: _____

Summative Clinical Skill Assessment (S-CSAT)

Equipment and resources: Simulated patient/mannequin; sample oral medications of various forms: tablet, liquid, spray; hand decontamination agent; disposable gloves; clinical waste bag; method of documenting the results

Associated Clinical Skills: Infection control; Communication; Consent

Staff/Student being assessed: _____

- Completed Formative Clinical Skill Assessment (F-CSAT): **YES** **NO**
- Completed Performance Improvement Plan (PIP): **YES** **NO** **N/A**

Administering oral medications

Activity	Critical Action	Achieved Without Direction	
Prepares paramedic	Washes hands and dons protective gloves.	NO	YES
Confirms patient	Checks correct patient for medication/indication.	NO	YES
Confirms medication	Checks correct medication and in correct form for chosen route.	NO	YES
Confirms dose	Checks appropriate dose for indication/prescription.		
Confirms right time	Confirms correct time for administration.	NO	YES
Medication presentation	Withdraws medication and places into clean container for presentation. Breaks scored tablet if required.	NO	YES
Patient preparation	Informs patient about medication. Ensures consent.	NO	YES
Instructs administration method	Provides specific instruction to taking medication.	NO	YES
Confirms allergies/ sensitivities	Reconfirms patient has no allergies/sensitivities.	NO	YES

Administering oral medications continued

Activity	Critical Action	Achieved Without Direction	
Oral delivery	Ideally, sits patient upright. Hands patient medication and observes them place it in their mouth.	NO	YES
Sublingual/buccal delivery	Ensures patient places medication correctly for buccal or sublingual delivery, without swallowing.	NO	YES
Reports	Documents/hands over dose, delivery, time, effects of the drug.	NO	YES

Source: *Adapted from Elliott and Liu, 2010.*

Standard Achieved: (please circle one)

Competent (C)   Not Yet Competent* (NYC)

Staff/Student Name: _____

Assessor (please print name): _____

Signed (Assessor): _____

Date of Assessment: _____

Comments:

*If Not Yet Competent (NYC) a PIP needs to be completed and a repeat of the F-CSAT

Clinical findings

Patient reassessment/monitoring

It is important to monitor a patient after medication has been administered in order to assess for both desired and adverse effects. The latter may include but is not limited to allergies, hypotension, vomiting, arrhythmias and dizziness. The duration and frequency of monitoring will vary with the medication administered and any previous exposure to its actions. Where an adverse response is likely, more frequent and detailed monitoring is necessary.

Dose errors

Errors can be introduced where dose or volume approximations are required to be made during preparation. Measuring cups are less reliable than droppers, spoons or syringes. Dose instructions can also cause errors where the instructions can be ambiguous or unclear, such as using a size abbreviation such as 'ts' or 'tbs' to refer to teaspoons or tablespoons (Gildon et al., 2016; Yin et al., 2010).

Paediatric patients

Children often fail to comply with medical assessment and the therapies provided. Reassuring the child, involving them in decision making, being honest and providing practical advice as to how to take medication can all help overcome their resistance.

The most common source of errors in administering paediatric medication occur in determining the dose, preparation and using an incorrect route of administration (Ghaleb et al., 2010; Gonzales, 2010). The most common errors are associated with weight-based calculations (Hoyle et al., 2012).

PRACTICE TIP!

Errors in medication dosage can occur when calculations are more complex, such as with children, emergency situations or where there are multiple patients. Where possible, use dose charts and confirm your calculations with a colleague.

PRACTICE TIP!

Giving a syrup or elixir orally to a child can be difficult at times. Use of a syringe is the preferred method of administration for measurement and delivery. If a parent is available, have them place the child in a comfortable position on their lap and have them give the child the medication. This can ease the child's anxiety.

TEST YOUR KNOWLEDGE QUESTIONS

1. **List five solid forms of oral medication.**
    Capsules; lozenges; tablets; pills; caplets; ODT.

2. **List five liquid forms of oral medication.**
    Elixirs; emulsions; suspensions; syrups; sprays.

3. **What are the five traditional rights of medication administration?**
    Right patient; right medication; right route; right time; right dose.

4. **What other four rights can be added to the traditional five rights of medication administration?**
    Right documentation; right action; right form; right response.

5. **What are five factors that influence the absorption of oral medication?**
    Medication solubility; gastric emptying; food eaten; emotion; physical activity.

6. **How does drug absorption via sublingual, buccal and lower rectal administration differ from that of oral administration?**
    Medication taken up does not drain into the portal system and so initially bypasses the liver.

7. **What effect can diarrhoea have on the uptake of oral medication?**
    Increased motility can decrease absorption because of reduced exposure time in the small intestine. This may lead to an ineffective therapeutic effect.

8. **List two factors that influence duration and frequency of patient monitoring required after oral drug administration.**
    The medication administered; previous medication exposure.

9. **What are the four gastrointestinal areas where medication can be absorbed?**
    Oral cavity; stomach; small intestine; colon/rectum.

10. **Which important instruction must be added when administering sublingual or buccal medication?**
    Leave medication placed in the mouth and do not chew or swallow.

References

Elliott, M. and Liu, Y., 2010. The nine rights of medication administration: an overview. *British Journal of Nursing*, 19(5).

Ensign, L.M., Cone, R. and Hanes, J., 2012. Oral drug delivery with polymeric nanoparticles: the gastrointestinal mucus barriers. *Advanced Drug Delivery Reviews*, 64(6), 557–570.

Ghaleb, M.A., Barber, N., Franklin, B.D. and Wong, I.C.K., 2010. The incidence and nature of prescribing and medication administration errors in paediatric inpatients. *Archives of Disease in Childhood*, adc158485.

Gildon, B.L., Condren, M., Phillips, C., Votruba, A. and Swar, S., 2016. Appropriateness of oral medication delivery devices available in community pharmacies. *Journal of the American Pharmacists Association*, 56(2), 137–140.

Gonzales, K., 2010. Medication administration errors and the pediatric population: a systematic search of the literature. *Journal of Pediatric Nursing*, 25(6), 555–565.

Hoyle Jr, J.D., Davis, A.T., Putman, K.K., Trytko, J.A. and Fales, W.D., 2012. Medication dosing errors in pediatric patients treated by emergency medical services. *Prehospital Emergency Care*, 16(1), 59–66.

Lakshmi Prasanna, J., Deepthi, B. and Rama Rao, N., 2012. Rectal drug delivery: A promising route for enhancing drug absorption. *Asian Journal of Research in Pharmaceutical Sciences*, 2(4), 143–149.

Narang, N. and Sharma, J., 2011. Sublingual mucosa as a route for systemic drug delivery. *International Journal of Pharmacy and Pharmaceutical Sciences*, 3(Suppl 2), 18–22.

Philip, A.K. and Philip, B., 2010. Colon targeted drug delivery systems: a review on primary and novel approaches. *Oman Medical Journal*, 25(2), 79.

Yin, H.S., Mendelsohn, A.L., Wolf, M.S., Parker, R.M., Fierman, A., van Schaick, L., Bazan, I.S., Kline, M.D. and Dreyer, B.P., 2010. Parents' medication administration errors: role of dosing instruments and health literacy. *Archives of Pediatrics & Adolescent Medicine*, 164(2), 181–186.

Bibliography

Bryant, B.J. and Knights, K.M., 2015. *Pharmacology for health professionals*, 4th edn. Sydney: Elsevier.

Curtis, K. and Ramsden, C., 2016. *Emergency and trauma care: for nurses and paramedics*, 2nd Australian and New Zealand edn. Sydney: Elsevier.

Sanders, M.J., 2010. *Sanders' paramedic textbook*, 3rd edn. St. Louis: Elsevier/Mosby.

4.2 | Administering intranasal medications

James Pearce and Liam Langford

Chapter objectives

At the end of this chapter the reader will be able to:

1. Describe the clinical rationale for administering intranasal (IN) medications
2. Identify the indications and contraindications for IN medication administration
3. Demonstrate the safe and effective use of a nasal mucosal atomising device (MAD Nasal)

Resources required for this assessment

- Standardised patient/mannequin with IN capabilities
- Hand decontamination agent
- Appropriate vial/ampoule for administration
- Drawing-up needle
- 1 mL syringe (preferably Luer lock)
- MAD Nasal
- Method of documenting results

Skill matrix

This assessment requires:

- Infection control (CS 1.3)
- Communication (CS 1.5)
- Consent (CS 1.6)
- Administering oral medications (CS 4.1)
- Preparing injections (CS 4.4)

This assessment is a component of:

- Medication administration (Chapter 4)

Introduction

Medications can be delivered via the intranasal (IN) route using several different methods, including sniffing, spraying, droppers and atomisers. This chapter focuses on the MAD Nasal, which is commonly used for IN medication administration by Australasian paramedics.

The IN route is ideal for prehospital and emergency use. Medications can be given rapidly, avoiding any delay in establishing intravenous access. There is no risk of needlestick injury to the paramedic. It is safe and effective for a variety of medications and clinical situations (Bailey et al., 2017; Corrigan et al., 2015; Rickard et al., 2007). The IN route is non-invasive and well tolerated by patients, and using it is a relatively easy skill to master.

In Australasian ambulance services, the IN route is currently used for various medications and clinical conditions. These include (but are not limited to) adrenaline for epistaxis (Wellington Free Ambulance, 2019), fentanyl for pain management (St John New Zealand, 2017; Ambulance Victoria, 2018), naloxone for opiate overdose (SA Ambulance Service, 2017) and midazolam for seizures (NSW Ambulance, 2016).

IN medication administration is discussed in this chapter.

Anatomy and physiology

The external nasal openings are called nostrils or nares (singular: naris), which internally lead to the vestibules

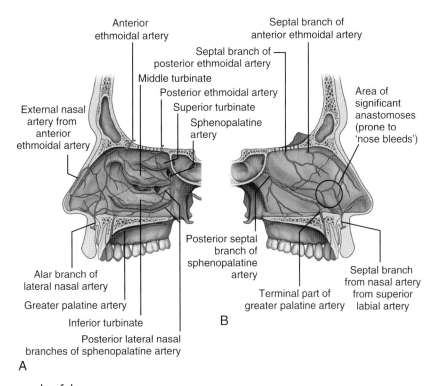

Figure 4.2.1 Vascular supply of the nose

Arterial supply of the nasal cavities. (a) Lateral wall of the right nasal cavity. (b) Septum (medial wall of right nasal cavity).
Source: Ramakrishnan, V.R. and Scholes, M.A., 2016, ENT secrets, 4th edn (Chapter 23, Figure 23-1), Elsevier.

in the anterior nasal cavity. The nasal cavity is divided into right and left halves by the nasal septum. Each half normally has three nasal turbinates (conchae). These create turbulence as air enters, helping warm, filter and humidify the inhaled air.

Lining the nasal cavity are the respiratory mucosa (lower two thirds) and olfactory mucosa (upper third). The respiratory mucosa contains highly vascular tissue with a rich blood supply (Fig. 4.2.1). It is innervated by branches of the trigeminal nerve (cranial nerve V). The olfactory mucosa is where the sense of smell arises. Olfactory nerve axons (cranial nerve I) project through the cribriform plate of the ethmoid bone and terminate in exposed endings in the olfactory epithelium.

Clinical rationale

The highly vascular nasal cavity tissue allows medication to be readily absorbed into surrounding capillaries. From here, medications can be transported into the systemic circulation and to target organs, thus avoiding first-pass metabolism by the liver.

The turbinate structures increase the surface area, allowing greater absorption. This nasal cavity surface area is limited. Where possible, administer <0.5 mL per nostril to avoid oversaturation and the formation of droplets and to optimise the efficiency of absorption (Rech et al., 2016). Alternating between nares allows enough time for the medication to be absorbed. Consider breaking larger single doses into two smaller doses, half in each nostril.

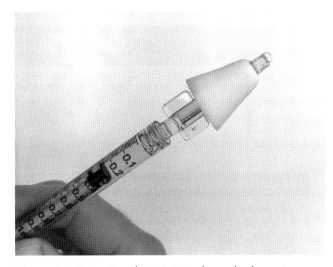

Figure 4.2.2 A primed MAD Nasal attached to a Luer-lock syringe

There is some evidence of a nose–brain pathway via the olfactory or trigeminal nerves directly into the brain and/or cerebrospinal fluid (Pardeshi and Belgamwar, 2013; Thorne et al., 2004). Although contentious, it remains theoretically possible for emergency medications to be taken up into the cerebrospinal fluid by this route.

The MAD Nasal (Fig. 4.2.2) has a soft, cone-shaped plug that is gently pressed into the nostril to form a seal and prevent the escape of fluid. The attached syringe is quickly pressed to create pressure. As fluid passes through the MAD Nasal, atomised droplets form that are 30–100 microns in size, ideal for mucosal absorption. The device works with the patient in any position.

The MAD Nasal has a 'dead space' of 0.06 mL which must be initially primed with 0.1 mL of medication on first use only. When priming the MAD Nasal, a small drop will be expelled. This drop will be 0.04 mL in volume. This leaves 0.06 mL of medication in the MAD Nasal device. The expelled drop plus volume in the primed MAD Nasal equates to 0.1 mL.

Indications

There are numerous reasons for administering drugs via the IN route, including an inability to gain IV access, paediatric patients, patient convenience, ease of administration and safety considerations in avoiding the use of needles.

To maximise spray entry into the nasal cavity, angle the atomiser so that it is aligned slightly above the top of the ear on the same side as the naris (Fig. 4.2.3).

Clinical skill assessment process

The following section outlines the clinical skill assessment tools that should be used to determine a student's ability to

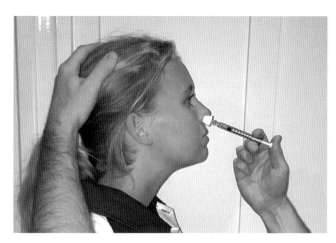

Figure 4.2.3 Inserting the MAD Nasal into the naris

demonstrate safe and accurate administration of intranasal medication.
1. Clinical Skill Work Instruction
2. Formative Clinical Skill Assessment (F-CSAT)
3. Performance Improvement Plan (PIP)
4. Summative Clinical Skill Assessment (S-CSAT)
(5. Direct Observation of Procedural Skills (DOPS) – see Chapter 1.1)

Clinical Skill Work Instruction

Equipment and resources: Standardised patient/mannequin with nasal access; hand decontamination agent; appropriate medication vial/ampoule; drawing-up needle; 1 mL syringe (preferably Luer lock); MAD Nasal; method of documenting results

Associated Clinical Skills: Infection control; Communication; Consent; Preparing injections

Administering intranasal medications

Activity	Critical Action	Rationale
Personal protection	Don PPE as appropriate.	Infection control.
Prepare medication	Select correct medication and ensure volume/dosage calculation is correct; cross-check with colleague.	The patient receives the right medication and dosage.
	Attach drawing-up needle to 1 mL Luer-lock syringe.	Ready to aspirate medication.
	Draw up medication to required volume/dosage plus 0.1 mL to prime MAD Nasal. Ensure no air bubbles are present.	0.1 mL extra is required to account for the dead space within the MAD Nasal.
	Disconnect syringe from drawing-up needle.	No longer required.
	Attach MAD Nasal to syringe. Twist Luer lock to secure.	High pressure develops during atomisation.
	Advance syringe plunger 0.1 mL to prime the MAD Nasal (approx. 0.04 mL will drip out).	Fills 0.06 mL dead space in the MAD Nasal.

Administering intranasal medications continued

Activity	Critical Action	Rationale
Prepare patient	Blow nose if a small amount of blood/mucus is present.	Excess mucus/blood reduces absorption.
	Advise patient to breathe through mouth during administration.	To avoid swallowing medication, the patient should **not** sniff or inhale during atomisation.
	Secure patient by gently holding their occiput with your free hand.	To reduce patient recoil.
Administer medication	Insert conical plug into patient's naris, ensuring a firm but gentle fit.	Ensures seal with nostril and maximises patient comfort and paramedic access.
	Angle the atomiser slightly above a line intersecting the top of the ear on the same side as the naris.	Ensures maximal nasal cavity coverage and absorption.
	Depress plunger briskly to atomise medication.	Brisk plunger compression ensures atomisation of medication.
Remove from naris	Remove MAD Nasal from naris. Detach MAD Nasal from syringe and store it in the original packaging or discard it as clinical waste.	Keeps MAD Nasal clean for next use.
Larger volume administration	Larger volumes can be divided between both nostrils. Excluding MAD Nasal priming, repeat above steps to administer the second half of required dose.	MAD Nasal is already primed, so no extra volume is required. Halving the volume between naris increases absorption.
Report	Document/hand over medication dose, route, effect and complete medication register.	For continuity of care and formal recording.

Formative Clinical Skill Assessment (F-CSAT)

Equipment and resources: Standardised patient/mannequin with nasal access; hand decontamination agent; appropriate medication vial/ampoule; drawing-up needle; 1 mL syringe (preferably Luer lock); MAD Nasal; method of documenting results

Associated Clinical Skills: Infection control; Communication; Consent; Preparing injections

Staff/Student being assessed: _____

Administering intranasal medications

Activity	Critical Action	Performance				
Personal protection	Dons PPE as appropriate.	0	1	2	3	4
Prepares medication	Selects correct medication and ensures volume/dosage calculation is correct. Cross-checks with colleague.	0	1	2	3	4
	Attaches drawing-up needle to 1 mL Luer-lock syringe.	0	1	2	3	4
	Draws up required medication volume/dosage, plus 0.1 mL to prime MAD Nasal. Ensures no air bubbles are present.	0	1	2	3	4

Administering intranasal medications continued

Activity	Critical Action	Performance				
	Disconnects syringe from drawing-up needle.	0	1	2	3	4
	Attaches MAD Nasal to syringe. Twists to secure Luer lock.	0	1	2	3	4
	Advances syringe plunger 0.1 mL to prime the MAD Nasal.	0	1	2	3	4
Prepares patient	Has patient blow nose if blood or mucus are present.	0	1	2	3	4
	Advises patient to breathe through mouth during administration.	0	1	2	3	4
	Secures patient by gently holding their occiput with free hand.	0	1	2	3	4
Administers medication	Inserts soft, conical plug into naris, ensuring a firm but gentle fit.	0	1	2	3	4
	Aims atomiser just above the top of the ear on the same side as the naris.	0	1	2	3	4
	Depresses plunger briskly to atomise medication.	0	1	2	3	4
Removes from naris	Removes MAD Nasal from naris. Detaches MAD Nasal device from syringe and stores in its original packaging or discards it correctly.	0	1	2	3	4
Larger volume administration	Excluding MAD Nasal priming, repeats above steps to administer second half of required dose.	0	1	2	3	4
Reports	Documents/hands over dose, route, effect and completes medication register.	0	1	2	3	4

Standard Achieved: (please circle one)

Competent (C)   Not Yet Competent* (NYC)

Staff/Student Name: _____

Assessor (please print name): _____

Signed (Assessor): _____

Date of Assessment: _____

Comments:

*If Not Yet Competent (NYC) a PIP needs to be completed and a repeat of the F-CSAT

Formative Clinical Skill Assessment (F-CSAT) Key

Skill level	Standard of procedure	Quality of performance	Outcome	Level of assistance required
4 Safe for unsupervised practice	Safe Accurate Behaviour is appropriate to context	Confident Accurate Expedient	Achieved intended outcome	No supporting cues* required
3 Requires supervision	Safe Accurate Behaviour is appropriate to context	Confident Accurate Takes longer than required	Achieved intended outcome	Requires occasional supportive cues*

Skill level	Standard of procedure	Quality of performance	Outcome	Level of assistance required
2 Requires assistance	Safe Accurate Behaviour generally appropriate to context	Lacks certainty	Would not have achieved outcome without support	Requires frequent verbal and occasional physical directives in addition to supportive cues*
1 Requires direction	Safe only with guidance Not completely accurate	Unskilled Inefficient	Would not have achieved outcome without support	Requires continuous verbal and frequent physical directive cues*
0 Unsafe	Unsafe Unable to demonstrate behaviour Lack of insight into behaviour appropriate to context	Unskilled	Would not have achieved outcome	Requires continuous verbal and continuous physical directive cues*

*Refers to physical directives or verbal supportive cues

Performance Improvement Plan (PIP)

Please document the agreed education plan and completion timelines for areas assessed as less than 4.

This plan should be presented to assessor prior to commencement of summative assessment.

Where was supervisor support required?	Student summary of deficit. (Why was there a problem?)	Improvement Plan	Completed (Y/N)

Staff/Student Name: _____

Staff/Student Signature: _____

Educator Name: _____

Educator Signature: _____

Summative Clinical Skill Assessment (S-CSAT)

Equipment and resources: Standardised patient/mannequin with nasal access; hand decontamination agent; appropriate medication vial/ampoule; drawing-up needle; 1 mL syringe (preferably Luer lock); MAD Nasal; method of documenting results

Associated Clinical Skills: Infection control; Communication, Consent; Preparing injections

Staff/Student being assessed: _____

- Completed Formative Clinical Skill Assessment (F-CSAT):   **YES   NO**

- Completed Performance Improvement Plan (PIP):   **YES   NO   N/A**

Administering intranasal medications

Activity	Critical Action	Achieved Without Direction	
Personal protection	Dons PPE as appropriate.	NO	YES
Prepares medication	Selects correct medication and ensures volume/dosage calculation is correct. Cross-checks with colleague.	NO	YES
	Attaches drawing-up needle to 1 mL Luer-lock syringe.	NO	YES
	Draws up required medication volume/dosage, plus 0.1 mL to prime MAD Nasal. Ensures no air bubbles are present.	NO	YES
	Disconnects syringe from drawing-up needle.	NO	YES
	Attaches MAD Nasal to syringe. Twists to secure Luer lock.	NO	YES
	Advances syringe plunger 0.1 mL to prime the MAD Nasal.	NO	YES
Prepares patient	Has patient blow nose if blood or mucus are present.	NO	YES
	Advises patient to breathe through mouth during administration.	NO	YES
	Secures patient by gently holding their occiput with free hand.	NO	YES
Administers medication	Inserts soft, conical plug into naris, ensuring a firm but gentle fit.	NO	YES
	Aims atomiser just above the top of the ear on the same side as the naris.	NO	YES
	Depresses plunger briskly to atomise medication.	NO	YES
Removes from naris	Removes MAD Nasal from naris. Detaches MAD Nasal device from syringe and stores in its original packaging or discards it correctly.	NO	YES
Larger volume administration	Excluding MAD Nasal priming, repeats above steps to administer second half of required dose.	NO	YES
Reports	Documents/hands over dose, route, effect and completes medication register.	NO	YES

Standard Achieved: (please circle one)

Competent (C)   Not Yet Competent* (NYC)

Staff/Student Name: _____

Assessor (please print name): _____

Signed (Assessor): _____

Date of Assessment: _____

Comments:

*If Not Yet Competent (NYC) a PIP needs to be completed and a repeat of the F-CSAT

Clinical findings

IN medication administration has contraindications and precautions for effective use.

Contraindications

IN administration is contraindicated for:

- nasal occlusion (e.g. excessive blood or mucus) whereby nasal mucosa uptake is unreliable
- nasal mucosa destruction (e.g. trauma, cocaine use, airway burns)
- nasal turbinate hypertrophy.

Precautions

The plunger must be depressed briskly for medication atomisation to occur. If it is done too slowly, medication will dribble into the nasopharynx and not be absorbed. This is uncomfortable for the patient and is not clinically effective.

Many medications intended for IN use are provided in increased concentration or contain a substance that enhances mucosal adhesion. Examples include midazolam, naloxone and fentanyl. Low-concentration drugs, such as many IV medication preparations, may not allow sufficient drug uptake in time to be effective.

While it is physically possible to aspirate medication directly through the MAD Nasal device by attaching a drawing-up needle or vial access cannula on the tip of the MAD, **this should not be done**. As medication is drawn up, air bubbles may form within the chamber, causing inadequate MAD Nasal priming and insufficient or incorrect dosing.

The MAD Nasal can be reused, but only for the same patient with the same medication and if the device is stored cleanly between doses (e.g. in its original packaging).

PRACTICE TIP!

Always depress the plunger briskly so the medication atomises correctly. Slow depression dribbles medication into the nasopharynx without absorption or effectiveness, and causes discomfort. Practise using the MAD Nasal with saline or water and discharging it into the air at different speeds for comparison.

PRACTICE TIP!

Some medications can result in a short stinging feeling or metallic taste after IN administration. Advising the patient about this slight discomfort beforehand will allow you to maintain a good rapport.

PRACTICE TIP!

When preparing IN medication, the dose may require calculation. Practise calculating doses to ensure your proficiency when under stress.

TEST YOUR KNOWLEDGE QUESTIONS

1. **What is the volume of 'dead space' of the MAD Nasal device?**
    0.06 mL. Prime the device with 0.1 mL of medication on first use.

2. **Why is a Luer-lock syringe preferred when using the MAD Nasal?**
    During atomisation, high pressures develop in the syringe. The Luer-lock hub provides superior syringe attachment.

3. **Does administering IN medications avoid first-pass liver metabolism?**
    Yes. The intranasal route allows medication absorption directly into the systemic circulatory system.

4. **Are all medications safe and effective when administered via the IN route?**
    No. Only medications with certain pharmacological properties are appropriate for IN use.

5. **Is the patient encouraged to 'sniff' during IN medication administration?**
    No. Ideally, the patient should breathe through their mouth during administration.

6. **Should medication be drawn up through the MAD Nasal device?**
    No. Air bubbles may form, causing inadequate priming and insufficient or incorrect dosing.

7. **If the dead space of the MAD Nasal is only 0.06 mL, why draw up 0.1 mL?**
    0.1 mL is generally the smallest amount that can be accurately drawn up. Only a small amount (0.04 mL) is wasted in the process.

8. **Is the MAD Nasal reusable?**
    Yes, but only for the same patient, using the same medication, and if stored hygienically.

9. **Why is it best practice to alternate between nares when administering intranasal medication?**
    The limited nasal surface area is easily saturated, reducing efficacy. Alternating between nares improves the absorption of the medication.

10. **Why are nasal occlusion, nasal mucosa destruction and nasal turbinate hypertrophy contraindicated in intranasal medication administration?**
    All impede the nasal cavity's ability to receive or absorb the required medication/dose.

References

Ambulance Victoria, 2018. *Clinical practice guidelines*, revised edn. Retrieved from: https://s3-ap-southeast-2.amazonaws.com/prod.assets.ambulance.vic.gov.au/wp-content/uploads/2018/03/latest-clinical-practice-guidelines.pdf

Bailey, A.M., Baum, R.A., Horn, K., Lewis, T., Morizio, K., Schultz, A., Weant, K. and Justice, S.N., 2017. Review of intranasally administered medications for use in the emergency department. *Journal of Emergency Medicine*, 53(1), 38–48.

Corrigan, M., Wilson, S.S. and Hampton, J., 2015. Safety and efficacy of intranasally administered medications in the emergency department and prehospital settings. *American Journal of Health-System Pharmacy*, 72(18), 1544–1554.

NSW Ambulance, 2016. *NSW Ambulance protocols and pharmacology: seizures*. Retrieved from: https://itunes.apple.com/au/app/nsw-ambulance-protocols/id1103576564?mt=8

Pardeshi, C.V. and Belgamwar, V.S., 2013. Direct nose to brain drug delivery via integrated nerve pathways bypassing the blood–brain barrier: an excellent platform for brain targeting. *Expert Opinion on Drug Delivery*, 10(7), 957–972.

Rech, M.A., Barbas, B., Chaney, W., Greenhalgh, E. and Turck, C., 2016. When to pick the nose: out-of-hospital and emergency department intranasal administration of medications. *Annals of Emergency Medicine*, 70(2), 203–211.

Rickard, C., O'Meara, P., McGrail, M., Garner, D., McLean, A. and Le Lievre, P., 2007. A randomized controlled trial of intranasal fentanyl vs intravenous morphine for analgesia in the prehospital setting. *American Journal of Emergency Medicine*, 25(8), 911–917.

SA Ambulance Service, 2017. *Narcotic overdose – paramedic*. Retrieved from: http://saaselearning.com.au/moodle/static/paramedic-cpgs.html

St John New Zealand, 2017. *Clinical procedures and guidelines: comprehensive edition 2016–2018*. Retrieved from: https://www.stjohn.org.nz/globalassets/documents/health-practitioners/cpg_comprehensive_web170525.pdf

Thorne, R.G., Pronk, G.J., Padmanabhan, V. and Frey, W.H., 2004. Delivery of insulin-like growth factor-I to the rat brain and spinal cord along olfactory and trigeminal pathways following intranasal administration. *Neuroscience*, 127(2), 481–496.

Wellington Free Ambulance, 2019. *Clinical procedures and guidelines: comprehensive edition 2019–2022*. Retrieved from: https://www.wfa.org.nz/assets/What-we-do/b8a3986cc7/WFA-CPG-Comprehensive-2019-2022.pdf

Using metered dose inhalers

Dianne Inglis

Chapter objectives

At the end of this chapter the reader will be able to:

1. Describe the rationale for using pressurised metered dose inhalers (pMDI)
2. Demonstrate the correct use of pMDIs and spacers
3. Identify and manage difficulties with pMDI use

Resources required for this assessment

- Standardised patient
- pMDI, spacer
- Disposable gloves
- Method of documenting the results

Skill matrix

This assessment requires:

- Infection control (CS 1.3)
- Communication (CS 1.5)
- Consent (CS 1.6)
- Patient assessment skills (Chapter 2, CS 2.6, 2.7, 2.8, 2.9, 2.10)

This assessment is a component of:

- Medication administration (Chapter 4)

Introduction

The pressurised metered dose inhaler (pMDI) has been available for over 50 years (Bell and Newman, 2007; Stein et al., 2014; Versteeg et al., 2006). Its principal use is to reliably administer multi-dose medications to asthmatics. Also called an 'inhaler' or 'puffer', the pDMI provides a method of drug delivery that allows targeting of the receptor site within the lungs themselves. This chapter discusses the effective use of pMDIs.

Anatomy and physiology

After entering the upper airway, airflow passes the larger bronchi and many bifurcations before reaching the terminal bronchioles and alveoli. These descending airways contain various receptors that can be activated by inhaled medication. However, they are not uniformly spread throughout the lungs. Beta receptor (e.g. salbutamol) sites are in the bronchioles, with very few in the bronchi, while muscarinic receptors (e.g. ipratropium bromide) are found in greater numbers in the bronchi (Labiris and Dolovich, 2003a).

A diminishing airway size means that particles must be smaller to gain entry. Particle sizes must be less than 10 micrometres (μm) to reach the lower airway. Small particles progress further but deliver less medication; larger particles deliver more medication but do not travel as far. Particles deposit medication by colliding with airways, gravity or diffusion. Airway inflammation and bronchospasm reduce airflow and the delivery of medication (Labiris and Dolovich, 2003a).

Delivering medication into the lungs offers rapid drug uptake and onset of action with fewer systemic side effects. The lungs have a large absorption area, with the bronchioles and alveoli receiving the entire blood circulation through it and bypassing first-pass metabolism in the liver. Medication is absorbed through the airway epithelium (Labiris and Dolovich, 2003a).

Clinical rationale

A pMDI is made up of a number of components (Fig. 4.3.1), including propellant, medication, a metering valve to consistently deliver the required amount of medication and the actuator to atomise the liquid (Newman, 2005; Myrdal et al., 2014; Stein et al., 2014). The canister itself is pressurised and contains sufficient dissolved (liquid) or suspended (solid) medication for repeated therapies (Newman, 2005; Stein et al., 2014). This canister sits within a plastic outer boot. When pressed downwards, the actuator valve releases the medication spray.

For pulmonary inhaled medication to work, aerosol therapy must form a particle stream that is able to reach sites within the smallest distal airways. Chlorofluorocarbon – the propellant that was originally used – has been replaced with hydrofluoroalkane (Cripps et al., 2000; McDonald and Martin, 2000). This change, combined with a smaller exit valve, has reduced the size of the atomised particles, improving the delivery of medication deep into the bronchi (Bell and Newman, 2007; Kleinstreuer et al., 2007; Versteeg et al., 2006). Particles must be small (around 5 μm). Too large and they will not penetrate beyond the upper airway; too small and they may be exhaled again before adhering to the airway (Labiris and Dolovich, 2003b; Lewis et al., 2016).

A principal difficulty with the use of pMDIs is the cognitive and physical ability of the patient to align activation and inhalation (Bensch et al., 2001; Geller, 2005; Scarfone et al., 2002). Aerosol spray is delivered at high speed to assist atomisation (Labiris and Dolovich, 2003b; Myrdal et al., 2014), which results in much of the medication not actually entering the lungs (Bell and Newman, 2007; Bensch et al., 2001; Biswas et al., 2017). The patient's inhalation technique influences how much

medication reaches the lungs, although even poor use can still prove partly effective (Leach et al., 2005; Levy et al., 2013). Incorrect use can lead to poor control of asthma (Levy et al., 2013). Education in the correct use of the device is critical for improving its reliability (Bosnic-Anticevich et al., 2010; Kim et al., 2009; Khassawneh et al., 2008; Levy et al., 2013; Melani et al., 2004; Self et al., 2016; Shaw et al., 2016).

Adding a spacer to the pMDI removes the need for coordination. Spacers are hollow containers that attach to the pMDI and catch the expelled medication, which can then be inhaled directly from the spacer. This allows increased time for evaporation of the propellant and the formation of smaller droplets for inhalation, reducing the speed of expulsion/delivery of the medication (Bensch et al., 2001; Cripps et al., 2000; Labiris and Dolvich, 2003b; Versteeg et al., 2006). The combination of these factors improves the effectiveness of the pMDI, allowing for more collection and availability of smaller droplets (Demirkan et al., 2000; Melani et al., 2004; Stein et al., 2014). However, spacers are not necessary if the pMDI is used correctly, so they are optional rather than essential (Newman, 2004). They are not intended for use with suspended (solid) medication inhalers.

Children have greater difficulty than adults with using pMDIs and achieving the reliable delivery of medication (Bensch et al., 2001; Kamps et al., 2000; Scarfone et al., 2002). The use of a spacer increases the clinical benefit in young paediatric patients compared to nebuliser therapy for acute asthma wheezing (Benito-Fernández et al., 2004; Castro-Rodriguez and Rodrigo, 2004; Delgado et al., 2003; Kamps et al., 2000; Kleinstreuer et al., 2007; Levy et al., 2013; Rubilar et al., 2000).

Emergency administration may require guidance on the correct use of the pMDI and addition of a spacer. Slow inspiration maximises the intake of medication, and this is further improved by holding the breath if possible (Scarfone et al., 2002), although this may not be possible in cases of severe breathing difficulty. Shaking the pMDI *immediately* before use improves medication/propellant mixing and delivery, particularly suspension-based medications (Hatley et al., 2017). If shaking is omitted when using a spacer, the dose of medication delivered will be less than it should be (Berlinski et al., 2018).

Using a pMDI

Remove the cap from the mouthpiece. Vigorously shake the inhaler several times just before use. Exhale fully. Holding the canister upright, place the inhaler mouthpiece into the mouth past the teeth and close the lips around it to create a seal. Tilt the head slightly backwards for a clear open airway (Fig. 4.3.2).

When ready, begin a slow and prolonged inhalation through the mouth. Avoid rapid inspiration, which reduces the intake of medication. Press downwards once on the canister to activate the atomizer while continuing to inhale. Do not keep the canister held down. The pMDI will release a 'puff' of medication that, if not concurrently

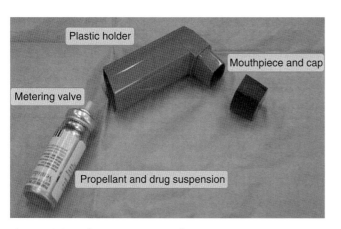

Figure 4.3.1 The components of a pMDI

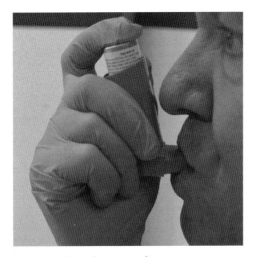

Figure 4.3.2 Holding the pMDI for use

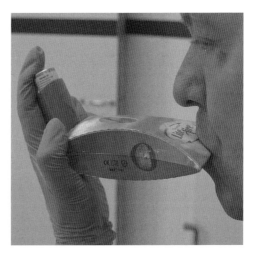

Figure 4.3.3 Holding the pMDI and spacer for use

inhaled, will adhere to the oropharynx instead and offer no clinical benefit. Continue inhaling until a full breath has been taken then hold for 5–10 seconds (if possible), allowing time for the medication to be deposited (Labiris and Dolovich, 2003b). Remove the device from the mouth and exhale slowly.

Using a spacer

If necessary, assemble the spacer. Remove the cap from the pMDI and shake the device. Press the mouthpiece into the inlet port on the spacer. Hold the spacer with one hand while holding the upright pMDI steady with the other. Exhale fully and place the lips on the spacer mouthpiece (Fig. 4.3.3). If using a mask, press it to the face to minimise leaks. Depress the inhaler canister to fill the spacer with one puff of medication. With the head tilted slightly backwards, take a slow and prolonged inhalation through the mouth. Remove the spacer from mouth/face and exhale.

The size of the medication dose cannot be varied. To provide increased dosing, more puffs must be added on subsequent breaths. Allow 30 seconds between medication

inhalations. One puff is delivered per breath. Adding multiple puffs causes the medication to adhere to the spacer and it will not be available for inhalation.

While puffers and reusable spacers should normally be wiped or rinsed after use, paramedic administration typically involves single-use/disposable items, so this is not applicable. The amount of medication contained within a pMDI is limited. However, this does not concern paramedics since there will be sufficient for a single patient episode, after which the puffer will be discarded.

Clinical skill assessment process

The following section outlines the clinical skill assessment tools that should be used to determine a student's ability to demonstrate the effective use of a metered dose inhaler.
1. Clinical Skill Work Instruction
2. Formative Clinical Skill Assessment (F-CSAT)
3. Performance Improvement Plan (PIP)
4. Summative Clinical Skill Assessment (S-CSAT)
(5. Direct Observation of Procedural Skills (DOPS) – see Chapter 1.1)

Clinical Skill Work Instruction

Equipment and resources: Standardised patient; pMDI and spacer; disposable gloves; method of documenting results

Associated Clinical Skills: Infection control; Communication; Consent; Patient assessment skills

Using metered dose inhalers

Activity	Critical Action	Rationale
Personal protection	Don PPE as required.	For infection control.

Using metered dose inhalers continued

Activity	Critical Action	Rationale
Prepare patient	Sit patient upright.	Assists inspiration/breathing.
	Assess for breathing difficulty and pMDI suitability.	To ensure pMDI is best option.
	Explain procedure. Obtain informed consent. Instruct patient how to use a pMDI correctly.	Understanding correct use is necessary for effectiveness.
pMDI use	Remove pMDI mouthpiece. Shake inhaler vigorously several times immediately before use. Hand it to the patient.	Mixes medication to assist with correct dosing.
	Have patient hold pMDI in dominant hand, with canister upright.	Ready for chamber compression.
	Have patient exhale fully.	Increases inspiratory effort.
	Have patient place pMDI mouthpiece into their mouth past their teeth, with lips closed around it. Tilt head back slightly.	Optimises inhalation.
	Have patient begin slow prolonged inhalation through the mouth.	To begin airflow as medication arrives.
	Have patient press downwards once on the chamber to activate atomiser while continuing to inhale a full breath.	Airflow encourages medication inhalation.
	Have patient hold breath for 5–10 seconds (if possible).	Allows time for deposition.
	Have patient remove device from mouth and exhale slowly.	Allows time for deposition.
pMDI use with spacer	Remove pMDI mouthpiece. Shake inhaler vigorously several times immediately before use.	Mixes medication to assist with correct dosing.
	Assemble spacer if necessary. Attach mask if used. Insert pMDI into spacer inlet. Hand it to the patient.	To make device ready for use.
	Have patient hold pMDI in dominant hand with chamber upright. Hold spacer with other hand.	To make device ready for use.
	Have patient exhale fully.	Increases inspiratory effort.
	Have patient place spacer mouthpiece into their mouth past their teeth, with lips closed around it. If using a mask, press against face to minimise any leak. Tilt head slightly back slightly.	Optimises inhalation.
	Have patient press downwards once on the chamber to activate atomiser into chamber.	Fills chamber with medication dose.
	Have patient begin slow and prolonged inhalation through the mouth until a full breath is achieved.	To inhale aerosol medication.
	Have patient hold breath for 5–10 seconds if they can.	Allows time for deposition.
	Have patient remove device from mouth and exhale slowly.	Allows time for deposition.
Reassess	Assess breathing for effectiveness.	To assess outcome.
Report	Document/hand over administration dose/time.	Accurate record kept and continuity of patient care.

Formative Clinical Skill Assessment (F-CSAT)

Equipment and resources: Standardised patient; pMDI and spacer; disposable gloves; method of documenting results

Associated Clinical Skills: Infection control; Communication; Consent; Patient assessment skills

Staff/Student being assessed: _____

Using metered dose inhalers

Activity	Critical Action	Participant Performance				
Personal protection	Dons PPE as required.	0	1	2	3	4
Prepares patient	Sits patient upright.	0	1	2	3	4
	Assesses patient for breathing difficulty and pMDI suitability.	0	1	2	3	4
	Explains procedure. Obtains informed consent. Instructs patient how to use a pMDI correctly.	0	1	2	3	4
pMDI use	Removes pMDI mouthpiece. Shakes inhaler immediately before use. Hands to patient.	0	1	2	3	4
	Has patient hold pMDI with canister upright.	0	1	2	3	4
	Has patient exhale fully.	0	1	2	3	4
	Has patient place pMDI into mouth correctly, with head tilted.	0	1	2	3	4
	Has patient begin slow, prolonged inhalation through mouth.	0	1	2	3	4
	Has patient press downwards once on canister while continuing full breath inhalation.	0	1	2	3	4
	Has patient hold breath for 5–10 seconds if possible.	0	1	2	3	4
	Has patient remove device and exhale slowly.	0	1	2	3	4
pMDI use with spacer	Removes pMDI mouthpiece. Shakes inhaler immediately before use.	0	1	2	3	4
	Assembles spacer/attaches mask if necessary. Inserts pMDI into spacer inlet. Hands device to patient.	0	1	2	3	4
	Has patient correctly hold pMDI and spacer.	0	1	2	3	4
	Has patient exhale fully.	0	1	2	3	4
	Has patient place spacer mouthpiece into mouth correctly, with head tilted.	0	1	2	3	4
	Has patient activate the pMDI once into the spacer.	0	1	2	3	4
	Has patient begin slow and prolonged inhalation until full breath is achieved.	0	1	2	3	4
	Has patient hold breath for 5–10 seconds if possible.	0	1	2	3	4
	Has patient remove device and exhale slowly.	0	1	2	3	4
Reassesses	Assesses breathing and airway patency for effectiveness.	0	1	2	3	4
Reports	Documents/hands over administration dose/time.	0	1	2	3	4

Standard Achieved: (please circle one)

Competent (C)   Not Yet Competent* (NYC)

Staff/Student Name: _____

Assessor (please print name): _____

Signed (Assessor): _____

Date of Assessment: _____

Comments:

*If Not Yet Competent (NYC) a PIP needs to be completed and a repeat of the F-CSAT

Formative Clinical Skill Assessment (F-CSAT) Key

Skill level	Standard of procedure	Quality of performance	Outcome	Level of assistance required
4 Safe for unsupervised practice	Safe Accurate Behaviour is appropriate to context	Confident Accurate Expedient	Achieved intended outcome	No supporting cues*required
3 Requires supervision	Safe Accurate Behaviour is appropriate to context	Confident Accurate Takes longer than required	Achieved intended outcome	Requires occasional supportive cues*
2 Requires assistance	Safe Accurate Behaviour generally appropriate to context	Lacks certainty	Would not have achieved outcome without support	Requires frequent verbal and occasional physical directives in addition to supportive cues*
1 Requires direction	Safe only with guidance Not completely accurate	Unskilled Inefficient	Would not have achieved outcome without support	Requires continuous verbal and frequent physical directive cues*
0 Unsafe	Unsafe Unable to demonstrate behaviour Lack of insight into behaviour appropriate to context	Unskilled	Would not have achieved outcome	Requires continuous verbal and continuous physical directive cues*

*Refers to physical directives or verbal supportive cues

Performance Improvement Plan (PIP)

Please document the agreed education plan and completion timelines for areas assessed as less than 4.

This plan should be presented to assessor prior to commencement of summative assessment.

Where was supervisor support required?	Student summary of deficit. (Why was there a problem?)	Improvement Plan	Completed (Y/N)

Staff/Student Name: _____

Staff/Student Signature: _____

Educator Name: _____

Educator Signature: _____

Summative Clinical Skill Assessment (S-CSAT)

Equipment and resources: Standardised patient; pMDI and spacer; disposable gloves; method of documenting results

Associated Clinical Skills: Infection control; Communication; Consent; Patient assessment skills

Staff/Student being assessed: _____

- Completed Formative Clinical Skill Assessment (F-CSAT):   **YES   NO**
- Completed Performance Improvement Plan (PIP):   **YES   NO   N/A**

Using metered dose inhalers

Activity	Critical Action	Achieved Without Direction	
Personal protection	Dons PPE as required.	NO	YES
Prepares patient	Sits patient upright.	NO	YES
	Assesses patient for breathing difficulty and pMDI suitability.	NO	YES
	Explains procedure. Obtains informed consent. Instructs patient how to use a pMDI correctly.	NO	YES

Using metered dose inhalers continued

Activity	Critical Action	Achieved Without Direction	
pMDI use	Removes pMDI mouthpiece. Shakes inhaler immediately before use. Hands to patient.	NO	YES
	Has patient hold pMDI with canister upright.	NO	YES
	Has patient exhale fully.	NO	YES
	Has patient place pMDI into mouth correctly, with head tilted.	NO	YES
	Has patient begin slow, prolonged inhalation through mouth.	NO	YES
	Has patient press downwards once on canister while continuing full breath inhalation.	NO	YES
	Has patient hold breath for 5–10 seconds if possible.	NO	YES
	Has patient remove device and exhale slowly.	NO	YES
pMDI use with spacer	Removes pMDI mouthpiece. Shakes inhaler immediately before use.	NO	YES
	Assembles spacer/attaches mask if necessary. Inserts pMDI into spacer inlet. Hands device to patient.	NO	YES
	Has patient correctly hold pMDI and spacer.	NO	YES
	Has patient exhale fully.	NO	YES
	Has patient place spacer mouthpiece into mouth correctly, with head tilted.	NO	YES
	Has patient activate the pMDI once into the spacer.	NO	YES
	Has patient begin slow and prolonged inhalation until full breath is achieved.	NO	YES
	Has patient hold breath for 5–10 seconds if possible.	NO	YES
	Has patient remove device and exhale slowly.	NO	YES
Reassesses	Assesses breathing and airway patency for effectiveness.	NO	YES
Reports	Documents/hands over administration dose/time.	NO	YES

Standard Achieved: (please circle one)

Competent (C) Not Yet Competent* (NYC)

Staff/Student Name: _____

Assessor (please print name): _____

Signed (Assessor): _____

Date of Assessment: _____

Comments:

*If Not Yet Competent (NYC) a PIP needs to be completed and a repeat of the F-CSAT

Clinical findings

pMDI complications

The most common problem encountered when using a pDMI is a failure to align inhalation with the delivery of the medication. Using a spacer, along with patient education, helps overcome this difficulty.

Slow, deep inhalation is necessary to deliver the medication to the receptor site. Insufficient inspiration and an inability to hold the breath is common during breathing difficulty. Any difficulty the patient experiences in cooperating can reduce the effectiveness of the therapy. Patients with severe breathing difficulty may simply not be able to use the pMDI correctly.

A failure to shake the pMDI repeatedly between breaths can reduce the dose delivered.

The use of a pDMI can occasionally cause cough or oral thrush, usually due to steroid medication (Versteeg et al., 2006). Once the medication has been administered, rinse the mouth to remove unwanted medication from the oropharynx.

PRACTICE TIP!

Don't underestimate the importance of shaking a pMDI before each activation, even if it means continually taking the spacer/inhaler back from the patient to do so.

PRACTICE TIP!

Emergency pMDI use may involve a patient who is unable to comply with instructions due to breathing difficulty, distraction or altered consciousness. If the patient is too unwell to use a pMDI correctly, choose an alternative therapy.

PRACTICE TIP!

Despite its apparent ease, using a pMDI can prove difficult in an emergency. Pre-instruction and continued coaching is necessary even for experienced users.

TEST YOUR KNOWLEDGE QUESTIONS

1. **What is the main reason for a pMDI to be ineffective?**
   The patient's inability to inhale just as the medication is being expelled.

2. **How does a spacer improve the delivery of medication?**
   It removes the need to coincide medication expulsion with inhalation, and it allows the propellant to evaporate, reducing the particle size.

3. **Why is only one puff released into a spacer each time?**
   Otherwise the medication adheres to the spacer wall.

4. **Why is it important for the patient to hold their breath after inhalation?**
   It increases the time for medication deposition on the airway walls.

5. **What is the advantage of a pMDI for particle size?**
   It produces the correct size of particles each time in order to reach targeted airways.

6. **Why is it important to shake the pMDI immediately before use?**
   To mix the contents and ensure medication as well as propellant is delivered.

7. **Why is pulmonary-delivered medication effective?**
   Medication is delivered to targeted receptors in the lungs.

8. **Is it always necessary to use a spacer?**
   Not if the patient can correctly use the pMDI.

9. **What should you do if the patient cannot use the pMDI correctly?**
   Either get them to use a spacer or turn to an alternative therapy.

10. **What is the method of delivering repeated puffs of medication?**
    One puff per breath; shake the pMDI again; wait 30 seconds between doses.

References

Bell, J. and Newman, S., 2007. The rejuvenated pressurised metered dose inhaler. *Expert Opinion on Drug Delivery*, 4(3), 215–234.

Benito-Fernández, J., González-Balenciaga, M., Capapé-Zache, S., Vázquez-Ronco, M.A. and Mintegi-Raso, S., 2004. Salbutamol via metered-dose inhaler with spacer versus nebulization for acute treatment of pediatric asthma in the emergency department. *Pediatric Emergency Care*, 20(10), 656–659.

Bensch, G., Lapidus, R.J., Levine, B.E., Lumry, W., Yegen, Ü., Kiselev, P. and Della Cioppa, G., 2001. A randomized, 12-week, double-blind, placebo-controlled study comparing formoterol dry powder inhaler with albuterol metered-dose inhaler. *Annals of Allergy, Asthma & Immunology*, 86(1), 19–27.

Berlinski, A., von Hollen, D., Pritchard, J.N. and Hatley, R.H., 2018. Delay between shaking and actuation of a hydrofluoroalkane fluticasone pressurized metered-dose inhaler. *Respiratory Care*, 63(3), 289–293.

Biswas, R., Hanania, N.A. and Sabharwal, A., 2017. Factors determining in vitro lung deposition of albuterol aerosol delivered by Ventolin metered-dose inhaler. *Journal of Aerosol Medicine and Pulmonary Drug Delivery*, 30(4), 256–266.

Bosnic-Anticevich, S.Z., Sinha, H., So, S. and Reddel, H.K., 2010. Metered-dose inhaler technique: the effect of two educational interventions delivered in community pharmacy over time. *Journal of Asthma*, 47(3), 251–256.

Castro-Rodriguez, J.A. and Rodrigo, G.J., 2004. β-agonists through metered-dose inhaler with valved holding chamber versus nebulizer for acute exacerbation of wheezing or asthma in children under 5 years of age: a systematic review with meta-analysis. *Journal of Pediatrics*, 145(2), 172–177.

Cripps, A.M.M.R., Riebe, M., Schulze, M. and Woodhouse, R., 2000. Pharmaceutical transition to non-CFC pressurized metered dose inhalers. *Respiratory Medicine*, 94, S3–S9.

Delgado, A., Chou, K.J., Silver, E.J. and Crain, E.F., 2003. Nebulizers vs metered-dose inhalers with spacers for bronchodilator therapy to treat wheezing in children aged 2 to 24 months in a pediatric emergency department. *Archives of Pediatrics & Adolescent Medicine*, 157(1), 76–80.

Demirkan, K., Tolley, E., Mastin, T., Soberman, J., Burbeck, J. and Self, T., 2000. Salmeterol administration by metered-dose inhaler alone vs metered-dose inhaler plus valved holding chamber. *Chest*, 117(5), 1314–1318.

Geller, D.E., 2005. Comparing clinical features of the nebulizer, metered-dose inhaler, and dry powder inhaler. *Respiratory Care*, 50(10), 1313–1322.

Hatley, R.H., Parker, J., Pritchard, J.N. and von Hollen, D., 2017. Variability in delivered dose from pressurized metered-dose inhaler formulations due to a delay between shake and fire. *Journal of Aerosol Medicine and Pulmonary Drug Delivery*, 30(1), 71–79.

Kamps, A.W., van Ewijk, B., Roorda, R.J. and Brand, P.L., 2000. Poor inhalation technique, even after inhalation instructions, in children with asthma. *Pediatric Pulmonology*, 29(1), 39–42.

Kim, S.H., Kwak, H.J., Kim, T.B., Chang, Y.S., Jeong, J.W., Kim, C.W., Yoon, H.J. and Jee, Y.K., 2009. Inappropriate techniques used by internal medicine residents with three kinds of inhalers (a metered dose inhaler, Diskus, and Turbuhaler): changes after a single teaching session. *Journal of Asthma*, 46(9), 944–950.

Khassawneh, B.Y., Al-Ali, M.K., Alzoubi, K.H., Batarseh, M.Z., Al-Safi, S.A., Sharara, A.M. and Alnasr, H.M., 2008. Handling of inhaler devices in actual pulmonary practice: metered-dose inhaler versus dry powder inhalers. *Respiratory Care*, 53(3), 324–328.

Kleinstreuer, C., Shi, H. and Zhang, Z., 2007. Computational analyses of a pressurized metered dose inhaler and a new drug–aerosol targeting methodology. *Journal of Aerosol Medicine*, 20(3), 294–309.

Labiris, N.R. and Dolovich, M.B., 2003a. Pulmonary drug delivery. Part I: physiological factors affecting therapeutic effectiveness of aerosolized medications. *British Journal of Clinical Pharmacology*, 56(6), 588–599.

Labiris, N.R. and Dolovich, M.B., 2003b. Pulmonary drug delivery. Part II: the role of inhalant delivery devices and drug formulations in therapeutic effectiveness of aerosolized medications. *British Journal of Clinical Pharmacology*, 56(6), 600–612.

Leach, C.L., Davidson, P.J., Hasselquist, B.E. and Boudreau, R.J., 2005. Influence of particle size and patient dosing technique on lung deposition of HFA-beclomethasone from a metered dose inhaler. *Journal of Aerosol Medicine*, 18(4), 379–385.

Lewis, D.A., O'Shea, H., Church, T.K., Brambilla, G., Traini, D. and Young, P.M., 2016. Exploring the impact of sample flowrate on in vitro measurements of metered dose inhaler performance. *International Journal of Pharmaceutics*, 514(2), 420–427.

Levy, M.L., Hardwell, A., McKnight, E. and Holmes, J., 2013. Asthma patients' inability to use a pressurised metered-dose inhaler (pMDI) correctly correlates with poor asthma control as defined by the global initiative for asthma (GINA) strategy: a retrospective analysis. *Primary Care Respiratory Journal*, 22, 406–411.

McDonald, K.J. and Martin, G.P., 2000. Transition to CFC-free metered dose inhalers – into the new millennium. *International Journal of Pharmaceutics*, 201(1), 89–107.

Melani, A.S., Zanchetta, D., Barbato, N., Sestini, P., Cinti, C., Canessa, P.A., Aiolfi, S. and Neri, M., 2004. Inhalation technique and variables associated with misuse of conventional metered-dose inhalers and newer dry powder inhalers in experienced adults. *Annals of Allergy, Asthma & Immunology*, 93(5), 439–446.

Myrdal, P.B., Sheth, P. and Stein, S.W., 2014. Advances in metered dose inhaler technology: formulation development. *AAPS PharmSciTech*, 15(2), 434–455.

Newman, S.P., 2004. Spacer devices for metered dose inhalers. *Clinical Pharmacokinetics*, 43(6), 349–360.

Newman, S.P., 2005. Principles of metered-dose inhaler design. *Respiratory Care*, 50(9), 1177–1190.

Rubilar, L., Castro-Rodriguez, J.A. and Girardi, G., 2000. Randomized trial of salbutamol via metered-dose inhaler with spacer versus nebulizer for acute wheezing in children less than 2 years of age. *Pediatric Pulmonology*, 29(4), 264–269.

Scarfone, R.J., Capraro, G.A., Zorc, J.J. and Zhao, H., 2002. Demonstrated use of metered-dose inhalers and peak flow meters by children and adolescents with acute asthma exacerbations. *Archives of Pediatrics & Adolescent Medicine*, 156(4), 378–383.

Self, T.H., Hoth, L.M., Bolin, J.M. and Stewart, C., 2016. Metered-dose inhaler technique per the Global Initiative for Asthma and Expert Panel Report 3: Why do pharmaceutical companies have one critical difference? *Annals of Allergy, Asthma & Immunology*, 117(1), 101–102.

Shaw, N., Le Souëf, P., Turkovic, L., McCahon, L., Kicic, A., Sly, P.D., Devadason, S. and Schultz, A., 2016. Pressurised metered dose inhaler-spacer technique in young children improves with video instruction. *European Journal of Pediatrics*, 175(7), 1007–1012.

Stein, S.W., Sheth, P., Hodson, P.D. and Myrdal, P.B., 2014. Advances in metered dose inhaler technology: hardware development. *AAPS PharmSciTech*, 15(2), 326–338.

Versteeg, H.K., Hargrave, G.K. and Kirby, M., 2006. Internal flow and near-orifice spray visualisations of a model pharmaceutical pressurised metered dose inhaler. *Journal of Physics: Conference Series*, 45(1), 207.

4.4 | Preparing injections

John Surgina

Chapter objectives

At the end of this chapter the reader will be able to:

1. Recognise different medication presentations and identify their suitability for safe injection
2. Demonstrate the correct method for preparing medication for injections
3. Describe the associated documentation/handover requirements

Resources required for this assessment

- Sharps container
- Medication ampoule/vial
- Disposable gloves
- Range of syringes
- Bevelled and non-bevelled needle
- Antiseptic swab
- Method of documenting results

Skill matrix

This assessment requires:

- Infection control (CS 1.3)
- Communication (CS 1.5)
- Consent (CS 1.6)
- Aseptic Non Touch Technique (ANTT®) (CS 2.20)
- Administering oral medications (CS 4.1)

This assessment is a component of:

- Medication administration (Chapter 4)

Introduction

The injection routes for prehospital medication include the subcutaneous, intramuscular, intravenous and intraosseous routes. Medication given by injection is irretrievable and can allow the entry of infection. Given the uncontrolled environment paramedics often work in, care in preparation and administration is needed. Hazards include needlestick injuries and incorrect medication or dose administration.

This chapter focuses on the safe preparation of medication for injections.

Anatomy and physiology

Intravenous medication is often administered prehospital, as this provides the most rapid and controllable uptake and action of the medication. The intraosseous route is an effective emergency alternative. Intramuscular injections are commonly used but act more slowly. Subcutaneous medication administration is slow and therefore less commonly used by paramedics.

The type of medication, rate of uptake and volume administered all impact on the route and method of preparation. Venous administration is rapid and may not have any volume stipulations; intramuscular administration varies with the muscle chosen (see Chapter 4.6); and subcutaneous administration is the most restricted, having the lowest blood supply and medication uptake (see Chapter 4.5). The choice of syringe will vary with the requirements.

Clinical rationale

Hygiene

Infection is a risk with all parenteral medication administration. Wash your hands and don clean gloves during preparation, using the aseptic method throughout (Ong et al., 2013; WHO, 2010).

Medication check

Checking the medication is a critical component of injection preparation. At least nine factors must be verified for patient safety (see Chapter 4.1). These include the traditional five rights of right patient, right medication, right route, right time and right dose. The dose should be calculated in advance to minimise the risk of error during preparation (Ong et al., 2013). Where medications require dissolution or dilution, first verify that the chosen fluid is appropriate, as not all fluids are compatible with all medications (Ong et al., 2013).

To these rights add the four further rights of right documentation, right medication action, right effects during reassessment and right form. The latter is particularly important, as some medication presentations are not intended for all parenteral routes. For example, medications intended for nebulised or intranasal routes are far too concentrated and may contain additives that are unsuitable for injection.

There are two main forms of medication presentation for injection: vials and ampoules.

Vials

Vials are plastic or glass bottles. They have a covered rubber port that must be penetrated to allow the removal of the contents.

Vials can be single- or multi-use. Multi-use vials carry an increased risk of improper medication disposal and excessive administration (Denholm, 2012). They should be discarded typically 24 hours after opening or as the manufacturer advises (WHO, 2010). Write the opening date on the vial.

Vial medication can be liquid for immediate removal or a crystalline powder, which requires the addition of liquid for dissolution.

Ampoules

Ampoules can be plastic or glass. They are sealed; plastic variants have a removable twist cap while glass variants have a glass cap that must be snapped off. The neck of both types is thinner than the rest of the ampoule, so the opening point is obvious. The neck of the glass ampoule is typically scored to facilitate breaking. This scoring is often enhanced on one side; where this is so, the ampoule is marked with a small dot to identify the point of weakness. There is a risk of injury due to the glass shattering or from exposure to the jagged edge (Bajwa and Kaur, 2012), so assistance devices are available to help avoid this. Some ampoules require a file to enhance the score and allow opening, but these are better avoided (WHO, 2010).

Medication inspection

Verify the quality of the contents, including the clarity, colour, foreign particles, volume within and expiry date, and have another paramedic confirm them where possible. Discard the medication if any of these qualities are unsatisfactory. If the container is coloured, the medication will need to be assessed by withdrawing the contents into a syringe during preparation.

Preparing a vial

To prepare a vial, first remove the covering cap protector to expose the stopper. Wipe the stopper with an antiseptic swab, allowing it to dry for >30 seconds (Hilliard et al., 2013; WHO, 2010).

Choose a sterile bevelled needle and syringe suited to the volume and type of medication. In all cases this must be a **new** syringe and needle, **never reused** (Paparella, 2011; Pugliese et al., 2010; WHO, 2010).

If the vial contains dry medication requiring dissolution, draw sterile fluid volume into the syringe from an appropriate ampoule/vial.

Pick up and invert the vial, and then insert the uncapped needle into and through the rubber stopper, keeping the bevel facing upwards (Fig. 4.4.1). Where the vial content is a dry substance, inject fluid into the vial to dissolve it and form a solution. Shake the vial with the needle still inserted until dissolution occurs.

With the needle tip in the lower neck of the vial, slowly withdraw the syringe plunger until the required medication is withdrawn. Then remove the needle/syringe from the vial, keeping it pointing upwards. Carefully depress the plunger until any air is expelled.

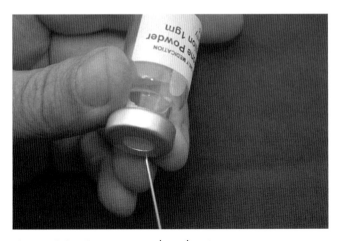

Figure 4.4.1 Preparing vial medication

Glass vials do not collapse when content is withdrawn. If using multi-dose vials or if more than a tiny volume is being withdrawn, an equivalent air volume as solution to be withdrawn must be injected into the vial first, to stop a vacuum forming during extraction (Perry et al., 2013).

Preparing an ampoule

Choose a sterile drawing-up (or bevelled) needle and syringe suited to the volume and type of medication. In all cases this must be a **new** syringe and needle, **never reused** (Paparella, 2011; Pugliese et al., 2010; WHO, 2010).

Hold the ampoule upright and lightly tap or rotate it until any medication trapped in the neck of the ampoule falls into the ampoule body. Clean the neck of the ampoule with an antiseptic wipe and allow to dry.

For glass ampoules, a purpose-intended cap breaker can be used to avoid hand holding. The cap breaker must fit completely over the ampoule cap.

Hold the ampoule body near the scored neck, with one hand between thumb and forefinger. Hold the cap near the score between thumb and forefinger of the other hand (or use the cap breaker if preferred). If there is a dot marked on the ampoule, face it towards you. Keep the two forefingers in contact with each other. With your arms held outstretched, snap open the cap by simultaneously pushing the top and bottom away from you, with the scored line opening towards you. Excess force, such as squeezing the thumb and forefinger, can shatter the ampoule, causing injury or the glass to contaminate the contents. A sterile cloth or swab can be used around the ampoule when breaking it to avoid lacerations to your hands (Fig. 4.4.2).

Inspect the ampoule for glass shards and contaminants. Discard it if any are detected.

Pick up the assembled needle, maintaining asepsis. Either hold the ampoule at an angle or place the ampoule on an upright surface, stabilising it with one hand. Insert the uncapped needle to the bottom of the ampoule and withdraw the required dose (Fig. 4.4.3).

Clearing the syringe of air bubbles

To remove any air bubbles, withdraw the syringe and hold it with the needle pointing upwards. Pull back slightly

on the plunger to withdraw all the medication from the needle shaft. Flick the syringe barrel lightly to force any air bubbles to the top of the syringe. Then slowly push the plunger forwards until the medication is in the needle hub and any air is expelled (Fig. 4.4.4).

Labelling

All syringes containing medication should be clearly labelled to identify the contents (Ong et al., 2013). This can be omitted if the syringe is immediately administered to the patient without leaving sight of the person preparing the medication. Ideally, the vial/ampoule should be provided with the syringe for verification and then any unused content discarded.

Documentation and handover

Registers should be completed when removing medication from storage, for compliance and tracking. These may

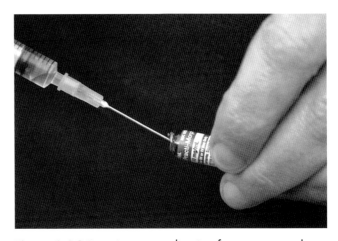

Figure 4.4.3 Drawing up medication from an ampoule

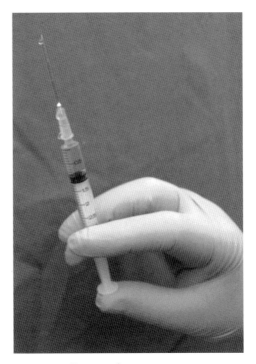

Figure 4.4.4 Expelling air from a syringe

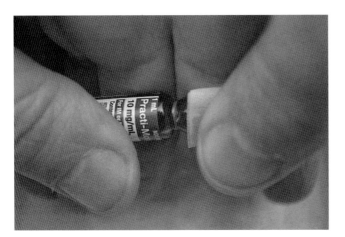

Figure 4.4.2 Opening an ampoule

vary depending on the classification/schedule of the medication.

The dose, time and route of administration should be clearly documented in the patient care record.

Clinical skill assessment process

The following section outlines the clinical skill assessment tools that should be used to determine a student's ability to demonstrate the safe and accurate preparation of injections.

1. Clinical Skill Work Instruction
2. Formative Clinical Skill Assessment (F-CSAT)
3. Performance Improvement Plan (PIP)
4. Summative Clinical Skill Assessment (S-CSAT)
(5. Direct Observation of Procedural Skills (DOPS) – see Chapter 1.1)

Clinical Skill Work Instruction

Equipment and resources: Sharps container; medication ampoule/vial; disposable gloves; range of syringes; bevelled and non-bevelled needle; antiseptic swab; method of documenting results; optional ampoule cap breaker

Associated Clinical Skills: Infection control; Communication; Consent; ANTT®; Administering oral medications

Preparing injections

Activity	Critical Action	Rationale
Verify medication	Choose prescribed medication, ensuring suitability for indication and route. Verify the colour, clarity, volume and expiry date of the contents. Confirm with a colleague.	To ensure right medication and fit for injection.
Prepare paramedic	Wash hands with suitable disinfectant or soap and water.	Decreases infection risk.
Prepare needle/ syringe	Select a syringe that is suitable for the medication. Attach a new, sterile needle suitable for the vial or ampoule. If medication requires dissolution or dilution, draw up the appropriate volume of diluent into syringe.	New needles are always used, as they are sterile items. Blunt drawing-up needles can be used for ampoules.
Open vial/ ampoule	Vial: Remove cap from vial to expose stopper. Clean the stopper with an antiseptic swab and allow >30 seconds to dry. Ampoule: Tap/swirl cap until content falls to bottom. Hold ampoule upright, one hand just below the neck score and the other just above it (or use a cap breaker if preferred). Any dot should face towards you. Keeping the forefingers together, apply gentle pressure with both hands away from the score until a break occurs. Monitor for risk of sharp injury and inspect for glass shards.	To open the vial/ampoule and allow removal of contents.
Draw medication from vial	Invert vial. Push uncapped needle tip through rubber bung into vial, keeping tip below fluid level. If dissolution is required, inject water into vial, keeping the needle in place, and gently shake. When solution is ready, withdraw syringe plunger to aspirate medication. Consider drawing equivalent air into syringe first and then pushing into vial.	Inverting pools fluid in the neck of the vial with air above the fluid. Solute may be required to dissolve a solid substance first. Prior injection of air prevents a vacuum forming.
Draw medication from ampoule	Hold ampoule at an angle or stabilised on a flat surface. Push uncapped needle tip to bottom of ampoule. Pull back on syringe plunger to aspirate medication.	To withdraw only the solution.
Expel air	Withdraw needle/syringe. Hold with tip upwards. Pull plunger back slightly. Flick syringe side to bring air bubbles to the tip. Gently push the plunger to expel air through the needle without expelling the contents.	Ensures no air enters the injection site.
Label syringe	Attach medication label to syringe. Accompany with ampoule/ vial for verification.	Identifies the syringe contents clearly.

Preparing injections continued

Activity	Critical Action	Rationale
Hold for use	Keep syringe tip covered with drawing-up or injection needle. Place syringe on clean surface or suitable dish, ready for use. Do not recap needle.	To maintain asepsis and avoid needlestick injuries.
Report	Document medication preparation appropriately. Inform receiver if preparer is not administering medication.	Medications can require regulatory and administrative documentation.

Formative Clinical Skill Assessment (F-CSAT)

Equipment and resources: Sharps container; medication ampoule/vial; disposable gloves; range of syringes; bevelled and non-bevelled needle; antiseptic swab; method of documenting results; optional ampoule cap breaker

Associated Clinical Skills: Infection control; Communication; Consent; ANTT®; Administering oral medications

Staff/Student being assessed: _____

Preparing injections

Activity	Critical Action	Performance				
Verifies medication	Chooses prescribed medication, ensuring suitability for indication and route. Verifies colour, clarity, volume and expiry date of contents. Confirms with colleague.	0	1	2	3	4
Washes hands	Washes hands using disinfectant solution or soap and water.	0	1	2	3	4
Prepares needle/ syringe	Selects suitable syringe. Attaches suitable new, sterile needle. Draws up appropriate diluent volume into syringe if needed.	0	1	2	3	4
Opens vial/ ampoule	Vial: removes cap. Cleans stopper with antiseptic swab and allows >30 seconds to dry. Ampoule: ensures cap empty of content. Holds ampoule correctly, using cap breaker if preferred. Applies correct method until break occurs. Monitors for risk of sharp injury and inspects for glass shards.	0	1	2	3	4
Draws medication from vial	Inverts vial. Correctly inserts needle. If dissolution is required, correctly injects water into vial and gently shakes. Injects air beforehand if necessary. Correctly withdraws syringe plunger to aspirate medication.	0	1	2	3	4
Draws medication from ampoule	Holds ampoule at an angle or stabilises on a flat surface. Correctly inserts needle and aspirates medication.	0	1	2	3	4
Expels air	Withdraws syringe. Correctly expels air without expelling contents.	0	1	2	3	4
Labels syringe	Attaches medication label to syringe. Accompanies with ampoule/vial for verification.	0	1	2	3	4
Holds for use	Keeps syringe tip covered with appropriate needle. Places syringe on clean surface or suitable dish, ready for use. Does not recap needle.	0	1	2	3	4
Reports	Documents medication preparation appropriately. Informs receiver of content if required.	0	1	2	3	4

Standard Achieved: (please circle one)

Competent (C)   Not Yet Competent* (NYC)

Staff/Student Name: _____

Assessor (please print name): _____

Signed (Assessor): _____

Date of Assessment: _____

Comments:

*If Not Yet Competent (NYC) a PIP needs to be completed and a repeat of the F-CSAT

Formative Clinical Skill Assessment (F-CSAT) Key

Skill level	Standard of procedure	Quality of performance	Outcome	Level of assistance required
4 Safe for unsupervised practice	Safe Accurate Behaviour is appropriate to context	Confident Accurate Expedient	Achieved intended outcome	No supporting cues* required
3 Requires supervision	Safe Accurate Behaviour is appropriate to context	Confident Accurate Takes longer than required	Achieved intended outcome	Requires occasional supportive cues*
2 Requires assistance	Safe Accurate Behaviour generally appropriate to context	Lacks certainty	Would not have achieved outcome without support	Requires frequent verbal and occasional physical directives in addition to supportive cues*
1 Requires direction	Safe only with guidance Not completely accurate	Unskilled Inefficient	Would not have achieved outcome without support	Requires continuous verbal and frequent physical directive cues*
0 Unsafe	Unsafe Unable to demonstrate behaviour Lack of insight into behaviour appropriate to context	Unskilled	Would not have achieved outcome	Requires continuous verbal and continuous physical directive cues*

*Refers to physical directives or verbal supportive cues

Performance Improvement Plan (PIP)

Please document the agreed education plan and completion timelines for areas assessed as less than 4.

This plan should be presented to assessor prior to commencement of summative assessment.

Where was supervisor support required?	Student summary of deficit. (Why was there a problem?)	Improvement Plan	Completed (Y/N)

Staff/Student Name: _____

Staff/Student Signature: _____

Educator Name: _____

Educator Signature: _____

Summative Clinical Skill Assessment (S-CSAT)

Equipment and resources: Sharps container; medication ampoule/vial; disposable gloves; range of syringes; bevelled and non-bevelled needle; antiseptic swab; method of documenting results; optional ampoule cap breaker

Associated Clinical Skills: Infection control; Communication; Consent; ANTT®; Administering oral medications

Staff/Student being assessed: _____

• Completed Formative Clinical Skill Assessment (F-CSAT):   **YES   NO**

• Completed Performance Improvement Plan (PIP):   **YES   NO   N/A**

Preparing injections

Activity	Critical Action	Achieved Without Direction	
Verifies medication	Chooses prescribed medication, ensuring suitability for indication and route. Verifies colour, clarity, volume and expiry date of contents. Confirms with colleague.	NO	YES
Washes hands	Washes hands using disinfectant solution or soap and water.	NO	YES
Prepares needle/syringe	Selects suitable syringe. Attaches suitable new, sterile needle. Draws up appropriate diluent volume into syringe if needed.	NO	YES
Opens vial/ampoule	Vial: removes cap. Cleans stopper with antiseptic swab and allows >30 seconds to dry. Ampoule: ensures cap empty of content. Holds ampoule correctly, using cap breaker if preferred. Applies correct method until break occurs. Monitors for risk of sharp injury and inspects for glass shards.	NO	YES
Draws medication from vial	Inverts vial. Correctly inserts needle. If dissolution is required, correctly injects water into vial and gently shakes. Injects air beforehand if necessary. Correctly withdraws syringe plunger to aspirate medication.	NO	YES
Draws medication from ampoule	Holds ampoule at an angle or stabilises on flat surface. Correctly inserts needle and aspirates medication.	NO	YES
Expels air	Withdraws syringe. Correctly expels air without expelling content.	NO	YES

Preparing injections continued

Activity	Critical Action	Achieved Without Direction	
Labels syringe	Attaches medication label to syringe. Accompanies with ampoule/vial for verification.	NO	YES
Holds for use	Keeps syringe tip covered with appropriate needle. Places syringe on clean surface or suitable dish ready for use. Does not recap needle.	NO	YES
Reports	Documents medication preparation appropriately. Informs receiver of content if required.	NO	YES

Standard Achieved: (please circle one)

Competent (C)   Not Yet Competent* (NYC)

Staff/Student Name: _____

Assessor (please print name): _____

Signed (Assessor): _____

Date of Assessment: _____

Comments:

*If Not Yet Competent (NYC) a PIP needs to be completed and a repeat of the F-CSAT

Clinical findings

Preparing the quantity of medication

To reduce the risk of medication errors, draw up the required dose only and discard the excess properly. Where any drug is discarded, it must be made known to the person administering the medication, if they are not the preparer, to help account for the actual syringe content. Administer the medication as soon as practicable. If there is to be a delay, draw up the entire volume. Store the needle-capped syringe in a clean dish for delivery (WHO, 2010).

Diluting the medication

If diluent is to be added to medication in a syringe, such as for small bolus intravenous injections, draw up the necessary diluent first and then add the medication to ensure the volume is correct.

PRACTICE TIP!

To help maintain asepsis, ensure the prepared syringe is stored on a clean, covered surface or in a container with a protective cap left covering the tip.

PRACTICE TIP!

Prepare the medication for injection into a syringe that has sufficient capacity for the entire medication and any dilution necessary.

PRACTICE TIP!

When the prepared syringe is not for immediate use, the entire ampoule/vial medication should be drawn up to account for the entire volume and provide assurance of the syringe contents. Content that is not required can be discarded immediately before use.

PRACTICE TIP!

During preparation, the correct medication, expiry date, dose required and route must be confirmed with a second paramedic wherever possible.

TEST YOUR KNOWLEDGE QUESTIONS

1. **What are the nine key points of medication selection?**
   Right patient; right medication; right dose; right administration time; right route; right documentation; right medication action; right effects during reassessment; right form.

2. **What inspections are necessary before preparation?**
   Confirm the medication's name, strength, expiry date, clarity and quality.

3. **What must be injected into a vial before liquid is withdrawn?**
   A small amount of air, to replace the liquid volume. If the medication is dry powder, a small liquid volume is first injected.

4. **What options are available to assist when opening an ampoule?**
   There is a small dot on the neck of some ampoules that denotes a weak area for ease of opening. Purpose devices are available to hold the ampoule during opening.

5. **How are the syringe contents identified after preparation?**
   The ampoule or vial is attached to the syringe with clear tape, with the label visible.

6. **What documentation is required when preparing medication?**
   Withdrawal notation in an appropriate medication register.

7. **What is done with the syringe once it has been prepared?**
   The tip is left covered with an appropriate needle. The syringe is placed on a clean surface or suitable dish, ready for use.

8. **How is air removed from the syringe during preparation?**
   Draw up with the needle tip kept carefully in the solution. Once the solution is in the syringe, hold the tip upright, pull back slightly on the plunger and then push forwards slowly to expel air without expelling the medication.

9. **Can medication for injection be prepared by one person alone?**
   It can, but for patient safety and to avoid medication error a second paramedic should always be employed in cross-checking.

10. **What are the labelling requirements for syringes containing medication?**
    They should be clearly labelled, identifying the contents. This can be omitted if the syringe content is administered immediately, without leaving sight of the person who prepared it. Provide the vial/ampoule for verification.

References

Bajwa S.J. and Kaur, J., 2012. Risk and safety concerns in anesthesiology practice: the present perspective. *Anesthesia: Essays and Researches*, 6, 14–20.

Denholm, B., 2012. Clinical issues, March 2012. *AORN Journal*, 95(3), 406–413.

Hilliard, J.G., Cambronne, E.D., Kirsch, J.R. and Aziz, M.F., 2013. Barrier protection capacity of flip-top pharmaceutical vials. *Journal of Clinical Anesthesia*, 25(3), 177–180.

Ong, W.M. and Subasyini, S., 2013. Medication errors in intravenous drug preparation and administration. *Medical Journal of Malaysia*, 68(1), 52–57.

Paparella, S., 2011. Safe injection practices: keeping safety in and the 'bugs' out. *Journal of Emergency Nursing*, 37(6), 564–566.

Perry, A.G., Potter, P.A. and Ostendorf, W., 2013. *Clinical nursing skills and techniques*, 8th edn (Chapter 20). St Louis: Elsevier Mosby.

Pugliese, G., Gosnell, C., Bartley, J.M. and Robinson, S., 2010. Injection practices among clinicians in United States health care settings. *American Journal of Infection Control*, 38(10), 789–798.

WHO (World Health Organization), 2010. *WHO best practices for injections and related procedures toolkit*. Retrieved from: https://apps.who.int/iris/handle/10665/44298

4.5 | Subcutaneous injection

John Surgina

Chapter objectives

At the end of this chapter the reader will be able to:

1. Discuss the rationale for subcutaneous (SC) injection
2. List the complications of SC injection
3. Demonstrate the safe administration of medication via SC injection

Resources required for this assessment

- Mannequin suitable for SC injection
- Hand decontamination agent
- Disposable gloves
- Needle, syringe
- Antiseptic swab
- Medication
- Sharps container
- Clinical waste bag
- Method of documenting the results

Skill matrix

This assessment requires:

- Infection control (CS 1.3)
- Consent (CS 1.6)
- Communication (CS 1.5)
- Aseptic Non Touch Technique (ANTT®) (CS 2.20)
- Administering oral medications (CS 4.1)
- Preparing injections (CS 4.4)

This assessment is a component of:

- Medication administration (Chapter 4)

Introduction

A subcutaneous injection involves delivery of a medication into the fatty and loose connective layer of tissue between the skin and underlying muscle. This chapter discusses the correct and safe method of administering subcutaneous injections.

Anatomy and physiology

The two skin layers, the epidermis and dermis, are supported by the hypodermis, or subcutaneous tissue, which is comprised predominantly of adipose and some loose connective tissue. In addition to being a fat store, it also serves to attach the skin to underlying structures, and insulate and protect these structures.

Below the subcutaneous tissue is a layer of muscle (intramuscular injection target site) and underlying structures. Vascular supply to subcutaneous tissue is via small vessel and much less than the blood supply available in the deeper muscle layer (Fig. 4.5.1).

While the thickness of skin in an adult is not significantly altered by demographic factors, subcutaneous tissue is influenced by factors such as anatomical location, age, body mass index (BMI) and gender (Derraik et al., 2014; Gibney et al., 2010).

Medication absorption via subcutaneous injection results in a slow but predictable rate of uptake.

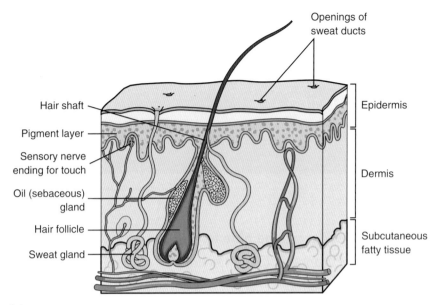

Figure 4.5.1 Layers of the integumentary system

The layers of the skin, with the relatively thin overlying epidermis and the deeper dermis dotted with skin appendages such as hair follicles and sebaceous glands.

Source: *Zellner, E.G. and Persing, J.A., 2017, Youmans and Winn neurological surgery, Figure 23-7, Elsevier, pp. e136–e149.*

Clinical rationale

The subcutaneous administration route is appropriate only for small volume, non-irritating, water-soluble medications.

The onset of action for medications administered via this route is delayed. If the intended treatment goal requires rapid onset, another route of administration should be considered.

Site selection

Multiple sites can be considered for subcutaneous injections (Fig. 4.5.2). The most common injection site is the abdomen, though care must be taken not to inject within 5 cm of the umbilicus to avoid the umbilical veins. Injection into the abdominal site can be less painful than injection into the thighs (Pourghaznein et al., 2014; Ogston-Tuck, 2014).

For patients who regularly administer medications via the subcutaneous route, it is recommended the site be rotated each time.

Areas with evidence of skin damage (burns, lacerations, scarring or recent injection site), inflammation, swelling, masses or infection should be avoided.

Skin fold

Pinching a fold of skin decreases the risk of administering medication into the intramuscular space, and should be performed any time the needle is considered longer than the distance between the dermis and underlying muscle (Frid et al., 2010; Hirsch et al., 2014; Hofman et al., 2010).

To correctly pinch a skin fold, lift the area of the injection using the index finger and thumb only (Fig. 4.5.3) (Frid et al., 2010; Ogston-Tuck, 2014).

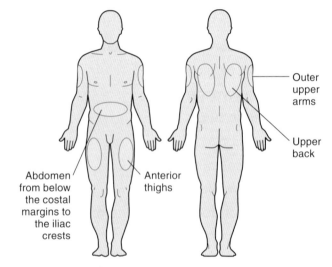

Figure 4.5.2 Subcutaneous injection sites

Source: *Koutoukidis, G., Stainton, K., Hughson, J., 2013, Tabbner's Nursing Care: Theory and Practice, 6th edn (Chapter 22, Figure 22.7), Elsevier.*

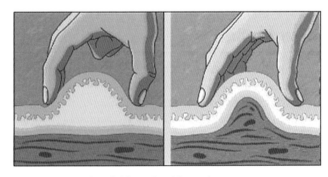

Figure 4.5.3 Skin fold method for subcutaneous injection

Left (correct technique) and right (incorrect technique).

Source: *Frid, A., Hirsch, L., Gaspar, R., Hicks, D., Kreugel, G., Liersch, J., Letondeur, C., Sauvanet, J.P., Tubiana-Rufi, N. and Strauss, K., 2010, New injection recommendations for patients with diabetes, Diabetes & Metabolism, 36, S3–S18.*

Needle selection and angle of injection

Needle length is important, as the needle must reach the subcutaneous tissue but not enter the intramuscular space.

Irrespective of patient demographics or BMI, a 4–8 mm long needle is adequate (Hirsch et al., 2014). Where the needle length is 4–8 mm, an injection angle of 90° is preferred. If the needle is longer than 8 mm, or the patient is thin or a child, using a skin fold and a 45° injection angle is recommended (Fig. 4.5.4). Ideally, a needle length <4 mm in children is preferred (Hofman et al., 2010; Lo Presti et al., 2012; Ogston-Tuck, 2014).

A 23–34 gauge needle can be used; however, a 25 gauge needle is recommended for adults.

Administration volume

The subcutaneous route is appropriate for administering only small volumes of medication (0.5–1 mL). If a larger volume is required, consider an alternative route or the use of multiple injection sites.

Slow injection and allowing 5 seconds before withdrawing the needle can reduce bruising (Akbari Sari et al., 2014; Pourghaznein et al., 2014). The speed of injection may not alter the level of pain the patient experiences, but increased volume will (Heise et al., 2014).

Prefilled syringes and pen needles

In addition to using a syringe and needle, the paramedic may be required to use a prefilled syringe or pen needle (e.g. an insulin pen).

An air bubble is intentionally included in prefilled subcutaneous injection syringes. This allows administration of the entire contents of the syringe. Before administration, ensure the air bubble is located against the plunger. This instruction relates **only** to the

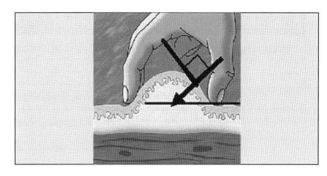

Figure 4.5.4 Correct angle of subcutaneous injection into a skin fold

When using a skin fold to aid injection into the subcutaneous tissue, insert the needle into the slope of the fold as indicated.

Source: Frid, A., Hirsch, L., Gaspar, R., Hicks, D., Kreugel, G., Liersch, J., Letondeur, C., Sauvanet, J.P., Tubiana-Rufi, N. and Strauss, K., 2010, New injection recommendations for patients with diabetes, Diabetes & Metabolism, 36, S3–S18.

administration of medication using a prefilled syringe via the subcutaneous route.

Clinical skill assessment process

The following section outlines the clinical skill assessment tools that should be used to determine a student's ability to demonstrate the safe and accurate administration of a medication via the subcutaneous route.

1. Clinical Skill Work Instruction
2. Formative Clinical Skill Assessment (F-CSAT)
3. Performance Improvement Plan (PIP)
4. Summative Clinical Skill Assessment (S-CSAT)
(5. Direct Observation of Procedural Skills (DOPS) – see Chapter 1.1)

Clinical Skill Work Instruction

Equipment and resources: Mannequin suitable for SC injection; hand decontamination agent; disposable gloves; needle and syringe; antiseptic swab; medication; sharps container; clinical waste bag; method of documenting results

Associated Clinical Skills: Infection control; Communication; Consent; ANTT®; Administering oral medications; Preparing injections

Subcutaneous injection

Activity	Critical Action	Rationale
Prepare patient	Discuss procedure with patient and obtain informed consent.	To reduce patient stress and gain cooperation.
	Arrange patient in relaxed and reclined position.	Reduces muscle tensing.
Prepare paramedic	Wash hands and don latex protective gloves.	Decreases infection risk.

Subcutaneous injection continued

Activity	Critical Action	Rationale
Prepare equipment	Place syringe in clean receptacle, with drug ampoule attached.	Identifies contents of syringe.
	Place sharps waste container conveniently within reach.	For safe sharps disposal.
Prepare injection site	Select, expose and inspect appropriate site. If previous injections, rotate injection sites.	Maximises likelihood of success and minimises potential risks.
	Prepare site with concentric circle antiseptic swabbing and allow area 30 seconds to dry.	Reduces infection risk.
	Using non-dominant hand, pinch area of injection using index finger and thumb (see Fig. 4.5.3). Avoid the muscle.	Using skin fold reduces risk of intramuscular injection.
Inject needle	Inject short needle at a 90° angle using a quick motion. If using a longer needle, insert at a 45° angle.	Avoids intramuscular injection.
Confirm correct placement	If appropriate, pull back slightly on syringe plunger to check for aspirated blood.	Confirms needle is not in a blood vessel.
Administer medication	Slowly push plunger and deliver medication. Do not massage the site following needle removal.	Administering medication slowly minimises pain. Massaging the injection site increases risk of haemorrhage and bruising.
Sharps and waste management	Remove needle and/or activate the safety device. Immediately dispose of device in a sharps container. Where required, cover the injection site. Dispose of clinical waste, remove gloves and wash hands.	Appropriate infection control and sharps management minimise risk of healthcare-associated infections.
Reassess	Assess patient for impact of medication.	Allows paramedic to assess response to medication.
Report and hand over	Record medication transaction to standard required by legislation and regulating bodies. Document/hand over drug, dose, route, time and patient response.	Government and health agencies regulate the acquisition, possession, administration and documenting of medications.

Formative Clinical Skill Assessment (F-CSAT)

Equipment and resources: Mannequin suitable for SC injection; hand decontamination agent; disposable gloves; needle and syringe; antiseptic swab; medication; sharps container; clinical waste bag; method of documenting results

Associated Clinical Skills: Infection control; Communication; Consent; ANTT®; Administering oral medications; Preparing injections

Staff/Student being assessed: _____

Subcutaneous injection

Activity	Critical Action	Performance				
Prepares patient	Discusses procedure with patient and obtains informed consent.	0	1	2	3	4
	Arranges patient in relaxed and reclined position.	0	1	2	3	4
Prepares paramedic	Washes hands and dons latex protective gloves.	0	1	2	3	4
Prepares equipment	Places syringe in clean receptacle, with drug ampoule attached.	0	1	2	3	4
	Places sharps waste container conveniently within reach.	0	1	2	3	4
Prepares injection site	Selects, exposes and inspects appropriate site. Where required, rotates injection sites.	0	1	2	3	4
	Prepares site with concentric circle antiseptic swabbing and allows area 30 seconds to dry.	0	1	2	3	4
	Using non-dominant hand, pinches area of injection using index finger and thumb. Avoids muscle.	0	1	2	3	4
Injects needle	Inserts short needle at 90° angle using a quick motion. If using a longer needle, inserts at 45° angle.	0	1	2	3	4
Confirms correct placement	If appropriate, pulls back slightly on syringe plunger to check for aspirated blood.	0	1	2	3	4
Administers medication	Slowly pushes plunger and delivers medication. Does not massage the site following removal of needle.	0	1	2	3	4
Sharps and waste management	Removes needle and/or activates the safety device. Immediately disposes in a sharps container. Where required, covers the injection site. Disposes of clinical waste, removes gloves and washes hands.	0	1	2	3	4
Reassesses	Assesses patient to identify impact of the medication.	0	1	2	3	4
Reports and hands over	Records medication transaction to standard required by legislation and regulating bodies. Documents/hands over drug, dose, route, time and patient response.	0	1	2	3	4

Standard Achieved: (please circle one)

Competent (C)   Not Yet Competent* (NYC)

Staff/Student Name: _____

Assessor (please print name): _____

Signed (Assessor): _____

Date of Assessment: _____

Comments:

*If Not Yet Competent (NYC) a PIP needs to be completed and a repeat of the F-CSAT

Formative Clinical Skill Assessment (F-CSAT) Key

Skill level	Standard of procedure	Quality of performance	Outcome	Level of assistance required
4 Safe for unsupervised practice	Safe Accurate Behaviour is appropriate to context	Confident Accurate Expedient	Achieved intended outcome	No supporting cues*required
3 Requires supervision	Safe Accurate Behaviour is appropriate to context	Confident Accurate Takes longer than required	Achieved intended outcome	Requires occasional supportive cues*
2 Requires assistance	Safe Accurate Behaviour generally appropriate to context	Lacks certainty	Would not have achieved outcome without support	Requires frequent verbal and occasional physical directives in addition to supportive cues*
1 Requires direction	Safe only with guidance Not completely accurate	Unskilled Inefficient	Would not have achieved outcome without support	Requires continuous verbal and frequent physical directive cues*
0 Unsafe	Unsafe Unable to demonstrate behaviour Lack of insight into behaviour appropriate to context	Unskilled	Would not have achieved outcome	Requires continuous verbal and continuous physical directive cues*

*Refers to physical directives or verbal supportive cues

Performance Improvement Plan (PIP)

Please document the agreed education plan and completion timelines for areas assessed as less than 4.

This plan should be presented to assessor prior to commencement of summative assessment.

Where was supervisor support required?	Student summary of deficit. (Why was there a problem?)	Improvement Plan	Completed (Y/N)

Staff/Student Name: _____

Staff/Student Signature: _____

Educator Name: _____

Educator Signature: _____

Summative Clinical Skill Assessment (S-CSAT)

Equipment and resources: Mannequin suitable for SC injection; hand decontamination agent; disposable gloves; needle and syringe; antiseptic swab; medication; sharps container; clinical waste bag; method of documenting results

Associated Clinical Skills: Infection control; Communication; Consent; ANTT®; Administering oral medications; Preparing injections

Staff/Student being assessed: _____

- Completed Formative Clinical Skill Assessment (F-CSAT): **YES** **NO**
- Completed Performance Improvement Plan (PIP): **YES** **NO** **N/A**

Subcutaneous injection

Activity	Critical Action	Achieved Without Direction	
Prepares patient	Discusses procedure with patient and obtains informed consent.	NO	YES
	Arranges patient in relaxed and reclined position.	NO	YES
Prepares paramedic	Washes hands and dons latex protective gloves.	NO	YES
Prepares equipment	Places syringe in clean receptacle, with drug ampoule attached.	NO	YES
	Places sharps waste container conveniently within reach.	NO	YES
Prepares injection site	Selects, exposes and inspects appropriate site. Where required, rotates injection.	NO	YES
	Prepares site with concentric circle antiseptic swabbing and allows area 30 seconds to dry.	NO	YES
	Using non-dominant hand, pinches area of injection using index finger and thumb. Avoids muscle.	NO	YES
Injects needle	Inserts short needle at 90° angle using a quick motion. If using a longer needle, inserts at 45° angle.	NO	YES
Confirms correct placement	If appropriate, pulls back slightly on syringe plunger to check for aspirated blood.	NO	YES
Administers medication	Slowly pushes plunger and delivers medication. Does not massage the site following removal of needle.	NO	YES
Sharps and waste management	Removes needle and/or activates the safety device. Immediately disposes in a sharps container. Where required, covers the injection site. Disposes of clinical waste, removes gloves and washes hands.	NO	YES
Reassesses	Assesses patient to identify impact of the medication.	NO	YES
Reports and hands over	Records medication transaction to standard required by legislation and regulating bodies. Documents/hands over drug, dose, route, time and patient response.	NO	YES

Standard Achieved: (please circle one)

Competent (C)   Not Yet Competent* (NYC)

Staff/Student Name: _____

Assessor (please print name): _____

Signed (Assessor): _____

Date of Assessment: _____

Comments:

*If Not Yet Competent (NYC) a PIP needs to be completed and a repeat of the F-CSAT

Clinical findings

Complications

Complications to consider include infection, pain, discomfort and bruising. This can vary with the medication administered and the injection technique. Patients who require ongoing subcutaneous injections may develop lesions, masses or scar tissue around the injection sites.

Arguably, the most obvious complication of subcutaneous injection is injection that is too deep and enters the muscle. Attention to needle length, angle of injection and skin pinching reduces the likelihood of this happening. The risk is greater with thigh injection than it is when injecting into the abdomen (Hirsch et al., 2014).

Since the absorption of medication is dependent on blood flow, patients with haemodynamic impairment will have compromised uptake. Blood flow from the network of vessels between the dermis and hypodermis is shunted into the central circulation. An alternative route of administration in patients presenting with signs of shock/poor perfusion should be used.

PRACTICE TIP!

Needlestick injuries are a serious issue. They can be prevented by undertaking risk assessments, clear communication and immediate safe sharps disposal after injection.

PRACTICE TIP!

Shorter needles have a lower rate of intramuscular injection than longer needles do, even when using the raised skin fold technique or injecting at a 45° angle.

TEST YOUR KNOWLEDGE QUESTIONS

1. **Describe subcutaneous tissue.**
   Subcutaneous tissue is predominantly made up of a layer of adipose tissue (fat) and some loose connective tissue serving to store fat. It attaches the skin to underlying structures, insulates the body and assists to protect underlying structures.

2. **For a subcutaneous injection, at what angle should the needle be inserted?**
   At 45° or 90°, depending on needle length and the estimated quantity of subcutaneous tissue.

3. **A 53-year-old female patient (weight 55 kg) could be administered 5 mL of medication via the subcutaneous route. True or false?**
   False. The subcutaneous route of administration is most appropriate for small volumes of medication (0.5–1 mL).

4. **Why is it important to gain the patient's consent before administering a medication via the subcutaneous route?**
   Patient consent is a central pillar of healthcare and is enshrined in providing legal, ethical and moral clinical care.

5. **Any medication can be administered via the subcutaneous route. True or false?**
   False. Only select water soluble medications can be administered via the subcutaneous route.

6. **List the safety considerations that must be addressed before, during and after administering a medication via the subcutaneous route.**
   Medication safety (i.e. drug checks); infection control procedures; sharps management.

7. **After inserting the needle and aspirating the syringe, you identify that blood is present in the syringe. What action should you take?**
   This indicates the needle is *not* situated in subcutaneous tissue. Remove the needle and safely dispose of the sharp. Prepare a new injection and repeat the process using a new injection site.

8. **What is the most common anatomical location for subcutaneous injection?**
   The abdomen (not less than 5 cm from the umbilicus).

9. **As a general rule, the injection site should *not* be massaged following a subcutaneous injection. True or false?**
   True. It will increase risk of haemorrhage and bruising.

10. **List five complications or adverse effects associated with the administration of a medication via the subcutaneous route.**
    Haematoma/bruise; pain or discomfort; soft tissue damage (scarring, hardening of tissue); infection; poorly absorbed medication; haemorrhage/bleeding.

References

Akbari Sari, A., Janani, L., Mohammady, M. and Nedjat, S., 2014. *Slow versus fast subcutaneous heparin injections for prevention of bruising and site-pain intensity*. Online: The Cochrane Library.

Derraik, J.G., Rademaker, M., Cutfield, W.S., Pinto, T.E., Tregurtha, S., Faherty, A., Peart, J.M., Drury, P.L. and Hofman, P.L., 2014. Effects of age, gender, BMI, and anatomical site on skin thickness in children and adults with diabetes. *PLOS ONE*, 9(1), e86637.

Frid, A., Hirsch, L., Gaspar, R., Hicks, D., Kreugel, G., Liersch, J., Letondeur, C., Sauvanet, J.P., Tubiana-Rufi, N. and Strauss, K., 2010. New injection recommendations for patients with diabetes. *Diabetes & Metabolism*, 36, S3–S18.

Gibney, M.A., Arce, C.H., Byron, K.J. and Hirsch, L.J., 2010. Skin and subcutaneous adipose layer thickness in adults with diabetes at sites used for insulin injections: implications for needle length recommendations. *Current Medical Research and Opinion*, 26(6), 1519–1530.

Heise, T., Nosek, L., Dellweg, S., Zijlstra, E., Præstmark, K.A., Kildegaard, J., Nielsen, G. and Sparre, T., 2014. Impact of injection speed and volume on perceived pain during subcutaneous injections into the abdomen and thigh: a single-centre, randomized controlled trial. *Diabetes, Obesity and Metabolism*, 16(10), 971–976.

Hirsch, L., Byron, K. and Gibney, M., 2014. Intramuscular risk at insulin injection sites – measurement of the distance from skin to muscle and rationale for shorter-length needles for subcutaneous insulin therapy. *Diabetes Technology & Therapeutics*, 16(12), 867–873.

Hofman, P.L., Derraik, J.G.B., Pinto, T.E., Tregurtha, S., Faherty, A., Peart, J.M., Drury, P.L., Robinson, E., Tehranchi, R., Donsmark, M. and Cutfield, W.S., 2010. Defining the ideal injection techniques when using 5-mm needles in children and adults. *Diabetes Care*, 33(9), 1940–1944.

Lo Presti, D., Ingegnosi, C. and Strauss, K., 2012. Skin and subcutaneous thickness at injecting sites in children with diabetes: ultrasound findings and recommendations for giving injection. *Pediatric Diabetes*, 13(7), 525–533.

Ogston-Tuck, S., 2014. Subcutaneous injection technique: an evidence-based approach. *Nursing Standard*, 29(3), 53–58.

Pourghaznein, T., Azimi, A.V. and Jafarabadi, M.A., 2014. The effect of injection duration and injection site on pain and bruising of subcutaneous injection of heparin. *Journal of Clinical Nursing*, 23(7–8), 1105–1113.

4.6 Intramuscular injection

Jeff Kenneally

Chapter objectives

At the end of this chapter the reader will be able to:

1. Describe the rationale for intramuscular (IM) injection
2. Demonstrate the method of choosing and locating IM injection sites
3. Demonstrate effective and safe IM injection
4. Accurately report on the performance of IM injection

Resources required for this assessment

- Simulated patient suitable for IM injection
- Disposable gloves
- Bevelled needles
- Syringes
- Antiseptic swabs
- Clinical waste bag
- Sharps container
- Method of documenting the results

Skill matrix

This assessment requires:

- Infection control (CS 1.3)
- Communication (CS 1.5)
- Consent (CS 1.6)
- Aseptic Non Touch Technique (ANTT®) (CS 2.20)
- Administering oral medications (CS 4.1)
- Preparing injections (CS 4.4)

This assessment is a component of:

- Medication administration (Chapter 4)

Introduction

Intramuscular (IM) injection is a common method of routine and emergency drug administration. This chapter discusses the safe and effective performance of this skill.

Anatomy and physiology

Skeletal muscle is key for movement and postural support. It receives blood from smaller arterioles and capillaries via larger arteries. Venous return is via venules and lymphatic drainage.

The skin, or cutaneous tissue, covers muscles and has several layers: the thin outer epidermis, underlying thicker dermis and deeper hypodermis.

The epidermis receives little blood supply, with only minute capillaries reaching its proximal edge. Arterioles, venules and capillaries permeate the dermis. Small arteries and veins are in the hypodermis connecting these smallest vessels. The hypodermis contains fat cells, while the deeper muscle tissue is more vascular (Chan et al., 2006).

Clinical rationale

IM injection is administration of medication from a syringe through a needle pushed deeply into a large muscle. The nature of the medication and the rate of uptake required dictate its choice (Barron and Cocoman, 2008; Nicoll and Hesby, 2002; Wynaden et al., 2015).

The greater the blood supply, the faster the drug uptake. IM injection is slower than intravenous and intraosseous routes but faster than subcutaneous. Conversely, slower uptake means a longer duration effect. Increased adipose tissue can cause muscle to be deeper, and some needle lengths are likely to reach only the subcutaneous level.

Injection site

IM injection requires a muscle large enough to accept the volume of drug injected and sufficient blood supply to take up the medication (Nicoll and Hesby, 2002). Five large muscles are commonly used: deltoid, dorsogluteal, ventrogluteal, vastus lateralis and rectus femoris (Barron and Cocoman, 2008; Petrofsky, 2012). Each have advantages and disadvantages.

Ventrogluteal

The ventrogluteal site is commonly used when the gluteus medius is the target muscle (Fig. 4.6.1). There is a lower likelihood of needle contact with major nerve or blood vessels at this site, which has thick muscle and thinner covering fat (Barron and Cocoman, 2008; Wynaden et al., 2015).

To locate it, position the patient laterally. Place your palm over the trochanter, with your index finger on the anterior iliac spine and middle finger at the posterior crest. The triangular opening between the fingers is the site.

Dorsogluteal

The dorsogluteal target muscle is the gluteus maximus (Figs 4.6.1 and 4.6.2). This site has a lower rate of drug absorption, higher risk of inadvertent sciatic nerve contact and greater likelihood of proximity to arteries than other lower limb IM options (Barron and Cocoman, 2008; Chan et al., 2006; Wynaden et al., 2015). Increased adipose cover often necessitates the use of a longer needle.

The site is located by dividing the buttock into four quadrants and using the upper, outer quadrant. Too high risks hitting bone; too low increases contact with the sciatic nerve. An alternative is to draw an imaginary line between the posterior iliac spine and greater trochanter. Superior and lateral to this line locates either the gluteus maximus or medius.

Vastus lateralis

The vastus lateralis suits deep IM injections as there is little chance of inadvertent major nerve or blood vessel contact (Figs 4.6.1 and 4.6.3). The site is between the greater trochanter and the femoral condyle on the lateral upper leg, in the middle third of the muscle (Barron and Cocoman, 2008).

Rectus femoris

The rectus femoris is near the vastus lateralis (Fig. 4.6.3), midway between iliac crest and kneecap on the anterior upper leg (Barron and Cocoman, 2008). Suitable for broad use, it is low risk and suitable for self-administration,

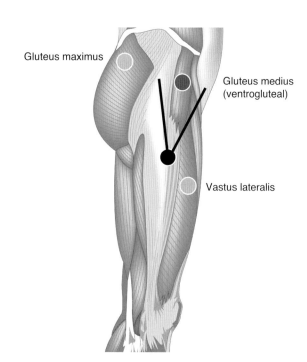

Figure 4.6.1 Ventrogluteal site

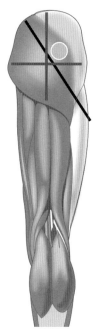

Figure 4.6.2 Dorsogluteal site

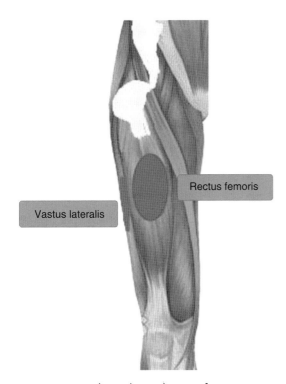

Figure 4.6.3 Vastus lateralis and rectus femoris sites

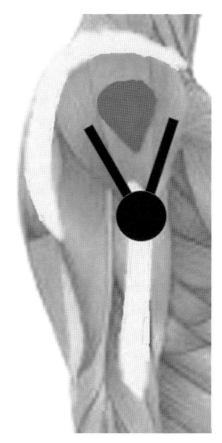

Figure 4.6.4 Deltoid site

particularly in emergencies such as anaphylaxis, where this is considered the ideal and preferred site (Simons et al., 2001).

Deltoid

The deltoid is in the upper limb (Fig. 4.6.4). It is relatively easy to gain access. It is smaller with less blood supply, reducing its versatility; volumes of injectable medication are limited to 1 mL (Barron and Cocoman, 2008). Axillary and radial nerves lie beneath this muscle and are vulnerable to inadvertent injection.

Locate the site by drawing an imaginary inverted triangle, with the base being where the shoulder meets the clavicle (the acromion process). Each end of the base is then brought down to a midline point just below the axilla level, with the arm hanging downwards. The injection site is the thickest triangle centre or 3–5 cm down from the acromion process. Completely expose the muscle for visualisation; merely rolling up a sleeve may partly conceal the muscle and prompt low injection.

Whichever of the above sites is selected, inspect the area for signs of unsuitability, including infection, injury or skin disease. The elderly and small children may have less muscle mass, making the vastus lateralis more desirable. For repeated injections, consider rotating the side and site.

Patient positioning

Make the muscle accessible, with the patient in a lying, sitting or standing position. Carry or support child patients with the site uppermost. Muscle relaxation can decrease pain (Nicoll and Hesby, 2002).

The choice of position depends on the site:

- *dorsogluteal:* prone positioning with internal femur rotation helps relax the gluteal muscles (Kara and Yapucu Güneş, 2016)
- *ventrogluteal and vastus lateralis:* lateral positioning, with the upper leg flexed by around 20°, allows the knee to lower and internally rotates the leg
- *rectus femoris:* supine positioning with leg flexed at the knee relaxes the muscle
- *deltoid:* placing the arm with the elbow bent and hand sitting on the opposite hip can relax the muscle.

Site preparation

Skin penetration can allow infection, so it is important to clean skin that is visibly dirty. Immunocompromised and older, at-risk patients require greater care.

Swab the skin with standard antiseptic agents such as antiseptic swabs, allowing the site 30 seconds to dry. Use concentrically larger circles until the site and swabs appear clean. Avoid palpating the site afterwards (Barron and Cocoman, 2008; Wynaden et al., 2005).

IM injection method

Patient consent is required for the administration of medication and the procedure.

Don latex medical gloves over clean hands. Locate a sharps waste receptacle for discarding the needle.

Position the patient, and then expose and clean the injection site (Nicoll and Hesby, 2002; Wynaden et al., 2005).

Select the appropriate syringe size for the drug volume. Attach a needle with a length that is suitable for the depth of the chosen muscle and the apparent amount of adipose tissue. A non-bevelled needle may be used for drawing up the drugs, but remove and replace it with a bevelled needle before injection. Attach the ampoule or label the syringe for identification. If necessary, discard any excess medication, leaving the correct dose in the syringe to reduce the risk of drug error.

Stabilise the injection site using the Z-track method (Barron and Cocoman, 2008; Kara and Yapucu Güneş, 2016; Wynaden et al., 2015; Wynaden et al., 2005). With the muscle exposed, identify the injection point. Place the fingertips of your non-dominant hand a few centimetres below the site, pressing firmly inwards and then away from the site, holding the skin taut. (As the needle is withdrawn after injection, releasing this hand allows the skin to move more than the underlying muscle. A Z-shaped needle track forms, reducing drug leakage and increasing uptake.)

With the skin taut, push the needle into the injection site quickly and firmly (Palma and Strohfus, 2013), at 90° to the skin. Hold the syringe like a dart several centimetres above the site before plunging forwards (Nicoll and Hesby, 2002; Wynaden et al., 2005). Alternatively, place the needle tip directly on the skin at the injection site and then firmly plunge it inwards. In either case, penetration is rapid, as the needle depth is close to the hub in one motion. Hold the syringe by the barrel to avoid inadvertently pushing the plunger (Nicoll and Hesby, 2002; Wynaden et al., 2005).

Hold the needle in place. Test to ensure the needle has not unintentionally penetrated a blood vessel. With the other hand, pull the plunger gently back for 2–3 seconds to ensure no blood appears through inadvertent penetration of the vessels. If blood appears, withdraw the needle without administering the drug and discard it. Repeat with a new syringe and drug preparation.

If the correct site and needle are used, the risk of inadvertent entry into the blood vessels is very low. However, many drugs carry significant implications if they are administered incorrectly, so prioritise safety and test the needle first, as described above (Barron and Cocoman, 2008; Sepah et al., 2014; Sisson, 2015; Wynaden et al., 2005).

Where no blood appears, depress the plunger to inject the drug (Sepah et al., 2014; Sisson, 2015). Administer the medication slowly, at 5–10 seconds per millilitre, to allow time for the muscle fibres to stretch and accommodate the volume (Nicoll and Hesby, 2002; Wynaden et al., 2005). Allow a few seconds for the drug to spread into the surrounding muscle. Withdraw the needle and immediately dispose of it into a sharps container. Note the time of administration.

Apply gentle pressure over the site for a few seconds to assist drug diffusion and uptake. Monitor the patient for effectiveness of and adverse reaction to the medication.

Occasionally, a small wound may occur at the injection site. Cover this with an adhesive dressing.

Clinical skill assessment process

The following section outlines the clinical skill assessment tools that should be used to determine a student's ability to demonstrate safe and accurate intramuscular injection.
1. Clinical Skill Work Instruction
2. Formative Clinical Skill Assessment (F-CSAT)
3. Performance Improvement Plan (PIP)
4. Summative Clinical Skill Assessment (S-CSAT)
(5. Direct Observation of Procedural Skills (DOPS) – see Chapter 1.1)

Clinical Skill Work Instruction

Equipment and resources: Simulated patient suitable for IM injection; syringes; bevelled needles; disposable gloves; sharps container; antiseptic swabs; clinical waste bag; method of documenting results

Associated Clinical Skills: Infection control; Communication; Consent; ANTT®; Administering oral medications; Preparing injections

Intramuscular injection

Activity	Critical Action	Rationale
Prepare paramedic	Wash hands and don latex protective gloves.	Decreases infection risk.

Intramuscular injection continued

Activity	Critical Action	Rationale
Prepare patient	Discuss procedure with patient. Obtain informed consent.	To reduce patient stress and gain cooperation.
	Select injection site appropriate to the patient and the drug involved.	Ensure muscle mass is suitable for volume and access.
	Expose site by removing clothing as necessary.	Provides visibility to ensure correct injection location.
	Position patient to expose and relax the muscle.	Decreases discomfort.
Prepare equipment	Select syringe for use.	To appropriately measure volume.
	Select and attach appropriate bevelled needle to syringe.	Non-bevelled needle can be discarded and replaced with clean needle for injection.
	Verify, prepare and draw drug into syringe.	Ensures right patient, drug and dose.
	Place syringe in clean receptacle with drug ampoule attached.	Identifies syringe contents.
	Place sharps waste container conveniently within reach.	For safe sharps disposal.
Inject drug	Anatomically locate the injection site.	Ensures nerves and blood vessels are avoided.
	Prepare site by antiseptic swabbing in concentric circles.	Reduces risk of infection.
	Use Z-track method to hold skin taut over site with non-dominant hand.	Reduces risk of drug leakage.
	Hold syringe in dominant hand. Push needle firmly and quickly into injection site, using either dart or push method, in one continuous motion until needle hub is reached.	Dart method begins approximately 10 cm above site. Push method begins with needle tip on skin.
	With needle injected, pull plunger back and inspect it for blood return.	Determines if needle is in blood vessel.
	If no blood returns into syringe, push plunger in to inject drug at rate of 1 mL per 5–10 seconds.	Allows muscle fibre to expand to accommodate drug.
	If blood does return, withdraw needle, discard, prepare new syringe and repeat.	Indicates needle has penetrated a blood vessel.
	Once drug has been injected, hold needle in place for several seconds.	To allow drug distribution.
	Withdraw needle quickly and discard immediately into sharps waste container.	For sharps safety.
Post injection	Release Z-track tension.	Reduces drug leakage.
	Press over site for 10 seconds.	To help distribute drug.
	Monitor patient for drug effectiveness and adverse effects.	Identifies adequate effect and alerts if present.
Report	Accurately document/hand over findings, including therapeutic benefit or adverse reaction.	Accurate record kept and patient care continuity.

Formative Clinical Skill Assessment (F-CSAT)

Equipment and resources: Simulated patient suitable for IM injection; syringes; bevelled needles; disposable gloves; sharps container; antiseptic swabs; clinical waste bag; method of documenting results

Associated Clinical Skills: Infection control; Communication; Consent; ANTT®; Administering oral medications; Preparing injections

Staff/Student being assessed: _____

Intramuscular injection

Activity	Critical Action	Participant Performance				
Prepares paramedic	Washes hands and dons gloves.	0	1	2	3	4
Prepares patient	Discusses procedure with patient. Obtains consent.	0	1	2	3	4
	Selects injection site.	0	1	2	3	4
	Exposes site by removing clothing as necessary.	0	1	2	3	4
	Positions patient to expose and relax muscle.	0	1	2	3	4
Prepares equipment	Selects desired syringe for use.	0	1	2	3	4
	Selects and attaches appropriate bevelled needle to syringe.	0	1	2	3	4
	Verifies, prepares and draws drug into syringe.	0	1	2	3	4
	Places syringe in clean receptacle with drug ampoule attached.	0	1	2	3	4
	Places sharps waste container conveniently within reach.	0	1	2	3	4
Injects drug	Anatomically locates injection site.	0	1	2	3	4
	Prepares site by antiseptic swabbing in concentric circles.	0	1	2	3	4
	Uses Z-track method to hold skin taut over site with non-dominant hand.	0	1	2	3	4
	Holds syringe in dominant hand. Pushes needle firmly and quickly into injection site, using either dart or push method, in one continuous motion until needle hub is reached.	0	1	2	3	4
	With needle in place, pulls plunger back, inspecting it for blood return.	0	1	2	3	4
	If there is no blood return, pushes plunger in to inject drug at 1 mL per 5–10 seconds.	0	1	2	3	4
	If blood returns, withdraws needle, discards, prepares new syringe and repeats.	0	1	2	3	4
	Once drug has been injected, holds needle in place for several seconds.	0	1	2	3	4
	Withdraws needle quickly and discards it immediately into sharps waste container.	0	1	2	3	4
Post injection	Releases Z-track tension.	0	1	2	3	4
	Presses over site for 10 seconds.	0	1	2	3	4
	Monitors patient for drug effectiveness and adverse effects.	0	1	2	3	4
Reports	Accurately documents/hands over findings.	0	1	2	3	4

Standard Achieved: (please circle one)

Competent (C)   Not Yet Competent* (NYC)

Staff/Student Name: _____

Assessor (please print name)**:** _____

Signed (Assessor)**:** _____

Date of Assessment: _____

Comments:

*If Not Yet Competent (NYC) a PIP needs to be completed and a repeat of the F-CSAT

Formative Clinical Skill Assessment (F-CSAT) Key

Skill level	Standard of procedure	Quality of performance	Outcome	Level of assistance required
4 Safe for unsupervised practice	Safe Accurate Behaviour is appropriate to context	Confident Accurate Expedient	Achieved intended outcome	No supporting cues* required
3 Requires supervision	Safe Accurate Behaviour is appropriate to context	Confident Accurate Takes longer than required	Achieved intended outcome	Requires occasional supportive cues*
2 Requires assistance	Safe Accurate Behaviour generally appropriate to context	Lacks certainty	Would not have achieved outcome without support	Requires frequent verbal and occasional physical directives in addition to supportive cues*
1 Requires direction	Safe only with guidance Not completely accurate	Unskilled Inefficient	Would not have achieved outcome without support	Requires continuous verbal and frequent physical directive cues*
0 Unsafe	Unsafe Unable to demonstrate behaviour Lack of insight into behaviour appropriate to context	Unskilled	Would not have achieved outcome	Requires continuous verbal and continuous physical directive cues*

*Refers to physical directives or verbal supportive cues

Performance Improvement Plan (PIP)

Please document the agreed education plan and completion timelines for areas assessed as less than 4.

This plan should be presented to assessor prior to commencement of summative assessment.

Where was supervisor support required?	Student summary of deficit. (Why was there a problem?)	Improvement Plan	Completed (Y/N)

Staff/Student Name: _____

Staff/Student Signature: _____

Educator Name: _____

Educator Signature: _____

Summative Clinical Skill Assessment (S-CSAT)

Equipment and resources: Simulated patient suitable for IM injection; syringes; bevelled needles; disposable gloves; sharps container; antiseptic swabs; clinical waste bag; method of documenting results

Associated Clinical Skills: Infection control; Communication; Consent; ANTT®; Administering oral medications; Preparing injections

Staff/Student being assessed: _____

- Completed Formative Clinical Skill Assessment (F-CSAT):   **YES**   **NO**
- Completed Performance Improvement Plan (PIP):   **YES**   **NO**   **N/A**

Intramuscular injection			
Activity	**Critical Action**	**Achieved Without Direction**	
Prepares operator	Washes hands and dons gloves.	NO	YES
Prepares patient	Discusses procedure with patient. Obtains consent.	NO	YES
	Selects appropriate injection site.	NO	YES
	Exposes site by removing clothing as necessary.	NO	YES
	Positions patient to expose and relax muscle.	NO	YES

Intramuscular injection continued

Activity	Critical Action	Achieved Without Direction	
Prepares equipment	Selects desired syringe for use.	NO	YES
	Selects and attaches appropriate bevelled needle to syringe.	NO	YES
	Verifies, prepares and draws drug into syringe.	NO	YES
	Places syringe in clean receptacle with drug ampoule attached.	NO	YES
	Places sharps waste container conveniently within reach.	NO	YES
Injects drug	Anatomically locates injection site.	NO	YES
	Prepares injection site by antiseptic swabbing in concentric circles.	NO	YES
	Uses Z-track method to hold skin taut over site with non-dominant hand.	NO	YES
	Holds syringe in dominant hand. Pushes needle firmly and quickly into injection site, using either dart or push method, in one continuous motion until needle hub is reached.	NO	YES
	With needle in place, pulls plunger back, inspecting it for blood return.	NO	YES
	If there is no blood return, injects drug at rate of 1 mL per 5–10 seconds.	NO	YES
	If blood returns, withdraws needle, prepares a new syringe and repeats.	NO	YES
	Once drug has been injected, holds needle in place for several seconds.	NO	YES
	Withdraws needle quickly and discards it immediately into sharps waste container.	NO	YES
Post injection	Releases Z-track tension.	NO	YES
	Holds pressure over site for 10 seconds.	NO	YES
	Monitors patient for drug effectiveness and adverse effects.	NO	YES
Reports	Accurately documents/hands over findings.	NO	YES

Standard Achieved: (please circle one)

Competent (C)   Not Yet Competent* (NYC)

Staff/Student Name: _____

Assessor (please print name): _____

Signed (Assessor): _____

Date of Assessment: _____

Comments:

*If Not Yet Competent (NYC) a PIP needs to be completed and a repeat of the F-CSAT

431

Clinical findings

Pain

Discuss pain as part of gaining informed consent. Pain can provoke unpleasant responses, particularly in children, and cause lasting apprehension (Barron and Cocoman, 2008).

Applying direct pressure to the site for several seconds just prior to injection and using Z-track site tension with a quick, single motion for penetration can make injections less painful.

The volume of injected medication causes muscle fibres to be stretched. Reducing the volume, injecting slowly into large muscles, correctly positioning the patient and relaxing the muscles can reduce pain (Nicoll and Hesby, 2002; Kara and Yapucu Güneş, 2016). Children also benefit from emotional support and being held.

Injury/complications

Nerve injury with IM injection is uncommon and can be avoided by locating the correct site. Other complications include infection, cellulitis, tissue necrosis, bleeding, tendonitis and even bone injury. Using correct methods for injection helps the paramedic avoid these issues (Barron and Cocoman, 2008).

Drug volume

The maximum injection volume varies with muscle size (see Table 4.6.1). No more than 3 mL in larger muscles should be considered for children.

Injection depth/needle length

IM needles pass through skin layers into the muscle. Factors influencing needle length include the amount of adipose tissue and the muscle size (Palma and Strohfus, 2013; Petrofsky, 2012; Wynaden et al., 2005; Wynaden et al., 2015).

A 23G needle is usual for adult IM drug injection. Smaller children and the elderly typically have smaller muscle mass, requiring shorter needles (25G).

Obesity increases subcutaneous space, necessitating the use of longer needles. IM injection requires muscle penetration of at least 5 mm. For obese patients, choose a less covered site or use a longer needle (21G). Dorsogluteal injections most commonly encounter adipose tissue, while this is less likely in deltoid injections (Palma and Strohfus, 2013).

PRACTICE TIP!

IM injection involves using multiple small and easily misplaced items. A clean pillowcase makes a more suitable surface on which to place items than random surfaces do. Though it is not aseptic, it is clean and orderly.

PRACTICE TIP!

Sharps safety is critical. Before injection, place a sharps container within immediate proximity to allow immediate disposal of syringes and needles. Call out the word 'sharp', or 'sharp out', before injection to heighten awareness of the exposed needle.

PRACTICE TIP!

Draw up the exact drug dose required into the syringe before injection. This reduces the risk of drug error, as it can be determined before and not during the injection. It also allows the drug administration to be safer, by immediately discarding the contaminated needle after the injection.

Table 4.6.1 Typical adult maximum volume per injection site	
Muscle	**Maximum volume**
Deltoid	1 mL
Ventrogluteal	3 mL
Dorsogluteal	4 mL
Rectus femoris	5 mL
Vastus lateralis	5 mL

TEST YOUR KNOWLEDGE QUESTIONS

1. **What are the five most suitable muscle sites for IM injection?**
    Dorsogluteal; deltoid; rectus femoris; vastus lateralis; ventrogluteal.

2. **What is the usual angle between the needle and skin during IM injection?**
    90°.

3. **Of the five IM injection sites, which carries the greatest risk of nerve or vascular injury?**
    The dorsogluteal site, as it has more immediate proximity to the underlying sciatic nerve.

4. **What maximum drug fluid volumes are usual for the five muscle sites during IM injection?**
    Deltoid 1 mL; ventrogluteal 3 mL; dorsogluteal 4 mL; rectus femoris 5 mL; vastus lateralis 5 mL.

5. **What needle gauge is recommended for adult and obese IM injection?**
    Adults: 23 gauge; obese adults: 21 gauge.

6. **Why is the plunger pulled back during IM injection?**
    To ensure the needle is not inadvertently within a blood vessel.

7. **What options help minimise pain during IM injection?**
    Reassurance/explanation; correct positioning of the patient and limb; correct needle size and drug volume for site; quick method of injection.

8. **What two injection methods can be used during needle penetration?**
    Plunge needle in from several centimetres above the skin; place needle against skin and push inwards.

9. **What complications can occur during IM injection?**
    Nerve injury; infection; cellulitis; tissue necrosis; bleeding; tendonitis; bone injury.

10. **What infectious risks are caused by IM injection?**
    Unclean preparation poses an infection risk to the patient; blood contact and needlestick injury pose a risk to the paramedic.

References

Barron, C. and Cocoman, A., 2008. Administering intramuscular injections to children: what does the evidence say? *Journal of Children's and Young People's Nursing*, 2(3), 138–144.

Chan, V.O., Colville, J., Persaud, T., Buckley, O., Hamilton, S. and Torreggiani, W.C., 2006. Intramuscular injections into the buttocks: are they truly intramuscular? *European Journal of Radiology*, 58(3), 480–484.

Kara, D. and Yapucu Güneş, Ü., 2016. The effect on pain of three different methods of intramuscular injection: a randomized controlled trial. *International Journal of Nursing Practice*, 22(2), 152–159.

Nicoll, L.H. and Hesby, A., 2002. Intramuscular injection: an integrative research review and guideline for evidence-based practice. *Applied Nursing Research*, 15(3), 149–162.

Palma, S. and Strohfus, P., 2013. Are IM injections IM in obese and overweight females? A study in injection technique. *Applied Nursing Research*, 26(4), e1–4.

Petrofsky, J.S., 2012. Resting blood flow in the skin: does it exist, and what is the influence of temperature, aging, and diabetes? *Journal of Diabetes Science and Technology*, 6(3), 674–685.

Sepah, Y., Samad, L., Altaf, A., Rajagopalan, N. and Khan, A.J., 2014. Aspiration in injections: should we continue or abandon the practice? *F1000Research*, 3, 157.

Simons, F.E.R., Gu, X. and Simons, K.J., 2001. Epinephrine absorption in adults: intramuscular versus subcutaneous injection. *Journal of Allergy and Clinical Immunology*, 108(5), 871–873.

Sisson, H., 2015. Aspirating during the intramuscular injection procedure: a systematic literature review. *Journal of Clinical Nursing*, 24(17–18), 2368–2375.

Wynaden, D., Landsborough, I., Chapman, R., McGowan, S., Lapsley, J. and Finn, M., 2005. Establishing best practice guidelines for administration of intra muscular injections in the adult: a systematic review of the literature. *Contemporary Nurse*, 20(2), 267–277.

Wynaden, D., Tohotoa, J., Omari, O.A., Happell, B., Heslop, K., Barr, L. and Sourinathan, V., 2015. Administering intramuscular injections: how does research translate into practice over time in the mental health setting? *Nurse Education Today*, 35(4), 620–624.

Bibliography

Craft, J., Gordon, C., Huether, S.E., McCance, K.L. and Brashers, V.L., 2015. *Understanding pathophysiology* (ANZ adaptation). Sydney: Elsevier.

McCance, K.L. and Huether, S.E., 2015. *Pathophysiology: the biologic basis for disease in adults and children*. Sydney: Elsevier.

4.7 | Intravenous access

Jeff Kenneally

Chapter objectives

At the end of this chapter the reader will be able to:

1. Describe the rationale for intravenous (IV) cannulation
2. Demonstrate the method of choosing IV cannulation sites
3. Demonstrate effective safe IV cannulation
4. Accurately report on IV cannulation

Resources required for this assessment

- Simulated patient/limb suitable for IV injection
- Disposable gloves, protective eyewear
- Intravenous cannulas
- Antiseptic swabs
- Tourniquet
- Adhesive dressing
- IV fitting or giving set
- Medical tape
- Gauze pad
- Clinical waste bag and sharps container
- Method of documenting results

Skill matrix

This assessment requires:

- Infection control (CS 1.3)
- Communication (CS 1.5)
- Consent (CS 1.6)
- Aseptic Non Touch Technique (ANTT®) (CS 2.20)

This assessment is a component of:

- Medication administration (Chapter 4)

Introduction

Intravenous (IV) access is invasive, providing direct venous access. It can be performed using a needle attached to a syringe. Alternatively, a purpose device can be inserted and left within a vein; this is called intravenous cannulation. This chapter discusses gaining peripheral intravenous needle access.

Anatomy and physiology

Peripheral blood vessels are located below the dermal and subcutaneous layers, above and within muscles. Veins are typically superficially prominent.

Within veins are a series of valves that allow blood flow forwards and prevent it from flowing backwards. Muscle

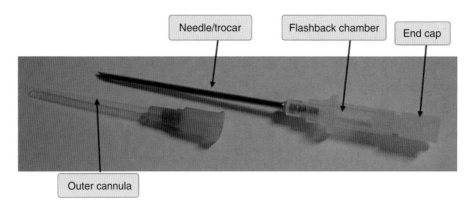

Figure 4.7.1 An intravenous cannula

Table 4.7.1 Representative IV cannula details				
IV hub colour	**Cannula gauge (G)**	**External diameter (mm)**	**Cannula length (mm)**	**Flow rate (mL/min)**
Orange	14	2.1	45	300
Grey	16	1.7	30–45	172–220
Green	18	1.3	30–45	76–105
Pink	20	1.0	25–30	54–65
Blue	22	0.8	25	31–35
Yellow	24	0.7	18	14–20

contractions compress the veins, thereby supporting blood flow; the veins then refill as the muscles relax.

Clinical rationale

IV cannulation involves a hollow trocar (needle) being pushed through the skin until the vein is penetrated. The trocar is removed, leaving the pliable outer catheter in situ (Fig. 4.7.1). This process allows the administration of drugs, blood products, fluids for rehydration and circulation expansion, parenteral nutrition and contrast radiological agents. It has no absolute contraindications; the major concern is the suitability of the substance being administered.

IV injection sites and cannula size

The usual location for IV cannulation is the arm. Using the patient's non-dominant arm reduces the impact of cannulation on their activities. Limb movement can be adversely affected if the cannula is placed near a joint. Veins can be found in the dorsum of the hand, wrist, forearm, antecubital fossae and bicep. Less common options include the external jugular, dorsum of feet, ankles and infant scalp veins (O'Grady et al., 2011).

Veins vary in size, as do IV cannulas. The size of the cannula used, measured by internal diameter (gauge; see Table 4.7.1) depends on its intended purpose.

The insertion of a larger sized cannula increases pain as, once it is inside a vein, blood flow must pass around the cannula. Use the smallest size possible, placing large cannulas only in large veins.

Larger IV cannulas (14–16G) are used for fluid or blood transfusion/donation. The flow rate of fluid through them is directly related to their radius. Medium (18–20G) cannulas have various uses, whereas small (22–24G) cannulas are mostly limited to paediatric care (O'Grady et al., 2011).

Locating a suitable vein can be difficult (Cuper et al., 2012; Nafiu et al., 2010; Sebbane et al., 2013). Adipose tissue makes veins less superficial, and vascular disease from hyperglycaemia or steroid use can make them fragile. Cold and shock cause vasoconstriction, while a warm temperature causes vasodilation.

A tourniquet used proximal to the cannulation site should impede venous return but not arterial flow, thereby allowing the engorgement of distal veins. Confirm the distal pulse after applying the tourniquet. Place the limb in a dependent position and have the patient slowly clench their fist to pump the muscles. Gentle finger tapping on a vein can increase its prominence.

Many patients have immediate vein options, while others will take longer for their veins to suitably fill. Apply the tourniquet early, while preparing the equipment (Fig. 4.7.2). Inspect both of the patient's arms before deciding on the best option.

Place the tourniquet over the mid-bicep. For the lower leg, place the tourniquet mid-calf. Apply it loosely and then pull it tighter, avoiding skin pinching by placing a finger

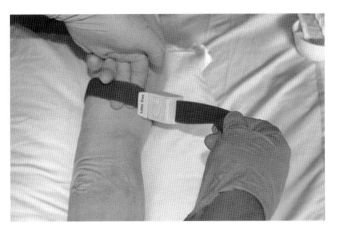

Figure 4.7.2 Applying a tourniquet

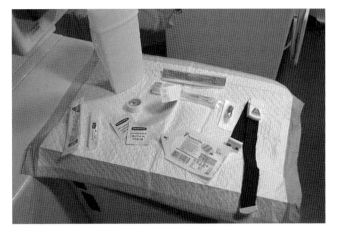

Figure 4.7.3 Laying out the IV equipment

beneath the tourniquet as it tightens. This is uncomfortable for the patient, so release it as soon as practicable.

Veins have a distinctive spongy feel when gentle downward pressure is placed on them with a finger. Ultrasound and infrared devices can locate superficial veins (Egan et al., 2013; Heinrichs et al., 2013; Perry et al., 2011). Valves are palpable as lumps that appear periodically along the length of the vein. Insert the IV between and not into the valves, to protect them.

Ideally, the veins should be long enough for the cannula to be completely pushed into. Changing direction while inserting a cannula creates the risk of the cannula not advancing or pushing through the vein wall. Some veins can be straightened using distal traction. Two veins bifurcating can provide a stable cannulation site.

Some sites are unsuitable for IV insertion, including when they are painful, red/swollen, infected, distal to injuries or in limbs with renal dialysis fistulae. The placement of the IV should not interfere with other therapies, such as splinting or bandaging, if these are required.

Method for performing IV cannulation

Ensure the patient gives their informed consent to the procedure. Support the limb using a pillow or rolled towel, with the vein accessible.

Topical analgesia can reduce pain (Beck et al., 2011; Page and Taylor, 2010; Schreiber et al., 2013; Yeoh and Lee, 2012). Consider the urgency of the situation against the delay required for analgesia to be effective. The underside of the forearm and the feet tend to be sensitive and painful when penetrated with a needle.

Adopt a position looking directly along the vein to avoid pushing the trocar across it. Ensure there is sufficient light.

Prepare all items in advance and lay them out on a clean or sterile surface (Fig. 4.7.3). IV preparation and insertion are aseptic (see Chapter 2.20). Place a sharps waste container in a convenient place for safe and rapid deposition. Wear protective eyewear to avoid blood splashes.

Clean the cannulation site with antiseptic swabs (O'Grady et al., 2011), using a circular process commencing around the site, extending outwards in increasing circles (Fig. 4.7.4). Repeat until the swabs come

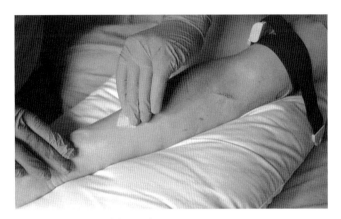

Figure 4.7.4 Swabbing the IV insertion site

away clean, and then allow 30 seconds for the skin to dry. Don't touch the site afterwards or it must be cleaned again.

Remove and discard the cannula sheath. No IV device should be recapped for risk of needlestick injury. Inform the patient and others that the procedure is occurring.

With the non-dominant hand, apply vein traction by pressing the skin several centimetres distal to the injection site, then pulling distally. This reduces sideway vein movement, which is worst in patients who are thin or have superficial veins (Sebbane et al., 2013). Traction must be maintained until the cannula is within the vein.

Place the tip bevel upwards onto or next to the vein. The angle of insertion required varies: visible/superficial veins need shallow angle of around 10° to avoid pushing through the wall of the opposite vein (Fig. 4.7.5a), while deeper veins may need an initial insertion angle of up to 35° from the skin (Fig. 4.7.5b).

Advance the tip of the trocar through the skin. Tougher skin, particularly in outdoor workers, can provide resistance. As the bevel penetrates the skin, observe the flashback chamber for blood. This might be sluggish with a small-gauge IV or if the patient is hypotensive.

Flashback indicates that the tip of the trocar has penetrated the vein. The cannula sits back from the tip, so advancing it a few more millimetres places it also inside the vein. Reduce the angle of the trocar to a few degrees above the skin, to avoid pushing through the opposite wall, while maintaining traction.

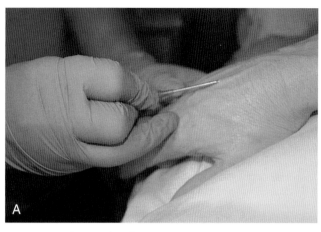
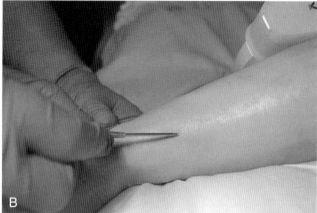

Figure 4.7.5 The angle of insertion
(a) Shallow angle for superficial veins. (b) Increased angle for deeper veins.

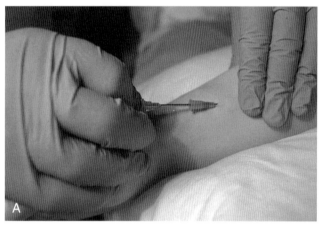
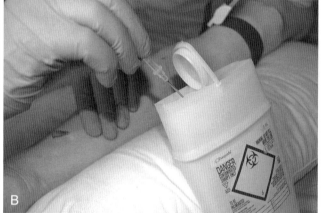

Figure 4.7.6 Withdrawing the trocar
(a) Removing the IV trocar with the cannula in situ. (b) Safely disposing of sharps.

If flashback stops prematurely, the trocar may have exited the vein. Pulling back slightly and advancing again may achieve success. If this is unsuccessful or doubtful, withdraw the trocar and discard it as a failed attempt.

There are two options for completing insertion:

Option 1: Continue advancing the flattened angle trocar/cannula into the vein several more millimetres. This allows the non-dominant hand to release the traction being held without the needle being pulled out of the vein with the released skin. This free hand is now available for advancing the cannula while the dominant hand holds the trocar.

Option 2: Do not advance the trocar further. Maintain traction with the non-dominant hand. Hold the trocar in its current position and advance the plastic cannula by pushing on the hub with the forefinger of the dominant hand. This takes dexterity; some devices have a raised lip to assist.

Advance the cannula hub fully inwards, with the trocar partly extending from the cannula. Unless you are withdrawing blood, release the tourniquet to avoid bleeding.

Place the first three fingers of the non-dominant hand over where the end of the cannula lies beneath the skin.

Press down to compress and stop blood from escaping. Withdraw the trocar, ensuring the cannula is not dragged out with it (Fig. 4.7.6a). Many newer IV cannula have features designed for safe withdrawal, including those that have an enclosing sheath over the needle with a metal-tipped cap.

Warn those nearby to remain clear and immediately drop the trocar into the sharps waste container (Fig. 4.7.6b).

Securely attach suitable fitting to the cannula such as bung, tap or giving set for intended use (Fig. 4.7.7a). Apply a clear adhesive dressing over cannula hub to secure and provide infection barrier (Fig. 4.7.7b).

Secure the hub to the skin with tape to ensure the cannula is not dislodged. Use an elastic bandage where the patient is diaphoretic or uncooperatively pulling at the IV. Tightness must not impede vascular flow.

No IV should be used if its patency is doubtful or in question. Before use, verify the IV's patency with a saline flush that can demonstrate freely injectable flow into the cannula. Resistance or swelling at the site suggests that the cannula is not placed correctly. Withdraw and discard a failed cannula, and then dress and apply pressure over the wound.

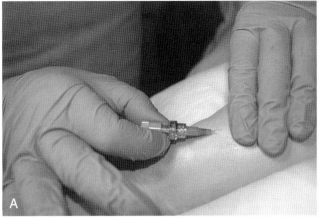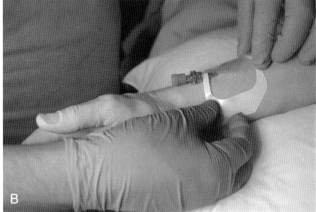

Figure 4.7.7 Securing the cannula hub
(a) Attaching the fitting to the cannula hub. (b) Applying an adhesive dressing.

Clinical skill assessment process

The following section outlines the clinical skill assessment tools that should be used to determine a student's ability to demonstrate safe and accurate intravenous access.
1. Clinical Skill Work Instruction
2. Formative Clinical Skill Assessment (F-CSAT)
3. Performance Improvement Plan (PIP)
4. Summative Clinical Skill Assessment (S-CSAT)
(5. Direct Observation of Procedural Skills (DOPS) – see Chapter 1.1)

Clinical Skill Work Instruction

Equipment and resources: Simulated patient/limb with injectable veins; disposable gloves and protective eyewear; IV cannulas; syringe; adhesive dressing; medical tape; IV fitting or giving set; clinical waste bag and sharps container; antiseptic swabs; gauze pad; bandage; tourniquet; method of documenting results

Associated Clinical Skills: Infection control; Communication; Consent; ANTT®

Intravenous access

Activity	Critical Action	Rationale
Personal protection	Don PPE as required.	Decreases risk of infection.
Prepare patient	Discuss procedure. Obtain informed consent.	To reduce patient stress and gain cooperation.
	Expose the limb and arrange it in a supported dependent position.	To visualise area and provide access.
	Apply tourniquet over bicep, ensuring pulse is palpable.	Tourniquet should be venous occlusive, not arterial.
	Determine site, using visualisation, palpation or both, and cannula size for intended use.	This may take several minutes for vein filling and tourniquets to multiple limbs.
Prepare equipment	Place sharps waste container in a convenient location.	For safe disposal of sharps.
	Lay out equipment on a clean surface, ensuring asepsis.	For orderliness and to avoid infection.
	Prepare cannulation site by swabbing in concentric circles. Allow 30 seconds to dry. Do not re-touch.	To reduce contamination.

Intravenous access continued

Activity	Critical Action	Rationale
Insert IV cannula	Hold cannula flashback chamber with dominant hand. Announce that sharp is in use. Remove cap and discard.	Dominant hand is used to guide insertion. To alert others of exposed sharp.
	Stabilise vein with distal traction using non-dominant hand.	To stop vein or skin moving when trocar inserted.
	Place tip either directly on top of vein or immediately beside it at appropriate angle for vein.	To identify insertion site.
	Push tip through skin at appropriate angle, with sufficient force to just enter the vein.	If force used is too hard, it can push through the vein.
	Observe for flashback. The trocar may need to be slightly advanced to enter the vein. When flashback is observed, stop advancing trocar and flatten angle to skin.	Indicates trocar is in the vein.
	Advance trocar a few more millimetres until plastic cannula is also in the vein. This distance can vary with bevel size.	Ensures that the cannula is also within the vein.
	Either feed off cannula with forefinger of dominant hand or continue to feed entire trocar further into the vein.	Advances cannula length into vein.
	Release traction, then release tourniquet.	Reduces pressure in the vein.
	Compress skin over cannula end with three fingers of non-dominant hand. Maintain pressure until cannula is capped.	To ensure blood does not flow from open IV hub.
	After warning others, withdraw trocar from cannula and immediately drop into sharps waste container.	For sharps safety and infection control.
Verify placement	Taking care to not dislodge cannula, gently flush with 5–10 mL saline. Look for free flow and no tissue swelling.	Identifies correct placement.
Secure IV cannula in place	Attach desired capping option to cannula end and twist in place. This may require pinching hub with non-dominant hand to stop twisting.	Includes bungs, 3-way taps and giving set fluid lines.
	Cover cannula hub with clear adhesive aseptic dressing.	Maintains asepsis of insertion site while allowing visibility.
	Secure cannula capping device with tape and/or bandage.	Secures cannula in place.
Report	Accurately document/hand over the procedure, including cannula size, location and patency verification.	Accurate record kept and continuity of patient care.

Formative Clinical Skill Assessment (F-CSAT)

Equipment and resources: Simulated patient/limb with injectable veins; disposable gloves and protective eyewear; IV cannulas; syringe; adhesive dressing; medical tape; IV fitting or giving set; clinical waste bag and sharps container; antiseptic swabs; gauze pad; bandage; tourniquet; method of documenting results

Associated Clinical Skills: Infection control; Communication, Consent; ANTT®

Staff/Student being assessed: _____

Intravenous access

Activity	Critical Action	Participant Performance				
Personal protection	Dons PPE.	O	1	2	3	4
Prepares patient	Discusses procedure. Obtains informed consent.	O	1	2	3	4
	Exposes limb and arranges it in a supported dependent position.	O	1	2	3	4
	Applies tourniquet over bicep, ensuring pulse is palpable.	O	1	2	3	4
	Determines cannulation site, using visualisation, palpation or both, and cannula size for intended use.	O	1	2	3	4
Prepares equipment	Places sharps waste container in convenient location.	O	1	2	3	4
	Lays out equipment on a clean surface, ensuring asepsis.	O	1	2	3	4
	Prepares site by swabbing in concentric circles. Allows 30 seconds to dry. Does not re-touch.	O	1	2	3	4
Inserts IV cannula	Holds cannula flashback chamber with dominant hand. Announces that sharp is in use. Removes protective cap and discards.	O	1	2	3	4
	Stabilises vein with distal traction using non-dominant hand.	O	1	2	3	4
	Places tip either directly on top of vein or immediately beside it, at appropriate angle for vein.	O	1	2	3	4
	Pushes tip through skin at appropriate angle, with sufficient force to just enter the vein.	O	1	2	3	4
	Observes for flashback. When flashback is observed, stops advancing trocar and flattens angle to skin.	O	1	2	3	4
	Advances trocar a few more millimetres until cannula is also in the vein.	O	1	2	3	4
	Either feeds off cannula with forefinger of dominant hand or continues to feed entire trocar further into the vein.	O	1	2	3	4
	Releases traction, then releases tourniquet.	O	1	2	3	4
	Compresses skin over cannula end with three fingers of non-dominant hand. Maintains pressure until cannula is capped.	O	1	2	3	4
	After warning others, withdraws trocar from cannula and immediately drops into sharps waste container.	O	1	2	3	4
Verifies placement	Taking care to not dislodge cannula, gently flushes with 5–10 mL saline. Looks for free flow and no tissue swelling.	O	1	2	3	4
Secures IV cannula in place	Attaches desired capping option to cannula end and twists in place.	O	1	2	3	4
	Covers hub with clear adhesive aseptic dressing.	O	1	2	3	4
	Secures capping device with tape and/or bandage.	O	1	2	3	4
Reports	Accurately documents/hands over the procedure, including cannula size, location and patency verification.	O	1	2	3	4

Standard Achieved: (please circle one)

Competent (C)   Not Yet Competent* (NYC)

Staff/Student Name: _____

Assessor (please print name): _____

Signed (Assessor): _____

Date of Assessment: _____

Comments:

*If Not Yet Competent (NYC) a PIP needs to be completed and a repeat of the F-CSAT

Formative Clinical Skill Assessment (F-CSAT) Key

Skill level	Standard of procedure	Quality of performance	Outcome	Level of assistance required
4 Safe for unsupervised practice	Safe Accurate Behaviour is appropriate to context	Confident Accurate Expedient	Achieved intended outcome	No supporting cues* required
3 Requires supervision	Safe Accurate Behaviour is appropriate to context	Confident Accurate Takes longer than required	Achieved intended outcome	Requires occasional supportive cues*
2 Requires assistance	Safe Accurate Behaviour generally appropriate to context	Lacks certainty	Would not have achieved outcome without support	Requires frequent verbal and occasional physical directives in addition to supportive cues*
1 Requires direction	Safe only with guidance Not completely accurate	Unskilled Inefficient	Would not have achieved outcome without support	Requires continuous verbal and frequent physical directive cues*
0 Unsafe	Unsafe Unable to demonstrate behaviour Lack of insight into behaviour appropriate to context	Unskilled	Would not have achieved outcome	Requires continuous verbal and continuous physical directive cues*

*Refers to physical directives or verbal supportive cues

Performance Improvement Plan (PIP)

Please document the agreed education plan and completion timelines for areas assessed as less than 4.

This plan should be presented to assessor prior to commencement of summative assessment.

Where was supervisor support required?	Student summary of deficit. (Why was there a problem?)	Improvement Plan	Completed (Y/N)

Staff/Student Name: _____

Staff/Student Signature: _____

Educator Name: _____

Educator Signature: _____

Summative Clinical Skill Assessment (S-CSAT)

Equipment and resources: Simulated patient/limb with injectable veins; disposable gloves and protective eyewear; IV cannulas; syringe; adhesive dressing; medical tape; IV fitting or giving set; clinical waste bag and sharps container; antiseptic swabs; gauze pad; bandage; tourniquet; method of documenting results

Associated Clinical Skills: Infection control; Communication, Consent; ANTT®

Staff/Student being assessed: _____

• Completed Formative Clinical Skill Assessment (F-CSAT):   **YES   NO**

• Completed Performance Improvement Plan (PIP):   **YES   NO   N/A**

Intravenous access

Activity	Critical Action	Achieved Without Direction	
Personal protection	Dons PPE.	NO	YES
Prepares patient	Discusses procedure. Obtains informed consent.	NO	YES
	Exposes limb and arranges it in a supported dependent position.	NO	YES
	Applies tourniquet over bicep, ensuring pulse is palpable.	NO	YES
	Determines cannulation site, using visualisation, palpation or both, and cannula size for intended use.	NO	YES
Prepares equipment	Places sharps waste container in convenient location.	NO	YES
	Lays out equipment on a clean surface, ensuring asepsis.	NO	YES
	Prepares site by swabbing in concentric circles. Allows 30 seconds to dry. Does not re-touch.	NO	YES
Inserts IV cannula	Holds cannula flashback chamber with dominant hand. Announces that sharp is in use. Removes protective cap and discards.	NO	YES
	Stabilises vein with distal traction using non-dominant hand.	NO	YES

Intravenous access continued

Activity	Critical Action	Achieved Without Direction	
	Places tip either directly on top of vein or immediately beside it, at appropriate angle for vein.	NO	YES
	Pushes tip through skin at appropriate angle, with sufficient force to just enter the vein.	NO	YES
	Observes for flashback. When flashback is observed, stops advancing trocar and flattens angle to skin.	NO	YES
	Advances trocar a few more millimetres until cannula is also in the vein.	NO	YES
	Either feeds off cannula with forefinger of dominant hand or continues to feed entire trocar further into the vein.	NO	YES
	Releases traction, then releases tourniquet.	NO	YES
	Compresses skin over cannula end with three fingers of non-dominant hand. Maintains pressure until cannula is capped.	NO	YES
	After warning others, withdraws trocar from cannula and immediately drops into sharps waste container.	NO	YES
Verifies placement	Taking care to not dislodge cannula, gently flushes with 5–10 ml saline. Looks for free flow and no tissue swelling.	NO	YES
Secures IV cannula in place	Attaches desired capping option to cannula end and twists in place.	NO	YES
	Covers hub with clear adhesive aseptic dressing.	NO	YES
	Secures capping device with tape and/or bandage.	NO	YES
Reports	Accurately documents/hands over the procedure, including cannula size, location and patency verification.	NO	YES

Standard Achieved: (please circle one)

Competent (C)   Not Yet Competent* (NYC)

Staff/Student Name: _____

Assessor (please print name): _____

Signed (Assessor): _____

Date of Assessment: _____

Comments:

*If Not Yet Competent (NYC) a PIP needs to be completed and a repeat of the F-CSAT

Clinical findings

Difficult insertion

Difficult veins are hard to predict (Cuper et al., 2012). Repeatedly punctured veins can scar and narrow from injury. Veins can become fragile and sclerotic from cardiovascular disease, diabetes or prolonged medication use, such as steroid administration. The skin, particularly in the elderly, can lose elasticity and tone, making it easier to cause bleeding/bruising. The loss of surrounding subcutaneous tissue can allow veins to move more easily and be less straight.

Handle older and fragile patients gently. Experiment with methods of traction to immobilise and straighten the vein. Use the smallest appropriate needle for the vein being considered, and attempt to insert it on top of the vein rather than beside it. Advance the needle and cannula slowly to respect the delicacy of the vein wall.

It is sometimes difficult to advance the cannula following successful venepuncture. In such cases, remove and discard the trocar and attach a saline-filled syringe to the hub. Gently flush to engorge the vein while advancing cannula, monitoring for patency.

If there is no insertion flashback, the tip may have missed the vein. The cannula may not advance if it has been misplaced into soft tissue.

Attempting relocation causes pain and delays treatment, so this should be brief. Remove the failed trocar, dress the wound and manage bleeding. Subsequent cannulation attempts should be on another limb or proximal to the failed attempt to avoid drug leakage into the tissue.

Pain

Reduce pain with distraction, referring to the illness and therapies rather than the procedure. Always forewarn the patient.

Topical anaesthetic agents or cold spray over the injection site take time for effect, and so are only useful if used in advance of the procedure (Beck et al., 2011; Hogan et al., 2014; Page and Taylor, 2010; Schreiber et al., 2013; Yeoh and Lee, 2012).

Infection and inflammation

Infection can be local or systemic. It occurs if the cannula is not aseptically inserted or if it is left in place for a long period (Rickard et al., 2012).

Signs of local infection include swelling, redness and pain. Aseptic approach is required during insertion and use (see Chapter 2.20). IV sites can be contaminated through moisture or environmental exposure (O'Grady et al., 2011; Rickard et al., 2012).

Embolism

Air bubbles can enter via the syringe or giving set. While smaller air bubbles break up and dissolve within the blood without causing harm, larger bubbles can cause pulmonary emboli or interfere with myocardial contraction. What constitutes problematic air volume is unclear, with estimates ranging from 1 to 8 mL/kg air to body weight.

Other embolisms include clots from the cannula. The cannula end can shear off if a trocar is reinserted, so this should never be allowed to occur.

Infiltration/extravasation

Incorrect IV placement allows drug leakage into the surrounding tissue, causing two broad problems: failure to provide therapy and injury to local tissue.

The area may swell, become red, taut or painful (O'Grady et al., 2011; Rickard et al., 2012). If this occurs, discontinue use and elevate the limb. Occasionally, necrosis can occur.

Arterial injection

Indications that injection has inadvertently entered an artery include brighter red blood flashback and rapid filling of the chamber. Bleeding can pulsate in the cannula hub.

If arterial injection is suspected, remove the cannula and apply direct pressure over the site for 10 minutes to manage haematoma.

Nerve injection

On rare occasions, a nerve can be injured. The cubital fossae median nerve, cutaneous forearm lateral nerve and superficial wrist radial nerve are vulnerable (Stevens et al., 2012). Inadvertent nerve injection can cause pain or numbness over the area.

PRACTICE TIP!

Veins on opposite limbs may present differently. Consider placing the tourniquet on both arms and allow time for venous filling. Examine both limbs before selecting the best option.

PRACTICE TIP!

The insertion of IV cannula requires numerous items. For cleanliness and orderliness, lay out a clean sheet or pillowcase to place them on during preparation.

PRACTICE TIP!

Sharps safety is paramount. The sharps waste container should be ready for use, placed nearby but not where it can be knocked over. If a container is not available, IV insertion should not occur.

PRACTICE TIP!

It can take a few minutes for the peripheral veins to engorge sufficiently for cannulation. Early tourniquet application during preparation helps maximise filling time.

PRACTICE TIP!

Patients with previous IV cannulation exposure may know they have difficult veins and may provide information on past successful attempts.

TEST YOUR KNOWLEDGE QUESTIONS

1. **What are the most suitable sites for IV injection/cannulation?**
   Dorsum of the hand; forearm; cubital fossae.

2. **What are the usual angles between the trocar and the skin during IV insertion?**
   10° on superficial veins; up to 35° on less superficial veins.

3. **List five indications for IV injection.**
   Drug administration; blood withdrawal and blood product administration; fluids for rehydration and blood volume expansion; parenteral nutrition; contrast radiological agents.

4. **What size IV cannulas are large and what are they used for?**
   14G and 16G; used for blood removal/transfusion and large volume fluid resuscitation.

5. **What size IV cannulas are small and what are they used for?**
   22 and 24G; use is limited to paediatric care.

6. **What infection complications can arise from IV cannulation?**
   Local site infection; systemic infection; paramedic blood splash; needlestick injury.

7. **Why is traction important during IV cannulation?**
   It reduces vein immobility, allowing easier penetration.

8. **How can vein valves be useful during cannulation?**
   The valves may be palpated when the vein cannot, identifying the vein line. Inserting between the valves can achieve success.

9. **How can IV patency be assessed?**
   Witnessing the chamber filling with flashback blood; the ease of cannula advancement into the vein; blood returning from placed cannula; the ease of flushing without resistance or swelling.

10. **How is a vein filled to allow IV cannulation?**
    Apply a tourniquet tightly enough for venous but not arterial occlusion; hang the limb dependent; have the patient squeeze a fist repeatedly; allow sufficient time.

References

Beck, R.M., Zbierajewski, F.J., Barber, M.K., Engoren, M. and Thomas, R., 2011. A comparison of the pain perceived during intravenous catheter insertion after injection with various local anesthetics. *AANA Journal*, 79(Suppl 4), S58–61.

Cuper, N.J., de Graaff, J.C., van Dijk, A.T., Verdaasdonk, R.M., van der Werff, D. and Kalkman, C.J., 2012. Predictive factors for difficult intravenous cannulation in pediatric patients at a tertiary pediatric hospital. *Pediatric Anesthesia*, 22(3), 223–229.

Egan, G., Healy, D., O'Neill, H., Clarke-Moloney, M., Grace, P.A. and Walsh, S.R., 2013. Ultrasound guidance for difficult peripheral venous access: systematic review and meta-analysis. *Emergency Medicine Journal*, 30(7), 521–526.

Heinrichs, J., Fritze, Z., Vandermeer, B., Klassen, T. and Curtis, S., 2013. Ultrasonographically guided peripheral intravenous cannulation of children and adults: a systematic review and meta-analysis. *Annals of Emergency Medicine*, 61(4), 444–454.

Hogan, M.E., Smart, S., Shah, V. and Taddio, A., 2014. A systematic review of vapocoolants for reducing pain from venipuncture and venous cannulation in children and adults. *Journal of Emergency Medicine*, 47(6), 736–749.

Nafiu, O.O., Burke, C., Cowan, A., Tutuo, N., Maclean, S. and Tremper, K.K., 2010. Comparing peripheral venous access between obese and normal weight children. *Pediatric Anesthesia*, 20(2), 172–176.

O'Grady, N.P., Alexander, M., Burns, L.A., Dellinger, E.P., Garland, J., Heard, S.O., Lipsett, P.A., Masur, H., Mermel, L.A., Pearson, M.L. and Raad, I.I., 2011. Summary of recommendations: guidelines for the prevention of intravascular catheter-related infections. *Clinical Infectious Diseases*, 52(9), 1087–1099.

Page, D.E. and Taylor, D.M., 2010. Vapocoolant spray vs subcutaneous lidocaine injection for reducing the pain of intravenous cannulation: a randomized, controlled, clinical trial. *British Journal of Anaesthesia*, 105(4), 519–525.

Perry, A.M., Caviness, A.C. and Hsu, D.C., 2011. Efficacy of a near-infrared light device in pediatric intravenous cannulation: a randomized controlled trial. *Pediatric Emergency Care*, 27(1), 5–10.

Rickard, C.M., Webster, J., Wallis, M.C., Marsh, N., McGrail, M.R., French, V., Foster, L., Gallagher, P., Gowardman, J.R., Zhang, L. and McClymont, A., 2012. Routine versus clinically indicated replacement of peripheral intravenous catheters: a randomised controlled equivalence trial. *Lancet*, 380(9847), 1066–1074.

Schreiber, S., Ronfani, L., Chiaffoni, G.P., Matarazzo, L., Minute, M., Panontin, E., Poropat, F., Germani, C. and Barbi, E., 2013. Does EMLA cream application interfere with the success of venipuncture or venous cannulation? A prospective multicenter observational study. *European Journal of Pediatrics*, 172(2), 265–268.

Sebbane, M., Claret, P.G., Lefebvre, S., Mercier, G., Rubenovitch, J., Jreige, R., Eledjam, J.J. and de La Coussaye, J.E., 2013. Predicting peripheral venous access difficulty in the emergency department using body mass index and a clinical evaluation of venous accessibility. *Journal of Emergency Medicine*, 44(2), 299–305.

Stevens, R.J., Mahadevan, V. and Moss, A.L., 2012. Injury to the lateral cutaneous nerve of forearm after venous cannulation: a case report and literature review. *Clinical Anatomy*, 25(5), 659–662.

Yeoh, C.N. and Lee, C.Y., 2012. Pain during venous cannulation: double-blind, randomized clinical trial of analgesic effect between topical amethocaine and eutectic mixture of local anesthetic. *Journal of Anaesthesiology, Clinical*, 28(2), 205–209.

Bibliography

Craft, J., Gordon, C., Huether, S.E., McCance, K.L. and Brashers, V.L., 2015. *Understanding pathophysiology* (ANZ adaptation). Sydney: Elsevier.

McCance, K.L. and Huether, S.E., 2015. *Pathophysiology: the biologic basis for disease in adults and children*. Sydney: Elsevier.

Chapter objectives

At the end of this chapter the reader will be able to:

1. Describe the rationale for intraosseous (IO) access
2. Demonstrate the method of locating IO access sites
3. Demonstrate effective and safe IO access performance using the EZ-IO®
4. Accurately report on IO access performance

Resources required for this assessment

- Mannequin/limb suitable for IO access
- Disposable gloves
- EZ-IO® drill and needles
- Needle stabiliser dressing
- Antiseptic swabs
- Medical tape
- Gauze pad
- Sharps waste container
- Saline flush and syringe
- Luer-lock 3-way tap
- Intravenous fluid bag and giving set
- Pressure bag
- Method of documenting the results

Skill matrix

This assessment requires:

- Infection control (CS 1.3)
- Communication (CS 1.5)
- Consent (CS 1.6)
- Aseptic Non Touch Technique (ANTT®) (CS 2.20)

This assessment is a component of:

- Medication administration (Chapter 4)

Introduction

Intraosseous (IO) access is an invasive method of drug administration for direct venous access. It requires a specialist-purpose needle.

This chapter describes IO access and the use of the EZ-IO°.

Anatomy and physiology

Bone is living tissue. Key long bone parts are the shaft (diaphysis) and the ends (epiphysis). Outside the bone is a periosteum layer that is important for bone healing and growth. Inside is a hollow medullary cavity. Red blood cells are produced at the marrow-filled ends of the long bones. Though red at birth, the marrow yellows with age due to the presence of fat. Marrow is also found in other bones, including the sternum, vertebrae and ribs.

Within the bone, Haversian canals run the length, keeping the inner spongy cavities from collapsing. Arteries and veins run within the canals, connecting directly to the systemic circulation.

While blood vessels vary in diameter with soft walls, bone-end marrow blood is retained within a rigid structure. This drains directly into the veins, including the proximal tibia into the popliteal vein, the distal tibia into the saphenous vein and the humeral head into the axillary vein.

Medullary cavity pressure is low at about 20–30 mmHg. Spicules within the cavity resist blood flow and may therefore require external pressure for intraosseous fluid flow.

Clinical rationale

Establishing IV access is not always possible. IO access is a quick and effective alternative (Dolister et al., 2013; Kurowski et al., 2014; Torres et al., 2013), using a needle placed into the marrow rich medullary cavity. It is commonly prompted by two circumstances (Lamhaut et al., 2010; Luck et al., 2010):

1. an extreme medical or traumatic emergency *and*
2. the actual or strong likelihood of difficulty gaining peripheral IV access.

This typically limits IO access to cardiac arrest, hypovolemic shock and other haemodynamic instability or severe respiratory difficulty (Dev et al., 2014).

Paediatric IV access is often difficult. For a child in extremis, IO access may be a first option with little IV site inspection (Kurowski et al., 2014; Lamhaut et al., 2010; Lewis and Wright, 2015). Make the decision for IO access quickly.

Adult IV access is perceived to be easier and is usually considered first. Early IO access when rapid intervention is required is reasonable (Lewis and Wright, 2015; Luck et al., 2010).

IO access enables rapid drug administration and resuscitation. A range of drugs and fluids can be administered via the IO route, including opioids, adrenaline, atropine, glucose, amiodarone and muscle

relaxants (Clemency et al., 2017; Dev et al., 2014; Gazin et al., 2011; Hoskins et al., 2012; Kurowski et al., 2014; Leidel et al., 2012; Lewis and Wright, 2015; Luck et al., 2010; Petitpas et al., 2016; Torres et al., 2013).

Device options

The numerous IO devices that are available differ in their method of insertion, though each places a needle directly into the bone marrow cavity (Lamhaut et al., 2010; Gazin et al., 2011; Leidel et al., 2012).

Early handheld devices required manual twisting to screw into the bone (Fig. 4.8.1). The success rate was reasonable but not reliable (Garside et al., 2016).

Bone Injection Gun (BIG)

The Bone Injection Gun (BIG) (Fig. 4.8.2) is spring loaded, driving a needle into the bone (Garside et al., 2016; Kurowski et al., 2014; Lewis and Wright, 2015; Petitpas et al., 2016; Weiser et al., 2012). The needle contained within the device body is available in adult and paediatric sizes.

FAST IO® needle

The FAST IO® needle is designed for insertion into the sternal manubrium (Garside et al., 2016; Lewis and Wright, 2015; Petitpas et al., 2016; Weiser et al., 2012). To guide location, an adhesive template is first placed over the target site.

The FAST IO® needle has multiple small needles that enter the bone, guiding the shallow insertion depth. The device acts as a handle. The needles are placed on the target site and pushed down firmly to inject. After discharge, a central solid needle with an outer plastic cannula is left in place.

EZ-IO®

The EZ-IO® is inserted using a handheld drill (Garside et al., 2016; Gazin et al., 2011; Kurowski et al., 2014; Lamhaut et al., 2010; Lewis and Wright, 2015; Petitpas et al., 2016; Weiser et al., 2012). It has three needle lengths: paediatric, adult and long (Kehrl et al., 2016).

The drill, with needle attached (Fig. 4.8.3), is positioned over the insertion site and the needle is drilled into the

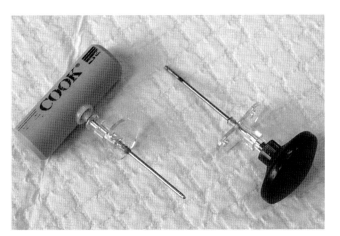

Figure 4.8.1 Manual IO needle

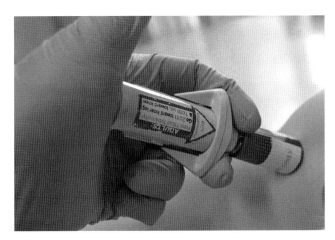

Figure 4.8.2 Bone Injection Gun

cavity. Though the drill can adjust the insertion depth, preselection of the correct size of needle is important.

IO sites and needle size

IO access is commonly obtained in the distal femur, proximal and distal tibia, proximal humerus or sternum (Dev et al., 2014; Luck et al., 2010; Torres et al., 2013).

Humerus

Humeral head location is convenient where the legs are obscured, such as in motor-vehicle entrapment. Subcutaneous tissue over this site typically requires a longer needle (Wampler et al., 2012).

To locate site, place the arm adducted and rotated inwards by bending at the elbow and placing the hand across the abdomen onto the opposite hip (Fig. 4.8.4).

Identify the acromion process – the prominent, hard point at the end of the scapula where it articulates with the clavicle. Run your fingers down 2 cm (adults) to locate the next hard prominent point, which is the greater tuberosity. This is the highest point of the humerus (Petitpas et al., 2016). Location of the humerus in children can be difficult, making this a better option for adults only.

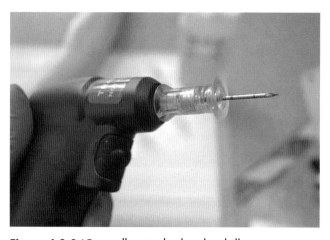

Figure 4.8.3 IO needle attached to the drill

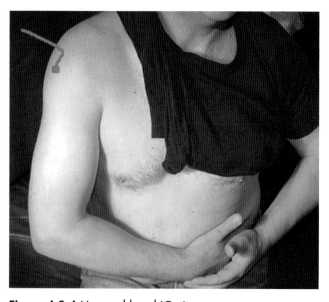

Figure 4.8.4 Humeral head IO site

Humeral venous return is through the superior vena cava, so blood flow is not adversely affected by pelvic or abdominal problems.

Sternum

The manubrium is the target (Petitpas et al., 2016). This is the upper portion of the sternum between the suprasternal notch and the sternal angle. Palpating the suprasternal notch first, move downwards 2 cm onto the manubrium. Insert the IO needle at 90° to the skin.

Sternum circulation includes mammary vein drainage. This site has prominent use in the military, where body armour offers protection.

The disadvantage of using the sternum is the shallow cavity overlying the heart and lungs. Only devices designed for this site can be used.

Proximal and distal tibia

The tibial sites are the proximal and distal bone ends (Petitpas et al., 2016) (Fig. 4.8.5).

The proximal end is commonly used, as it has an easily located flat plateau and less subcutaneous tissue. This site is located differently in small children compared to larger children and adults, due to the critical need to avoid causing injury to the bone-end growth plate.

Locate the tibial tuberosity on the anterior surface at the proximal tibia end. This is the hard, prominent bulge in the tibia just below the patella. From that point, move the fingers inferiorly 1–2 cm, then medially 1–2 cm, varying with the age of the patient. This is the tibial plateau (Dev et al., 2014; Petitpas et al., 2016).

For the distal tibia, locate the medial malleolus – the prominent ankle bone on the inner leg. Move 2–3 cm proximally then palpate the flat, lateral surface (see Fig. 4.8.5) (Petitpas et al., 2016). IO insertion is at 90° to the skin. The site can be better exposed by externally rotating the hip.

Distal femur

IO insertion at the distal femur is less common due to its greater amount of overlying tissue. Slightly flex the hip and externally rotate the leg. The knee is partially flexed to relax the quadriceps muscles. Locate the prominent medial and lateral external condyles, then the midline point on the anterior femur. Move 2–3 cm proximally and 1–2 cm medially.

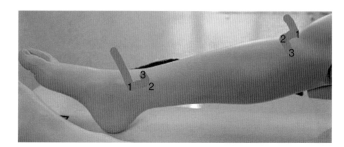

Figure 4.8.5 Distal and proximal tibial IO site

Method of insertion and use (EZ-IO®)

IO injection requires an aseptic procedure. With clean hands, don latex protective gloves (Petitpas et al., 2016).

Where possible, position the patient for limb support and site exposure (Fig. 4.8.6). Palpate applicable landmarks and identify the insertion point. Swab the site with antiseptic, moving in outwards, concentric circles (Petitpas et al., 2016).

Lay out the equipment, including a sharps container (Fig. 4.8.7). Select an appropriate needle for the site based on subcutaneous tissue depth rather than patient size. Attach the needle to the drill and remove the protective cap.

Place the tip of the needle against the site. Gently push forwards until it penetrates the skin and touches bone. One black line must be visible to ensure sufficient needle length remains for the penetration depth. If not, choose a longer needle or a different injection site. With the needle at 90° to the bone surface, squeeze the drill trigger while applying gentle forwards pressure (Fig. 4.8.8).

Cease drilling when the needle hub is almost against the skin. For children, a change in resistance may be felt, indicating that it is at the correct depth. The needle should stand firmly if correctly placed (Dev et al., 2014; Petitpas et al., 2016). Remove the drill from the needle. Remove the stylet from the needle by twisting counter-clockwise

(Fig. 4.8.9) and discard immediately into the sharps container.

Attach the stabiliser dressing over the needle hub to hold it securely in place against the skin. Attach a 10 mL syringe to the hub and aspirate the marrow. An inability to aspirate is common and should not be taken as a sign of failure (Dev et al., 2014; Petitpas et al., 2016).

Attach the primed Luer-lock 3-way extension tap to the needle hub. Flush with 3–5 mL of normal saline to verify patency, anticipating resistance. Secure the tap and giving set line to the limb with tape. While flow may occur, it may require a pressurised bag of up to 300 mmHg to overcome resistance (Dev et al., 2014; Lewis and Wright, 2015). Monitor for signs of extravasation.

When the procedure is complete, wipe the drill clean using an appropriate disinfectant solution and cloth.

Specific site contraindications

The following specific sites are contraindicated for IO insertion:

- traumatic limb injury, including fracture and burns, where structural integrity is compromised and extravasation is possible (Dev et al., 2014; Luck et al., 2010; Petitpas et al., 2016)
- limb vascular injury, where arterial delivery or venous return may be compromised

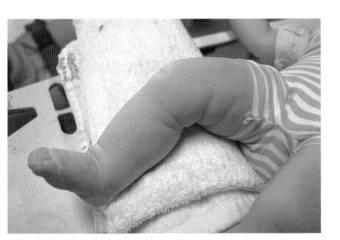

Figure 4.8.6 Supporting a limb for IO insertion

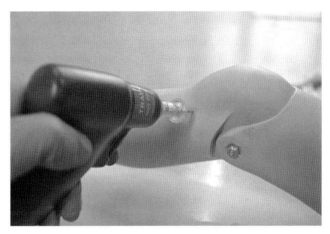

Figure 4.8.8 IO drilling

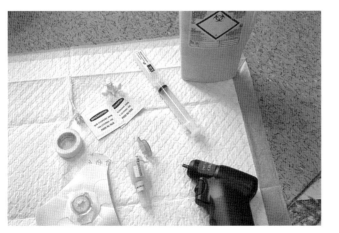

Figure 4.8.7 Laying out the equipment

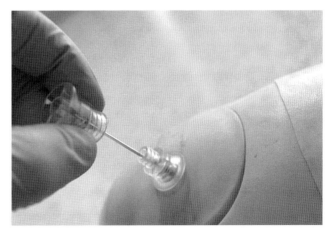

Figure 4.8.9 Removing the inner needle

- limb infection or inflammation, where disease could gain systemic access (Luck et al., 2010; Petitpas et al., 2016)
- brittle bones, including due to osteogenesis imperfecta or severe osteoporosis, as these are easily broken during IO insertion and less able to maintain a needle in place (Luck et al., 2010; Petitpas et al., 2016)
- underlying target sites that have peculiar unsuitability, including orthopaedic surgical pins.

Where anatomical landmarks cannot be identified, a blind hopeful attempt is not recommended.

Clinical skill assessment process

The following section outlines the clinical skill assessment tools that should be used to determine a student's ability to demonstrate safe and accurate intraosseous access.

1. Clinical Skill Work Instruction
2. Formative Clinical Skill Assessment (F-CSAT)
3. Performance Improvement Plan (PIP)
4. Summative Clinical Skill Assessment (S-CSAT)
(5. Direct Observation of Procedural SKILLS (DOPS) – see Chapter 1.1)

Clinical Skill Work Instruction

Equipment and resources: Mannequin/limb for IO injection; disposable gloves; EZ-IO® drill and needles; needle stabiliser dressing; antiseptic swabs; medical tape; gauze pad; sharps waste container; saline flush and syringe; Luer-lock 3-way tap; intravenous fluid bag and fluid administration set; pressure bag; method of documenting results

Associated Clinical Skills: Infection control; Communication; Consent; ANTT®

Staff/Student being assessed: _____

Intraosseous access

Activity	Critical Action	Rationale
Personal protection	Wash hands. Don PPE as required.	To decrease risk of infection.
Prepare patient	Discuss procedure. Obtain informed consent.	To reduce patient stress and gain cooperation.
	Position patient with limb supported and insertion site exposed.	To visualise area and provide access.
	Locate insertion site by palpating landmarks.	Ensures correct location.
	Swab insertion site.	To reduce risk of infection.
Prepare equipment	Select needle size.	To use correct length for site.
	Place sharps waste container in a convenient location.	For safe sharps disposal.
	Lay out equipment required on clean/aseptic surface, maintaining sterility.	For orderliness and to avoid infection.
	Attach needle to drill. Remove needle cap.	So it is ready for use.
Insert IO needle	Place needle against insertion site at 90° angle to bone surface.	To ensure correct angle for insertion.
	Gently pierce skin with needle tip until bone is touched, ensuring at least one line remains visible. If not, choose longer needle or alternative site.	To ensure medullary space is reached.
	Squeeze drill trigger while applying gentle forward pressure to rotate needle into medullary cavity.	To ensure slow and steady progression through the bone.
	Cease drilling when needle hub is almost against skin. For children, a change in resistance can indicate correct insertion.	To ensure it is correctly positioned in medullary cavity.
	Remove drill from needle.	To allow access to stylet.
	Remove stylet from needle by twisting counter-clockwise. Discard into a sharps container.	Leaves cannula in situ for use. For safe sharps disposal.

Intraosseous access continued

Activity	Critical Action	Rationale
Secure IO needle	Attach stabiliser dressing over needle hub.	Keeps cannula stable and in position.
	Aspirate blood/marrow by attaching a 10 mL syringe to needle and pulling plunger back.	This may not occur so is not essential to confirm placement.
	Connect primed Luer-lock 3-way extension tap to needle.	Allows fluid and drug administration.
Verify patency	Flush with 3–5 mL to verify needle patency, using 10 mL syringe containing normal saline attached to hub.	To ensure patency and no extravasation.
IO use	If patient is responsive and feels pain, consider local analgesia.	For patient comfort.
	Attach primed IV infusion set to 3-way tap.	To administer fluid and flush drugs.
	Commence infusion to assess fluid flow. If necessary, attach pressure bag to fluid bag. Inflate to about 300 mmHg.	Pressure assists fluid flows.
	Secure tap/IV giving set to limb with tape.	To avoid dislodgement.
	Monitor limb for extravasation.	Indicates cannula has been dislodged or is not sited correctly.
Report	Accurately document/hand over procedure, including needle size, location and patency.	Accurate record and continuity of patient care.

Source: *Adapted from EZ-IO® manufacturer's instructions.*

Formative Clinical Skill Assessment (F-CSAT)

Equipment and resources: Mannequin/limb for IO injection; disposable gloves; EZ-IO® drill and needles; needle stabiliser dressing; antiseptic swabs; medical tape; gauze pad; sharps waste container; saline flush and syringe; Luer-lock 3-way tap; intravenous fluid bag and fluid administration set; pressure bag; method of documenting results

Associated Clinical Skills: Infection control; Communication; Consent; ANTT®

Staff/Student being assessed: _____

Intraosseous access

Activity	Critical Action	Participant Performance				
Personal protection	Washes hands. Dons PPE.	0	1	2	3	4
Prepares patient	Discusses procedure. Obtains consent.	0	1	2	3	4
	Positions patient with limb supported and insertion site exposed.	0	1	2	3	4
	Locates insertion site by palpating landmarks.	0	1	2	3	4
	Swabs insertion site.	0	1	2	3	4
Prepares equipment	Selects needle size.	0	1	2	3	4
	Place sharps waste container in a convenient location.	0	1	2	3	4
	Lays out equipment, maintaining sterility.	0	1	2	3	4
	Attaches needle to drill. Removes needle cap.	0	1	2	3	4

Intraosseous access continued

Activity	Critical Action	Participant Performance				
Inserts IO needle	Places needle against insertion site at 90° angle to bone surface.	0	1	2	3	4
	Gently pierces skin with needle tip until bone is touched, ensuring at least one line remains visible. If not, chooses a longer needle or alternative site.	0	1	2	3	4
	Squeezes drill trigger while applying gentle forward pressure to rotate needle into medullary cavity.	0	1	2	3	4
	Ceases drilling when needle hub is almost against skin.	0	1	2	3	4
	Removes drill from needle.	0	1	2	3	4
	Removes stylet from needle by twisting counter-clockwise. Discards into a sharps container.	0	1	2	3	4
Secures IO needle	Attaches stabiliser dressing over needle hub.	0	1	2	3	4
	Aspirates blood/marrow by attaching a 10 mL syringe to the needle and pulling plunger back.	0	1	2	3	4
	Connects primed Luer-lock 3-way extension tap to needle.	0	1	2	3	4
Verifies patency	Flushes with 3–5 mL to verify needle patency, using 10 mL syringe containing normal saline.	0	1	2	3	4
IO use	If patient is responsive and feels pain, considers local analgesia.	0	1	2	3	4
	Attaches primed IV infusion set to 3-way tap.	0	1	2	3	4
	Commences infusion to assess fluid flow. If necessary, attaches pressure bag to fluid bag. Inflates to about 300 mmHg.	0	1	2	3	4
	Secures tap/IV giving set to limb with tape.	0	1	2	3	4
	Monitors limb for extravasation.	0	1	2	3	4
Reports	Accurately documents/hands over procedure, including needle size, location and patency.	0	1	2	3	4

Source: *Adapted from EZ-IO® manufacturer's instructions.*

Standard Achieved: (please circle one)

Competent (C)   Not Yet Competent* (NYC)

Staff/Student Name: _____

Assessor (please print name): _____

Signed (Assessor): _____

Date of Assessment: _____

Comments:

*If Not Yet Competent (NYC) a PIP needs to be completed and a repeat of the F-CSAT

Formative Clinical Skill Assessment (F-CSAT) Key

Skill level	Standard of procedure	Quality of performance	Outcome	Level of assistance required
4 Safe for unsupervised practice	Safe Accurate Behaviour is appropriate to context	Confident Accurate Expedient	Achieved intended outcome	No supporting cues*required
3 Requires supervision	Safe Accurate Behaviour is appropriate to context	Confident Accurate Takes longer than required	Achieved intended outcome	Requires occasional supportive cues*
2 Requires assistance	Safe Accurate Behaviour generally appropriate to context	Lacks certainty	Would not have achieved outcome without support	Requires frequent verbal and occasional physical directives in addition to supportive cues*
1 Requires direction	Safe only with guidance Not completely accurate	Unskilled Inefficient	Would not have achieved outcome without support	Requires continuous verbal and frequent physical directive cues*
0 Unsafe	Unsafe Unable to demonstrate behaviour Lack of insight into behaviour appropriate to context	Unskilled	Would not have achieved outcome	Requires continuous verbal and continuous physical directive cues*

*Refers to physical directives or verbal supportive cues

Performance Improvement Plan (PIP)

Please document the agreed education plan and completion timelines for areas assessed as less than 4.

This plan should be presented to assessor prior to commencement of summative assessment.

Where was supervisor support required?	Student summary of deficit. (Why was there a problem?)	Improvement Plan	Completed (Y/N)

Staff/Student Name: _____

Staff/Student Signature: _____

Educator Name: _____

Educator Signature: _____

Summative Clinical Skill Assessment (S-CSAT)

Equipment and resources: Mannequin/limb for IO injection; disposable gloves; EZ-IO® drill and needles; needle stabiliser dressing; antiseptic swabs; medical tape; gauze pad; sharps waste container; saline flush and syringe; Luer-lock 3-way tap; intravenous fluid bag and fluid administration set; pressure bag; method of documenting results

Associated Clinical Skills: Infection control; Communication; Consent; ANTT®

Staff/Student being assessed: _____

- Completed Formative Clinical Skill Assessment (F-CSAT): **YES** **NO**
- Completed Performance Improvement Plan (PIP): **YES** **NO** **N/A**

Intraosseous access

Activity	Critical Action	Achieved Without Direction	
Personal protection	Washes hands. Dons PPE.	NO	YES
Prepares patient	Discusses procedure. Obtains consent.	NO	YES
	Positions patient with limb supported and insertion site exposed.	NO	YES
	Locates insertion site by palpating landmarks.	NO	YES
	Swabs insertion site.	NO	YES
Prepares equipment	Selects needle size.	NO	YES
	Place sharps waste container in a convenient location.	NO	YES
	Lays out equipment required on a clean/aseptic surface, maintaining sterility.	NO	YES
	Attaches needle to drill. Removes needle cap.	NO	YES
Inserts IO needle	Places needle against insertion site at 90° angle to bone surface.	NO	YES
	Gently pierces skin with needle tip until bone is touched, ensuring at least one line remains visible. If not, chooses longer needle or alternative site.	NO	YES
	Squeezes drill trigger while applying gentle forward pressure to rotate needle into medullary cavity.	NO	YES
	Ceases drilling when needle hub is almost against skin.	NO	YES
	Removes drill from needle.	NO	YES
	Removes stylet from needle by twisting counter-clockwise. Discards into a sharps container.	NO	YES
Secures IO needle	Attaches stabiliser dressing over needle hub.	NO	YES
	Aspirates blood/marrow by attaching a 10 mL syringe to needle and pulling plunger back.	NO	YES
	Connects primed Luer-lock 3-way extension tap to needle.	NO	YES
Verifies patency	Flushes with 3–5 mL to verify needle patency, using 10 mL syringe containing normal saline.	NO	YES

Intraosseous access continued

Activity	Critical Action	Achieved Without Direction	
IO use	If patient is responsive and feels pain, considers local analgesia.	NO	YES
	Attaches primed IV infusion set to 3-way tap.	NO	YES
	Commences infusion to assess fluid flow. If necessary, attaches pressure bag to fluid bag. Inflates to about 300 mmHg.	NO	YES
	Secures tap/IV giving set to limb with tape.	NO	YES
	Monitors limb for extravasation.	NO	YES
Reports	Accurately documents/hands over procedure, including needle size, location and patency.	NO	YES

Source: *Adapted from EZ-IO® manufacturer's instructions.*

Standard Achieved: (please circle one)

Competent (C)   Not Yet Competent* (NYC)

Staff/Student Name: _____

Assessor (please print name)**:** _____

Signed (Assessor)**:** _____

Date of Assessment: _____

Comments:

*If Not Yet Competent (NYC) a PIP needs to be completed and a repeat of the F-CSAT

Clinical findings

Extravasation

Verify the patency of the intraosseous cannula before using it and then monitor this throughout. The signs of extravasation include site swelling. Compare the limb to the opposite one. If the patient is conscious, they may complain of pain at the insertion site or surrounding tissue if extravasation has occurred. If enough volume is injected, particularly under pressure, compartment syndrome can occur (Dev et al., 2014; Dolister et al., 2013; Lewis and Wright, 2015; Petitpas et al., 2016).

If the patency of the intraosseous needle is in doubt, do not use it. Remove it to ensure there is no further attempt to use it and cover the site with sterile adhesive dressing (Dev et al., 2014).

Infection

The IO route provides systemic access for infection, necessitating aseptic insertion and use. Infection can occur around the injection site.

Embolism

Increased bone cavity pressure can cause fat embolism. This is relatively common but clinically significant problems are rare (Dev et al., 2014; Petitpas et al., 2016).

Injection pain

IO needle insertion is typically not painful. However, fluid and drug administration can cause pain for conscious patients. Local anaesthetic 1–2% lidocaine, suitable for IV injection, can be administered through the needle before use and periodically (Dev et al., 2014; Garside et al., 2016; Petitpas et al., 2016).

Growth plate injury

Long bone ends have epiphyseal growth plates that, if injured, can affect growth. Incorrect IO placement can cause such injury, necessitating careful placement in children (Lewis and Wright, 2015).

PRACTICE TIP!

IO needle insertion can be disturbing to watch. Explaining the procedure to the patient and their family may provide reassurance.

PRACTICE TIP!

IO injection is an alternative to IV injection. In extremis, don't hesitate for long before considering it.

PRACTICE TIP!

Inserting an IO cannula requires numerous pieces of equipment. To keep them clean and orderly, lay them out on a clean surface, such as a pillowcase, during preparation.

TEST YOUR KNOWLEDGE QUESTIONS

1. **How does IO injection compare to the IV route?**
   Both provide alternative direct access to systemic circulation.

2. **What are two characteristics that prompt IO injection?**
   An extreme medical or traumatic emergency; the actual or strong likelihood of difficulty in gaining peripheral IV access.

3. **Which are usual sites for IO injection?**
   Manubrium of sternum; distal femur; proximal and distal tibia; proximal humerus.

4. **How long should you wait before considering IO insertion?**
   In some cases, immediate consideration is appropriate; otherwise, 1–2 minutes.

5. **What drug options are suitable for IO injection?**
   IV-suitable drugs, including opioids, adrenaline, atropine, glucose, muscle relaxants and amiodarone.

6. **What are the contraindications for IO injection?**
   Traumatic bone injury with damaged structural integrity; vascular limb injury; infection or inflammation in the limb; brittle bone disease; underlying target sites having peculiar unsuitability; where anatomical landmarks cannot be identified.

7. **Why might IO flow not occur and how is this remedied?**
   Due to incorrect placement; patency must be verified. Tubercule resistance within the marrow cavity; a pressure bag inflated up to 300 mmHg may be necessary for continued flow.

8. **Can marrow always be aspirated after insertion?**
   Not always. The ability to aspirate is a clue but is not essential to confirm placement.

9. **How is the pain caused by IO injection managed?**
   Pain is not normally caused during insertion, but instead when drugs are administered into the bone. Local lidocaine injected first can assist.

10. **What signs indicate IO needle extravasation?**
    Skin swelling; pain around the needle.

References

Clemency, B., Tanaka, K., May, P., Innes, J., Zagroba, S., Blaszak, J., Hostler, D., Cooney, D., McGee, K. and Lindstrom, H., 2017. Intravenous vs. intraosseous access and return of spontaneous circulation during out of hospital cardiac arrest. *American Journal of Emergency Medicine*, 35(2), 222–226.

Dev, S.P., Stefan, R.A., Saun, T. and Lee, S., 2014. Insertion of an intraosseous needle in adults. *New England Journal of Medicine*, 370(24), e35.

Dolister, M., Miller, S., Borron, S., Truemper, E., Shah, M., Lanford, M.R. and Philbeck T.E., 2013. Intraosseous vascular access is safe, effective and costs less than central venous catheters for patients in the hospital setting. *Journal of Vascular Access*, 14(3), 216–224.

Garside, G., Prescott, S. and Shaw, S., 2016. Intraosseous vascular access in critically ill adults – a review of the literature. *Nursing in Critical Care*, 21(3), 167–177.

Gazin, N., Auger, H., Jabre, P., Jaulin, C., Lecarpentier, E., Bertrand, C., Margenet, A. and Combes, X., 2011. Efficacy and safety of the EZ-IO™ intraosseous device: out-of-hospital implementation of a management algorithm for difficult vascular access. *Resuscitation*, 82(1), 126–129.

Hoskins, S.L., do Nascimento, P., Lima, R.M., Espana-Tenorio, J.M. and Kramer, G.C., 2012. Pharmacokinetics of intraosseous and central venous drug delivery during cardiopulmonary resuscitation. *Resuscitation*, 83(1), 107–112.

Kehrl, T., Becker, B.A., Simmons, D.E., Broderick, E.K. and Jones, R.A., 2016. Intraosseous access in the obese patient: assessing the need for extended needle length. *American Journal of Emergency Medicine*, 34(9), 1831–1834.

Kurowski, A., Timler, D., Evrin, T. and Szarpak, Ł., 2014. Comparison of 3 different intraosseous access devices for adult during resuscitation. Randomized crossover manikin study. *American Journal of Emergency Medicine*, 32(12), 1490–1493.

Lamhaut, L., Dagron, C., Apriotesei, R., Gouvernaire, J., Elie, C., Marx, J.S., Télion, C., Vivien, B. and Carli, P., 2010. Comparison of intravenous and intraosseous access by pre-hospital medical emergency personnel with and without CBRN protective equipment. *Resuscitation*, 81(1), 65–68.

Leidel, B.A., Kirchhoff, C., Bogner, V., Braunstein, V., Biberthaler, P. and Kanz, K.G., 2012. Comparison of intraosseous versus central venous vascular access in adults under resuscitation in the emergency department with inaccessible peripheral veins. *Resuscitation*, 83(1), 40–45.

Lewis, P. and Wright, C., 2015. Saving the critically injured trauma patient: a retrospective analysis of 1000 uses of intraosseous access. *Emergency Medicine Journal*, 32(6), 463–467.

Luck, R.P., Haines, C. and Mull, C.C., 2010. Intraosseous access. *Journal of Emergency Medicine*, 39(4), 468–475.

Petitpas, F., Guenezan, J., Vendeuvre, T., Scepi, M., Oriot, D. and Mimoz, O., 2016. Use of intra-osseous access in adults: a systematic review. *Critical Care*, 20(1), 102.

Torres, F., Galán, M.D., del Mar, A.M, Suárez, R., Camacho, C. and Almagro, V., 2013. Intraosseous access EZ-IO in a prehospital emergency service. *Journal of Emergency Nursing*, 39(5), 511–514.

Wampler, D., Schwartz, D., Shumaker, J., Bolleter, S., Beckett, R. and Manifold, C., 2012. Paramedics successfully perform humeral EZ-IO intraosseous access in adult out-of-hospital cardiac arrest patients. *American Journal of Emergency Medicine*, 30(7), 1095–1099.

Weiser, G., Hoffmann, Y., Galbraith, R. and Shavit, I., 2012. Current advances in intraosseous infusion–a systematic review. *Resuscitation*, 83(1), 20–26.

Bibliography

Craft, J., Gordon, C., Huether, S.E., McCance, K.L. and Brashers, V.L., 2015. *Understanding pathophysiology* (ANZ adaptation). Sydney: Elsevier.

McCance, K.L. and Huether, S.E., 2015. *Pathophysiology: the biologic basis for disease in adults and children*. Sydney: Elsevier.

4.9 | Oxygen therapy (mask and nasal cannula)

Jeff Kenneally

Chapter objectives

At the end of this chapter the reader will be able to:

1. Describe the physiological rationale for administering supplemental oxygen
2. Describe methods of varying the fraction of inspired oxygen
3. Safely and effectively use a nasal cannula or face mask to deliver supplemental oxygen
4. Identify when supplemental oxygen therapy may be harmful

Resources required for this assessment

- Standardised patient/mannequin
- Nasal cannula or oxygen therapy mask
- Oxygen source with flow meter
- Disposable gloves
- Method of documenting the results

Skill matrix

This assessment requires:

- Infection control (CS 1.3)
- Communication (CS 1.5)
- Consent (CS 1.6)
- Patient assessment skills (Chapter 2, CS 2.6, 2.7, 2.8, 2.9, 2.10)

This assessment is a component of:

- Medication administration (Chapter 4)

Introduction

There are many occasions where there is insufficient oxygen in the alveoli, blood or at cellular level. Supplemental oxygen therapy can often improve this. Oxygen, like any medication, must be administered for the right indications, in the right dose, with the right precautions and considerations. Oxygen therapy is discussed in this chapter.

Anatomy and physiology

The Krebs cycle is a chemical reaction sequence that produces adenosine triphosphate (ATP) for energy. Without oxygen (anaerobic), only two ATP molecules form by partly metabolising glucose to lactic acid (Burton et al., 2004). No further energy is produced.

With oxygen, one glucose molecule produces 38 ATP molecules. Hypoxia reduces energy production, leading to cellular process failures.

Atmospheric air pressure at sea level is 760 mmHg. Air is a mixture of gases, its total pressure the sum of the partial pressures of each component gas. In normal air, oxygen is 21% of 760 mmHg or about 160 mmHg.

$$\text{Ambient total air pressure\%}$$
$$= P\%(\text{Oxygen}) + P\%(\text{Nitrogen})$$

Only 2% of oxygen is transported dissolved in plasma, while 98% is bound to haemoglobin. Oxygen partial pressure drives alveolar to pulmonary circulation diffusion, haemoglobin attachment, and then release at the cellular level.

Clinical rationale

Normal arterial oxygen partial pressure is between 80 and 100 mmHg, correlating with pulse oximetry readings (SpO_2) 94% to 100%. Hypoxaemia is insufficient arterial oxygen and hypoxia is insufficient oxygen available at the cellular level.

Increasing alveolar oxygen partial pressure by displacing nitrogen with supplemental oxygen can reduce hypoxia (Bouroche and Bourgain, 2015). A flow meter attached to an oxygen source allows control of the delivery flow in litres per minute (L/min).

The air inhalation rate, known as peak inspiratory flow rate (PIFR), is normally around 30 L/min. The normal PIFR of oxygen is:

$$21\% \text{ of } 30 \text{ L/min} = 6.3 \text{ L/min oxygen}$$

Supplemental oxygen addition to inspired air increases the percentage or fraction of inspired oxygen (FiO_2). For example, if 4L/min supplemental oxygen therapy is provided, the PIFR now includes:

$$4 \text{ L/min of } 100\% \text{ oxygen}$$

The remainder of the 30 L/min PIFR contains 21% oxygen:

$$21\% \text{ of } (30 - 4 = 26) = 5.5 \text{ L/min}$$

Total oxygen PIFR equals:

$$5.5 + 4 = 9.5 \text{ L/min oxygen}$$

Supplemental oxygen therapy increases FiO_2, improving pulse oximetry and arterial partial pressure (Beasley et al., 2015; O'Driscoll et al., 2011).

FiO_2 varies with breathing. Faster or deeper breathing increases PIFR, reducing the impact of supplemental oxygen.

Where breathing is inadequate, PIFR must be increased through assisted ventilation (see Chapter 3.11) rather than simply increasing inspired FiO_2 with oxygen therapy.

Oxygen safety and hazards

Portable oxygen cylinders contain compressed gas. Before use, ensure that you understand the pressures within the cylinder and the volume and duration of the content available for use. Cylinder depletion will reduce or cease the flow and delivery of oxygen, reducing the effectiveness of the therapy for the patient and potentially leading to hypoxia and hypercapnoea.

Oxygen can support the combustion of flammable materials, so do not use it in a potentially flammable atmosphere.

All operators must be proficient in connecting cylinders to the oxygen regulator for the device they are using. Cylinder yokes must be free of dirt and grease. Cylinders must be stored and carried safely. Dropped or damaged cylinders or those with heat damage tags should not be used and instead returned to the supplier for assessment.

Oxygen therapy devices

Oxygen therapy can be divided into low and high gas flow. Commonly used low-flow options are nasal cannula and oxygen therapy masks (including non-rebreathing and nebuliser masks). The choice of device and oxygen flow rate varies with the clinical need. Improvement or deterioration may prompt a change of device or flow rate.

Nasal cannula

Nasal cannula deliver reliable small FiO_2 increases for minor hypoxia. They consist of tubing with two prongs on one end that sit one just inside each nostril, kept in place by a loop or elastic fitting around the head (Figs 4.9.1 to 4.9.3). The other tubing end attaches to the oxygen flow meter.

Standard nasal cannula flow rates range between 1 and 8 L/min. Flow rates >6 L/min are uncomfortable (Beasley et al., 2015). Higher, non-humidified flow rates dry the nasal passages, occasionally causing nose bleeds.

Nasal cannula are useful for chronic hypoxemic states that require long-term use, such as COPD, allowing

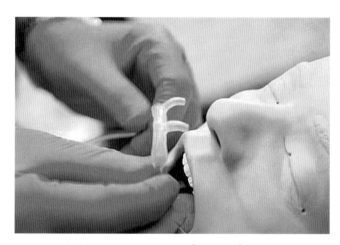

Figure 4.9.1 Fitting prongs into the nostrils

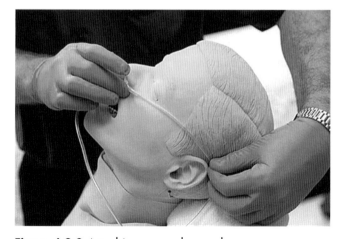

Figure 4.9.2 Attaching a nasal cannula

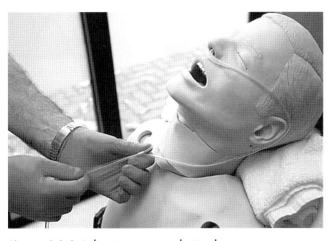

Figure 4.9.3 Adjusting a cannula in place

FiO$_2$ (%)	L/min flow rate
0.24 (24%)	1
0.30 (30%)	2
0.35 (35%)	3
0.40 (40%)	4
0.45 (45%)	5
0.48 (48%)	6

Table 4.9.1 Typical nasal cannula flow rates

Source: *Wettstein et al., 2005.*

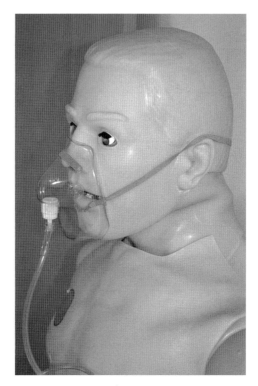

Figure 4.9.4 Oxygen mask

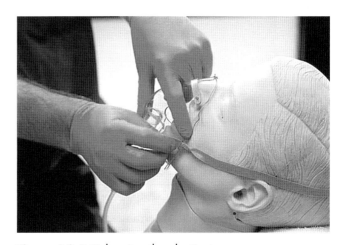

Figure 4.9.5 Tightening the elastic strap

eating, drinking and speaking freely. The only significant impediment is the risk of nasal injury or infection.

Inspired oxygen fractions at different flow rates for a nasal cannula are unpredictable and vary with the rate/depth of breathing and whether the mouth is open or closed (see Table 4.9.1). For nasal cannula use, the patient should only require a small FiO$_2$ increase. For larger increases, use an alternative delivery system.

Commence oxygen flow before application to avoid inadvertently delivering excess flow. Other than loss of therapy, nasal cannula will not cause problems if oxygen flow is turned off while they are left in place.

Oxygen mask

Simple oxygen face masks come in adult and paediatric sizes. A contoured triangular top sits over the nose and has a mouldable malleable strip. The bottom is wider and rounded to fit the chin. A front nipple attaches tubing to an oxygen flow meter (Fig. 4.9.4).

Fit the mask by placing it over the nose and then the chin. The elastic strip attached to either side of the mask is loosened, and then stretched over the patient's head and tightened to fit (Fig. 4.9.5).

On either side of the mask are holes that allow air to be drawn in during inhalation and escape with exhalation.

The holes are small, allowing inflowing oxygen in the mask to flush out exhaled carbon dioxide. To be effective, minimum mask flow is 5 L/min.

Oxygen masks permit higher FiO$_2$ values than nasal cannula and are used for more severe hypoxaemia. FiO$_2$ varies at different flow rates (see Table 4.9.2).

Non-rebreather masks have soft bags attached, creating an oxygen reservoir (Fig. 4.9.6). Higher oxygen flow rates ranging from 10 to 15 L/min (Beasley et al., 2015) allow FiO$_2$ fractions approaching 100% (see Table 4.9.3).

The nebuliser mask is like the non-rebreather mask only with a nebuliser bowl instead of a reservoir bag (Fig. 4.9.7). Oxygen passes through any liquid in the bowl, forming tiny aerosol drops for inhalation. Nebulisation requires at least 6 L/min, preferably a 8 L/min flow (O'Driscoll et al., 2011).

Table 4.9.2 Oxygen mask flow rates

FiO₂ (%)	L/min flow rate
0.35 (35%)	5
0.5 (50%)	8
0.6 (60%)	10

Source: *Beasley et al., 2015.*

Table 4.9.3 Non-rebreather mask flow rates

FiO₂ (%)	L/min flow rate
0.9 (90%)	10
1.0 (100%)	15

Source: *Branson and Johannigman, 2013.*

Figure 4.9.6 Oxygen non-rebreather mask with reservoir bag

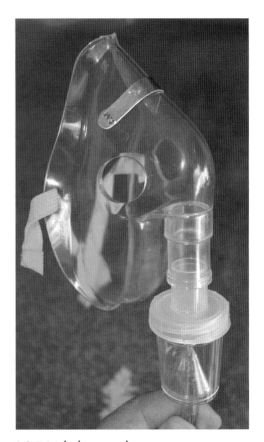

Figure 4.9.7 Nebuliser mask

Clinical skill assessment process

The following section outlines the clinical skills assessment tools that should be used to determine a student's ability to demonstrate safe and accurate oxygen therapy using nasal cannula and mask.

1. Clinical Skill Work Instruction
2. Formative Clinical Skill Assessment (F-CSAT)
3. Performance Improvement Plan (PIP)
4. Summative Clinical Skill Assessment (S-CSAT)
(5. Direct Observation of Procedural Skills (DOPS) – see Chapter 1.1)

Clinical Skill Work Instruction

Equipment and resources: Patient or mannequin; nasal cannula or oxygen mask; oxygen source with flow meter; disposable gloves; method of documenting results

Associated Clinical Skills: Infection control; Communication; Consent; Patient assessment skills

Oxygen therapy (mask and nasal cannula)

Activity	Critical Action	Rationale
Assess need	Assess respiratory status, disease and pulse oximetry to determine appropriate device and flow rate.	Ensures appropriate delivery system is selected.

Oxygen therapy (mask and nasal cannula) continued

Activity	Critical Action	Rationale
Prepare patient	Administer oxygen therapy in any position, including upright, supine or lateral. Most patients with breathing difficulty prefer an upright posture.	Maintains patient comfort.
	Explain the oxygen therapy device to be used.	To gain cooperation and compliance.
Prepare equipment	Unpack device and straighten tubing.	Removes kinks.
	Loosen head elastic strap to its fullest length.	Allows easier application.
	If using a nebuliser mask, add drug to bowl and attach to mask. Attach oxygen tubing to nebuliser.	So medication is ready to nebulise.
	Attach oxygen tubing to flow meter. Set flow rate. Acknowledge minimum flow rate for device.	Oxygen flow is required before application.
	If the mask has an oxygen reservoir bag, allow it to fill before use.	To optimise oxygen availability.
	Ensure malleable mask nose clip is wide enough to easily fit over nose.	Ensures comfort.
Apply cannula	If cannula is the non-elastic type, move the neck clip away from the nasal prongs.	Allows easier application.
	Place elastic over the head, seating on the occiput. If the cannula is non-elastic, loop tubing around both ears, leaving prongs near the nose.	To ensure proper location before tightening.
	Insert one prong in each nostril.	To ensure proper location before tightening.
	Adjust elastic or push up plastic clip on the tubing to tighten cannula in place. Confirm cannula comfortable and evenly in each nostril.	To maintain cannula in correct position.
Apply mask	Place mask over the nose and lower it to cover chin. Ensure mask sits neatly over nose and symmetrically over face.	For comfort and to ensure optimal oxygen delivery.
	Gently pinch malleable nose clip to mould mask to face.	To reduce leaks and eye irritation.
	Adjust elastic to hold mask in place. Confirm comfortable fit.	For patient comfort and compliance.
	If there is a reservoir bag, ensure it remains at least partly filled. If there is a nebuliser, ensure it is appropriately misting.	Ensures adequate delivery of oxygen or medication.
Reassess	Assess effectiveness, including pulse oximetry.	To determine if correct option has been chosen.
Report	Accurately document/hand over device used, flow rate and time commenced.	Accurate record kept and continuity of patient care.

Formative Clinical Skill Assessment (F-CSAT)

Equipment and resources: Patient or mannequin; nasal cannula or oxygen mask; oxygen source with flow meter; disposable gloves; method of documenting results

Associated Clinical Skills: Infection control; Communication; Consent; Patient assessment skills

Staff/Student being assessed: _____

Oxygen therapy (mask and nasal cannula)

Activity	Critical Action	Participant Performance				
Assesses need	Assesses respiratory status, disease and pulse oximetry and determines appropriate device and flow rate.	0	1	2	3	4
Prepares patient	Recognises oxygen therapy can be administered in any position, with most patients with breathing difficulty preferring an upright posture.	0	1	2	3	4
	Explains oxygen therapy device to be used.	0	1	2	3	4
Prepares equipment	Unpacks device and straightens tubing.	0	1	2	3	4
	Loosens head elastic strap to its fullest length.	0	1	2	3	4
	If using nebuliser mask, adds drug to bowl and attaches to mask. Attaches oxygen tubing to nebuliser.	0	1	2	3	4
	Attaches oxygen tubing to flow meter. Sets flow rate. Acknowledges minimum flow rate for device.	0	1	2	3	4
	If the mask has an oxygen reservoir bag, allows it to fill before use.	0	1	2	3	4
	Ensures malleable mask nose clip is wide enough to easily fit over nose.	0	1	2	3	4
Applies cannula	If cannula is non-elastic type, moves the neck clip away from nasal prongs.	0	1	2	3	4
	Places elastic over the head, seating on occiput. If cannula is non-elastic, loops cannula tubing around both ears, leaving prongs near the nose.	0	1	2	3	4
	Inserts one prong in each nostril.	0	1	2	3	4
	Adjusts elastic or pushes up plastic clip on the tubing to tighten cannula in place. Confirms cannula comfortable and evenly in each nostril.	0	1	2	3	4
Applies mask	Places mask over the nose and lowers it to cover chin. Ensures mask sits neatly over nose and symmetrically over face.	0	1	2	3	4
	Gently pinches malleable nose clip to mould mask to face.	0	1	2	3	4
	Adjusts elastic to hold mask in place. Confirms comfortable fit.	0	1	2	3	4
	If there is a reservoir bag, ensures it remains at least partly filled. If there is a nebuliser, ensures it is appropriately misting.	0	1	2	3	4
Reassesses	Assesses effectiveness, including pulse oximetry.	0	1	2	3	4
Reports	Accurately documents/hands over the device used, flow rate and time commenced.	0	1	2	3	4

Standard Achieved: (please circle one)

Competent (C)   Not Yet Competent* (NYC)

Staff/Student Name: _____

Assessor (please print name): _____

Signed (Assessor): _____

Date of Assessment: _____

Comments:

*If Not Yet Competent (NYC) a PIP needs to be completed and a repeat of the F-CSAT

Formative Clinical Skill Assessment (F-CSAT) Key

Skill level	Standard of procedure	Quality of performance	Outcome	Level of assistance required
4 Safe for unsupervised practice	Safe Accurate Behaviour is appropriate to context	Confident Accurate Expedient	Achieved intended outcome	No supporting cues*required
3 Requires supervision	Safe Accurate Behaviour is appropriate to context	Confident Accurate Takes longer than required	Achieved intended outcome	Requires occasional supportive cues*
2 Requires assistance	Safe Accurate Behaviour generally appropriate to context	Lacks certainty	Would not have achieved outcome without support	Requires frequent verbal and occasional physical directives in addition to supportive cues*
1 Requires direction	Safe only with guidance Not completely accurate	Unskilled Inefficient	Would not have achieved outcome without support	Requires continuous verbal and frequent physical directive cues*
0 Unsafe	Unsafe Unable to demonstrate behaviour Lack of insight into behaviour appropriate to context	Unskilled	Would not have achieved outcome	Requires continuous verbal and continuous physical directive cues*

*Refers to physical directives or verbal supportive cues

Performance Improvement Plan (PIP)

Please document the agreed education plan and completion timelines for areas assessed as less than 4.

This plan should be presented to assessor prior to commencement of summative assessment.

Where was supervisor support required?	Student summary of deficit. (Why was there a problem?)	Improvement Plan	Completed (Y/N)

Staff/Student Name: _____

Staff/Student Signature: _____

Educator Name: _____

Educator Signature: _____

Summative Clinical Skill Assessment (S-CSAT)

Equipment and resources: Patient or mannequin; nasal cannula or oxygen mask; oxygen source with flow meter; disposable gloves; method of documenting results

Associated Clinical Skills: Infection control; Communication; Consent; Patient assessment skills

Staff/Student being assessed: _____

• Completed Formative Clinical Skill Assessment (F-CSAT): **YES   NO**

• Completed Performance Improvement Plan (PIP): **YES   NO   N/A**

Oxygen therapy (mask and nasal cannula)

Activity	Critical Action	Achieved Without Direction	
Assesses need	Assesses respiratory status, disease and pulse oximetry and determines appropriate device and flow rate.	NO	YES
Prepares patient	Recognises oxygen therapy can be administered in any position, with most patients with breathing difficulty preferring an upright posture.	NO	YES
	Explains oxygen therapy device to be used.	NO	YES

Oxygen therapy (mask and nasal cannula) continued

Activity	Critical Action	Achieved Without Direction	
Prepares equipment	Unpacks device and straightens tubing.	NO	YES
	Loosens head elastic strap to its fullest length.	NO	YES
	If using nebuliser mask, adds drug to bowl and attaches to mask. Attaches oxygen tubing to nebuliser.	NO	YES
	Attaches oxygen tubing to flow meter. Sets flow rate. Acknowledges maximum flow rate for device.	NO	YES
	If the mask has an oxygen reservoir bag, allows it to fill before use.	NO	YES
	Ensures malleable mask nose clip is wide enough to easily fit over nose.	NO	YES
Applies cannula	If cannula is non-elastic type, moves the neck clip away from nasal prongs.	NO	YES
	Places elastic over the head, seating on occiput. If cannula is non-elastic, loops cannula tubing around both ears, leaving prongs near the nose.	NO	YES
	Inserts one prong in each nostril.	NO	YES
	Adjusts elastic or pushes up plastic clip on the tubing to tighten cannula in place. Confirms comfort and sitting evenly in each nostril.	NO	YES
Applies mask	Places mask over the nose and lowers it to cover chin. Ensures mask sits neatly over nose and symmetrically over face.	NO	YES
	Gently pinches malleable nose clip to mould mask to face.	NO	YES
	Adjusts elastic to hold mask in place. Confirms comfortable fit.	NO	YES
	If there is a reservoir bag, ensures it remains at least partly filled. If there is a nebuliser, ensures it is appropriately misting.	NO	YES
Reassesses	Assesses effectiveness, including pulse oximetry.	NO	YES
Reports	Accurately documents/hands over device used, flow rate and time commenced.	NO	YES

Standard Achieved: (please circle one)

Competent (C)   Not Yet Competent* (NYC)

Staff/Student Name: _____

Assessor (please print name)**:** _____

Signed (Assessor)**:** _____

Date of Assessment: _____

Comments:

*If Not Yet Competent (NYC) a PIP needs to be completed and a repeat of the F-CSAT

Clinical findings

Stroke and acute coronary syndrome

Hypoxia can occur naturally, triggering a normal physiological response. Hyperoxia is unnatural, being caused by supplemental oxygen. It causes vasoconstriction, reducing coronary and cerebral artery blood flow and worsening ischemia during acute coronary syndrome or stroke (Beasley et al., 2015; Branson and Johannigman, 2013; Cornet et al., 2013; Sepehrv and Ezekowitz, 2016).

COPD

COPD involves inadequate alveoli ventilation, carbon dioxide (CO_2) retention and hypoxemia. Localised pulmonary vascular constriction occurs, intending to reduce blood flow to the alveoli (Branson and Johannigman, 2013; Cornet et al., 2013; Abdo and Heunks, 2012).

Supplemental oxygen increases alveolar oxygen, causing vascular flow to return to the alveoli. In COPD, ventilation is unimproved so CO_2 removal does not occur in these alveoli. Blood returns into circulation with retained CO_2 (Abdo and Heunks, 2012; Branson and Johannigman, 2013; Cornet et al., 2013).

For COPD patients, pulse oximetry of 88–92% is a level of hypoxaemia that is commonly accepted without intervention (Austin et al., 2010; Beasley et al., 2015; O'Driscoll et al., 2011).

Paraquat and bleomycin

Paraquat is a fast-acting toxic herbicide. It combines with oxygen to form reactive oxygen species (ROS) that are able to damage cells, particularly mitochondria. As such lower levels than normal of available oxygen are beneficial, SpO_2 <88% prompts oxygen intervention (Beasley et al., 2015; Gawarammana and Buckley, 2011).

Bleomycin is an antibiotic used to attack the DNA of tumours. It is associated with significant lung injury with even minimal administration of supplemental oxygen (Reinert et al., 2013).

Breathlessness

Breathlessness is a feeling of difficulty breathing. Oxygen administration does not relieve breathlessness in the absence of hypoxemia (Austin et al., 2010; Beasley et al., 2015; Branson and Johannigman, 2013).

Oxygen toxicity

Short-term oxygen therapy is usually safe. Longer term therapy can cause pulmonary and central nervous problems, including confusion, disorientation, visual disturbances, eye injury and seizures. Pulmonary endothelial damage can cause atelectasis and impaired gas exchange (Branson and Johannigman, 2013; Cornet et al., 2013).

The principal mechanism of oxygen toxicity is excessive harmful ROS. Normal antioxidants are overwhelmed, leaving ROS to react with other cell chemicals. Cell membrane lipids are vulnerable (Martin and Grocott, 2013; Sepehrv and Ezekowitz, 2016).

Other hypoxia

Anaemic hypoxia involves insufficient haemoglobin despite sufficient alveolar oxygen. Supplemental oxygen therapy may not assist.

Haemoglobin may be unable to perform its function. Carbon monoxide binds preferentially with haemoglobin over oxygen. High-flow oxygen therapy can eventually displace it. Methemoglobinemia has altered iron compared to haemoglobin, and has greater affinity for oxygen.

Stagnant hypoxia involves slowed blood flow to cells, depleting oxygen. Supplemental oxygen may offer benefit.

Histotoxic hypoxia is the impaired ability of cells to use oxygen. The most common cause is cyanide poisoning. ATP-producing enzymes are inhibited, reducing usefulness of oxygen in energy production. Supplemental oxygen therapy is of little assistance.

Warming/humidification

Compressed oxygen is dry and cold, resulting in dry mucosa and difficulty removing secretions. This is more significant with longer oxygen administration.

PRACTICE TIP!

Oxygen therapy does not assist with the removal of carbon dioxide. If spontaneous breathing inadequately ventilates the alveoli, oxygen therapy must be replaced by assisted ventilation.

PRACTICE TIP!

Hyperoxia is unnatural. It can pose serious problems and worsen the outcomes of some acute and chronic conditions. Oxygen therapy should have a clinical indication, as with any other drug. Pulse oximetry provides no clue to hyperoxic states. It is, however, key to the need to commence and guide therapy where hypoxia exists.

PRACTICE TIP!

Oxygen therapy was long considered 'the good gas' that 'can do no harm'. This is no longer so. Supplemental oxygen is now a medication administered in a prescribed manner for appropriate indications.

TEST YOUR KNOWLEDGE QUESTIONS

1. **What are the two impediments to nasal cannula use?**
   Nasal injury; infection.

2. **What measurable values define hypoxaemia?**
   Arterial oxygen partial pressure <80 mmHg or oxygen saturation <94%.

3. **What oxygen flow rates are used through standard nasal cannula?**
   1–8 L/min, with the usual maximum being 6 L/min.

4. **What is the minimum standard oxygen mask flow rate and why?**
   5 L/min; to ensure exhaled carbon dioxide is flushed out of the mask and not rebreathed.

5. **What other non-hypoxemic forms of hypoxia exist?**
   Anaemic, stagnant, histotoxic hypoxemia; dysfunctional haemoglobin, including carbon monoxide poisoning and methemoglobinemia.

6. **What flow rates are used with non-rebreather masks and what FiO_2 do these correlate with?**
   10 L/min = FiO_2 0.9 through to 15 L/min = FiO_2 1.0.

7. **What is the purpose of the holes in the sides of oxygen masks?**
   They allow air to be drawn in from or exhaled to the atmosphere, yet are small enough for oxygen to accumulate in the mask.

8. **Why should an oxygen therapy device be connected to oxygen flow first?**
   A nasal cannula could be uncomfortable if the flow is set too high. A mask could allow re-breathing if it is not already filling with oxygen.

9. **What advantages does a nasal cannula have over other oxygen devices?**
   It can be used long term, allowing the patient to eat, drink and speak freely.

10. **Is oxygen therapy appropriate when a patient is hypoventilating?**
    No. Inadequate respiratory rate or tidal volume is replaced with assisted ventilation.

References

Abdo, W.F. and Heunks, L.M., 2012. Oxygen-induced hypercapnia in COPD: myths and facts. *Critical Care*, 16(5), 1.

Austin, M.A., Wills, K.E., Blizzard, L., Walters E.H. and Wood-Baker, R., 2010. Effect of high flow oxygen on mortality in chronic obstructive pulmonary disease patients in prehospital setting: randomised controlled trial. *BMJ*, 341, c5462.

Beasley, R., Chien, J., Douglas, J., Eastlake, L., Farah, C., King, G., Moore, R., Pilcher, J., Richards, M., Smith, S. and Walters, H., 2015. Thoracic Society of Australia and New Zealand oxygen guidelines for acute oxygen use in adults: 'swimming between the flags'. *Respirology*, 20(8), 1182–1191.

Bouroche, G. and Bourgain, J.L., 2015. Pre-oxygenation and general anesthesia: a review. *Minerva Anestesiologica*, 81, 910–920.

Branson, R.D. and Johannigman, J.A., 2013. Pre-hospital oxygen therapy. *Respiratory Care*, 58(1), 86–97.

Burton, A.B., Stokes, K. and Hall, G.M., 2004. Physiological effects of exercise. *Continuing Education in Anaesthesia, Critical Care & Pain*, 4(6), 185–188.

Cornet, A.D., Kooter, A.J., Peters M.J. and Smulders Y.M., 2013. The potential harm of oxygen therapy in medical emergencies. *Critical Care*, 17(2), 1.

Gawarammana, I.B. and Buckley, N.A., 2011. Medical management of paraquat ingestion. *British Journal of Clinical Pharmacology*, 72(5), 745–757.

Martin, D.S. and Grocott, M.P., 2013. III. Oxygen therapy in anaesthesia: the yin and yang of O2. *British Journal of Anaesthesia*, 111(6), 867–871.

O'Driscoll, B.R., Howard, L.S. and Davison, A.G., 2011. Emergency oxygen use in adult patients: concise guidance. *Clinical Medicine*, 11(4), 372–375.

Reinert, T., da Rocha Baldotto, C.S., Nunes, A.P. and de Souza Scheliga, A.A., 2013. Bleomycin induced lung injury. *Journal of Cancer Research*, https://doi.org/10.1155/2013/480608.

Sepehrv, N. and Ezekowitz, J.A., 2016. Oxygen therapy in patients with acute heart failure: friend or foe? *JACC: Heart Failure*, 4(10), 783–790.

Wettstein, R.B., Shelledy, D.C. and Peters, J.I., 2005. Delivered oxygen concentrations using low-flow and high-flow nasal cannulas. *Respiratory Care*, 50(5), 604–609.

Bibliography

Craft, J., Gordon, C., Huether, S.E., McCance, K.L. and Brashers, V.L., 2015. *Understanding pathophysiology* (ANZ adaptation). Sydney: Elsevier.

McCance, K.L. and Huether, S.E., 2015. *Pathophysiology: the biologic basis for disease in adults and children*. Sydney: Elsevier.

Chapter objectives

At the end of this chapter the reader will be able to:

1. Describe how continuous positive airway pressure (CPAP) works during breathing
2. Describe the component parts of a CPAP system
3. Demonstrate the effective administration of CPAP
4. Recognise the limitations and complications of CPAP to allow safe administration

Resources required for this assessment

- Standardised patient/mannequin
- Disposable gloves, protective eyewear, respiratory mask
- CPAP therapy device, including mask, head harness and pressure generator
- Oxygen source
- Method of documenting the results

Skill matrix

This assessment requires:

- Infection control (CS 1.3)
- Communication (CS 1.5)
- Consent (CS 1.6)
- Patient assessment (Chapter 2, CS 2.1, 2.2, 2.4, 2.6, 2.7, 2.8, 2.10)
- Airway and ventilation (Chapter 3, CS 3.7, 3.6, 3.11)

This assessment is a component of:

- Medication administration (Chapter 4)

Introduction

Continuous positive airway pressure (CPAP) offers therapeutic benefit for some respiratory distress conditions. Understanding how it works enables identification of those patients who will gain benefit from CPAP and those whose condition may potentially be worsened by it. CPAP is discussed in this chapter.

Anatomy and physiology

Adult tidal volume is about 500 mL. This includes the dead space volume that is not involved with gas exchange, which makes up about one-third of tidal volume. For gas exchange to occur, the alveoli must be ventilated. The more alveoli that are inflated, the greater the total lung volume.

The other lung variable is pressure. For airflow, there must be a high to low pressure gradient.

Boyle's law describes an inverse relationship between pressure and volume: as lung volume increases, pressure decreases. Respiratory muscle contraction increases chest and lung size. A pressure gradient is created and air flows inwards from the now higher atmospheric pressure to the lower lung pressure.

Expiration is primarily passive, resulting from elastic chest recoil. As the respiratory muscles relax, lung volume decreases and the lung pressure rises above atmospheric pressure, encouraging outwards flow. If needed, abdominal and external intercostal muscles can add some expiratory force.

Air contains a mix of oxygen, nitrogen and carbon dioxide, the proportions of which change as gases move in and out of the alveoli. Sea-level atmospheric pressure is 760 mmHg. With gas mixtures, total pressure is the sum of the partial pressures of each gas, with ambient air containing about 21% (160 mmHg) oxygen and 78% (593 mmHg) nitrogen. Other gases make up the remaining 1%, with carbon dioxide a nominal 0.04%.

Gases exert pressure on the container in which they are held, including gas within the alveoli and air within the atmosphere:

$$\text{Ambient total pressure }\%$$
$$= P\%(\text{Oxygen}) + P\%(\text{Nitrogen})$$

In air, oxygen partial pressure is 21% of 760 mmHg, or about 160 mmHg. This drives diffusion into pulmonary circulation. Lowering air pressure or oxygen partial pressure results in less diffusion. Raising air pressure or increasing oxygen partial pressure increases diffusion rate into the circulation.

Clinical rationale

Patients in respiratory failure have difficulty maintaining adequate arterial oxygen and/or carbon dioxide levels. If this difficulty is due to an insufficient respiratory rate or tidal volume, it must be corrected using intermittent positive pressure ventilation (IPPV). For spontaneous respiration, support includes supplemental oxygen therapy or non-invasive ventilation, including CPAP.

The most common way to increase oxygen diffusion is to increase the fraction of inspired oxygen (FiO$_2$). Oxygen partial pressure can be increased by replacing nitrogen:

$$\text{Ambient total pressure}$$
$$= \uparrow P\%(\text{Oxygen}) + \downarrow P\%(\text{Nitrogen})$$

This can be achieved through supplemental oxygen therapy, using options ranging from low-flow nasal cannula to high-flow bag/valve/mask devices.

Maximum oxygen partial pressure is 100% of ambient air pressure. This can increase diffusion, reducing hypoxia:

$$\text{Ambient total pressure} = P100\%(\text{Oxygen})$$

While oxygen therapy increases the oxygen available it does little to support inspiration, expiration and work of breathing. Oxygen diffusion can also be increased by increasing inspired total air pressure. Since the diffusion gradient is a factor of inspired oxygen fraction and total air pressure, oxygen partial pressure also rises:

$$\uparrow \text{Increased total pressure}$$
$$= \uparrow\uparrow P\%(\text{Oxygen}) + \uparrow\uparrow P\%(\text{Nitrogen})$$

The maximum increase possible in oxygen delivery is to increase the total inspired air pressure and fraction of oxygen (Bledsoe et al., 2012):

$$\uparrow \text{Increased total air pressure}$$
$$= \uparrow\uparrow\uparrow P\%(\text{Oxygen}) + \downarrow P\%(\text{Nitrogen})$$

CPAP is a non-invasive ventilation method that increases air pressure throughout the respiratory cycle, affecting inspiration and expiration (Bledsoe et al., 2012).

Inspiratory positive airway pressure
CPAP does not change the gradient between inspired air pressure and alveoli. Instead, it raises both pressures equally, increasing airway pressure, alveolar ventilation and oxygen delivery for the same work of breathing (Fig. 4.10.1).

CPAP supports spontaneous breathing. The patient must create the lower inspiratory alveolar pressure for airflow. CPAP is not positive pressure ventilation and it will not force chest expansion as IPPV does.

Expiratory positive airway pressure
CPAP provides continuous expiratory positive airway pressure, maintaining the increase in airway pressure during expiration (Miro et al., 2004). Expiratory resistance helps hold the bronchioles and alveoli open, improving air escape and the time available for gas exchange (Dib et al., 2012; Ferrer et al., 2012; Miro et al., 2004).

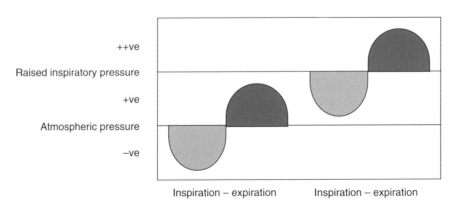

Figure 4.10.1 Inspiration and expiration at normal atmospheric pressure versus raised inspiratory pressure

Alveolar inflation support

The alveoli collapse during expiration, reducing the time available for gas exchange to occur. If they are collapsed, the alveoli must be reinflated. This requires energy and increases the work of breathing (Dib et al., 2012; Bledsoe et al., 2012; Ferrer et al., 2012; Miro et al., 2004). Maintaining alveolar inflation therefore improves oxygenation and ventilation.

Alveoli are normally covered by lipoprotein surfactant liquid to reduce surface tension. Surface tension is created where liquid molecules attract each other when contacting air. The greater the surface tension, the harder it is for the alveoli to inflate. Surfactant breaks apart easily, making the alveoli easier to inflate.

Some conditions, particularly pulmonary oedema, drowning, aspiration or infection can cause infiltration into the alveoli, washing out surfactant. The work of reinflating the alveoli then increases (Agarwal et al., 2010; DiBardino and Wunderink, 2015; Ferrer et al., 2012; BTS, 2002; Raghavendran et al., 2011).

Smaller airway support

During some illnesses, including chronic obstructive pulmonary disease (COPD) and asthma, the bronchioles and smaller bronchi become obstructed (Miro et al., 2004). As air escapes during expiration, air above the obstruction escapes readily. The obstructed airway collapses inwards, trapping alveolar air, reducing air escape and increasing intra-alveolar pressure. Slowing air escape from larger airways, as CPAP does, means obstructed airways are less likely to collapse inwards and facilitates alveolar air escape.

CPAP has a caveat for the management of COPD. Increased intra-alveolar pressure dictates a lower CPAP than where alveolar collapse is the problem, and the potential for barotrauma increases.

Using the CPAP device

Numerous systems are available that are capable of producing reliable CPAP. High oxygen flow rates may be necessary to entrain large airflow rates to support pressure delivery.

The components that make up the CPAP system include a delivery mask, head harness, pressure generation method and high-flow oxygen supply. The mask is critical. Nasal or full-face masks are available. The latter are typically used in emergencies as they do not rely on the patient cooperating by keeping their mouth closed. The disadvantages of a full-face mask include the difficulties they create in drinking, eating, talking or clearing airway secretions.

CPAP masks are not unlike those used for IPPV. A low-pressure cuff allows an effective seal, although, unlike IPPV, the CPAP mask can accommodate a slight leak in use. Pressurised air/oxygen is entrained inwards while venting off exhaled breath to the atmosphere. High gas flow supports exhaled air removal.

Assemble the device before use. Attach the oxygen source and confirm the device is functioning correctly. Applying a CPAP mask that is non-functioning to a patient could increase their distress and worsen hypoxia or hypercapnoea.

The CPAP device must have a means of measuring and adjusting airway pressure to ensure it is correct and suited to the patient's condition. Pressures usually range between 2.5 and 12.5 cm/H_2O, with 5–10 cm/H_2O being the most common. Set the desired pressure before initiating the therapy. This might be determined by adjusting the inwards oxygen flow or changing the attachable positive end expiratory pressure (PEEP) valves (Ferrer et al., 2012).

Occasionally it may be necessary to suction fluid or secretion from a patient's mouth before beginning therapy, or later by removing the mask.

Typical therapy commences with lower pressure, increasing as necessary until a benefit is achieved but before any complications occur. Alveoli diseases, such as pulmonary oedema, tend to tolerate and require relatively higher pressures to reinflate on inspiration. Bronchiole diseases that result in airway collapse and gas trapping on expiration typically require lower pressures (Ferrer et al., 2012).

Applying the mask to a patient's face can take a few minutes if they are anxious, distressed or dislike having their face covered. The mask may be held in place by the paramedic until it is accepted by the patient. Patients are positioned sitting upright, to maximise alveolar recruitment.

Once the mask has been accepted and is functioning, secure it with the head harness. The harness is attached to the mask at multiple points by straps. It extends around the back of the patient's head, holding it in place without great pressure to achieve a balance between comfort and effectiveness (Fig. 4.10.2a and b).

Many CPAP systems are disposable. Used items should be disposed of in standard infectious waste systems, being mindful they may be covered in body fluid. Reusable components should be appropriately cleaned.

Clinical skill assessment process

The following section outlines the clinical skill assessment tools that should be used to determine a student's ability to demonstrate the safe and accurate use of CPAP.
1. Clinical Skill Work Instruction
2. Formative Clinical Skill Assessment (F-CSAT)
3. Performance Improvement Plan (PIP)
4. Summative Clinical Skill Assessment (S-CSAT)
(5. Direct Observation of Procedural Skills (DOPS) – see Chapter 1.1)

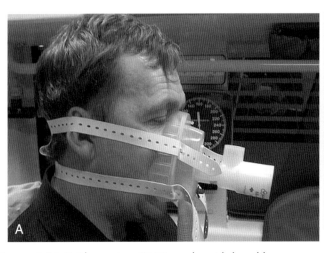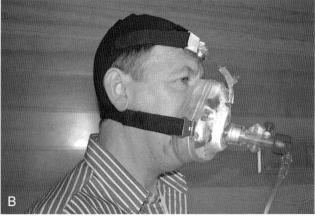

Figure 4.10.2 Alternative CPAP masks with head harness
(a) PEEP valve device with clip-on head harness. (b) CPAP determined by oxygen flow rate with head-covering harness.

Clinical Skill Work Instruction

Equipment and resources: Standardised patient/mannequin; disposable gloves, protective eyewear and respiratory mask; CPAP therapy device, including mask, head harness and pressure generator; oxygen source; method of documenting the results

Associated Clinical Skills: Infection control; Communication; Consent; Patient assessment skills; Airway and ventilation skills

Continuous positive airway pressure

Activity	Critical Action	Rationale
Prepare paramedic	Don appropriate personal protection, including eyewear and respiratory mask.	Airway procedures are high risk for infection transmission.
	The therapy can be fitted from beside or behind the patient.	Patient access for mask application can vary.
Prepare patient	Explain the procedure to the patient.	Compliance and consent is required.
	The patient is typically positioned sitting upright.	Patients in respiratory distress typically prefer this position. It helps pulmonary vascular drainage and alveoli inflation.
	Suction froth or fluid from airway if necessary before applying the mask and beginning the therapy.	Fluid often comes from the lungs and cannot be removed by prolonged suction attempts.
Prepare equipment	Assemble CPAP system for use, including the appropriate PEEP valve.	To ensure device is ready for application.
	Attach to oxygen source and adjust flow to desired rate. Inspect for correct functioning for use.	The device must be operating correctly before application. Flow rate may vary CPAP pressure.

Continuous positive airway pressure continued

Activity	Critical Action	Rationale
Apply face mask seal	Hold mask over patient's nose and mouth, positioning it to gain an effective seal. This may require fitting the mask against one cheek first, then over bridge of nose, then into other cheek. The therapy can be fitted from beside or behind the patient.	To ensure proper fit.
	Allow patient to become accustomed to the mask. Provide reassurance and explanation.	To increase compliance and reduce anxiety.
	Apply head harness evenly to maintain effective seal. Adjust as necessary until mask is functioning without being too tight.	Ensures effectiveness and comfort.
	Ensure airflow is constant and desired PEEP reading is attained.	To achieve desired effect.
Reassess patient	Reassess continuously to monitor effectiveness of therapy, including consciousness and pulse oximetry.	For early recognition of changes in patient's condition.
	If patient's condition deteriorates due to respiratory failure or life-threatening complications, remove therapy and respond appropriately.	In order to work, CPAP requires effective, spontaneous ventilation.
Report	Accurately document/hand over the findings.	Accurate record kept and patient care continuity.

Formative Clinical Skill Assessment (F-CSAT)

Equipment and resources: Standardised patient/mannequin; disposable gloves, protective eyewear and respiratory mask; CPAP therapy device, including mask, head harness and pressure generator; oxygen source; method of documenting the results

Associated Clinical Skills: Infection control; Communication; Consent; Patient assessment skills; Airway and ventilation skills

Staff/Student being assessed: _____

Continuous positive airway pressure

Activity	Critical Action	Participant Performance				
Prepares paramedic	Dons appropriate personal protection, including eyewear and respiratory mask.	0	1	2	3	4
	Acknowledges therapy can be fitted from beside or behind patient.	0	1	2	3	4
Prepares patient	Explains the procedure to the patient.	0	1	2	3	4
	Positions patient sitting upright.	0	1	2	3	4
	Suctions froth or fluid from the airway if necessary before applying mask application and beginning therapy.	0	1	2	3	4
Prepares equipment	Assembles CPAP system for use, including PEEP valve if included.	0	1	2	3	4
	Attaches to an oxygen source and adjusts flow to desired rate. Inspects device for correct functioning for use.	0	1	2	3	4

Continuous positive airway pressure continued

Activity	Critical Action	Participant Performance				
Applies face mask seal	Holds face mask over patient's nose and mouth, positioning it to gain an effective seal. If necessary, fits against one cheek first, then over bridge of nose, then onto other cheek.	0	1	2	3	4
	Allows patient to become accustomed to mask. Provides reassurance and explanation.	0	1	2	3	4
	Applies head harness evenly to maintain effective seal. Adjusts as necessary until mask is functioning without being too tight.	0	1	2	3	4
	Ensures airflow is constant and desired pressure reading is attained.	0	1	2	3	4
Reassesses patient	Reassesses patient continuously to monitor effectiveness of therapy, including consciousness and pulse oximetry.	0	1	2	3	4
	If patient's condition deteriorates due to respiratory failure or life-threatening complications, removes therapy and responds appropriately.	0	1	2	3	4
Reports	Accurately documents/hands over the findings.	0	1	2	3	4

Standard Achieved: (please circle one)

Competent (C)   Not Yet Competent* (NYC)

Staff/Student Name: _____

Assessor (please print name): _____

Signed (Assessor): _____

Date of Assessment: _____

Comments:

*If Not Yet Competent (NYC) a PIP needs to be completed and a repeat of the F-CSAT

Formative Clinical Skill Assessment (F-CSAT) Key

Skill level	Standard of procedure	Quality of performance	Outcome	Level of assistance required
4 Safe for unsupervised practice	Safe Accurate Behaviour is appropriate to context	Confident Accurate Expedient	Achieved intended outcome	No supporting cues* required
3 Requires supervision	Safe Accurate Behaviour is appropriate to context	Confident Accurate Takes longer than required	Achieved intended outcome	Requires occasional supportive cues*

Skill level	Standard of procedure	Quality of performance	Outcome	Level of assistance required
2 Requires assistance	Safe Accurate Behaviour generally appropriate to context	Lacks certainty	Would not have achieved outcome without support	Requires frequent verbal and occasional physical directives in addition to supportive cues*
1 Requires direction	Safe only with guidance Not completely accurate	Unskilled Inefficient	Would not have achieved outcome without support	Requires continuous verbal and frequent physical directive cues*
0 Unsafe	Unsafe Unable to demonstrate behaviour Lack of insight into behaviour appropriate to context	Unskilled	Would not have achieved outcome	Requires continuous verbal and continuous physical directive cues*

*Refers to physical directives or verbal supportive cues

Performance Improvement Plan (PIP)

Please document the agreed education plan and completion timelines for areas assessed as less than 4.

This plan should be presented to assessor prior to commencement of summative assessment.

Where was supervisor support required?	Student summary of deficit. (Why was there a problem?)	Improvement Plan	Completed (Y/N)

Staff/Student Name: _____

Staff/Student Signature: _____

Educator Name: _____

Educator Signature: _____

Summative Clinical Skill Assessment (S-CSAT)

Equipment and resources: Standardised patient/mannequin; disposable gloves, protective eyewear and respiratory mask; CPAP therapy device, including mask, head harness and pressure generator; oxygen source; method of documenting the results

Associated Clinical Skills: Infection control; Communication; Consent; Patient assessment skills; Airway and ventilation skills

Staff/Student being assessed: _____

- Completed Formative Clinical Skill Assessment (F-CSAT):   **YES   NO**

- Completed Performance Improvement Plan (PIP):   **YES   NO   N/A**

Title: 4.10 Continuous positive airway pressure

Activity	Critical Action	Achieved Without Direction	
Prepares paramedic	Wears appropriate personal protection, including eyewear and respiratory mask.	NO	YES
	Acknowledges therapy can be fitted from beside or behind patient.	NO	YES
Prepares patient	Explains the procedure to the patient.	NO	YES
	Positions patient sitting upright.	NO	YES
	Suctions froth or fluid from the airway if necessary before applying mask and beginning therapy.	NO	YES
Prepares equipment	Assembles CPAP system for use, including PEEP valve if included.	NO	YES
	Attaches to an oxygen source and adjusts flow to desired rate. Inspects device for correct functioning for use.	NO	YES
Applies face mask seal	Holds face mask over patient's nose and mouth, positioning it to gain an effective seal. If necessary, fits mask against one cheek first, then over bridge of nose, then onto other cheek.	NO	YES
	Allows the patient to become accustomed to mask. Provides reassurance and explanation.	NO	YES
	Applies head harness evenly to maintain effective seal. Adjusts as necessary until mask is functioning without being too tight.	NO	YES
	Ensures airflow is constant and desired pressure reading is attained.	NO	YES
Reassesses patient	Reassesses patient continuously to monitor effectiveness of therapy, including consciousness and pulse oximetry.	NO	YES
	If patient's condition deteriorates due to respiratory failure or life-threatening complications, removes therapy and responds appropriately.	NO	YES
Reports	Accurately documents/hands over the findings.	NO	YES

Standard Achieved: (please circle one)

Competent (C)   Not Yet Competent* (NYC)

Staff/Student Name: _____

Assessor (please print name): _____

Signed (Assessor): _____

Date of Assessment: _____

Comments:

*If Not Yet Competent (NYC) a PIP needs to be completed and a repeat of the F-CSAT

Clinical findings

Respiratory failure or altered consciousness

The effectiveness of CPAP relies on adequate spontaneous breathing. Where the latter is insufficient to maintain consciousness, CPAP offers no benefit. Consciousness offers a crude guide to whether breathing is adequate. Drowsiness and a score below 13 on the Glasgow Coma Scale indicates spontaneous ventilation is unlikely to be sufficient for CPAP to be used.

Where this happens, IPPV is necessary to support breathing. Though CPAP can help avoid intubation, there will still be occasions when intubation may be needed. CPAP is not an alternative to IPPV or intubation (BTS, 2002).

Agitation and lack of cooperation

Patients can become anxious, combative and uncooperative from hypoxia or hypercapnoea. They may struggle against the paramedic's efforts, pushing the CPAP mask away and making it difficult to apply and maintain the mask.

Reassurance and gentle arm restraint can allow CPAP to provide benefit from and acceptance of the therapy. Where the patient remains combative, administering sedation carries risks, including cardiovascular compromise through vasodilation, airway reflex reduction and, importantly, reduced respiratory effort (BTS, 2002).

Facial irritation

Eye, membrane and skin irritation can be caused by airflow. This may be annoying and prompt attempts to remove the mask (BTS, 2002).

Facial trauma

Facial injuries and burns make using CPAP difficult and cause so much discomfort that it may not be maintainable (BTS, 2002).

Active vomiting

Using full-face CPAP may be difficult, if not impossible, if the patient vomits. In such cases, therapy must be discontinued and the mask removed (BTS, 2002).

Elevated intrathoracic pressure: reduction in inferior venous return

Normal breathing contributes to the effectiveness of circulation, with inspiratory intrathoracic pressure reduction leading to increased venous return and pulmonary vascular filling. Ventilation and perfusion increase during inspiration.

Like IPPV, CPAP increases intrathoracic pressure, potentially compromising venous return and cardiac output. Patients susceptible to a reduction in venous return can be adversely affected, including hypovolemia, vasodilation or arrhythmia. A reduction in venous return might help in some cases, including for left ventricular

failure (Simpson and Bendall, 2011; Ducros et al., 2011; Vital et al., 2013).

Provided the pressure applied is not too high, CPAP does not commonly cause a problem. If it does cause cardiovascular compromise, a plan to improve blood pressure or reduce the CPAP delivery pressure must be considered (Dib et al., 2012).

Elevated intrathoracic pressure: reduction in superior venous return

Not all venous return is from the inferior vena cava, as some returns via the superior vena cava. Impaired drainage into the chest can raise jugular venous congestion, affecting cerebral blood flow raising intracranial pressure (Ducros et al., 2011; Vital et al., 2013). The situations in which CPAP could worsen this problem include stroke and other central nervous emergencies.

Elevated intrathoracic pressure: barotrauma

Excessive alveoli pressure can cause pulmonary barotrauma and air entering the pleural space. Weakened lung tissue is particularly susceptible. Vulnerable lung tissue is found in diseases such as COPD and acute respiratory distress syndrome (ARDS).

While it is unlikely that CPAP alone will cause barotrauma, using it for conditions in which air is already within the pleural space is risky because pneumothorax can turn into tension pneumothorax (BTS, 2002; Ducros et al., 2011; Vital et al., 2013).

Cardiac arrhythmia

While CPAP is not associated with causing cardiac arrhythmia, its application in the presence of them is risky. Arrhythmias reduce cardiac output, which is problematic if CPAP further reduces venous return and ventricular filling (Ducros et al., 2011; Vital et al., 2013).

Elevated intra-gastric pressure

Airway reflexes diminish with altered consciousness. Loss of oesophageal and cardiac sphincter tone make it easier for air to enter the stomach and gastric content to escape.

There is a small risk of increasing intragastric pressure during CPAP. This can cause patient discomfort if gastric distention occurs. It can also inflate the stomach, making it difficult for the diaphragm to move during inspiration, particularly in the child patient. Regurgitation of gastric content can cause aspiration (Ducros et al., 2011; Vital et al., 2013).

PRACTICE TIP!

CPAP is not IPPV. Unless there is effective spontaneous breathing, CPAP will not be able to offer any benefit. Whenever spontaneous breathing is inadequate to maintain consciousness, IPPV must replace CPAP.

PRACTICE TIP!

Patients typically show clinical signs of improvement when receiving CPAP therapy. To be able to determine its effectiveness, assess the patient's physical and vital signs before beginning the therapy, so that any improvements can then be objectively qualified.

PRACTICE TIP!

Despite the effectiveness of CPAP, some patients demonstrate initial agitation and reluctance to accept a mask over their face. Reassurance and patient coaching can prove critical to overcoming this resistance.

TEST YOUR KNOWLEDGE QUESTIONS

1. **What is the fundamental difference between the indications for IPPV and CPAP?**
    CPAP requires adequate spontaneous breathing, which it can support but not replace. IPPV is administered where spontaneous breathing is absent or insufficient to maintain consciousness, and substitutes for breathing.

2. **What are the two ways in which oxygen partial pressure can be increased?**
    Supplemental oxygen to displace nitrogen; increasing the overall pressure of inspired air.

3. **List five common indications for emergency CPAP therapy.**
    COPD; acute pulmonary oedema; gastric aspiration; pneumonia; near drowning; ARDS.

4. **What is the common pressure range used for CPAP therapy?**
    5–10 cm/H_2O, with an outer range of 2.5–12.5 cm/H_2O.

5. **How does CPAP offer benefit during acute pulmonary oedema?**
    Washing out alveolar surfactant can lead to alveolar collapse, decreased gas exchange and increasing work of breathing to reopen the alveoli. CPAP maintains alveolar inflation, increases gas exchange time, decreases work of breathing and opposes pulmonary hydrostatic pressure, and can reduce venous return and ventricular preload.

6. **How does CPAP offer benefit during COPD exacerbations?**
    COPD involves smaller, narrowed airways that can collapse during expiration, leading to gas trapping, reduced alveolar ventilation and increased work of breathing to reopen the airways. CPAP can hold open smaller airways during expiration, increasing expiratory airflow and alveolar ventilation and decreasing work to reopen them again.

7. **How can CPAP adversely affect cardiac output?**
    CPAP can increase intrathoracic pressure, leading to decreased venous return and reduced cardiac output.

8. **How critical is gaining a face mask seal during CPAP?**
    Unlike the IPPV mask, the CPAP mask can tolerate small leaks during use.

9. **What should be confirmed on the CPAP system before application?**
    The oxygen is connected and flowing and the level of the CPAP is set at the desired amount.

10. **List three conditions where CPAP might offer benefit but carry a risk of worsening the patient's condition.**
    Low ventricular preload, such as hypovolemia, arrhythmia or hypotension; raised intracranial pressure problems, such as stroke; existing barotrauma.

References

Agarwal, R., Aggarwal, A.N. and Gupta, D., 2010. Role of noninvasive ventilation in acute lung injury/acute respiratory distress syndrome: a proportion meta-analysis. *Respiratory Care*, 55(12), 1653–1660.

Bledsoe, B.E., Anderson E., Hodnick R., Johnson L., Johnson S. and Dievendorf, E., 2012. Low–fractional oxygen concentration continuous positive airway pressure is effective in the prehospital setting. *Prehospital Emergency Care*, 16(2), 217–221.

BTS (British Thoracic Society), 2002. Non-invasive ventilation in acute respiratory failure. *Thorax*, 57(3), 192–211.

Dib, J.E., Matin, S.A. and Luckert, A., 2012. Prehospital use of continuous positive airway pressure for acute severe congestive heart failure. *Journal of Emergency Medicine*, 42(5), 553–558.

DiBardino, D.M. and Wunderink, R.G., 2015. Aspiration pneumonia: a review of modern trends. *Journal of Critical Care*, 30(1), 40–48.

Ducros, L., Logeart, D., Vicaut, E., Henry, P., Plaisance, P., Collet, J.P., Broche, C., Gueye, P., Vergne, M., Goetgheber, D. and

Pennec, P.Y., 2011. CPAP for acute cardiogenic pulmonary oedema from out-of-hospital to cardiac intensive care unit: a randomised multicentre study. *Intensive Care Medicine*, 37(9), 1501–1509.

Ferrer, M., Cosentini, R. and Nava, S., 2012. The use of non-invasive ventilation during acute respiratory failure due to pneumonia. *European Journal of Internal Medicine*, 23(5), 420–428.

Miro, A.M., Pinsky, M.R. and Rogers, P.L., 2004. Effects of the components of positive airway pressure on work of breathing during bronchospasm. *Critical Care*, 8(2), R72.

Raghavendran, K., Nemzek, J., Napolitano, L.M. and Knight, P.R., 2011. Aspiration-induced lung injury. *Critical Care Medicine*, 39(4), 818.

Simpson, P.M. and Bendall, J.C., 2011. Prehospital non-invasive ventilation for acute cardiogenic pulmonary oedema: an evidence-based review. *Emergency Medicine Journal*, 28(7), 609–612.

Vital, F.M., Ladeira, M.T. and Atallah, Á.N., 2013. *Non-invasive positive pressure ventilation (CPAP or bilevel NPPV) for cardiogenic pulmonary oedema*. Online: The Cochrane Library.

Bibliography

Craft, J., Gordon, C., Huether, S.E., McCance, K.L. and Brashers, V.L., 2015. *Understanding pathophysiology* (ANZ adaptation). Sydney: Elsevier.

Mal, S., McLeod, S., Iansavichene, A., Dukelow A. and Lewell, M., 2014. Effect of out-of-hospital noninvasive positive-pressure support ventilation in adult patients with severe respiratory distress:

a systematic review and meta-analysis. *Annals of Emergency Medicine*, 63(5), 600–607.

McCance, K.L. and Huether, S.E., 2015. *Pathophysiology: the biologic basis for disease in adults and children*. Sydney: Elsevier.

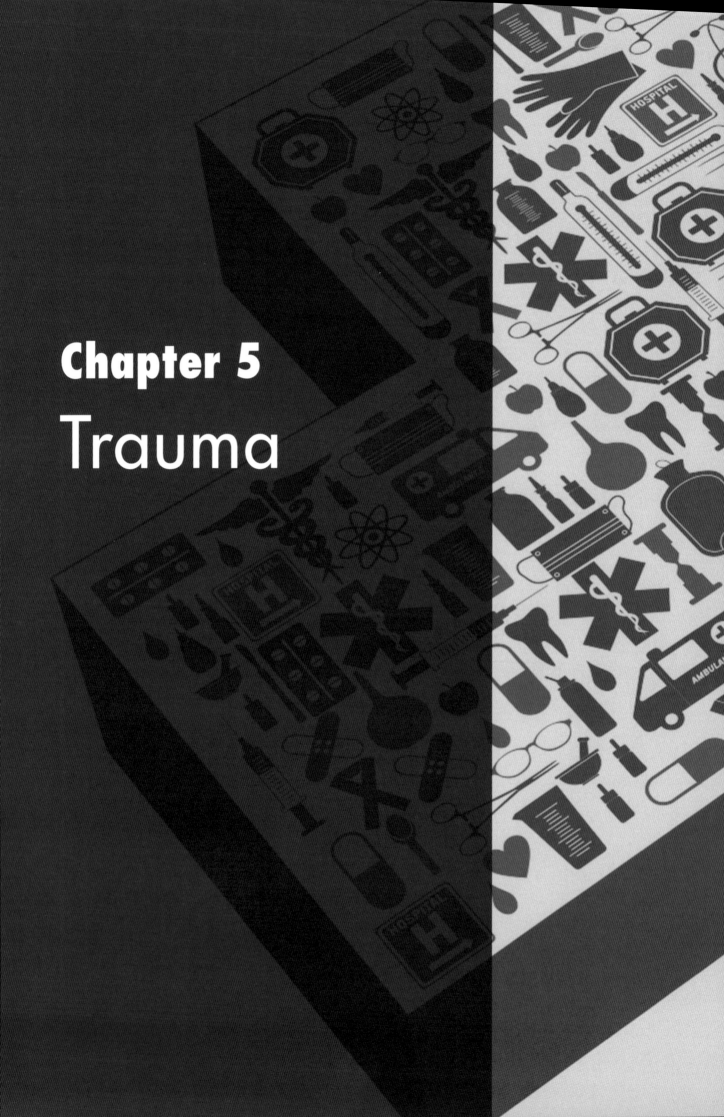

Chapter 5
Trauma

5.1 | Trauma assessment

Dianne Inglis and Jeff Kenneally

Chapter objectives

At the end of this chapter the reader will be able to:

1. Describe the rationale behind trauma assessment
2. Demonstrate trauma assessment
3. Accurately report trauma assessment findings

Resources required for this assessment

- Standardised patient/mannequin
- Hand decontamination agent
- Disposable gloves, goggles, mask, gown
- Method of documenting results

Skill matrix

This assessment requires:

- Infection control (CS 1.3)
- Communication (CS 1.5)
- Consent (CS 1.6)
- Patient assessment skills (Chapter 2)
- Pelvic splint application (CS 5.8)
- Cervical collar application (CS 5.7)
- Log roll (CS 7.1)

This assessment is a component of:

- Trauma (Chapter 5)

Introduction

Trauma can be used to describe emotional or psychological experiences that are distressing or disturbing. It can also be used to describe physical injuries provided from external forces. The two may coexist. This chapter focuses on the latter.

In many ways, assessing the patient for trauma is easier than for medical complaints. Although major trauma is frequently concealed internally, within the body, many clues for assessing trauma come from what has been seen to happen and simple examination: does it look broken, does it feel broken and does it hurt? This chapter discusses trauma assessment, from mild and localised to major multi-trauma. It should be considered in conjunction with the other assessments referred to throughout the chapter.

Anatomy and physiology

Trauma assessment involves comprehensive external examination of the patient. A broad knowledge and understanding of anatomy and physiology are required, including of the nervous, respiratory, cardiovascular and musculoskeletal systems.

This chapter refers extensively to other more specific chapters in this workbook, including those in Chapter 2, Patient assessment; Chapter 3, Airway and ventilation; Chapter 5, Trauma; and Chapter 7, Manual handling.

Clinical rationale

Trauma assessment involves an algorithmic approach, prioritising findings in their order of urgency. This begins with establishing the nature of the trauma, identifying any immediate threats to life and then systematically assessing the patient. Emergency trauma management is chaotic and prone to errors, including missed assessment findings (Gruen et al., 2006).

Mechanism of injury

The 'mechanism of injury' concept provides a general statement to the type of event involved – essentially, what has happened. Although the patient has experienced an incident, there is no certainty they have actually sustained injury. Major examples of injury mechanisms include where a pedestrian has been struck, motor vehicle collisions and falls from height; variables such as speed or height are critical.

The mechanism is established through visual examination on arrival and by interviewing witnesses or patients. A major injury mechanism has the potential to cause major traumatic injuries, while lesser mechanisms help describe the lesser injuries anticipated. On the other hand, higher risk patients incur injury more easily with even lesser mechanisms. Falls from a standing height, for instance, can lead to severe injury and even fatality in the aged/elderly (Ayoung-Chee et al., 2014; Carpenter et al., 2017; Lee et al., 2015; Rowbotham and Blau, 2017; Sammy et al., 2016). Other at-risk groups include children (McCarthy et al., 2016; Wright, 2015), pregnant women (Augustin et al., 2018; Huls and Detlefs, 2018) and those who already have significant comorbidities (Mitchell et al., 2016; Stawicki et al., 2015).

Dangers

The term 'trauma' implies an event that is potentially threatening to others. Before approaching any trauma patient, first ensure that any major hazard is negated or the patient is safely moved away from it. The trauma patient should not be approached until this is done. A range of lesser hazards are also often present, including broken glass, jagged edges, debris and fuels and the patient's blood. Paramedics' PPE may include hard helmets, high-visibility clothing and tough gloves during any rescue phase; the equipment needed will then change to standard universal precautions during patient assessment.

Primary (life-threat) survey

The initial assessment identifies immediate threats to life. Advanced trauma life support begins with an RABCDE algorithm (Kirkpatrick et al., 2008; Thim et al., 2012; Wilson and Clebone, 2014), prioritising lifesaving treatments. The first element of RABCDE is only necessary for patients who appear to be unconscious, as it essentially determines whether the patient is alive or not.

Despite any urgency, the presence and extent of any injuries at this point is unknown. Move the patient only as necessary and as little as possible. At the same time, be mindful of any non-purposeful noises, including gurgling from the escape of lung air caused by the patient being moved rather than by their own respiratory efforts.

R: Determine if the patient is in any way responsive, using a purposeful verbal question or command (e.g. call loudly, 'Can you hear me?' or 'Open your eyes'), shaking the patient's shoulders or applying painful stimuli sufficient to rouse any person who is not deeply unconscious.

A: If the patient remains unresponsive, position the head in the neutral anatomical position (see Chapter 3.2), using gentle, controlled movement. Inspect the *airway* for externally visible obstruction, including blood, vomitus or facial trauma.

B: Determine if the patient is making any effective *breathing* effort by looking and feeling for chest movement and listening for audible breathing sounds. Distinguish this from infrequent agonal gasping that is not effective breathing.

C: Assess *circulation* for palpable radial or carotid pulse/ major haemorrhage.

D: Assess the patient's *disability*/neurological status using AVPU (see Chapter 2.2).

E: *Expose* the patient in order to conduct the assessment, considering the *environment* they are in.

A hot environment can expose the patient to dehydration or burning from the surface on which they are found, whereas a cold environment (especially if wet or windy) can exacerbate body temperature loss. Either is undesirable for trauma patients (Beilman et al., 2009; Tsuei and Kearney, 2004; Wang et al., 2005). Many patients will already be exposed to an adverse environment before paramedics arrive, and this may have to be addressed before or during assessment. The assessment itself entails the removal of clothing, exposing the patient to environment and privacy concerns. It is therefore important to find a balance between exposing the patient for assessment and keeping as much of them covered as possible.

Patients who are unresponsive and have no effective breathing or palpable pulse are in traumatic cardiac arrest, and require immediate resuscitation without continuing the assessment.

Where there are signs of life, including breathing and a pulse, assess the patient for major external haemorrhage after checking their pulse. This does not extend to every visible injury, only those that can lead to short-term exsanguination. Controlling any major external haemorrhage before continuing with trauma assessment and resuscitation is critical (Kirkpatrick et al., 2008).

Survey of vital signs

Abnormal vital signs can immediately disclose seriously unwell patients. Compromised perfusion, respiratory distress or altered consciousness all suggest significant injuries. Assess vital signs early and quickly as a baseline for monitoring trends in patient condition and to identify patients whose injuries are urgent. Complete the assessment of each group of vital signs (e.g. perfusion) together and then make a clear statement of the result (e.g. inadequate perfusion) (see Chapter 2).

Injury pattern

The term 'injury pattern' describes the type of force applied and its actual points of contact with the patient. Trauma transfers energy, causing damage or injury when tissue tolerance or capacity is exceeded. Energy variables include the type, amount and duration of force. The resulting injury also varies with the type of tissue impacted.

The pattern of injury can in part be determined by what the patient has endured. For instance, a person sitting in the driver's seat of a car running head-on into a solid object will continue forwards (notwithstanding seatbelts or airbags), potentially striking windscreen (head), steering wheel (chest/abdomen), dashboard (knees/legs/pelvis) and pedals or firewall (feet/ankles). Some injury patterns are complex, including explosions and vehicle rollovers.

Three types of trauma are caused by force:
1. Penetrating trauma, including lower force stabbing and impalement, and higher force projectiles including gunshot and explosive objects
2. Blunt trauma (kinetic energy), which is by far the most common
3. Burns (thermal energy), including flame, chemical and high-voltage electricity.

To this can be added specific injuries that are otherwise difficult to classify by type of force but are still urgent due to their potential for major haemorrhage and injury complications. These include limb amputations, crush injury/syndrome, multiple long-bone (femur/tibia/humerus) fractures and suspected pelvic fracture.

An assessment of the injury pattern is obtained from direct observation of the scene, how the patient was found, the history described by the patient and witnesses and from the injuries themselves.

Physical assessment

While the assessment of an injury pattern is applied to particular regions of the body, a physical (whole body/head to toe/secondary) assessment considers each region in turn.

Commence at the patient's head and work inferiorly. Repeat generalised elements for all regions, applying specific elements to individual regions only. The generalised elements are as follows:
1. Ask the patient if there is any pain in that region.
2. Visually inspect the region for abnormality, including swelling, deformity, abrasions/lacerations/bruising/bleeding or burns.

3. Palpate the region for tenderness or deformity. Specific assessment elements include:
- the face, where the orbits, cheeks, mandible and teeth are specifically considered. Facial trauma is important given its relationship to airway and the senses. Assess facial nerves, particularly the eyes and pupillary responses (see Chapter 2.12)
- the remainder of the head, including lateral and posterior. Inspect the ears for injury and any blood or fluid escaping from them
- the neck, for injury and critical elements passing through it. Consider jugular venous distension or tracheal position, suggesting a significant chest injury
- the chest, including comparing symmetry and movement bilaterally, auscultating air entry and audible sounds (see Chapter 2.8) and assessing for palpable emphysema or presence of sucking chest wounds
- the abdomen, including for wall rigidity, distension, guarding or evisceration (see Chapter 2.17)
- the pelvis (see Chapter 5.8). Pelvic springing is unreliable and unnecessary. Log rolling should be avoided or the patient should only be rolled partly, to minimise injury aggravation
- the legs and arms, particularly for limb symmetry, shortening, inward or outward rotation, function, sensation, distal colour, palpable pulses, temperature and amputation/degloving injuries
- finally, the back, including spinal column and posterior chest and abdomen (retroperitoneal). Log roll the patient with suitable spinal care (see Chapter 7.1) and hold laterally to allow physical assessment.

Also perform a spinal motor/sensation examination and cervical spine clearance assessment (see Chapters 2.13 and 5.7). This can be completed as a separate entity or integrated throughout during limb assessment.

Clinical skill assessment process

The following section outlines the clinical skill assessment tools that should be used to determine a student's ability to demonstrate safe and accurate trauma assessment.
1. Clinical Skill Work Instruction
2. Formative Clinical Skill Assessment (F-CSAT)
3. Performance Improvement Plan (PIP)
4. Summative Clinical Skill Assessment (S-CSAT)
(5. Direct Observation of Procedural Skills (DOPS) – see Chapter 1.1)

Clinical Skill Work Instruction

Equipment and resources: Standardised patient/mannequin; disposable gloves, goggles, mask and gown; hand decontamination agent; method of documenting results

Associated Clinical Skills: Infection control; Communication; Consent; Patient assessment skills; Pelvic splint application; Cervical collar application; Log roll

Trauma

Activity	Critical Action	Rationale
Injury mechanism	Identify nature of trauma from visual cues and history provided. Recognise major trauma criteria if present.	Establishing what happened identifies the potential for injury.
Personal protection	If hazards are present at the scene, either remove patient or manage hazard. Do not proceed further unless safe.	Scene hazards must not compromise safety.
	Don PPE as required for situation and procedure. Consider burnt clothing, chemical exposure, haemorrhage.	PPE requirements vary with hazards and patient condition.
Patient preparation	If patient is conscious, provide introduction, reassurance and explanation of assessment. Obtain informed consent.	Gain cooperation.
Primary survey: RABCDE	If patient does not appear conscious: *Response:* grasp patient's shoulders. Gently shake and call out to elicit any response. *Airway:* observe for abnormal head position. Return to neutral anatomical position where possible. Observe for visible facial blood, vomitus or trauma obstruction. *Breathing:* observe chest movement, audible breathing, breath felt. *Circulation:* assess for palpable carotid/radial pulse.	Identifies signs of life or threat to life. Provides cervical spine precautions before patient movement.
	Assess for visible major external haemorrhage.	Prompts immediate control.
	Disability: assess neurological status using AVPU. *Expose/Environment:* remove or protect patient from adverse exposure as soon as practicable. Expose patient being mindful of environment/need for privacy.	Heat or cold can worsen a trauma patient's condition. Exposure is required to complete the assessment.
Vital signs	Assess and determine: • perfusion status • respiratory status • conscious state, using GCS; identify any altered behaviour, including agitation and confusion • tympanic temperature, pulse oximetry, ECG/cardiac monitor.	Abnormal vital signs define the patient requiring urgent care and paramedic intervention.
	Identify abnormalities and urgency.	Abnormal vital signs betray a major underlying injury.
Injury pattern	Perform physical head-to-toe examination using body region approach. For each region: • ask if there is any pain • inspect for visible abnormality, including swelling, deformity, abrasions/laceration/bruising/bleeding or burns • palpate for tenderness, deformity. Consider trauma type: • blunt • penetrating/impalement • burns (thermal/chemical/electrical). Assess: • face – eyes, orbits, cheeks, mandible, teeth; cranial nerve assessment, including pupils • head – lateral/posterior; ears, including for presence of blood/fluid • neck – jugular venous distension, tracheal position • chest – bilateral movement, symmetry, auscultate air entry, emphysema, sucking chest wound • abdomen – wall rigidity, distension, guarding, evisceration • pelvis – priapism, haematuria • limbs (legs and arms) – distal colour, pulse present, temperature, sensation, motor function, limb symmetry, angulation, rotation, amputation/degloving • back – log roll patient with spinal care.	A systematic look/listen/feel approach over the whole body, with variations suited to each region, is included to identify all abnormalities.

Trauma continued

Activity	Critical Action	Rationale
	Identify injury pattern. Identify any major trauma.	Turn findings into prompts for decision making.
Spinal assessment	Assess sensory and motor function. Assess and determine need for cervical spine care.	Can be performed separately or during head-to-toe examination.
Mechanism modifiers	Identify factors heightening trauma urgency: • children • aged/elderly • pregnancy • significant comorbidities.	These patient groups are at greater risk.
Reassess	Do not rely on single/first assessment. Repeat periodically to identify new findings or any changes.	Traumatic injuries can progress and worsen or appear later.
Report	Document/hand over incident description and clinical findings.	Provides accurate record for care continuity.

Source: *Adapted from Thim et al., 2012.*

Formative Clinical Skill Assessment (F-CSAT)

Equipment and resources: Standardised patient/mannequin; disposable gloves, goggles, mask and gown; hand decontamination agent; method of documenting results

Associated Clinical Skills: Infection control; Communication; Consent; Patient assessment skills; Pelvic splint application; Cervical collar application; Log roll

Staff/Student being assessed: _____

Trauma

Activity	Critical Action	Performance				
Injury mechanism	Identifies trauma nature. Recognises any major trauma criteria.	0	1	2	3	4
Personal protection	Identifies and responds to scene hazards. Dons PPE.	0	1	2	3	4
Patient preparation	If patient does not appear conscious: • assesses response • returns head to neutral anatomical position • observes for airway obstructions • assesses for breathing, palpable pulse, major external haemorrhage, disability using AVPU • removes or protects patient from adverse exposure as soon as practicable. Exposes patient, being mindful of environment/privacy.	0	1	2	3	4
Vital signs	Assesses perfusion, respiratory and conscious-state status using GCS/altered behaviour, tympanic temperature, pulse oximetry, ECG monitor. Identifies abnormalities and urgency.	0	1	2	3	4
Injury pattern	Performs physical head-to-toe examination using body region approach: face, head, neck, chest, abdomen, pelvis, limbs and back. Identifies injury pattern and major trauma.	0	1	2	3	4

Trauma continued

Activity	Critical Action	Performance				
Spinal assessment	Assesses sensory and motor function and need for cervical care.	0	1	2	3	4
Mechanism modifiers	Identifies factors heightening trauma urgency.	0	1	2	3	4
Reassesses	Repeats assessment periodically.	0	1	2	3	4
Reports	Documents/hands over incident description and findings.	0	1	2	3	4

Source: *Adapted from Thim et al., 2012.*

Standard Achieved: (please circle one)

Competent (C)   Not Yet Competent* (NYC)

Staff/Student name: _____

Assessor (please print name): _____

Signed (Assessor): _____

Date of Assessment: _____

Comments:

*If Not Yet Competent (NYC) a PIP needs to be completed and a repeat of the F-CSAT

Formative Clinical Skill Assessment (F-CSAT) Key

Skill level	Standard of procedure	Quality of performance	Outcome	Level of assistance required
4 Safe for unsupervised practice	Safe Accurate Behaviour is appropriate to context	Confident Accurate Expedient	Achieved intended outcome	No supporting cues* required
3 Requires supervision	Safe Accurate Behaviour is appropriate to context	Confident Accurate Takes longer than required	Achieved intended outcome	Requires occasional supportive cues*
2 Requires assistance	Safe Accurate Behaviour generally appropriate to context	Lacks certainty	Would not have achieved outcome without support	Requires frequent verbal and occasional physical directives in addition to supportive cues*
1 Requires direction	Safe only with guidance Not completely accurate	Unskilled Inefficient	Would not have achieved outcome without support	Requires continuous verbal and frequent physical directive cues*
0 Unsafe	Unsafe Unable to demonstrate behaviour Lack of insight into behaviour appropriate to context	Unskilled	Would not have achieved outcome	Requires continuous verbal and continuous physical directive cues*

*Refers to physical directives or verbal supportive cues

Performance Improvement Plan (PIP)

Please document the agreed education plan and completion timelines for areas assessed as less than 4.

This plan should be presented to assessor prior to commencement of summative assessment.

Where was supervisor support required?	Student summary of deficit. (Why was there a problem?)	Improvement Plan	Completed (Y/N)

Staff/Student Name: _____

Staff/Student Signature: _____

Educator Name: _____

Educator Signature: _____

Summative Clinical Skill Assessment (S-CSAT)

Equipment and resources: Standardised patient/mannequin; disposable gloves, goggles, mask and gown; hand decontamination agent; method of documenting results

Associated Clinical Skills: Infection control; Communication; Consent; Patient assessment skills; Pelvic splint application; Cervical collar application; Log roll

Staff/Student being assessed: _____

- Completed Formative Clinical Skill Assessment (F-CSAT):   **YES   NO**
- Completed Performance Improvement Plan (PIP):   **YES   NO   N/A**

Trauma				
Activity	**Critical Action**		**Achieved Without Direction**	
Injury mechanism	Identifies trauma nature. Recognises any major trauma criteria.		NO	YES
Personal protection	Identifies and responds to scene hazards. Dons PPE.		NO	YES
Patient preparation	If patient does not appear conscious: • assesses response • returns head to neutral anatomical position • observes for airway obstructions • assesses for breathing, palpable pulse, major external haemorrhage, disability using AVPU • removes or protects patient from adverse exposure as soon as practicable. Exposes patient, being mindful of environment/privacy.		NO	YES

Trauma continued

Activity	Critical Action	Achieved Without Direction	
Vital signs	Assesses perfusion, respiratory and conscious-state status using GCS/ altered behaviour, tympanic temperature, pulse oximetry, ECG monitor. Identifies abnormalities and urgency.	NO	YES
Injury pattern	Performs physical head-to-toe examination using body region approach: face, head, neck, chest, abdomen, pelvis, limbs and back. Identifies injury pattern and major trauma.	NO	YES
Spinal assessment	Assesses sensory, motor function and need for cervical care.	NO	YES
Mechanism modifiers	Identifies factors heightening trauma urgency.	NO	YES
Reassesses	Repeats assessment periodically.	NO	YES
Reports	Documents/hands over incident description and findings.	NO	YES

Source: Adapted from Thim et al., 2012.

Standard Achieved: (please circle one)

Competent (C)   Not Yet Competent* (NYC)

Staff/Student Name: _____

Assessor (please print name): _____

Signed (Assessor): _____

Date of Assessment: _____

Comments:

*If Not Yet Competent (NYC) a PIP needs to be completed and a repeat of the F-CSAT

Clinical findings

Inability to examine the patient

In some cases, assessing the trauma patient can be difficult and the assessment must be modified accordingly. Patients trapped in vehicles or who are otherwise partly inaccessible may have to be partially assessed pending further extrication. Achieve whatever is possible in the presenting circumstances.

Distracting injury

Patients with severe or painful injuries can be difficult to assess. The injury can distract the paramedic, causing them to focus on it rather than on the overall assessment. Acknowledge the injury and explain to the patient the need to complete the assessment. The injury can also distract the patient, who may become uncooperative or unable to acknowledge lesser symptoms that may still be important.

PRACTICE TIP!

Physical assessment requires visualising exposed skin, and therefore the removal of clothing. When removing/cutting clothing, consider the potential for causing pain, aggravating the injury and exposing the patient to an adverse environment, as well as their need for dignity/ privacy. Expose the patient by body region only, or re-cover them with blankets as soon as practicable.

PRACTICE TIP!

Trauma assessment involves a high likelihood of contact with blood or bodily fluid. Ensure suitable PPE is used and change protective gloves during assessment to avoid the spread of infection.

PRACTICE TIP!

Reassess patients and don't rely on your original findings. Trauma patients are dynamic. In particular, injuries are more likely to go undetected in patients with altered consciousness (Buduhan and McRitchie, 2000).

TEST YOUR KNOWLEDGE QUESTIONS

1. **What patient groups are at higher risk during any mechanism of injury?**
   The aged/elderly; children; pregnant women; those with significant comorbidities.

2. **What are the two ways in which patients can be exposed to environmental concerns?**
   Prior to ambulance arrival; during examination and removal of clothing.

3. **At what point is a major haemorrhage check performed in trauma assessment?**
   In the primary survey, between circulation and disability.

4. **Why are vital signs assessed early and quickly?**
   To provide a baseline for monitoring trends in patient condition and to identify patients whose injuries are urgent.

5. **What are the three types of injury pattern force?**
   Blunt; penetrating; thermal.

6. **What are the three generalised elements of physical trauma assessment?**
   Determine patient pain in any region; visually inspect the region for abnormality; palpate the region for tenderness/deformity.

7. **How is a distracting injury dealt with during trauma assessment?**
   By acknowledging it and explaining to the patient the need to complete the assessment.

8. **How is injury pattern determined?**
   From direct observation of the scene, how the patient was found, the history described by the patient and witnesses and, in part, from the injuries themselves.

9. **What specific injuries are considered during assessment of the injury pattern?**
   Limb amputations; crush injury/syndrome; multiple long-bone (femur/tibia/humerus) fractures; suspected pelvic fracture.

10. **What features are considered when assessing limbs during trauma assessment?**
    Limb symmetry; shortening; inward or outward rotation; function; sensation; distal colour; palpable pulses; temperature; amputation/degloving injuries.

References

Augustin, S.M., Almenoff, M. and Sparks, A., 2018. Trauma during pregnancy. In *The diagnosis and management of the acute abdomen in pregnancy.* Cham: Springer, pp. 209–216.

Ayoung-Chee, P., McIntyre, L., Ebel, B.E., Mack, C.D., McCormick, W. and Maier, R.V., 2014. Long-term outcomes of ground-level falls in the elderly. *Journal of Trauma and Acute Care Surgery*, 76(2), 498–503.

Beilman, G.J., Blondet, J.J., Nelson, T.R., Nathens, A.B., Moore, F.A., Rhee, P., Puyana, J.C., Moore, E.E. and Cohn, S.M., 2009. Early hypothermia in severely injured trauma patients is a significant risk factor for multiple organ dysfunction syndrome but not mortality. *Annals of Surgery*, 249(5), 845–850.

Buduhan, G. and McRitchie, D.I., 2000. Missed injuries in patients with multiple trauma. *Journal of Trauma and Acute Care Surgery*, 49(4), 600–605.

Carpenter, C.R., Arendts, G., Hullick, C., Nagaraj, G., Cooper, Z. and Burkett, E., 2017. Major trauma in the older patient: evolving trauma care beyond management of bumps and bruises. *Emergency Medicine Australasia*, 29(4), 450–455.

Gruen, R.L., Jurkovich, G.J., McIntyre, L.K., Foy, H.M. and Maier, R.V., 2006. Patterns of errors contributing to trauma mortality: lessons learned from 2594 deaths. *Annals of Surgery*, 244(3), 371.

Huls, C.K. and Detlefs, C., 2018, February. Trauma in pregnancy. *Seminars in Perinatology*, 42(1), 13–20.

Kirkpatrick, A.W., Ball, C.G., D'amours, S.K. and Zygun, D., 2008. Acute resuscitation of the unstable adult trauma patient: bedside diagnosis and therapy. *Canadian Journal of Surgery*, 51(1), 57.

Lee, H., Bein, K.J., Ivers, R. and Dinh, M.M., 2015. Changing patterns of injury associated with low-energy falls in the elderly: a 10-year analysis at an Australian Major Trauma Centre. *ANZ Journal of Surgery*, 85(4), 230–234.

McCarthy, A., Curtis, K. and Holland, A.J., 2016. Paediatric trauma systems and their impact on the health outcomes of severely injured children: an integrative review. *Injury*, 47(3), 574–585.

Mitchell, R.J., Cameron, C.M. and McClure, R., 2016. Quantifying the hospitalised morbidity and mortality attributable to traumatic injury using a population-based matched cohort in Australia. *BMJ Open*, 6(12), e013266.

Rowbotham, S.K. and Blau, S., 2017. The circumstances and characteristics of fatal falls in Victoria, Australia: a descriptive study. *Australian Journal of Forensic Sciences*, 49(4), 403–420.

Sammy, I., Lecky, F., Sutton, A., Leaviss, J. and O'Cathain, A., 2016. Factors affecting mortality in older trauma patients – a systematic review and meta-analysis. *Injury*, 47(6), 1170–1183.

Stawicki, S.P., Kalra, S., Jones, C., Justiniano, C.F., Papadimos, T.J., Galwankar, S.C., Pappada, S.M., Feeney, J.J. and Evans, D.C., 2015. Comorbidity polypharmacy score and its clinical utility: a pragmatic practitioner's perspective. *Journal of Emergencies, Trauma, and Shock*, 8(4), 224.

Thim, T., Krarup, N.H.V., Grove, E.L., Rohde, C.V. and Løfgren, B., 2012. Initial assessment and treatment with the Airway, Breathing, Circulation, Disability, Exposure (ABCDE) approach. *International Journal of General Medicine*, 5, 117.

Tsuei, B.J. and Kearney, P.A., 2004. Hypothermia in the trauma patient. *Injury*, 35(1), 7–15.

Wang, H.E., Callaway, C.W., Peitzman, A.B. and Tisherman, S.A., 2005. Admission hypothermia and outcome after major trauma. *Critical Care Medicine*, 33(6), 1296–1301.

Wilson, C.T. and Clebone, A., 2014. Initial assessment and management of the trauma patient. In *Anesthesia for trauma*. New York: Springer, pp. 1–14.

Wright, J.L., 2015. Pediatric trauma priorities. In *Emergency medical services: clinical practice and systems oversight*, 2nd edn. New Jersey: Wiley, pp. 393–396.

Control of severe haemorrhage

Paul Burke

Chapter objectives

At the end of this chapter the reader will be able to:

1. Describe the rationale for controlling severe haemorrhage
2. Differentiate between compressible and non-compressible haemorrhages
3. Demonstrate arterial tourniquet use
4. Demonstrate haemostatic dressing use
5. Accurately report on findings

Resources required for this assessment

- Mannequin capable of simulating severe haemorrhage
- Arterial tourniquet
- Haemostatic dressing
- Disposable gloves and safety glasses
- Clinical waste bag
- Method of documenting results

Skill matrix

This assessment requires:
- Infection control (CS 1.3)
- Communication (CS 1.5)
- Consent (CS 1.6)
- Trauma assessment (CS 5.1)

This assessment is a component of:
- Trauma (Chapter 5)

Introduction

The patient with severe haemorrhage presents with imminent life threat, requiring urgent management. Bleeding or its consequences (including coagulopathy) are reported to be responsible for approximately 40% of trauma deaths (Curry et al., 2011). Following management of the airway, breathing and lack of circulation, haemorrhage control is a priority for primary survey. Guidelines on traumatic cardiac arrest manage haemorrhage before or at the same time as commencing chest compressions (Lockey et al., 2013). The prehospital management of severe haemorrhage, which is discussed in this chapter, aims to stop the haemorrhage long enough to get the patient to definitive surgical care.

Anatomy and physiology

Severe haemorrhage can be arterial or venous. Arterial bleeding is pulsatile and bright red in colour, while venous bleeding is non-pulsatile and a darker, maroon colour. Their distinction may indicate the urgency of the situation, as a patient with an arterial bleed will deteriorate into cardiac arrest faster than a patient with a venous bleed. This classification is useful when considering treatment options, allowing the paramedic to distinguish whether the haemorrhage is compressible or non-compressible.

All external bleeding should initially be managed by direct pressure, with other measures employed subsequently if the bleeding is not controlled (ANZCOR, 2017). Compressible bleeding is likely to involve the extremities, which are accessible and therefore allow external compression to be applied. Non-compressible bleeding, on the other hand, tends to originate in the torso and is significantly more challenging to manage (Kisat et al., 2013).

Clinical rationale

Identifying severe haemorrhage

Identifying patients suffering severe haemorrhage is not simple and requires clinical judgment. The Australian and New Zealand Committee on Resuscitation (ANZCOR) guideline suggests bleeding should be managed as severe or life threatening in scenarios involving:

- fully or partially amputated limbs proximal to the wrist or ankle
- shark attack, propeller cuts or similar mechanism resulting in major trauma
- bleeding that is not controlled by direct pressure
- patients showing signs of shock, further clarified as pale and sweaty with a heart rate >100 or capillary refill >2 seconds and/or with altered consciousness (ANZCOR, 2017).

While these criteria provide some guidance, they are not specific. The amount of blood visible at the scene is often reported on, but this is an unreliable way to estimate blood loss (Frank et al., 2010).

An Australian study showed that older age, greater experience and practising at higher clinical levels was associated with a greater belief by paramedics in their ability to estimate visible blood loss (Harris et al., 2017). This belief is potentially harmful, as it may lead to undertreatment of patients who are suffering severe haemorrhage or to overtreatment of those who are not.

While it is difficult to accurately assess the actual volume of blood loss, the presence of severe haemorrhage will be evident either from a combination of visual cues and presentation or during patient assessment through the discovery of wound/s and changes in vital signs.

Once the haemorrhage site is identified, classification of the wound as compressible or non-compressible will dictate the next step in treatment. For a compressible wound, direct pressure/dressing should be applied to the site (ANZCOR, 2017; Bulger et al., 2014). If the wound is non-compressible, or direct pressure is ineffective, treatment moves to the next step based on the anatomical location of the injury.

Arterial tourniquets

For severe limb wound haemorrhage, an arterial tourniquet should be applied proximal to the wound (ANZCOR, 2017; Bulger et al., 2014; Engle and Fruendt, 2017; Rossaint et al., 2016). If bleeding persists, a second tourniquet should be applied, ideally proximal to the first (ANZCOR, 2017; Engle and Fruendt, 2017).

The efficacy of arterial tourniquets has been established in military and now civilian use. There are several types of tourniquet available, with either a windlass or turnkey device working to tighten the tourniquet once it has been applied, allowing adjustment until blood flow is cut off.

Venous tourniquets will not generate adequate pressure to stop blood flow. In the absence of a commercially manufactured arterial tourniquet, an improvised tourniquet can be applied, ideally with a rod or stick inserted so that it can be tightened similarly to the windlass in commercial devices.

Haemostatic dressings

For severe haemorrhage from non-compressible wounds or if direct pressure is ineffective in locations that are not amenable to tourniquet placement, a haemostatic dressing should be applied (ANZCOR, 2017; Bulger et al., 2014; Engle and Fruendt, 2017).

As for arterial tourniquets, haemostatic dressings have migrated from military into civilian use. The dressings are impregnated with one of a number of chemicals that promote haemostasis. The two most common types contain either kaolin, a mineral-based compound, or chitosan derived from crustacean shells. Both types of dressing have been proven effective, and there is currently no clear recommendation for one type over the other.

The chemical is activated by contact with blood. The dressing must therefore be placed in contact with the bleeding vessel if possible, in order to stem the haemorrhage at its source.

Once a limb wound haemorrhage has been identified, and if direct pressure has failed (or is unable to be applied due to size or nature of the wound), an arterial tourniquet should be applied.

Applying a tourniquet

Prepare the patient

Ideally, tourniquets should not be applied until the limb and wound are fully exposed. Where possible, tourniquets should not be applied over clothing.

Apply tourniquet proximal to the wound

Wrap the tourniquet around the limb, proximal to the wound. Tourniquets can be applied partially assembled by looping them over a limb, taking care not to twist the band as it is passed over the limb. While there is no ideal distance proximal to the wound, contemporary guidelines recommend applying the tourniquet as close to it as possible, 5–7 cm above the wound (Engle and Fruendt, 2017; Queensland Ambulance Service, 2018).

Secure the tourniquet

Secure the tourniquet, tightening it to the point where fingers cannot be slipped between it and skin.

Tighten the tourniquet

Whether using a windlass or turnkey mechanism, tighten until bleeding stops or distal pulse is no longer palpable. Secure the mechanism (Fig. 5.2.1) and note the time the tourniquet was applied.

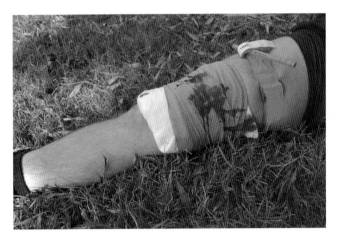

Figure 5.2.1 Application of an arterial tourniquet

Applying a haemostatic dressing

Where the haemorrhage is non-compressible and direct pressure has failed to control it, a haemostatic dressing should be applied.

Choose the correct dressing

The options available for haemostatic dressing include rolled gauze and pads of various sizes. Rolled gauze is ideal for small or multiple penetrating wounds, such as stab wounds or small-calibre gunshot wounds. Small pads suit small, non-life-threatening wounds or haemorrhages such as nose bleeds (although nasal tampons are purpose-built dressings for these types of bleeds). Large pads suit large, open wounds such as shotgun blasts or significant explosive injuries that require large surface area packing.

Clean out the wound

Before applying the haemostatic dressing, clean out any pooled blood with regular gauze. This maximises the chance of direct contact with the dressing at the site of the bleeding. Actively bleeding wounds pool again quickly, so a rapid transition should be made between cleaning out the wound and placing the haemostatic dressing in situ.

Insert the dressing

The chemicals in haemostatic dressings require contact with blood to activate the haemostatic mechanism and assist with clotting. Dressings placed on the wound surface will not stop bleeding at the source. They must be actively and invasively inserted into the wound to activate clotting at the source of the bleeding. This involves the paramedic gathering an amount of dressing at the wound entry point and driving their fingers or whole hand (depending on hole size) into the wound, to push the dressing as close as possible to the site of the bleeding. For multiple smaller wounds, the rolled gauze can be unrolled and lengths inserted into each wound.

Pack the wound

The wound should then be packed with the remaining dressing as compactly as possible. Direct pressure is then applied for 2–3 minutes, to ensure the dressing controls the haemorrhage effectively.

Clinical skill assessment process

The following section outlines the clinical skill assessment tools that should be used to determine a student's ability to demonstrate the control of severe haemorrhage.
1. Clinical Skill Work Instruction
2. Formative Clinical Skill Assessment (F-CSAT)
3. Performance Improvement Plan (PIP)
4. Summative Clinical Skill Assessment (S-CSAT)
(5. Direct Observation of Procedural Skills (DOPS) – see Chapter 1.1)

Clinical Skill Work Instruction

Equipment and resources: Mannequin capable of simulating severe haemorrhage; arterial tourniquet; haemostatic dressing; disposable gloves and safety glasses; clinical waste bag; method of documenting results

Associated Clinical Skills: Infection control; Communication; Consent; Trauma assessment

Control of severe haemorrhage

Activity	Critical Action	Rationale
Personal protection	Don gloves and eyewear as minimum PPE.	Contact with blood is high risk.
Prepare patient	Place the patient supine. Explain the procedure.	Placing the patient supine reduces the risk of further bleeding.
Assess injury	Expose relevant part of the patient, maintaining their dignity as appropriate. Identify severe haemorrhage. Apply direct dressing/pressure to wound.	Failing to expose the wound potentially impacts ability to control haemorrhage.

Control of severe haemorrhage continued

Activity	Critical Action	Rationale
Compressible limb wound: Apply arterial tourniquet	Identify compressible limb wound that is not responding to direct pressure. Select arterial tourniquet.	Incorrect wound assessment may lead to inappropriate management.
	Apply tourniquet around limb proximal to the wound. Tighten until fingers cannot be slipped between the tourniquet and the skin.	Ensures tightening of device will be quickly and effectively achieved.
	Use tightening mechanism to stop bleeding and/or cut off peripheral pulse.	Stopping arterial flow is indicative of ceasing blood flow to the limb and stopping haemorrhage.
Non-compressible wound: Apply appropriate dressing	Identify non-compressible wound. Select haemostatic dressing.	Incorrect assessment of wound may lead to inappropriate management.
	Clean out wound and apply appropriate type of haemostatic dressing based on type of wound/s.	Dressing needs direct contact with wound. Different haemostatic dressings are appropriate for different wounds.
	Insert dressing into wound as far as possible to activate haemostatic chemical at site of bleed. Pack remaining dressing into wound.	Failing to insert dressing appropriately reduces the effectiveness of the haemostatic agent.
Reassess	Confirm haemorrhage has ceased.	Provides indication that primary survey issue is being managed.
Ongoing care	Identify reassessment points: if used, tourniquet is visible; reassess after each patient movement. If bleeding continues, apply second tourniquet proximal to first. For dressing, observe wound. If bleeding continues, remove dressing and replace in same manner. Consider analgesia.	Ongoing reassessment is required.
Report	Record/hand over details of wound, blood loss and control applied.	Accurate record kept and continuity of patient care.

Formative Clinical Skill Assessment (F-CSAT)

Equipment and resources: Mannequin capable of simulating severe haemorrhage; arterial tourniquet; haemostatic dressing; disposable gloves and safety glasses; clinical waste bag; method of documenting results

Associated Clinical Skills: Infection control; Communication; Consent; Trauma assessment

Staff/Student being assessed: _____

Control of severe haemorrhage

Activity	Critical Action	Participant Performance				
Personal protection	Dons gloves and eyewear as minimum PPE.	0	1	2	3	4
Prepares patient	Places patient supine. Explains procedure.	0	1	2	3	4

Control of severe haemorrhage continued

Activity	Critical Action	Participant Performance				
Assesses injury	Exposes relevant part of patient, maintaining patient's dignity as appropriate. Identifies severe haemorrhage. Applies direct dressing/pressure to wound.	0	1	2	3	4
Compressible limb wound: Applies tourniquet	Identifies compressible limb wound that is not responding to direct pressure. Selects arterial tourniquet.	0	1	2	3	4
	Applies tourniquet around limb proximal to wound. Tightens until fingers cannot be slipped between tourniquet and the skin.	0	1	2	3	4
	Utilises tightening mechanism to stop bleeding and/or cut off peripheral pulse.	0	1	2	3	4
Non-compressible wound: Applies appropriate dressing	Identifies non-compressible wound. Selects haemostatic dressing.	0	1	2	3	4
	Cleans out wound and applies appropriate type of haemostatic dressing based on wound/s type.	0	1	2	3	4
	Inserts dressing into wound as far as possible to activate haemostatic chemical at site of bleed. Packs remaining dressing into wound.	0	1	2	3	4
Reassesses	Confirms haemorrhage has ceased.	0	1	2	3	4
Ongoing care	Identifies reassessment points – if used, tourniquet is visible; reassesses after each patient movement. If bleeding continues, applies second tourniquet proximal to first. For dressing, observes wound. If bleeding continues, removes dressing and replaces it in same manner. Considers analgesia.	0	1	2	3	4
Reports	Records/hands over details of wound, blood loss and control applied.	0	1	2	3	4

Standard Achieved: (please circle one)

Competent (C)   Not Yet Competent* (NYC)

Staff/Student Name: _____

Assessor (please print name): _____

Signed (Assessor): _____

Date of Assessment: _____

Comments:

*If Not Yet Competent (NYC) a PIP needs to be completed and a repeat of the F-CSAT

Formative Clinical Skill Assessment (F-CSAT) Key

Skill level	Standard of procedure	Quality of performance	Outcome	Level of assistance required
4 Safe for unsupervised practice	Safe Accurate Behaviour is appropriate to context	Confident Accurate Expedient	Achieved intended outcome	No supporting cues*required
3 Requires supervision	Safe Accurate Behaviour is appropriate to context	Confident Accurate Takes longer than required	Achieved intended outcome	Requires occasional supportive cues*
2 Requires assistance	Safe Accurate Behaviour generally appropriate to context	Lacks certainty	Would not have achieved outcome without support	Requires frequent verbal and occasional physical directives in addition to supportive cues*
1 Requires direction	Safe only with guidance Not completely accurate	Unskilled Inefficient	Would not have achieved outcome without support	Requires continuous verbal and frequent physical directive cues*
0 Unsafe	Unsafe Unable to demonstrate behaviour Lack of insight into behaviour appropriate to context	Unskilled	Would not have achieved outcome	Requires continuous verbal and continuous physical directive cues*

*Refers to physical directives or verbal supportive cues

Performance Improvement Plan (PIP)

Please document the agreed education plan and completion timelines for areas assessed as less than 4.

This plan should be presented to assessor prior to commencement of summative assessment.

Where was supervisor support required?	Student summary of deficit. (Why was there a problem?)	Improvement Plan	Completed (Y/N)

Staff/Student Name: _____

Staff/Student Signature: _____

Educator Name: _____

Educator Signature: _____

Summative Clinical Skill Assessment (S-CSAT)

Equipment and resources: Mannequin capable of simulating severe haemorrhage; arterial tourniquet; haemostatic dressing; disposable gloves and safety glasses; clinical waste bag; method of documenting results

Associated Clinical Skills: Infection control; Communication; Consent; Trauma assessment

Staff/Student being assessed: _____

- Completed Formative Clinical Skill Assessment (F-CSAT):   **YES   NO**
- Completed Performance Improvement Plan (PIP):   **YES   NO   N/A**

Control of severe haemorrhage

Activity	Critical Action	Achieved Without Direction	
Personal protection	Dons gloves and eyewear as minimum PPE.	NO	YES
Prepares patient	Places patient supine. Explains procedure.	NO	YES
Assesses injury	Exposes relevant part of patient, maintaining patient's dignity as appropriate. Identifies severe haemorrhage. Applies direct dressing/ pressure to wound.	NO	YES
Compressible limb wound: Applies tourniquet	Identifies compressible limb wound that is not responding to direct pressure. Selects arterial tourniquet.	NO	YES
	Applies tourniquet around the limb proximal to wound. Tightens until fingers cannot be slipped between tourniquet and the skin.	NO	YES
	Utilises tightening mechanism to stop bleeding and/or cut off peripheral pulse.	NO	YES
Non-compressible wound: Applies appropriate dressing	Identifies non-compressible wound. Selects haemostatic dressing.	NO	YES
	Cleans out wound and applies appropriate type of haemostatic dressing based on wound/s type.	NO	YES
	Inserts dressing into wound as far as possible to activate haemostatic chemical at site of bleed. Packs remaining dressing into wound.	NO	YES
Reassesses	Confirms haemorrhage has ceased.	NO	YES
Ongoing care	Identifies reassessment points – if used, tourniquet is visible; reassesses after each patient movement. If bleeding continues, applies second tourniquet proximal to first. For dressing, observes wound. If bleeding continues, removes dressing and replaces it in same manner. Considers analgesia.	NO	YES
Reports	Records/hands over details of wound, blood loss and control applied.	NO	YES

Standard Achieved: (please circle one)

Competent (C)   Not Yet Competent* (NYC)

Staff/Student Name: _____

Assessor (please print name): _____

Signed (Assessor): _____

Date of Assessment: _____

Comments:

*If Not Yet Competent (NYC) a PIP needs to be completed and a repeat of the F-CSAT

Clinical findings

Persistent bleeding

If bleeding persists after a first tourniquet has been applied, confirm the tightness of the tourniquet. If it is correct, a second tourniquet should be applied, ideally proximal to the first, following the same method.

Where a haemostatic dressing has been applied, reassess the wound. If the bleeding is controlled, place a clean, sterile dressing (gauze or a combination) over the top of the wound and secure it. If the bleeding is not controlled, the haemostatic dressing must be completely removed and a second haemostatic dressing inserted as for the original, as close as possible to the site of the bleeding. To be effective, haemostatic dressings must be in immediate contact with the source of the bleeding.

All wounds need to be periodically reassessed to ensure bleeding remains controlled.

Ongoing tourniquet care

The key points for ongoing care of the tourniquet are as follows:

- The tourniquet must be visible once applied and not covered by dressings or clothing.
- Once applied, tourniquets should not be removed until definitive haemorrhage control care arrives.
- The exception is if the tourniquet was initially applied because there were multiple patients and the available resources were overwhelmed. If it is anticipated that the wound can be controlled using basic haemorrhage control measures, a trial removal may occur to manage the bleeding with direct pressure and dressings. If removing the tourniquet proves unsuccessful, replace it rapidly and make no further attempts at removal.

- The tourniquet and wound should be checked every time the patient is moved to ensure bleeding has not recommenced.
- Conscious patients may require analgesia to tolerate the tourniquet.
- If the tourniquet is in situ for a prolonged period, prepare to manage potential crush injury on its removal.

Pacagnella et al. (2013) concluded there are no specific vital signs findings that correlate to the volume of blood loss. However, vital signs change as bleeding progresses, and the shock index (heart rate divided by systolic blood pressure) is an accurate indicator of blood loss compensation.

PRACTICE TIP!

Severe haemorrhage is a primary survey issue. It overrides progression to secondary assessment items and requires management as an urgent priority.

PRACTICE TIP!

Regularly practising the physical skills and decision making involved in high-stress, low-volume cases such as severe haemorrhage can make it easier to manage these events and make them less stressful when they are encountered.

PRACTICE TIP!

Heavy clothing, and especially dark-coloured material, can soak up and camouflage significant blood loss. Similarly, it may be more challenging to identify bleeding in dark environments or in patients with dark skin. For trauma patients, particularly those presenting in a state of altered consciousness, particularly following trauma, complete a thorough, palpable, head-to-toe assessment, with appropriate exposure, to identify any concealed wounds. Inspect your gloves for blood that may not be visible.

PRACTICE TIP!

Severe haemorrhage carries a high risk of contamination by body fluid. Paramedics must approach with appropriate PPE and decontaminate themselves thoroughly afterwards.

TEST YOUR KNOWLEDGE QUESTIONS

1. **What are the classifications of severe haemorrhage that guide treatment?**
   Compressible or non-compressible.

2. **What is the initial treatment for all haemorrhage?**
   Direct pressure.

3. **What is the likely site of a compressible haemorrhage?**
   Accessible limb wounds.

4. **What is the likely site of a non-compressible haemorrhage?**
   Usually torso wounds, or an inaccessible wound.

5. **How is the volume of blood loss assessed?**
   A combination of visual cues, patient presentation and vital signs (specifically, shock index) may indicate severe haemorrhage.

6. **Where should an arterial tourniquet be positioned?**
   Proximal to the injury. There is no ideal distance, but recommendations include 5–7 cm or as close as possible.

7. **What is the correct action to take if the tourniquet does not stop the bleeding?**
   Apply another tourniquet, ideally proximal to the first one.

8. **What is the correct method of haemostatic dressing application?**
   Insert the dressing into the wound to contact the site of bleeding directly, so that the haemostatic agent activates.

9. **What is the definitive management of severe haemorrhage?**
   Surgery. Even if the bleeding is controlled, patients need urgent transport to hospital.

10. **Which patients may have severe haemorrhage that is not obvious?**
    Patients wearing heavy, dark clothing; patients in dark environments; patients with dark skin.

References

Anzcor (Australian and New Zealand Committee on Resuscitation), 2017. *ANZCOR Guideline 9.1.1: First aid for management of bleeding.* Retrieved from https://resus.org.au/guidelines

Bulger, E.M., Snyder, D., Schoelles, K., Gotschall, C., Dawson, D., Lang, E., Sanddal, N.D., Butler, F.K., Fallat, M., Taillac, P., Salomone, J.P., Seifarth, W., Betzner, M.J., Johannigman, J. and McSwain, N., 2014. An evidence-based prehospital guideline for external hemorrhage control: American College of Surgeons Committee on Trauma. *Prehospital Emergency Care*, 18, 163–173.

Curry, N., Hopewell, S., Dorée, C., Hyde, C., Brohi, K. and Stanworth, S., 2011. The acute management of trauma haemorrhage: a systematic review of randomized controlled trials. *Critical Care*, 15, R92.

Engle, W. and Fruendt, J.C., 2017. *Tactical combat casualty care handbook*, version 5. Kansas: Centre for Army Lessons Learned (CALL).

Frank, M., Schmucker, U., Stengel, D., Fischer, L., Lange, J., Grossjohann, R., Ekkernkamp, A. and Matthes, G., 2010. Proper estimation of blood loss on scene of trauma: tool or tale? *Journal of Trauma, Injury, Infection and Critical Care*, 69(5), 1191–1195.

Harris, W., Rotheram, A., Pearson, S., Lucas, P., Edwards, D., Bowerman, L. and Williams, A.M., 2017. Paramedic confidence in estimating external blood loss. *Australasian Journal of Paramedicine*, 14(3).

Lockey, D.J., Lyon, R.M. and Davies, G.E., 2013. Development of a simple algorithm to guide the effective management of traumatic cardiac arrest. *Resuscitation*, 84, 738–742.

Kisat, M., Morrison, J.J., Hashmi, Z.G., Efron, D.T., Rasmussen, T.E. and Haider, A.H., 2013. Epidemiology and outcomes of non-compressible torso haemorrhage. *Journal of Surgical Research*, 184, 414–421.

Pacagnella, R.C., Souza, J.P., Durocher, J., Perel, P., Blum, J., Winikoff, B. and Gülmezoglu, A.H., 2013. A systematic review of the relationship between blood loss and clinical signs. *PLOS ONE*, 8(3), e57594.

Queensland Ambulance Service, 2018. *Clinical practice guidelines.* Retrieved from: https://www.ambulance.qld.gov.au/docs/clinical/cpp/CPP_Arterial%20tourniquet.pdf

Rossaint, R., Bouillon, B., Cerny, V., Coats, T.J., Duranteau, J., Fernández-Mondéjar, E., Filipescu, D., Hunt, B.J., Komadina, R., Nardi, G., Neugebauer, E.A.M., Ozier, Y., Riddez, L., Schultz, A., Vincent, J.L. and Spahn, D.R., 2016. The European guideline on management of major bleeding and coagulopathy following trauma, 4th edn. *Critical Care*, 20, 100.

5.3 | Chest decompression

Matt Rose

Chapter objectives

At the end of this chapter the reader will be able to:

1. Describe the anatomy and physiology related to chest trauma
2. Define simple and tension pneumothorax
3. Identify the signs and symptoms of tension pneumothorax
4. Perform a needle decompression

Resources required for this assessment

- Standardised mannequin suited to chest trauma
- Hand decontamination agent
- Disposable gloves, safety glasses, face mask
- High-concentration oxygen therapy
- Large-bore 14G IV cannula
- Alcohol wipes, adhesive dressings
- Clinical waste bag
- Sharps container
- Method of documenting results

Skill matrix

This assessment requires:
- Infection control (CS 1.3)
- Communication (CS1.5)
- Consent (CS 1.6)
- Using Antiseptic Non Touch Technique (ANTT®) (CS 2.20)
- Trauma assessment (CS 5.1)

This assessment is a component of:
- Trauma (Chapter 5)

Introduction

Chest injuries are a leading cause of traumatic deaths in Australia and New Zealand (Curtis et al., 2012). Thoracic trauma is responsible for 25% of all trauma deaths and contributes to a further 25% of traumatic deaths (Cameron et al., 2014).

Identifying chest injuries forms a core component of major trauma patient assessment. This chapter discusses the anatomy and physiology relevant to thoracic trauma, pneumothorax, tension pneumothorax and needle chest decompression.

Anatomy and physiology

The thoracic cavity is surrounded by the thoracic cage, which is comprised of the sternum, ribs, thoracic spine, back and chest musculature, and bordered at its base by the diaphragm (Marieb and Hoehn, 2013). It contains the lungs, tracheobronchial tree, oesophagus, heart and other major vascular structures. It further divides into two pleural cavities, each surrounding a lung, the mediastinum and the pericardial cavity, which contains the heart (Martini et al., 2012).

The pleural cavities are lined by a thin, double-layered serous pleural membrane, the inner chest wall (parietal pleura) and the lung surfaces (visceral pleura) (Marieb and Hoehn, 2013). A clear, serous fluid separates and lubricates the pleurae.

A slight negative pressure within the intrapleural space keeps the external lung surface in contact with the interior aspect of the chest wall. Without this negative pressure, the spongy and elastic lung tissue would recoil and collapse (Marieb and Hoehn, 2013). During inspiration, expansion of the pleural cavity reduces intrapulmonary pressure, causing atmospheric air to rush in, inflating the lung and pushing the inner pleura against the outer pleura. During expiration, chest recoil reduces lung size, venting air to the atmosphere and pressing the outer pleura towards the inner pleura (Marieb and Hoehn, 2013).

Clinical rationale

Pneumothorax

Blunt or penetrating trauma can breach either pleural layer, allowing air and/or blood to enter the intrapleural space (Curtis and Ramsden, 2016). If pleural volume increases, lung volume decreases, reducing gas exchange and causing hypoxia.

Blunt trauma may result in laceration through rib fracture, while penetrating trauma may directly lacerate the visceral pleura. If the volume of air entering is self-limiting, or exits at the same rate as it enters, simple pneumothorax results (Curtis and Ramsden, 2016).

Tension pneumothorax

Tension pneumothorax is a life-threatening emergency requiring immediate intervention via a chest tube or needle decompression. It occurs when a breach in the pleura forms a 'one-way valve', whereby air enters the pleural cavity but cannot be released (Cameron et al., 2014). It may be caused by laceration to lung tissue or an open chest wall injury, allowing air entry into the intrapleural space.

Tension pneumothorax can cause rapid deterioration, shock and death. The progressive increase of air trapped in the intrapleural space compresses the lung, increasing respiratory distress and hypoxia (Curtis and Ramsden, 2016). A continued increase in pressure exerts force on nearby structures, including the heart, trachea and vena cava. This pressure on the vena cava reduces venous return to the heart, causing a rapid deterioration to cardiogenic shock and cardiac arrest (Curtis and Ramsden, 2016).

Presentation

A patient with tension pneumothorax typically presents with reduced or absent breath sounds on the affected side, signs of shock and evidence of blunt or penetrating thoracic injury (Curtis and Ramsden, 2016). The lateral chest and anterior axilla can be auscultated to avoid misinterpretation of transmitted lung sounds (Lee et al., 2007).

Alternatively, patients can present in an altered conscious state accompanying respiratory failure. In such cases, they will usually require assisted ventilation using positive pressure methods. The implementation of this essential and lifesaving intervention can greatly increase the likelihood of pneumothorax becoming tension pneumothorax, causing hypotension and eventuating in cardiac arrest (Roberts et al., 2015).

If there is any suspicion of tension pneumothorax associated with difficulty in breathing and hypotension, needle chest decompression is recommended, with the benefits outweighing the risks (Aylwin et al., 2008; Blackwell, 2016). Low SpO_2 despite supplemental oxygen is a strong sign that tension pneumothorax may be present (Blackwell, 2016). Needle decompression is part of traumatic cardiac arrest resuscitation (Mistry et al., 2009).

The following may indicate traumatic tension pneumothorax (Roberts et al., 2015). Less reliable/detectable signs (present in fewer than 10% of cases) are:
- distended jugular veins
- surgical emphysema (more common during assisted ventilation)
- asymmetry of chest
- absent or hyper-resonant chest sounds on the affected side (more common during assisted ventilation
- tracheal deviation (uncommon and very late).

More reliable/detectable signs (present in greater than 30% of cases) are:
- chest pain
- increasing respiratory distress/dyspnoea
- complaining of shortness of breath
- decreasing perfusion (particularly or worsening with assisted ventilation)
- decreasing conscious state.

Management

Provide high-flow oxygen; waiting for decreasing SpO_2 can be detrimental. Position the patient upright if perfusion allows. Ensure an intensive-care paramedic is present to provide back up. IV access should not delay needle chest decompression.

Needle decompression

The fastest and easiest procedure for decompressing tension pneumothorax is needle decompression ('needle thoracostomy'). A large-bore IV cannula, 14G and 45 mm long, is inserted into the affected side in the second intercostal space at the mid-clavicular line (Fig. 5.3.1) to allow air release (Curtis and Ramsden, 2016; Welch and Saltarelli, 2018; Wernick et al., 2015). A 16G, 30 mm cannula is preferred for children <8 years.

At times, 45 mm needles may not be long enough to penetrate the chest wall to the pleura (Ball et al., 2010; Clemency et al., 2015; Greene and Callaway, 2016; Kaserer et al., 2017; Laan et al., 2016; Wernick et al., 2015). Increased body mass increases the needle length required, with the obese requiring a 6–8 cm needle (Aho et al., 2016; Ozen et al., 2016; Powers et al., 2014).

Inserting a needle into the chest carries a risk of haemorrhage. The internal mammary artery, subclavian

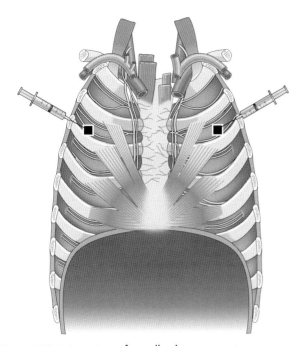

Figure 5.3.1 Location of needle decompression

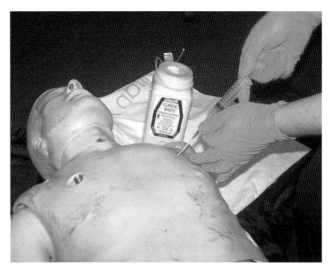

Figure 5.3.2 Set-up for syringe/cannula

and intercostal vessels and pulmonary artery are vulnerable (Wernick et al., 2015). Poorly angled, the needle can injure the heart (Zahoor et al., 2015). Insertion must not be medial of the mid-clavicular line and not above the second intercostal space. Further, it must be immediately above the third rib due to the location of the intercostal artery along the inferior rib surface.

The needle must be inserted 90° to the chest wall, angled towards the patient's spine (Fig. 5.3.2). The chest wall provides considerable resistance. An initial scalpel incision can be made if necessary. It can be difficult to hold a long IV needle and provide sufficient insertion force. If the insertion is successful, a rush of air escaping may be heard as the needle is withdrawn.

Alternatively, to allow sufficient needle force, attach a 10 mL syringe to the distal IV cannula end to form a handle. Prefill the syringe with a few millilitres of sterile saline or water to allow the plunger to be withdrawn during insertion. Air should bubble back once the needle enters the pleural space.

Alternative needle insertion sites include the fourth or fifth intercostal space in the mid-axillary line and the anterior axillary line (Bach and Sølling, 2015; Chang et al., 2014; Greene and Callaway, 2016; Inaba et al., 2015; Laan et al., 2016; Welch and Saltarelli, 2018; Wernick et al., 2015). Though these sites are arguably more reliable

for decompression, there is conflicting evidence regarding needle failure during patient movement (Leatherman et al., 2017; Zahoor et al., 2015).

There is also a risk of iatrogenic cardiac injury at these sites, and the safety of using long needles is in question (Lesperance et al., 2018). Arm adduction on the affected side is necessary to allow access to the chest. Finger thoracostomy is often preferred at these sites to ensure safe decompression. The advantages of these sites are widely recognised and their use is increasingly advocated, including in the paediatric patient where the risk of myocardial injury is greater at the second intercostal space site (Galvagno et al., 2019; Rashid, 2018; Terboven et al., 2019).

Despite the urgency of the situation, ensure asepsis (Aylwin et al., 2008) and the safe disposal of sharps, including containers that are sufficiently deep for long needles. Secure the cannula in place with adhesive dressings, ensuring it cannot kink.

Clinical skill assessment process

The following section outlines the clinical skill assessment tools that should be used to determine a student's ability to demonstrate safe and accurate chest decompression.
1. Clinical Skill Work Instruction
2. Formative Clinical Skill Assessment (F-CSAT)
3. Performance Improvement Plan (PIP)
4. Summative Clinical Skill Assessment (S-CSAT)
(5. Direct Observation of Procedural Skills (DOPS) – see Chapter 1.1)

Clinical Skill Work Instruction

Equipment and resources: Standardised mannequin for chest trauma; hand decontamination agent; disposable gloves, safety glasses and face mask; high-concentration oxygen therapy; large-bore 14G IV cannula; alcohol wipes and adhesive dressings; clinical waste bag; sharps container; method of documenting results

Associated Clinical Skills: Infection control; Communication; Consent, Using ANTT®; Trauma assessment

Chest decompression

Activity	Critical Action	Rationale
PPE	Don gloves, safety glasses, respiratory mask.	Infection control.
Confirm tension pneumothorax	State signs and symptoms, indicating tension pneumothorax.	Identify when the procedure is required.
Oxygen therapy	Administer high-concentration oxygen therapy (or ensure assisted ventilation is occurring if patient is in respiratory failure).	To increase the inspired oxygen fraction.
Prepare patient	Sufficiently expose the chest. Patient can be positioned sitting upright or supine. Explain procedure. Obtain informed consent.	Unhindered chest visualisation allows for both assessment and location of the insertion site. Despite the life-threatening nature of the injury, consent is not assumed if the patient is conscious.
Prepare equipment	Attach 14G cannula (16G if <8 years) to 10 mL syringe containing 3–4 mL saline.	To reach pleural space. Provides a handle.
Locate insertion site	Palpate second intercostal space at the mid-clavicular line (above the third rib), or alternatively the fifth intercostal space at mid- or anterior axillary line if used. Adduct patient's arm to allow access.	Allows effective needle decompression. Reduces risk of piercing the neurovascular bundle or heart.
Prepare site	Swab with alcohol-based wipe or equivalent. Allow to dry.	To decrease risk of infection.
Insert needle	Insert needle into skin at 90° to the chest wall immediately above third rib. Proceed until a 'give' is felt or air bubbles are observed in syringe. Have colleague observe findings.	Directs the needle towards the intrapleural space. The 'give' and/or air bubbles indicate entry into the parietal pleura.
Remove needle	Leave cannula in place. Remove needle and discard.	Allows for continued air release.
Secure catheter	Secure cannula to chest with adhesive dressings, ensuring not to kink or block it.	Reduces the risk of blocking catheter.
Monitor patient	Reassess patient for signs of improvement.	To ensure procedure has been successful.
Report	Accurately document/hand over details of indications, procedure and responses.	Accurate record kept and continuity of patient care.

Formative Clinical Skill Assessment (F-CSAT)

Equipment and resources: Standardised mannequin for chest trauma; hand decontamination agent; disposable gloves, safety glasses and face mask; high-concentration oxygen therapy; large-bore 14G IV cannula; alcohol wipes and adhesive dressings; clinical waste bag; sharps container; method of documenting results

Associated Clinical Skills: Infection control; Communication; Consent, Using ANTT®; Trauma assessment

Staff/Student being assessed: _____

Chest decompression

Activity	Critical Action	Performance				
PPE	Dons PPE.	0	1	2	3	4
Confirms tension pneumothorax	States signs and symptoms indicating tension pneumothorax.	0	1	2	3	4
Oxygen therapy	Administers high-concentration oxygen therapy (or ensures assisted ventilation occurring if patient is in respiratory failure).	0	1	2	3	4
Prepares patient	Sufficiently exposes chest. Explains procedure. Obtains informed consent.	0	1	2	3	4
Prepares equipment	Attaches 14G cannula to 10 mL syringe containing 3–4 mL saline.	0	1	2	3	4
Locates insertion site	Palpates second intercostal space at the mid-clavicular line (above the third rib), or alternatively the fifth intercostal space at mid- or anterior axillary line if used. Adducts patient's arm to allow access.	0	1	2	3	4
Prepares site	Swabs with alcohol-based wipe or equivalent. Allows to dry.	0	1	2	3	4
Inserts needle	Inserts needle into the skin at 90° to the chest in the lower part of the intercostal space. Proceeds until a 'give' is felt or a release of air is observed. Has colleague observe findings.	0	1	2	3	4
Removes needle	Leaves cannula in place. Removes needle and discards.	0	1	2	3	4
Secures catheter	Secures cannula to chest, ensuring not to kink or block it.	0	1	2	3	4
Monitors patient	Reassesses patient for signs of improvement.	0	1	2	3	4
Reports	Accurately documents/hands over details of indications, procedure and responses.	0	1	2	3	4

Standard Achieved: (please circle one)

Competent (C)   Not Yet Competent* (NYC)

Staff/Student: _____

Assessor (please print name)**:** _____

Signed (Assessor)**:** _____

Date of Assessment: _____

Comments:

*If Not Yet Competent (NYC) a PIP needs to be completed and a repeat of the F-CSAT

Formative Clinical Skill Assessment (F-CSAT) Key

Skill level	Standard of procedure	Quality of performance	Outcome	Level of assistance required
4 Safe for unsupervised practice	Safe Accurate Behaviour is appropriate to context	Confident Accurate Expedient	Achieved intended outcome	No supporting cues*required
3 Requires supervision	Safe Accurate Behaviour is appropriate to context	Confident Accurate Takes longer than required	Achieved intended outcome	Requires occasional supportive cues*
2 Requires assistance	Safe Accurate Behaviour generally appropriate to context	Lacks certainty	Would not have achieved outcome without support	Requires frequent verbal and occasional physical directives in addition to supportive cues*
1 Requires direction	Safe only with guidance Not completely accurate	Unskilled Inefficient	Would not have achieved outcome without support	Requires continuous verbal and frequent physical directive cues*
0 Unsafe	Unsafe Unable to demonstrate behaviour Lack of insight into behaviour appropriate to context	Unskilled	Would not have achieved outcome	Requires continuous verbal and continuous physical directive cues*

*Refers to physical directives or verbal supportive cues

Performance Improvement Plan (PIP)

Please document the agreed education plan and completion timelines for areas assessed as less than 4.

This plan should be presented to assessor prior to commencement of summative assessment.

Where was supervisor support required?	Student summary of deficit. (Why was there a problem?)	Improvement Plan	Completed (Y/N)

Staff/Student Name: _____

Staff/Student Signature: _____

Educator Name: _____

Educator Signature: _____

Summative Clinical Skill Assessment (S-CSAT)

Equipment and resources: Standardised mannequin for chest trauma; hand decontamination agent; disposable gloves, safety glasses, face mask; high-concentration oxygen therapy; large-bore 14G IV cannula; alcohol wipes and adhesive dressings; clinical waste bag; sharps container; method of documenting results

Associated Clinical Skills: Infection control; Communication; Consent, Using ANTT®; Trauma assessment

Staff/Student being assessed: _____

- Completed Formative Clinical Skill Assessment (F-CSAT):   **YES**   **NO**
- Completed Performance Improvement Plan (PIP):   **YES**   **NO**   **N/A**

Chest decompression

Activity	Critical Action	Achieved Without Direction	
PPE	Dons PPE.	NO	YES
Confirms tension pneumothorax	States signs and symptoms indicating tension pneumothorax.	NO	YES
Oxygen therapy	Administers high-concentration oxygen therapy (or ensures assisted ventilation occurring if patient is in respiratory failure).	NO	YES
Prepares patient	Sufficiently exposes chest. Explains procedure. Obtains informed consent.	NO	YES
Prepares equipment	Attaches 14G cannula to 10 mL syringe containing 3–4 mL saline.	NO	YES
Locates insertion site	Palpates second intercostal space at the mid-clavicular line (above the third rib), or alternatively fifth intercostal space at mid- or anterior axillary line if used. Adducts patient's arm to allow access.	NO	YES

Chest decompression continued

Activity	Critical Action	Achieved Without Direction	
Prepares site	Swabs with alcohol-based wipe or equivalent. Allows to dry.	NO	YES
Inserts needle	Inserts needle into the skin at 90° to the chest in the lower part of the intercostal space. Proceeds until a 'give' is felt or a release of air is heard. Has colleague observe findings.	NO	YES
Removes needle	Leaves cannula in place. Removes needle and discards.	NO	YES
Secures catheter	Secures cannula to chest, ensuring not to kink or block.	NO	YES
Monitors patient	Reassesses patient for signs of improvement.	NO	YES
Reports	Accurately documents/hands over details of indications, procedure and responses.	NO	YES

Standard Achieved: (please circle one)

Competent (C)   Not Yet Competent* (NYC)

Staff/Student Name: _____

Assessor (please print name)**:** _____

Signed (Assessor)**:** _____

Date of Assessment: _____

Comments:

*If Not Yet Competent (NYC) a PIP needs to be completed and a repeat of the F-CSAT

Clinical findings

Needle/catheter decompression should release air from the pneumothorax, improving perfusion as venous return increases and respiration as air entry increases. Following the insertion of the needle, air may be heard to escape (Ball et al., 2010) or may bubble in the syringe; a small amount of blood may escape too.

No improvement in patient condition

A lack of improvement in the patient's condition following the procedure may indicate that the presentation was not a result of a tension pneumothorax.

It could also mean the needle length was insufficient or that it was incorrectly inserted. Removal and reinsertion is the only option in such event. If it was not secured correctly, the original catheter may have partly withdrawn and stopped working.

The catheter may kink after the needle is removed, or become blocked by a clot of blood or plug of tissue (Jones and Hollingsworth, 2002). In such cases, flush the catheter with a few millilitres of sterile saline to unplug it.

Air may enter the pleural space quicker than it can escape via the needle, thereby maintaining the tension within the pleural space (Jones and Hollingsworth, 2002). This more commonly occurs during positive pressure ventilation where air is forced into the lungs under pressure (Wernick et al., 2015).

Bilateral tension pneumothorax may be encountered, which may be difficult to differentiate from a single-sided injury. It can also sometimes be difficult to identify which side the injury is on. Injury to the second lung can explain why there is little or no response to the initial management. Where the injury side is uncertain or both lungs are believed affected, decompress both sides. Bilateral decompression should be initiated on the right side first. Right-sided tension pneumothorax can shift the mediastinum towards the left. Since the heart sits predominantly in the left chest, any further movement places it at risk during left needle decompression.

Bleeding from catheter

Blood loss can be caused by an incorrect method of needle insertion (Rawlins et al., 2003; Wernick et al., 2015). If a significant amount of blood escapes from the catheter, cap it to stem the blood loss.

PRACTICE TIP!

Each rib has a neurovascular bundle, containing nerves, arteries and lymph vessels, running along its inferoposterior surface. Aiming just above the third rib superior surface limits the chances of piercing this bundle.

PRACTICE TIP!

There are five steps to correctly inserting a decompression needle:

1. Second intercostal space; 2. Mid-clavicular line; 3. Above the rib below; 4. Right angle to the chest wall; 5. Towards the spine (the chest wall is curved – angle the needle slightly to compensate).

PRACTICE TIP!

Assess for tension pneumothorax in all blunt or penetrating thoracic or multi-trauma, especially if the patient has increasing respiratory distress and poor perfusion.

PRACTICE TIP!

Tension pneumothorax decompression treats an immediate threat to life and must be performed expediently.

PRACTICE TIP!

Always wear suitable PPE when attending traumatic injuries, due to the risk of exposure to bodily fluids.

TEST YOUR KNOWLEDGE QUESTIONS

1. **The lungs and chest wall are lined by two thin, serous membranes What are they called?**
    The visceral and parietal pleura.

2. **What needle size/length is required for needle decompression?**
    14G/45 mm, or 16G/30 mm for children <8 years.

3. **What is the importance of intrapleural negative pressure?**
    It keeps the external lung surface in contact with the internal chest wall, stopping the spongy and elastic lung tissue from recoiling and shrinking.

4. **What happens if the decompression needle is too short?**
    It will not reach the affected pleural space.

5. **Why is needle insertion just above the rib?**
    Each rib has a neurovascular bundle along its inferoposterior surface. Aiming just above the superior surface of the third rib limits the chances of piercing this bundle.

6. **How can tension pneumothorax affect cardiac output?**
    Increasing intrapleural pressure increases pressure on the vena cava, reducing venous return to the heart, affecting cardiac output and causing rapid deterioration to cardiogenic shock and cardiac arrest.

7. **List six 'soft signs' of tension pneumothorax.**
    Distended jugular veins; surgical emphysema; asymmetry of chest; absent or hyper-resonant chest sounds on affected side; signs of hypoxia; tracheal deviation (uncommon and very late).

8. **List three 'hard signs' of tension pneumothorax.**
    Increasing respiratory distress; decreasing perfusion; decreasing conscious state.

9. **How is suspected bilateral tension pneumothorax managed?**
    Decompress both sides, starting with the right side. Right-sided tension pneumothorax can cause left mediastinum shift, placing the heart at risk during left needle decompression.

10. **List five key steps for anatomical location for needle decompression.**
    Second intercostal space; mid-clavicular line; above the rib below; right angle to the chest wall; towards the spine.

References

Aho, J.M., Thiels, C.A., El Khatib, M.M., Ubl, D.S., Laan, D.V., Berns, K.S., Habermann, E.B., Zietlow, S.P. and Zielinski, M.D., 2016. Needle thoracostomy: clinical effectiveness is improved using a longer angiocatheter. *Journal of Trauma and Acute Care Surgery*, 80(2), 272–277.

Aylwin, C.J., Brohi, K., Davies, G.D. and Walsh, M.S., 2008. Pre-hospital and in-hospital thoracostomy: indications and complications. *Annals of the Royal College of Surgeons of England*, 90(1), 54–57.

Bach, P.T. and Sølling, C., 2015. Failed needle decompression of bilateral spontaneous tension pneumothorax. *Acta Anaesthesiologica Scandinavica*, 59(6), 807–810.

Ball, C.G., Wyrzykowski, A.D., Kirkpatrick, A.W., Dente, C.J., Nicholas, J.M., Salomone, J.P., Rozycki, G.S., Kortbeek, J.B. and Feliciano, D.V., 2010. Thoracic needle decompression for tension pneumothorax: clinical correlation with catheter length. *Canadian Journal of Surgery*, 53(3), 184.

Blackwell, T., 2016. *Prehospital care of the adult trauma patient.* Retrieved from: www.uptodate.com

Cameron, P., Jelinek, G., Kelly, A., Brown, A. and Little, M., 2014. *Textbook of adult emergency medicine*, 4th edn. Edinburgh: Churchill Livingstone/Elsevier.

Clemency, B.M., Tanski, C.T., Rosenberg, M., May, P.R., Consiglio, J.D. and Lindstrom, H.A., 2015. Sufficient catheter length for pneumothorax needle decompression: a meta-analysis. *Prehospital and Disaster Medicine*, 30(3), 249–253.

Chang, S.J., Ross, S.W., Kiefer, D.J., Anderson, W.E., Rogers, A.T., Sing, R.F. and Callaway, D.W., 2014. Evaluation of 8.0-cm needle at the fourth anterior axillary line for needle chest decompression of tension pneumothorax. *Journal of Trauma and Acute Care Surgery*, 76(4), 1029–1034.

Curtis, K. and Ramsden, C., 2016. *Emergency and trauma care: for nurses and paramedics*, 2nd edn. Sydney: Elsevier.

Curtis, K., Caldwell, E., Delprado, A. and Munro, B., 2012. Traumatic injury in Australia and New Zealand. *Australasian Emergency Nursing Journal*, 15(1), 45–54.

Galvagno, S.M., Nahmias, J.T. and Young, D.A., 2019. Advanced Trauma Life Support⁺ update 2019: management and applications for adults and special populations. *Anesthesiology Clinics*, 37(1),13–32.

Greene, C. and Callaway, D.W., 2016. Needle thoracostomy for decompression of tension pneumothorax. In *Interventional critical care*. Cham: Springer, pp. 171–178.

Inaba, K., Karamanos, E., Skiada, D., Grabo, D., Hammer, P., Martin, M., Sullivan, M., Eckstein, M. and Demetriades, D., 2015. Cadaveric comparison of the optimal site for needle decompression of tension pneumothorax by prehospital care providers. *Journal of Trauma and Acute Care Surgery*, 79(6), 1044–1048.

Jones, R. and Hollingsworth, J., 2002. Tension pneumothoraces not responding to needle thoracocentesis. *Emergency Medicine Journal*, 19(2), 176–177.

Kaserer, A., Stein, P., Simmen, H.P., Spahn, D.R. and Neuhaus, V., 2017. Failure rate of prehospital chest decompression after severe thoracic trauma. *American Journal of Emergency Medicine*, 35(3), 469–474.

Laan, D.V., Vu, T.D.N., Thiels, C.A., Pandian, T.K., Schiller, H.J., Murad, M.H. and Aho, J.M., 2016. Chest wall thickness and decompression failure: a systematic review and meta-analysis comparing anatomic locations in needle thoracostomy. *Injury*, 47(4), 797–804.

Leatherman, M.L., Held, J.M., Fluke, L.M., McEvoy, C.S., Inaba, K., Grabo, D., Martin, M.J., Earley, A.S., Ricca, R.L. and Polk, T.M., 2017. Relative device stability of anterior versus axillary needle decompression for tension pneumothorax during casualty movement: preliminary analysis of a human cadaver model. *Journal of Trauma and Acute Care Surgery*, 83(1), S136–S141.

Lee, C., Revell, M., Porter, K. and Steyn, R., 2007. The prehospital management of chest injuries: a consensus statement. Faculty of Pre-hospital Care, Royal College of Surgeons of Edinburgh. *Emergency Medicine Journal*, 24, 220–224.

Lesperance, R.N., Carroll, C.M., Aden, J.K., Young, J.B. and Nunez, T.C., 2018. Failure rate of prehospital needle decompression for tension pneumothorax in trauma patients. *American Surgeon*, 84(11), 1750–1755.

Marieb, E. and Hoehn, K., 2013. *Human anatomy & physiology*, 9th edn. San Francisco: Pearson.

Martini, F., Nath, J. and Bartholomew, E., 2012. *Fundamentals of anatomy & physiology*, 9th edn. San Francisco: Pearson.

Mistry, N., Bleetman, A. and Roberts, K.J., 2009. Chest decompression during the resuscitation of patients in prehospital traumatic cardiac arrest. *Emergency Medicine Journal*, 26(10), 738–740.

Ozen, C., Akoglu, H., Ozdemirel, R.O., Omeroglu, E., Ozpolat, C.U., Onur, O., Buyuk, Y. and Denizbasi, A., 2016. Determination of the chest wall thicknesses and needle thoracostomy success rates at second and fifth intercostal spaces: a cadaver-based study. *American Journal of Emergency Medicine*, 34(12), 2310–2314.

Powers, W.F., Clancy, T.V., Adams, A., West, T.C., Kotwall, C.A. and Hope, W.W., 2014. Proper catheter selection for needle thoracostomy: a height and weight-based criteria. *Injury*, 45(1), 107–111.

Rashid, M.A., 2018. Tension pneumothorax: are current techniques and guidelines safe? *Journal of Cardiothoracic Trauma*, 3(1), 19.

Rawlins, R., Brown, K., Carr, C. and Cameron, C., 2003. Life threatening haemorrhage after anterior needle aspiration of pneumothoraces. A role for lateral needle aspiration in emergency decompression of spontaneous pneumothorax. *Emergency Medicine Journal*, 20(4), 383–384.

Roberts, D.J., Leigh-Smith, S., Faris, P.D., Blackmore, C., Ball, C.G., Robertson, H.L., Dixon, E., James, M.T., Kirkpatrick, A.W., Kortbeek, J.B. and Stelfox, H.T., 2015. Clinical presentation of patients with tension pneumothorax: a systematic review. *Annals of Surgery*, 261(6), 1068–1078.

Terboven, T., Leonhard, G., Wessel, L., Viergutz, T., Rudolph, M., Schöler, M., Weis, M. and Haubenreisser, H., 2019. Chest wall thickness and depth to vital structures in paediatric patients – implications for prehospital needle decompression of tension pneumothorax. *Scandinavian Journal of Trauma, Resuscitation and Emergency Medicine*, 27(1), 45.

Welch, J.L. and Saltarelli, N., 2018. Tension pneumothorax: lateral needle decompression. *Visual Journal of Emergency Medicine*, 10, 118–119.

Wernick, B., Hon, H.H., Mubang, R.N., Cipriano, A., Hughes, R., Rankin, D.D., Evans, D.C., Burfeind Jr, W.R., Hoey, B.A., Cipolla, J. and Galwankar, S.C., 2015. Complications of needle thoracostomy: a comprehensive clinical review. *International Journal of Critical Illness and Injury Science*, 5(3), 160.

Zahoor, B.A., Scalea, T.M., Noorbakhsh, M.R. and Bruns, B.R., 2015. Penetrating cardiac injury as the result of pre-hospital needle decompression. *Heart, Lung and Circulation*, 24, e69–e72.

Chapter objectives

At the end of this chapter the reader will be able to:

1. Describe the anatomy and physiology relevant to body region impalement
2. Understand the clinical implications of an impaled object
3. Provide prehospital management of an impaled object

Resources required for this assessment

- Mannequin with impaled object
- Hand decontamination agent
- Disposable gloves, eyewear, mask
- Various gauze, combine pads, bandages, splints
- Clinical waste bag
- Method of documenting results

Skill matrix

This assessment requires:

- Infection control (CS 1.3)
- Communication (CS 1.5)
- Consent (CS 1.6)
- Trauma assessment (CS 5.1)

This assessment is a component of:

- Trauma (Chapter 5)

Introduction

Impalement injuries are rare and occur from a variety of mechanisms including falls, motor vehicle accidents or by projected or falling objects. In the civilian context, mechanisms can range from industrial or farming equipment to household or gardening equipment (Curtis and Ramsden, 2016). Impalement injuries can be divided into two categories:

- type 1: injuries that are the result of the human body hitting a stationary object
- type 2: injuries that are the result of a moving object penetrating the stationary body (Powitzky et al., 2008).

This chapter discusses the management of impaled objects to the head, face, neck and eyes, the thoracoabdominal region and limbs.

Anatomy and physiology

The anatomy and physiology relevant to impalement injuries varies depending on the body region(s) affected. Impalement/penetrating injuries have the potential to impair any or all the organs and systems.

The face and neck contain many vital body structures, including major blood vessels and nerves, the larynx, trachea, oesophagus and cervical spine. They are relatively superficial, in close proximity to each other and difficult to avoid in penetrating trauma.

The thoracic and abdominal cavities contain organs capable of generating massive haemorrhage, including the heart, liver and great vessels. The abdomen is filled with the bowel, stomach and pancreas which contain digestive juices, faeces and bacteria, all of which are capable of causing injury and disease in the surrounding body tissue if they are released.

The limbs, particularly the legs, contain major arteries and veins that are easily capable of causing major haemorrhage if ruptured.

Clinical rationale

While the management of impalement injuries presents prehospital challenges, there is uniform agreement that the impaled object should be left in place until surgical management at a tertiary trauma centre is available (Kuhajda et al., 2014; Malla et al., 2014).

Do not allow the spectacular nature and uniqueness of the impalement injury to distract from following the appropriate procedures (Powitzky et al., 2008). Ensure a thorough patient assessment is performed, providing management as appropriate.

The impaling object should be left in place and secured by paramedics so that it will not dislodge during transport to an appropriate trauma centre where surgical support is available in a controlled environment (Karmy-Jones et al., 2014). The time between injury and definitive surgical intervention is directly related to increased adverse outcomes (Rossaint et al., 2016).

Impalements to head, face, neck or eyes

Penetrating impalements to the head and neck are rare, representing 5–10% of all trauma cases. They present unique challenges given the serious injury they cause to vital structures (Powitzky et al., 2008) including the airway, neurological and vascular systems.

Objects impaled in the skull, ear or eye should not be removed, but instead secured in place and protected from movement (Henry et al., 2010; Pante and Pollak, 2010).

Removing an object from the eye may cause permanent damage (Henry et al., 2010). Stabilise the object with a dressing built up around it to prevent it from moving and any pressure from being transmitted to the eye (Henry et al., 2010). Place a protective barrier (plastic cup, cardboard cone or other improvised item) over the affected eye and object and secure it in place with a bulky dressing. The unaffected eye should also be covered to limit unnecessary reflex movement of the affected eye (Pante and Pollak, 2010).

Impaled objects in the soft tissue of the mouth should be stabilised in place unless it interferes with the patient's breathing or the ability to manage the airway. Impaled objects posing catastrophic threat to the airway may be removed (from the same direction in which they entered) while applying direct pressure to the wound to control haemorrhage (Pante and Pollak, 2010).

Objects impaled in the neck should be stabilised in place and protected from movement unless they are obstructing, or impeding, airway management (Pante and Pollak, 2010).

Impalements to thoracoabdominal regions

Thoracoabdominal impalements are one of the most severe types of penetrating trauma (Malla et al., 2014). They are uncommon in civilian practice (Edwin et al., 2009) and generally occur during motorbike and car accidents (Karmy-Jones et al., 2014; Stamatios et al., 2016).

Major blood vessels may tamponade by the penetrating object itself. The object should not be removed, as this could lead to catastrophic bleeding (Stamatios et al., 2016). These impalements require surgical attention with the impaling object left in situ during transport (Edwin et al., 2009; Kuhajda et al., 2014). The only exception is if the impaled object interferes with the ability to perform cardiopulmonary resuscitation (Henry et al., 2010).

The general principles of trauma care apply to thoracic or abdominal impalements, with attention given to airway, breathing and circulation (Edwin et al., 2009). The abdomen should not be palpated or percussed, as these actions may produce additional organ injury (NAEMT, 2016).

Impalements to limbs

Penetrating limb trauma may be disabling but is rarely life threatening. The exception is where major blood vessels are injured (Hardcastle et al., 2012). Tourniquets may be required to control massive arterial haemorrhage (Hardcastle et al., 2012; Rossaint et al., 2016), with rapid transport to hospital if the limb's viability is in threat (see Chapter 5.2).

As external movement of the object is mirrored by internal movement and tissue injury, the object must be secured in situ to immobilise it during transfer and transport (Hardcastle et al., 2012). Perform a thorough limb assessment for neurovascular compromise.

Clinical skill assessment process

The following section outlines the clinical skill assessment tools that should be used to determine a student's ability to demonstrate the safe and accurate management of impalement injuries.
1. Clinical Skill Work Instruction
2. Formative Clinical Skill Assessment (F-CSAT)
3. Performance Improvement Plan (PIP)
4. Summative Clinical Skill Assessment (S-CSAT)
(5. Direct Observation of Procedural Skills (DOPS) – see Chapter 1.1)

Clinical Skill Work Instruction

Equipment and resources: Mannequin with impaled object; hand decontamination agent; disposable gloves, eyewear and mask; various gauze, combine pads, bandages and splints; clinical waste bag; method of documenting results

Associated Clinical Skills: Infection control; Communication; Consent; Trauma assessment

Management of impaled objects

Activity	Critical Action	Rationale
Wear appropriate PPE	Don PPE (gloves, safety glasses and mask, as appropriate).	To decrease the risk of infection.
Prepare patient	Reassure the patient. Explain procedure. Expose and support injured area.	To reduce patient stress. To gain consent. To visualise whole injury.
Prepare dressing	Select and prepare gauze, combine pads and bandages as appropriate. Prepare a rigid improvised item for splinting the object (such as plastic cup or cardboard cone, as required).	Dressing controls haemorrhage, reduces infection risk and provides stabilisation of impaling object.
Apply dressing	Apply dressing so that it: • compresses any haemorrhage • does not put pressure on object • supports and stabilises object.	Provides haemorrhage control and prevents any further injury by immobilising impaled object.
Provide splinting	If limb impalement, splint the limb.	To prevent further movement of the limb or object and reduce further injury.
	If head or torso is impaled, provide anatomical splinting and support to prevent movement of patient or object during transport.	Reduces movement of the patient's torso or head by limiting limb movement throughout.
	If eye is impaled, cover object with plastic cup, cardboard cone or other improvised item and cover unaffected eye.	Reduces movement of both the object and the affected eye and prevents unnecessary pressure being placed on the eye.
Monitor patient	Reassess vital signs, pain and bleeding during transport.	Ongoing patient assessment required to monitor for patient deterioration.
Report	Accurately document/hand over details of injury, procedure and responses.	Accurate record keeping and continuity of care.

Formative Clinical Skill Assessment (F-CSAT)

Equipment and resources: Mannequin with impaled object; hand decontamination agent; disposable gloves, eyewear and mask; various gauze, combine pads, bandages and splints; clinical waste bag; method of documenting results

Associated Clinical Skills: Infection control; Communication; Consent; Trauma assessment

Staff/Student being assessed: _____

Management of impaled objects

Activity	Critical Action	Performance				
Wears appropriate PPE	Dons PPE.	0	1	2	3	4
Prepares patient	Reassures, explains procedure and exposes injured area.	0	1	2	3	4
Prepares dressing	Selects and prepares gauze, combine pads and bandages as appropriate.	0	1	2	3	4
Applies dressing	Applies dressing in such a way that it: • compresses any haemorrhage • does not put pressure on object • supports and stabilises the object.	0	1	2	3	4
Provides splinting	If limb impalement, splints limb. If head or torso impalement, provides anatomical splinting and support to prevent movement of patient or object during transport. If eye impalement, covers object with plastic cup, cardboard cone or other improvised item and covers unaffected eye.	0	1	2	3	4
Monitors patient	Reassesses vital signs, pain and bleeding during transport.	0	1	2	3	4
Reports	Accurately documents/hands over details of injury, procedure and responses.	0	1	2	3	4

Standard Achieved: (please circle one)

Competent (C)   Not Yet Competent* (NYC)

Staff/Student Name: _____

Assessor (please print name)**:** _____

Signed (Assessor)**:** _____

Date of Assessment: _____

Comments:

*If Not Yet Competent (NYC) a PIP needs to be completed and a repeat of the F-CSAT

Formative Clinical Skill Assessment (F-CSAT) Key

Skill level	Standard of procedure	Quality of performance	Outcome	Level of assistance required
4 Safe for unsupervised practice	Safe Accurate Behaviour is appropriate to context	Confident Accurate Expedient	Achieved intended outcome	No supporting cues*required
3 Requires supervision	Safe Accurate Behaviour is appropriate to context	Confident Accurate Takes longer than required	Achieved intended outcome	Requires occasional supportive cues*
2 Requires assistance	Safe Accurate Behaviour generally appropriate to context	Lacks certainty	Would not have achieved outcome without support	Requires frequent verbal and occasional physical directives in addition to supportive cues*
1 Requires direction	Safe only with guidance Not completely accurate	Unskilled Inefficient	Would not have achieved outcome without support	Requires continuous verbal and frequent physical directive cues*
0 Unsafe	Unsafe Unable to demonstrate behaviour Lack of insight into behaviour appropriate to context	Unskilled	Would not have achieved outcome	Requires continuous verbal and continuous physical directive cues*

*Refers to physical directives or verbal supportive cues

Performance Improvement Plan (PIP)

Please document the agreed education plan and completion timelines for areas assessed as less than 4.

This plan should be presented to assessor prior to commencement of summative assessment.

Where was supervisor support required?	Student summary of deficit. (Why was there a problem?)	Improvement Plan	Completed (Y/N)

Staff/Student Name: _____

Staff/Student Signature: _____

Educator Name: _____

Educator Signature: _____

Summative Clinical Skill Assessment (S-CSAT)

Equipment and resources: Mannequin with impaled object; hand decontamination agent; disposable gloves, eyewear and mask; various gauze, combine pads, bandages and splints; clinical waste bag; method of documenting results

Associated Clinical Skills: Infection control; Communication; Consent; Trauma assessment

Staff/Student being assessed: _____

- Completed Formative Clinical Skill Assessment (F-CSAT):   **YES   NO**
- Completed Performance Improvement Plan (PIP):   **YES   NO   N/A**

Management of impaled objects

Activity	Critical Action	Achieved Without Direction	
Wears appropriate PPE	Dons PPE.	NO	YES
Prepares patient	Reassures, explains procedure and exposes injured area.	NO	YES
Prepares dressing	Selects and prepares gauze, combine pads and bandages as appropriate.	NO	YES
Applies dressing	Applies dressing in such a way that it: • compresses any haemorrhage • does not put pressure on object • supports and stabilises the object.	NO	YES
Provides splinting	If limb impalement, splints limb. If head or torso impalement, provides anatomical splinting and support to prevent movement of patient or object during transport. If eye impalement, covers object with plastic cup, cardboard cone or other improvised item and covers unaffected eye.	NO	YES
Monitors patient	Reassesses vital signs, pain and bleeding during transport.	NO	YES
Reports	Accurately documents/hands over details of injury, procedure and responses.	NO	YES

Standard Achieved: (please circle one)

Competent (C)   Not Yet Competent* (NYC)

Staff/Student Name: _____

Assessor (please print name): _____

Signed (Assessor): _____

Date of Assessment: _____

Comments:

*If Not Yet Competent (NYC) a PIP needs to be completed and a repeat of the F-CSAT

Clinical findings

Rescue

Rescue of the patient with impaled penetrating trauma can be difficult. Where the penetrating object is too large to allow patient transfer, reduce its size, such as by cutting, to allow it to be left in situ (Powitzky et al., 2008). Minimise movement and heat generation during such a rescue.

If the patient is suspended by the impaling object, immediate action should be taken to release the pressure, to prevent gravitational force causing further injury (Powitzky et al., 2008).

Scene delay

Severe penetrating injury is associated with poorer outcomes when longer prehospital delays are incurred. The time it will take to deliver the patient to definitive care must be balanced against the management provided (Funder et al., 2011; Rossaint et al., 2016; Swaroop et al., 2013). While lifesaving procedures may be performed, including tension pneumothorax decompression (Kuhajda et al., 2014), other advanced life-support procedures, particularly fluid resuscitation, should not be allowed to create delay (Kudo et al., 2017; Newgard et al., 2015; Rossaint et al., 2016). Analgesia may be necessary for the patient to be moved in comfort.

Applying spinal care for penetrating trauma patients causes delay and is not usually necessary (Haut et al., 2010; Stuke et al., 2011).

PRACTICE TIP!

The impaled object should never be removed in the prehospital setting as it can tamponade vessels and removal may lead to massive haemorrhage. The only exceptions to this rule are if the object is obstructing the airway or the ability to manage the airway, or if the patient is in cardiac arrest and the object is interfering with chest compressions.

PRACTICE TIP!

Movement of the object outside of the body is mirrored by movement inside the body and can cause further internal injury. It is therefore important to stabilise the impaling object before transfer and transport.

PRACTICE TIP!

Rescue will involve communication with various emergency service personnel. Communicate early for adequate back up and resources. Early notification to the trauma centre allows the hospital to be prepared.

TEST YOUR KNOWLEDGE QUESTIONS

1. **What is a type 1 penetrating injury?**
   An injury resulting from the human body hitting a *stationary object*.

2. **What is a type 2 penetrating injury?**
   An injury resulting from a *moving object* penetrating the stationary body.

3. **With a penetrating eye injury, why should the unaffected eye also be covered?**
   To limit reflexive movement of the affected eye.

4. **Describe the unique dressing required to splint a penetrating eye injury.**
   Place a protective barrier (plastic cup, cardboard cone or other improvised item) over the affected eye and object and secure it in place with a bulky dressing.

5. **Why is prehospital removal of impaled objects not recommended?**
   The penetrating object may be providing tamponade. If removed, it may allow for massive bleeding, haemorrhagic shock and death.

6. **In what rare circumstance would an impaled object in the mouth or neck be removed in the prehospital setting?**
   If there is a catastrophic threat to the patient's airway.

7. **In what rare circumstance would an impaled object in the chest or abdomen be removed in the prehospital setting?**
   If the object is interfering with the ability to perform cardiopulmonary resuscitation.

8. **How can stabilising the impaling object limit further internal injuries?**
   Any movement of the object outside of the body is mirrored inside the body and can therefore cause further internal injury.

9. **It is important to palpate the abdomen with an impaled object to determine the exact location and depth of the object. True or false?**
   False. The abdomen should not be palpated or percussed, as these actions may produce additional organ injury.

10. **What actions would you take if the penetrating object is too large to manage or transport the patient?**
    The object should be cut or reduced, while taking care to leave it in situ.

References

Curtis, K. and Ramsden, C., 2016. *Emergency and trauma care: for nurses and paramedics*, 2nd edn. Sydney: Elsevier.

Edwin, F., Tettey, M., Sereboe, L., Aniteye, E., Kotei, D., Tamatey, M., Entsuamensah, K., Delia, I. and Frimpong-Boateng, K., 2009. Case reports: impalement injuries of the chest. *Ghana Medical Journal*, 43(2) 86–89.

Funder, K.S., Petersen, J.A. and Steinmetz, J., 2011. On-scene time and outcome after penetrating trauma: an observational study. *Emergency Medicine Journal*, 28(9), 797–801.

Hardcastle, T., Venter, C. and Hollander, D., 2012. Penetrating extremity trauma – vascular aspects. In Rogers, R., Scalea, T., Wallis, L. and Geduld, H. (eds), *Vascular emergencies*, Cambridge: Cambridge University Press, pp. 137–147.

Haut, E.R., Kalish, B.T., Efron, D.T., Haider, A.H., Stevens, K.A., Kieninger, A.N., Cornwell III, E.E. and Chang, D.C., 2010. Spine immobilization in penetrating trauma: more harm than good? *Journal of Trauma and Acute Care Surgery*, 68(1), 115–121.

Henry, M., Stapleton, E. and Edgerly, D., 2012. *EMT prehospital care*, 4th edn. St. Louis: Mosby/Elsevier.

Karmy-Jones, R., Namias, N., Coimbra, R., Moore, E.E., Schreiber, M., McIntyre Jr, R., Croce, M., Livingston, D.H., Sperry, J.L., Malhotra, A.K. and Biffl, W.L., 2014. Western Trauma Association critical decisions in trauma: penetrating chest trauma. *Journal of Trauma and Acute Care Surgery*, 77(6), 994–1002.

Kudo, D., Yoshida, Y. and Kushimoto, S., 2017. Permissive hypotension/hypotensive resuscitation and restricted/controlled resuscitation in patients with severe trauma. *Journal of Intensive Care*, 5(1), 11.

Kuhajda, I., Zarogoulidis, K., Kougioumtzi, I., Huang, H., Li, Q., Dryllis, G., Kioumis, I., Pitsiou, G., Machairiotis, N., Katsikogiannis, N. and Papaiwannou, A., 2014. Penetrating trauma. *Journal of Thoracic Disease*, 6(Suppl 4), S461.

Malla, G., Basnet, B., Vohra, R., Herrforth, C., Adhikari, S. and Bhandari, A., 2014. Thoraco-abdominal impalement injury: a case report. *BMC Emergency Medicine*, 14, 7.

NAEMT (National Association of Emergency Medical Technicians), 2016. *PHTLS: Prehospital trauma life support*, 8th edn. St. Louis: Moseby/Elsevier.

Newgard, C.D., Meier, E.N., McKnight, B., Drennan, I.R., Richardson, D., Brasel, K., Schreiber, M., Kerby, J.D., Kannas, D., Austin, M. and Bulger, E.M., 2015. Understanding traumatic shock: out-of-hospital hypotension with and without other physiologic compromise. *Journal of Trauma and Acute Care Surgery*, 78(2), 342.

Pante, M. and Pollak, A., 2010. *Advanced assessment and treatment of trauma*. Sudbury: Jones and Bartlett.

Powitzky, R., Cordero, J., Robinson, M., Helmer, R. and Halldorsson, A., 2008. Spectacular impalement through face and neck: a case report and literature review. *Journal of Trauma Injury, Infection and Critical Care*, 65(6).

Rossaint, R., Bouillon, B., Cerny, V., Coats, T.J., Duranteau, J., Fernández-Mondéjar, E., Filipescu, D., Hunt, B.J., Komadina, R., Nardi, G. and Neugebauer, E.A., 2016. The European guideline on management of major bleeding and coagulopathy following trauma. *Critical Care*, 20(1), 100.

Stamatios, A., Ioannis, M., Dimitrios, K., Andreas, F., Styliani, P., Dimitrios, K. and Constantinos, T., 2016. A rare case of transabdominal impalement after a fall from a ladder. *International Journal of Surgery Case Reports*, 22, 40–43.

Stuke, L.E., Pons, P.T., Guy, J.S., Chapleau, W.P., Butler, F.K. and McSwain, N.E., 2011. Prehospital spine immobilization for penetrating trauma – review and recommendations from the Prehospital Trauma Life Support Executive Committee. *Journal of Trauma and Acute Care Surgery*, 71(3), 763–770.

Swaroop, M., Straus, D.C., Agubuzu, O., Esposito, T.J., Schermer, C.R. and Crandall, M.L., 2013. Pre-hospital transport times and survival for hypotensive patients with penetrating thoracic trauma. *Journal of Emergencies, Trauma, and Shock*, 6(1), 16.

Bibliography

Martini, F., Nath, J. and Bartholomew, E., 2012. *Fundamentals of anatomy & physiology*, 9th edn. San Francisco: Pearson Education.

5.5 | Crash helmet removal

Joe Karlek

Chapter objectives

At the end of this chapter the reader will be able to:

1. Identify the indications to remove a crash helmet
2. Demonstrate the safe removal of a crash helmet

Resources required for this assessment

- Standardised patient or mannequin
- Motorcycle helmet
- Hand decontamination agent
- Disposable gloves
- Clinical waste bag
- Method of documenting the results

Skill matrix

This assessment requires:
- Infection control (CS 1.3)
- Communication (CS 1.5)
- Consent (CS 1.6)
- Trauma assessment (CS 5.1)
- Cervical collar application (CS 5.6)

This assessment is a component of:
- Trauma (Chapter 5)

Introduction

Crash helmets are synonymous with motorcycle riding and some motor sports, and the benefits of wearing them are almost intuitive. However, although helmets are worn for the purposes of safety, they can inhibit the prompt and effective assessment and management of those wearing them. Paramedics must be competent in the removal of crash helmets so that treatment is not delayed or injury made more severe. This chapter discusses the safe removal of motorcycle helmets.

Anatomy and physiology

Closed head injuries experienced by motorcycle riders include coup and contra-coup, concussion, shearing of blood vessels, intracranial haemorrhage and meningeal bleeding (Fernandes and de Sousa, 2013; Singleton,

2017). These injuries vary in severity and are related to the level of deceleration experienced by the rider. The face and cervical spine are similarly vulnerable in motorcycle trauma wherever head trauma can occur. Spinal injury is relatively uncommon, and it is unclear whether wearing a helmet is beneficial or a contributing factor (Branfoot, 1994; Liu et al., 2008; Rice et al., 2016).

Crash helmets have been found to be an effective method of reducing cerebral injury and mortality (McIntosh et al., 2013; Rice et al., 2016; Singleton, 2017; Sung et al., 2016). A 2008 Cochrane review found that crash helmets are effective at reducing mortality and head injury by 42% and 69% respectively (Liu et al., 2008). The scalp, skull and intracranial contents are better able to tolerate collision forces when a crash helmet is worn, due to the distribution of forces.

Crash helmets typically enclose the head and face, extending over the occiput to the point of the upper spine to offer protection against head, neck and facial injury. Unsurprisingly, injuries to these areas can be difficult to manage with a helmet in place.

Clinical rationale

A crash helmet has four distinct components: a hard outer shell, inner lining, comfort padding and chin strap. These components work collectively but in different ways to protect the head when it is involved in a collision. The outer shell and inner lining are directly related to dealing with the forces experienced by the head during a crash. The chin strap maintains the helmet in position and prevents its dislodgement. The padding is primarily for the rider's comfort, but in newer models it can be removed easily to aid helmet removal.

The hard outer shell is designed to spread the impact force over a larger surface area and prevent sharp objects penetrating the helmet. This spread across the helmet allows the inner liner to absorb these forces by crumpling, reducing the amount of force that actually reaches the skull and brain (Coelho et al., 2013; Fernandes and de Sousa, 2013; Fernandes et al., 2013). The energy involved in a motorcycle collision can be extreme due to the speeds involved and the lack of safety features on a motorcycle compared to a modern car.

Most conscious and ambulant patients remove their own crash helmet before the emergency services arrive. The patient who is still wearing their helmet may need assistance in its removal. Bystanders often elect against removing the helmet (Branfoot, 1994) for fear of exacerbating injury.

Removing the helmet allows more effective communication and patient assessment. Failure to do so interferes with all airway procedures and the assessment and management of other injuries (Branfoot, 1994). Full head enclosure leads to rebreathing exhaled gas, and hypoxia/hypercarbia can occur (Brühwiler et al., 2005).

Helmet removal can cause notable movement of the cervical spine. This should be opposed by a second paramedic providing manual in-line stabilisation (Branfoot, 1994). Once the helmet has been removed, a cervical collar can be applied if indicated. It is important not to discard the helmet or leave it at the scene, as it can provide insights into the impact for the Emergency Department and may be deemed evidence by the police.

Several styles of motorcycle helmets are available:

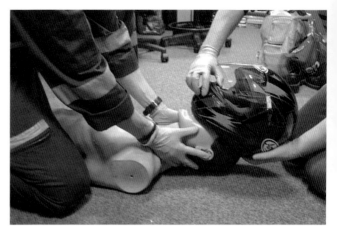

Figure 5.5.1 Removing a helmet occiput first

- full-face helmets, which are designed to cover the entire head, face and neck
- modified full-face helmets with a flip-open or removable face/chin
- open-face helmets that have no face or chin coverage
- motocross helmets, which are like full-face helmets but are designed to be worn with goggles; they may have an attached visor.

Since the helmet is designed to fit reasonably tightly, it will take some manipulative effort to remove. The best strategy is to release or cut the chin strap, flex the lower sides to loosen it if possible, then rotate the helmet off over the face. It will not likely pull straight off in an upwards fashion as the chin piece may snare on the patient's nose. By the helmet rotating back upwards and over towards the front, this can be avoided. As the helmet is removed, the second paramedic providing manual in-line stabilisation will have to be prepared to support the head and prevent the occiput from falling (Fig. 5.5.1).

Clinical skill assessment process

The following section outlines the clinical skill assessment tools that should be used to determine a student's ability to demonstrate the safe removal of a crash helmet.

1. Clinical Skill Work Instruction
2. Formative Clinical Skill Assessment (F-CSAT)
3. Performance Improvement Plan (PIP)
4. Summative Clinical Skill Assessment (S-CSAT)
(5. Direct Observation of Procedural Skills (DOPS) – see Chapter 1.1)

Clinical Skill Work Instruction

Equipment and resources: Standardised patient or mannequin; motorcycle helmet; hand decontamination agent; disposable gloves; clinical waste bag; method of documenting results

Associated Clinical Skills: Infection control; Communication; Consent; Trauma assessment; Cervical collar application

Crash helmet removal

Activity	Critical Action	Rationale
Personal protection	Don PPE as required.	For infection control.
Prepare patient	Position patient supine if circumstances allow. Helmet can be removed from any position if patient cannot be moved.	Removal is easiest if the patient is supine.
	Second paramedic maintains spinal immobilisation.	Spinal immobilisation is likely to be required.
	Explain procedure to patient. Open helmet visor if possible to facilitate communication.	Gain consent and cooperation.
Prepare helmet for removal	Identify and unclip or, if necessary, cut away chin strap. Remove glasses if patient is wearing them.	Removal of the helmet is inhibited while the chin strap is in situ. Glasses may cause injury if not removed.
Manual in-line stabilisation	Assistant places one hand under patient's occiput for support. Their other hand supports the mandible above the neck to provide spinal immobilisation.	Support must be from below to allow helmet removal.
Remove chin pads	Pull on release tabs if helmet has this feature for emergency removal.	Removing chin pads provides more room and easier removal.
Remove helmet	Grip base of helmet at the lateral edges and apply outward pressure to open the helmet. Gently pull chin piece upwards slightly, towards the nose. Rotate the posterior helmet base from occiput over the head in line with the spine. Once the rear has been part-way removed, rotate the front by tilting chin portion over the nose. Remove helmet fully.	Pulling helmet opening apart helps avoid catching the ears, tilting it avoids the nose and occiput. Maintain direction of removal with that of spine to prevent unnecessary cervical spine movement.
Head support	Provide occipital support with padding. Second paramedic provides manual in-line spinal immobilisation (see Chapter 5.7), replacing anterior/posterior support with lateral support.	Spinal immobilisation is maintained throughout the procedure.
Replace glasses	Replace glasses if removed during procedure and patient requires them.	Inability to see may be distressing.
Retain helmet	Retain helmet for review by Emergency Department staff and the police.	The helmet provides information in relation to pattern of injury and it may also be evidence.
Report	Document/hand over whether a helmet was worn/removed and deliver helmet if retained.	Accurate record kept and continuity of patient care.

Formative Clinical Skill Assessment (F-CSAT)

Equipment and resources: Standardised patient or mannequin; motorcycle helmet; hand decontamination agent; disposable gloves; clinical waste bag; method of documenting results

Associated Clinical Skills: Infection control; Communication; Consent; Trauma assessment; Cervical collar application

Staff/Student being assessed: _____

Crash helmet removal

Activity	Critical Action	Performance				
Personal protection	Dons PPE as required.	O	1	2	3	4
Prepares patient	Positions supine if circumstances allow.	O	1	2	3	4
	Second paramedic maintains spinal immobilisation.	O	1	2	3	4
	Explains procedure to patient. Opens helmet visor if possible to facilitate communication.	O	1	2	3	4
Prepares helmet for removal	Identifies and unclips or, if necessary, cuts away chin strap. Removes glasses if worn.	O	1	2	3	4
Manual in-line stabilisation	Assistant places one hand under patient's occiput for support. Their other hand supports the mandible above the neck to provide spinal immobilisation.	O	1	2	3	4
Removes chin pads	Pulls on release tabs if helmet has this feature for emergency removal.	O	1	2	3	4
Removes helmet	Grips base of helmet at lateral edges and applies outward pressure to open helmet. Gently pulls chin piece upwards slightly towards the nose. Rotates posterior helmet base from occiput over the head, in line with the spine. Once rear has been part-way removed, rotates the front by tilting chin portion over the nose. Removes helmet fully.	O	1	2	3	4
Head support	Provides occipital support with padding. Second paramedic provides manual in-line spinal immobilisation (see Chapter 5.7), replacing anterior/posterior support with lateral support.	O	1	2	3	4
Replaces glasses	Replaces glasses if removed during procedure and patient requires them.	O	1	2	3	4
Retains helmet	Retains helmet for review by Emergency Department staff and police.	O	1	2	3	4
Reports	Documents/hands whether a helmet was worn/removed and delivers helmet if retained.	O	1	2	3	4

Standard Achieved: (please circle one)

Competent (C)   Not Yet Competent* (NYC)

Staff/Student Name: _____

Assessor (please print name): _____

Signed (Assessor): _____

Date of Assessment: _____

Comments:

*If Not Yet Competent (NYC) a PIP needs to be completed and a repeat of the F-CSAT

Formative Clinical Skill Assessment (F-CSAT) Key

Skill level	Standard of procedure	Quality of performance	Outcome	Level of assistance required
4 Safe for unsupervised practice	Safe Accurate Behaviour is appropriate to context	Confident Accurate Expedient	Achieved intended outcome	No supporting cues*required
3 Requires supervision	Safe Accurate Behaviour is appropriate to context	Confident Accurate Takes longer than required	Achieved intended outcome	Requires occasional supportive cues*
2 Requires assistance	Safe Accurate Behaviour generally appropriate to context	Lacks certainty	Would not have achieved outcome without support	Requires frequent verbal and occasional physical directives in addition to supportive cues*
1 Requires direction	Safe only with guidance Not completely accurate	Unskilled Inefficient	Would not have achieved outcome without support	Requires continuous verbal and frequent physical directive cues*
0 Unsafe	Unsafe Unable to demonstrate behaviour Lack of insight into behaviour appropriate to context	Unskilled	Would not have achieved outcome	Requires continuous verbal and continuous physical directive cues*

*Refers to physical directives or verbal supportive cues

Performance Improvement Plan (PIP)

Please document the agreed education plan and completion timelines for areas assessed as less than 4.

This plan should be presented to assessor prior to commencement of summative assessment.

Where was supervisor support required?	Student summary of deficit. (Why was there a problem?)	Improvement Plan	Completed (Y/N)

Staff/Student Name: _____

Staff/Student Signature: _____

Educator Name: _____

Educator Signature: _____

Summative Clinical Skill Assessment (S-CSAT)

Equipment and resources: Standardised patient or mannequin; motorcycle helmet; hand decontamination agent; disposable gloves; clinical waste bag; method of documenting results

Associated Clinical Skills: Infection control; Communication; Consent; Trauma assessment; Cervical collar application

Staff/Student being assessed: _____

- Completed Formative Clinical Skill Assessment (F-CSAT): **YES** **NO**
- Completed Performance Improvement Plan (PIP): **YES** **NO** **N/A**

Crash helmet removal

Activity	Critical Action	Achieved Without Direction	
Personal protection	Dons PPE as required.	NO	YES
Prepares patient	Positions supine if circumstances allow.	NO	YES
	Second paramedic maintains spinal immobilisation.	NO	YES
	Explains procedure to patient. Opens helmet visor if possible to facilitate communication.	NO	YES
Prepares helmet for removal	Identifies and unclips or, if necessary, cuts away chin strap. Removes glasses if worn.	NO	YES
Manual in-line stabilisation	Assistant places one hand under patient's occiput for support. Their other hand supports the mandible above the neck to provide spinal immobilisation.	NO	YES
Removes chin pads	Pulls on release tabs if helmet has this feature for emergency removal.	NO	YES
Removes helmet	Grips base of helmet at lateral edges and applies outward pressure to open helmet. Gently pulls chin piece upwards slightly, towards the nose. Rotates posterior helmet base from occiput over the head, in line with the spine. Once rear has been part-way removed, rotates the front by tilting chin portion over the nose. Removes helmet fully.	NO	YES
Head support	Provides occipital support with padding. Second paramedic provides manual in-line spinal immobilisation (see Chapter 5.7), replacing anterior/posterior support with lateral support.	NO	YES
Replaces glasses	Replaces glasses if removed during procedure and patient requires them.	NO	YES
Retains helmet	Retains helmet for review by Emergency Department staff and police.	NO	YES
Reports	Documents/hands over helmet if a helmet was worn/removed and delivers helmet if retained.	NO	YES

Standard Achieved: (please circle one)

Competent (C)   Not Yet Competent* (NYC)

Staff/Student Name: _____

Assessor (please print name): _____

Signed (Assessor): _____

Date of Assessment: _____

Comments:

*If Not Yet Competent (NYC) a PIP needs to be completed and a repeat of the F-CSAT

Clinical findings

Basic options
Opening the visor, if there is one, allows better communication, removal of the patient's glasses if worn and rudimentary facial/airway access. It may also help to avoid rebreathing.

Head support
The second paramedic providing head stabilisation is likely to have to make several adjustments throughout. The first position involves the helmet resting on the ground. This will change to providing support from below the head/neck during helmet removal, likely sitting beside the patient. The last is a traditional in-line stabilisation position superior to the patient's head. Removal should occur at a pace that allows the support person to adjust their position each time to enable their role.

Minimise movement
It is difficult to stop all head movement, even if resistance is concerted. Gentle and small helmet removal movements can assist, using progressive back and forward gains rather than one direct attempt at removal.

> **PRACTICE TIP!**
>
> Some helmets allow the removal of components including ear padding, fold-up chin pieces or even frontal pieces. If any of these features are present, make use of them first. If possible, ask the rider for any tips or strategies for removing the helmet. They are familiar with the device and may offer useful suggestions.

> **PRACTICE TIP!**
>
> Before removing the helmet, double check that the patient's glasses have been removed and the strap is undone.

> **PRACTICE TIP!**
>
> Helmet removal is better if performed by two paramedics, with one supporting the head and resisting movement, and the other removing the helmet.

TEST YOUR KNOWLEDGE QUESTIONS

1. **List the styles of helmets you might encounter during practice.**
   Full-face; open-face; flip-up; motocross with detachable visor and goggles.

2. **What are the four main components of the helmet?**
   Hard outer shell; inner lining; comfort padding; chin strap.

3. **What is the purpose of the outer shell and inner lining?**
   To prevent penetration of objects and to distribute the force of the impact.

4. **How can the inner lining help the rescuer remove the helmet?**
   On newer helmets the inner lining can be removed, aiding removal of the helmet.

5. **What is the most common type of injury experienced by motorcycle riders?**
   Closed head injuries.

6. **List the specific injuries common to the type given in question 5.**
   Coup and contra-coup; shearing of blood vessels; bleeding between the meninges.

7. **What factor affecting the rider impacts most on a head injury?**
   The force of deceleration.

8. **Removing the helmet is important for what reasons?**
   Communication; airway management; patient assessment.

9. **What position should the patient be in for helmet removal?**
   Supine.

10. **Why should the helmet not be discarded?**
    It is helpful to the Emergency Department and may be deemed evidence by the police.

References

Branfoot, T., 1994. Motorcyclists, full face helmets and neck injuries: can you take the helmet off safely, and if so, how? *Journal of Accident and Emergency Medicine*, (11), 117–120.

Brühwiler, P.A., Stämpfli, R., Huber, R. and Camenzind, M., 2005. CO2 and O2 concentrations in integral motorcycle helmets. *Applied Ergonomics*, 36(5), 625–633.

Coelho, R.M., de Sousa, R.A., Fernandes, F.A.O. and Teixeira-Dias, F.M.V.H., 2013. New composite liners for energy absorption purposes. *Materials & Design*, 43, 384–392.

Fernandes, F.A.O. and de Sousa, R.A., 2013. Motorcycle helmets – a state of the art review. *Accident Analysis & Prevention*, 56, 1–21.

Fernandes, F.A., de Sousa, R.J.A., Willinger, R. and Deck, C., 2013. *Finite element analysis of helmeted impacts and head injury evaluation with a commercial road helmet.* Paper presented at the International Research Council on the Biomechanics of Injury (IRCOBI) conference, 11–13 September, Gothenburg, Sweden.

Liu, B.C., Ivers, R., Norton, R., Boufous, S., Blows, S. and Lo, S.K., 2008. *Helmets for preventing injury in motorcycle riders.* Online: The Cochrane Library.

McIntosh, A.S., Curtis, K., Rankin, T., Cox, M., Pang, T.Y., McCrory, P. and Finch, C.F., 2013. Associations between helmet use and brain injuries amongst injured pedal- and motor-cyclists: a case series analysis of trauma centre presentations. *Journal of the Australasian College of Road Safety*, 24(2), 11.

Rice, T.M., Troszak, L., Ouellet, J.V., Erhardt, T., Smith, G.S. and Tsai, B.W., 2016. Motorcycle helmet use and the risk of head, neck, and fatal injury: revisiting the Hurt Study. *Accident Analysis & Prevention*, 91, 200–207.

Singleton, M.D., 2017. Differential protective effects of motorcycle helmets against head injury. *Traffic Injury Prevention*, 18(4), 387–392.

Sung, K.M., Noble, J., Kim, S.C., Jeon, H.J., Kim, J.Y., Do, H.H., Park, S.O., Lee, K.R. and Baek, K.J., 2016. The preventive effect of head injury by helmet type in motorcycle crashes: a rural Korean single-center observational study. *BioMed Research International*, doi: 10.1155/2016/1849134.

Chapter objectives

At the end of this chapter the reader will be able to:

1. Describe the rationale for applying a cervical collar
2. Describe cervical spine care supporting cervical collar application
3. Demonstrate the application of a cervical collar

Resources required for this assessment

- Standardised patient or mannequin
- Cervical collar (soft or rigid) in a range of sizes
- Towel
- Disposable gloves, eyewear, respiratory mask
- Clinical waste bag
- Method of documenting results

Skill matrix

This assessment requires:

- Infection control (CS 1.3)
- Communication (CS 1.5)
- Consent (CS 1.6)
- Assessment of motor and sensory nerve function (CS 2.13)
- Head positioning (CS 3.2)
- Trauma assessment (CS 5.1)

This assessment is a component of:

- Trauma (Chapter 5)

Introduction

Management of potential cervical spinal injury (CSI) has long dominated prehospital trauma practice. It has evolved from the extensive spinal immobilisation of many trauma patients to current principles, which include clearance screening.

The cervical collar is synonymous with spinal care. It was a mainstay until 2016, when the International Liaison Committee of Resuscitation (ILCOR) and Australian and New Zealand Council on Resuscitation (ANZCOR) recommended that alternative measures, including manual in-line stabilisation, were preferable to using semi-rigid collars (ANZCOR, 2016).

This chapter discusses the use of cervical collars in prehospital spinal care.

Anatomy and physiology

The spine is separable into two divisions: structural (spinal column) and nervous (spinal cord). The spinal column comprises the vertebra, intervertebral discs, supportive muscles and ligaments and its blood supply. There are 33 vertebrae: 7 cervical, 12 thoracic, 5 lumbar, 5 fused sacral and 4 fused distal coccyx bones. The disc structure and musculoskeletal support allow a range of movements, including twisting, flexion and extension.

Posteriorly, the spinal column appears straight; left and right curvatures suggest abnormality. Laterally there are several normal spinal column curves. Cervical vertebrae are noted by an inward C-shaped curve, changing to a reverse outward C-shaped thoracic curve before slightly curving inwards in a C-shape again in the lumbar. Thoracic and lumbar vertebrae are supported by the trunk, offering greater strength than the cervical vertebrae but restricted range of motion.

The spinal cord runs from the brainstem down the length of the spine to the second lumbar vertebra, and is contained within the vertebrae throughout. Each vertebra corresponds to a spinal cord segment from which the peripheral sensory and motor nerves emanate.

Clinical rationale

The cervical spine is most vulnerable to injury, although the lower spine can also be injured. Spinal care involves the whole of the spine, not just the cervical spine. CSI commonly accompanies head, chest, limb injuries and altered consciousness (Sundstrøm et al., 2014).

The first indication that a CSI may have occurred is the mechanism of injury. Most major causes of trauma, including motor vehicle/cycle collisions, falls from height, diving and sporting accidents and blows to the head, are classic examples of CSI injury mechanisms (ANZCOR, 2016). Vulnerable groups, including the elderly, have an increased risk of injury from lesser mechanisms such as falls from standing height.

Multiple force directions can cause primary CSI:
- hyperextension – the spine is pushed backwards (from a frontal head strike or backward push)
- hyperflexion – the spine is pushed forwards (from a posterior head strike or forward push)
- compression – the spine is pushed downwards (from the head being pushed into a solid object or an object falling on the head)
- overstretching – the spine is pulled along its length (where the head is held and the body pulled)
- rotation – the spine is rotated in different directions (e.g. from a vehicle rollover) (Johnson et al., 2014; Iencean, 2003).

Extension of the original injury can occur hours to days later (Sundstrøm et al., 2014). This secondary injury can result from oedema or ongoing haemorrhage causing ischemia. There is potential for extension of the injury due to spinal movement during rescue, even without acute neurological symptoms; this issue underpins the debate regarding appropriate prehospital care. However, the high energy required to cause spinal injury is unlikely to be rivalled during rescue, and it is rare that further injury follows patient handling (Sundstrøm et al., 2014).

Cervical spine care is not applied to all trauma patients. Screening allows effective exclusion where it is unnecessary. Most commonly employed are the National Emergency XRadiography Utilisation Study (NEXUS) criteria and the Canadian C-Spine Rule (Hood and Considine, 2015). Both of these tools guide cervical spine imaging post trauma and have been modified for making decisions about immobilisation.

Effective screening means only those with CSI risk receive cervical spine care. It cannot be safely excluded:

- for patients with a major trauma injury mechanism or pattern of injury
- for patients showing evidence of spinal column/structure injury, betrayed by bony midline tenderness and pain
- if there is evidence of spinal cord injury, including neurological abnormalities such as altered sensation, movement, tingling or numbness, even if these are unilateral (see Chapter 2.13)
- for those at increased risk of injury risk, including the elderly (the Canadian C-Spine Rule indicates those who are ≥65 years, but local guidelines may differ on the precise age) and those with bony (e.g. osteoporosis) or neuromuscular disease (e.g. muscular dystrophy) where bony injury has increased the likelihood of CSI
- where there is any difficulty properly assessing the patient, including those who are unconscious or have altered consciousness (acute or chronic GCS score <15) or patients who are drug or alcohol impaired, or where there is major distracting injury, including fractures and burns.

For adult patients meeting any of these criteria, cervical spine care is appropriate (Sundstrøm et al., 2014). This can, though not always, include cervical collar application. The care of children, discussed later, is guided by different principles.

Head position
Return the head to the neutral anatomical position (see Chapter 3.2) with neither neck flexion nor extension.

Head support
A second paramedic kneels superiorly to the patient's head, encouraging head stillness. One hand is placed each side of the patient's head, with the fingers spread across the cheeks. Sufficient manual in-line axial traction force is provided to resist movement caused by the patient or the paramedic (Johnson et al., 2014). This is maintained, even during laryngoscopy, despite its possible adverse impact on glottis view (Gupta et al., 2017; Ilyas et al., 2014; Sridhar and Hagberg, 2014) (see Chapter 3.6).

Applying a cervical collar
Semi-rigid/hard cervical collars are more commonly used to reduce neck movement than soft collars. Cervical collars warn subsequent health carers that the patient has not been spinally cleared. They can hinder performance of other critical assessments or procedures (Sundstrøm et al., 2014).

Rigid collars
Rigid collars reduce neck movement by as much as 63% (Whitcroft et al., 2011) but sometimes less than this (Horodyski et al., 2011; Sundstrøm et al., 2014). Collars are provided in fixed sizes that range from paediatric to tall neck. Alternatively, adjustable options fit a range of neck sizes.

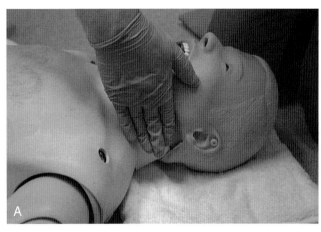
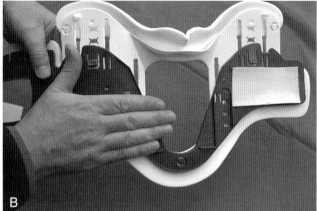

Figure 5.6.1 Measuring for cervical collar size
(a) Determining the distance to the jaw angle. (b) Measuring from the bottom of the plastic collar side.

Soft collars

Soft collars made from foam rubber lack the rigidity of hard collars. They can reduce neck movement by as little as 17% in many cases (Whitcroft et al., 2011), but this may still be sufficient (Sundstrøm et al., 2014). They too are provided in differing sizes and are measured and fitted for use.

Collar sizing

The cervical collar must be measured for fit. Different products may be sized differently. A common method is to place one hand, palm against the neck with the little finger against the clavicle. The distance to the jaw angle (number of fingers) is determined (Fig. 5.6.1a). This distance is then measured from the bottom of the plastic collar side (not the foam) (Fig. 5.6.1b). The fingers extend to the sizing point. If the collar is adjustable, lock in correct position.

Incorrectly sized collars either don't restrict movement sufficiently or, if too large, force the neck into a non-neutral position (Sundstrøm et al., 2014). Sizing and application errors are common (Kreinest et al., 2015). If the collar does not appear correctly sized, remove and apply a different size.

Method of application

The cervical collar can be fitted with the patient in any position, including seated, supine and standing. Flex the collar to loosen it before use. Remove any jewellery that can be trapped by the collar.

There are two methods of applying a collar. It can be placed against the anterior neck first, and then wrapped around the occiput and fastened on the other side. However, hair can be caught using this method, causing head movement. An alternative, less disruptive method is to pass the Velcro® collar end behind the neck first (Fig. 5.6.2), and then bend the collar into position and fasten it.

The collar must sit symmetrically without impinging on the patient's ears. The sternum contact should be flush against the skin. The chin piece should sit neatly beneath

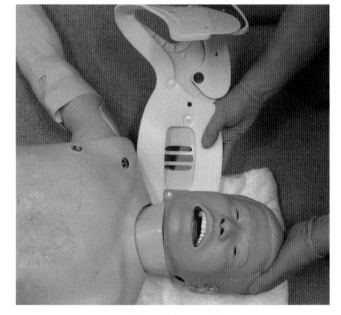

Figure 5.6.2 Passing the Velcro® end first

the chin (Fig. 5.6.3a and b), avoiding pressing into the soft underjaw or slipping off over the mouth. Provide manual in-line support as required (Fig. 5.6.3b).

Contraindications

Penetrating neck trauma is associated with significant vascular and airway injuries that are hampered by the application of a cervical collar. Cervical collars are not necessary for penetrating neck trauma (Kodadek et al., 2017; Klein et al., 2016; Sundstrøm et al., 2014; Turnock et al., 2016).

Occasionally, it may not be possible to return the neck to neutral anatomical alignment. Pain or resistance, abnormal cervical kyphosis or ankylosing spondylitis can compromise the neck position. In such cases, avoid cervical collars and support the neck as it is found or in a position of comfort (Papadopoulos et al., 1999).

Avoid cervical collars where they will interfere with critical airway devices, including in surgical airways and

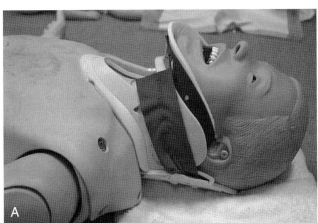
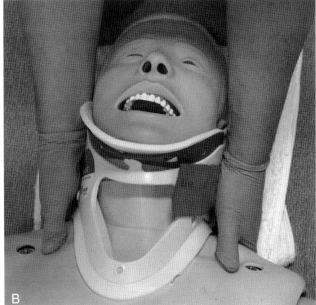

Figure 5.6.3 Cervical collar secured in position
(a) Lateral view. (b) Frontal view with manual in-line support provided.

tracheostomy or where facial or jaw injuries will not permit their application.

Clinical skill assessment process

The following section outlines the clinical skill assessment tools that should be used to determine a student's ability to demonstrate the accurate application of a cervical collar.

1. Clinical Skill Work Instruction
2. Formative Clinical Skill Assessment (F-CSAT)
3. Performance Improvement Plan (PIP)
4. Summative Clinical Skill Assessment (S-CSAT)
(5. Direct Observation of Procedural Skills (DOPS) – see Chapter 1.1)

Clinical Skill Work Instruction

Equipment and resources: Standardised patient or mannequin; cervical collars; towel; disposable gloves, eyewear and respiratory mask; clinical waste bag; method of documenting results

Associated Clinical Skills: Infection control; Communication; Consent; Assessment of motor and sensory function; Head positioning; Trauma assessment

Cervical collar application

Activity	Critical Action	Rationale
Personal protection	Don PPE as required.	To minimise exposure to infection.
Assess patient	Reassure the patient and explain the procedure. Advise them to hold their head motionless.	The patient's cooperation is required.
	Assess trauma and use a method of cervical spine screening.	To exclude unnecessary immobilisation.

Cervical collar application continued

Activity	Critical Action	Rationale
Position patient's head	Return patient's head to neutral anatomical position, provided there is no pain or resistance. Use occipital padding as necessary.	This is the natural neck position and places minimal pressure on the vertebrae and spinal cord. Pain/resistance caused by movement suggests injury that could be worsened in the process. Padding supports the adult head/neck from falling into partial extension.
Head stabilisation	Second paramedic kneels superiorly to patient's head. This person then provides manual in-line stabilisation using hands either side of patient's head. Encourage patient not to move.	To resist any movement of patient's head.
Apply cervical collar	Measure the collar for fit. Choose the correct size or lock in place an adjustable sized collar. Flex collar for use. Ensure any pre-use assembly is complete.	The correct size is required to maintain neutral immobilisation. Some devices have locking clips to activate before use.
	Remove any jewellery items that might interfere. Where possible, remove or cut away clothing, ensuring no head movement is caused.	Collars work best against the skin.
	Pass the Velcro® end beneath posterior neck until it clears the other side again, being careful to avoid catching on patient's hair or causing neck movement.	To position without moving patient's head.
	Bend front of collar over anterior neck. Bend sides in contour with patient's neck and push inwards until collar contacts chin and chest. Use hands to mould collar into a symmetrical shape, with the sides sitting on trapezius and under each ear.	To assist with correct best fit to patient.
	Hold collar in position with one hand. With second hand, pull Velcro® end around fully and attach to collar side. Tighten collar sides firmly.	Ensures correct and symmetrical fit, head in neutral position.
Confirm collar position	Inspect collar for tightness, symmetry, clearance from ears, patient discomfort, position of chin piece and contact with sternum. Adjust as necessary.	An incorrect position has adverse complications.
Continued manual stabilisation	Second paramedic moves hands to grasp patient's clavicles and gently squeezes forearms against patient's head.	To immobilise head and body as one aligned unit. Rolled up towel can be placed between arms and patient's head.
Report	Document/hand over spinal assessment results, collar size and effectiveness.	Accurate record kept and continuity of patient care.

Formative Clinical Skill Assessment (F-CSAT)

Equipment and resources: Standardised patient or mannequin; cervical collars; towel; disposable gloves, eyewear and respiratory mask; clinical waste bag; method of documenting results

Associated Clinical Skills: Infection control; Communication; Consent; Assessment of motor and sensory function; Head positioning; Trauma assessment

Staff/Student being assessed: _____

Cervical collar application

Activity	Critical Action	Performance				
Personal protection	Dons PPE as required.	0	1	2	3	4
Assesses patient	Reassures patient and explains method. Advises patient to hold head motionless.	0	1	2	3	4
	Assesses trauma and uses cervical spine screening method.	0	1	2	3	4
Positions patient's head	Returns head to neutral anatomical position provided there is no pain or resistance. Uses occipital padding as necessary.	0	1	2	3	4
Head stabilisation	Second paramedic kneels superiorly to patient's head. This person then provides manual in-line stabilisation. Encourages patient not to move.	0	1	2	3	4
Applies cervical collar	Measures collar for fit. Chooses correct size of collar or locks in place adjustable sized collar. Flexes collar and completes any pre-use assembly.	0	1	2	3	4
	Removes interfering jewellery items. Where possible, removes or cuts away clothing, ensuring no head movement is caused.	0	1	2	3	4
	Passes Velcro® end behind posterior neck until it clears the other side, avoiding catching patient's hair or moving neck.	0	1	2	3	4
	Brings front of collar over anterior neck. Contours sides with patient's neck and pushes inwards until collar contacts chin and chest. Moulds collar into a symmetrical shape, with sides sitting on trapezius and under each ear.	0	1	2	3	4
	Holds collar in position with one hand. With second hand, pulls Velcro® end around fully and attaches to side of collar. Tightens collar sides.	0	1	2	3	4
Confirms collar position	Inspects collar for tightness, symmetry, clearance from ears, patient discomfort, position of chin piece and sternum contact point. Adjusts collar as necessary.	0	1	2	3	4
Continued manual stabilisation	Second paramedic moves hands to grasp patient's clavicles and gently squeezes forearms against patient's head.	0	1	2	3	4
Reports	Documents/hands over spinal assessment results, collar size and effectiveness.	0	1	2	3	4

Standard Achieved: (please circle one)

Competent (C)   Not Yet Competent* (NYC)

Staff/Student Name: _____

Assessor (please print name)**:** _____

Signed (Assessor)**:** _____

Date of Assessment: _____

Comments:

*If Not Yet Competent (NYC) a PIP needs to be completed and a repeat of the F-CSAT

Formative Clinical Skill Assessment (F-CSAT) Key

Skill level	Standard of procedure	Quality of performance	Outcome	Level of assistance required
4 Safe for unsupervised practice	Safe Accurate Behaviour is appropriate to context	Confident Accurate Expedient	Achieved intended outcome	No supporting cues*required
3 Requires supervision	Safe Accurate Behaviour is appropriate to context	Confident Accurate Takes longer than required	Achieved intended outcome	Requires occasional supportive cues*
2 Requires assistance	Safe Accurate Behaviour generally appropriate to context	Lacks certainty	Would not have achieved outcome without support	Requires frequent verbal and occasional physical directives in addition to supportive cues*
1 Requires direction	Safe only with guidance Not completely accurate	Unskilled Inefficient	Would not have achieved outcome without support	Requires continuous verbal and frequent physical directive cues*
0 Unsafe	Unsafe Unable to demonstrate behaviour Lack of insight into behaviour appropriate to context	Unskilled	Would not have achieved outcome	Requires continuous verbal and continuous physical directive cues*

*Refers to physical directives or verbal supportive cues

Performance Improvement Plan (PIP)

Please document the agreed education plan and completion timelines for areas assessed as less than 4.

This plan should be presented to assessor prior to commencement of summative assessment.

Where was supervisor support required?	Student summary of deficit. (Why was there a problem?)	Improvement Plan	Completed (Y/N)

Staff/Student Name: _____

Staff/Student Signature: _____

Educator Name: _____

Educator Signature: _____

Summative Clinical Skill Assessment (S-CSAT)

Equipment and resources: Standardised patient or mannequin; cervical collars; towel; disposable gloves, eyewear and respiratory mask; clinical waste bag; method of documenting results

Associated Clinical Skills: Infection control; Communication; Consent; Assessment of motor and sensory function; Head positioning; Trauma assessment

Staff/Student being assessed: _____

- Completed Formative Clinical Skill Assessment (F-CSAT): **YES**   **NO**
- Completed Performance Improvement Plan (PIP): **YES**   **NO**   **N/A**

Cervical collar application

Activity	Critical Action	Achieved Without Direction	
Personal protection	Dons PPE as required.	NO	YES
Assesses patient	Reassures patient and explains method. Advises patient to hold head motionless.	NO	YES
	Assesses trauma and uses cervical spine screening method.	NO	YES
Positions patient's head	Returns head to neutral anatomical position, provided there is no pain or resistance. Uses occipital padding as necessary.	NO	YES
Head stabilisation	Second paramedic kneels superiorly to patient's head. This person then provides manual in-line stabilisation. Encourages patient not to move.	NO	YES
Applies cervical collar	Measures collar for fit. Chooses correct size of collar or locks in place adjustable sized collar. Flexes collar and completes any pre-use assembly.	NO	YES
	Removes interfering jewellery items. Where possible, removes or cuts away clothing, ensuring no head movement is caused.	NO	YES
	Passes Velcro® end beneath posterior neck until it clears the other side, avoiding catching patient's hair or moving neck.	NO	YES
	Bends front of collar over anterior neck. Contours sides with patient's neck and pushes inwards until collar contacts chin and chest. Moulds collar into a symmetrical shape, with sides sitting on trapezius and under each ear.	NO	YES
	Holds collar in position with one hand. With second hand, pulls Velcro® end around fully and attaches to side of collar. Tightens collar sides.	NO	YES
Confirms collar position	Inspects collar for tightness, symmetry, clearance from ears, patient discomfort, position of chin piece and sternum contact point. Adjusts collar as necessary.	NO	YES
Continued manual stabilisation	Second paramedic moves hands to grasp patient's clavicles and gently squeezes forearms against patient's head.	NO	YES
Reports	Documents/hands over spinal assessment results, collar size and effectiveness.	NO	YES

Standard Achieved: (please circle one)

Competent (C)   Not Yet Competent* (NYC)

Staff/Student Name: _____

Assessor (please print name): _____

Signed (Assessor): _____

Date of Assessment: _____

Comments:

*If Not Yet Competent (NYC) a PIP needs to be completed and a repeat of the F-CSAT

Clinical findings

Single rescuer

Fitting a cervical collar as a single rescuer undermines the concept of stabilisation while the device is fitted. Using a second operator for support when fitting a cervical collar minimises unwanted neck movement (Sundstrøm et al., 2014).

Airway procedures

Airway procedures are more difficult to perform with a cervical collar fitted. The mouth cannot be effectively opened to allow suctioning or laryngoscopy (Sundstrøm et al., 2014). Patients vomiting will be hindered from doing so, increasing the risk of aspiration. Supraglottic devices can be used where cervical collars are fitted (Mann et al., 2012; Sridhar and Hagberg, 2014).

Patient discomfort

Cervical collars are uncomfortable, frequently causing patients to move and attempt to remove them (Sundstrøm et al., 2014). Prior and ongoing explanation may help. It is possible that patient cooperation alone, or supported with towel/sandbag head support, may become a necessary alternative where the application of a collar is not tolerable.

Intracranial pressure

Cervical collars are implicated in increasing intracranial pressure by hindering neck venous drainage. This is problematic in head trauma (Karason et al., 2014; Maissan et al., 2017; Moscote-Salazar et al., 2018; Mobbs et al., 2002; Sundstrøm et al., 2014), which is typically when a cervical collar might be fitted. There is currently no clear method of identifying the point at which cervical collars begin causing intracranial pressure problems in prehospital practice. Consider removing a collar if it causes the patient irritation, indicated by increased agitation or attempts to remove it.

Impediments to application

Long hair makes it more difficult to pass the Velcro° posteriorly. Some ground surfaces, such as long grass, can also cause difficulties. Sliding one end of the collar beneath the patient's neck first before fitting it anteriorly can assist.

Clothing interferes with the contour of the cervical collar sitting against the patient's skin. Where possible, clothes should be cut or pulled away. However, cervical collars can still remain effective even where clothing items cannot be fully removed (Chi et al., 2005).

Children

Most paediatric spinal injuries are cervical, proportionately more so than in adults. While the injury mechanisms are similar, they are more likely to include falls and abuse. The upper cervical spine is more commonly injured in children <8 years due to their relatively larger head size, weaker supportive ligament/musculature and higher natural fulcrum point (Horn et al., 2017).

Younger children are more difficult to assess and communicate with (Baumann et al., 2015; Ramrattan et al., 2012). It is not easy to restrict their movement or gain their cooperation. Neutral anatomical alignment in children varies from that in adults, particularly in the smaller child (see Chapter 3.2).

The spinal column of the smaller child is capable of vertebral movement that is sufficient to cause injury to the spinal cord but which does not then appear during radiological assessment. This is referred to as spinal cord injury without radiological abnormality (SCIWORA) (Horn et al., 2017; Ramrattan et al., 2012). Prehospital spinal screening/clearance is typically not advocated in the paediatric patient because of this increased likelihood of injury and assessment difficulty.

PRACTICE TIP!

Different cervical collars can be assembled and sized differently. Ensure and maintain familiarity with multiple devices, particularly those used in your ambulance service.

PRACTICE TIP!

Cervical collar application is frequently performed on patients with other injuries that are more significant and urgent. The need to address spinal injury carefully and with caution must be balanced against these more pressing and potentially life-threatening demands.

PRACTICE TIP!

Since the cervical collar can be fitted with the patient in a variety of positions, training in applying the collar should be similarly varied.

TEST YOUR KNOWLEDGE QUESTIONS

1. **What patient head position is best suited for cervical spine care?**
   The neutral anatomical position.

2. **When should this position *not* be used?**
   When there is resistance to or pain from movement, or an abnormality such as kyphosis.

3. **What method of cervical collar measurement is commonly used?**
   Measuring the angle of the mandible to the clavicle, using the fingers of one hand.

4. **What problems can occur if the cervical collar is not sized correctly?**
   If it is too small, there may be inadequate immobilisation; if it is too large, the neck may be pushed into partial extension.

5. **Why is position of the collar chin piece important?**
   If the position is incorrect, the chin piece can press into the soft flesh of the underjaw or slip off over the mouth.

6. **Must patient clothing be removed for cervical collar application?**
   It should ideally be removed, to allow skin contact. However, collars still remain effective if this is not possible.

7. **List three contraindications for cervical collar application.**
   Penetrating neck trauma; unable to return neck to neutral; surgical airway interference; facial/jaw injuries.

8. **Can a cervical collar be applied if the neck cannot be returned to neutral?**
   No. Support the neck as it is found.

9. **List three complications of applying a cervical collar.**
   Unwanted neck movement; airway procedures more difficult due to closed mouth and risk of vomiting/aspiration; discomfort, pain or restlessness; raised intracranial pressure.

10. **List three ways in which paediatric cervical spine care differs from that for adults.**
    Harder to assess; higher cervical injury; possibility of SCIWORA; no prehospital exclusion; different neutral anatomical position.

References

ANZOR (Australian New Zealand Council on Resuscitation), 2016. *Guideline 9.1.6: Management of suspected spinal cord injury*. Retrieved from: https://resus.org.au/wpfb-file/anzcor-guideline-9-1-6-spinal-jan16-pdf

Baumann, F., Ernstberger, T., Neumann, C., Nerlich, M., Schroeder, G.D., Vaccaro, A.R. and Loibl, M., 2015. Pediatric cervical spine injuries: a rare but challenging entity. *Journal of Spinal Disorders & Techniques*, 28(7), E377.

Chi, C., Wu, F., Tsai, S., Wang, C. and Stern, S.A. 2005. Effect of hair and clothing on neck immobilization using a cervical collar. *American Journal of Emergency Medicine*, 23(3) 386–390.

Gupta, G., Bagdi, K., Virk, R.S., Garg, A. and Gupta, I., 2017. Assessment of difficulty during orotracheal intubation in patients with cervical spine immobilisation – a comparison of Macintosh and Truview laryngoscopes. *Journal of Pharmaceutical and Biomedical Sciences*, 7(11).

Hood, N. and Considine, J., 2015. Spinal immobilisaton in pre-hospital and emergency care: a systematic review of the literature. *Australasian Emergency Nursing Journal*, 18(3), 118–137.

Horn, A., Workman, M.I., Dix-Peek, S. and Dunn, R.N., 2017. Ligamentous integrity in Spinal Cord Injury without Radiographic Abnormality (SCIWORA): a case series. *SA Orthopaedic Journal*, 16(2), 32–38.

Horodyski, M., DiPaola, C.P., Conrad, B.P. and Rechtine, G.R., 2011. Cervical collars are insufficient for immobilizing an unstable cervical spine injury. *Journal of Emergency Medicine*, 41(5), 513.

Iencean, S.M., 2003. Classification of spinal injuries based on the essential traumatic spinal mechanisms. *Spinal Cord*, 41(7), 385.

Ilyas, S., Symons, J., Bradley, W.P.L., Segal, R., Taylor, H., Lee, K., Balkin, M., Bain, C. and Ng, I., 2014. A prospective randomised controlled trial comparing tracheal intubation plus manual in-line stabilisation of the cervical spine using the Macintosh laryngoscope vs the McGrath® Series 5 videolaryngoscope. *Anaesthesia*, 69(12), 1345–1350.

Johnson, M., Boyd, L., Grantham, H.J. and Eastwood, K., 2014. *Paramedic principles and practice ANZ*. Sydney: Harcourt, p. 608.

Karason, S., Reynisson, K., Sigvaldason, K. and Sigurdsson, G.H., 2014. Evaluation of clinical efficacy and safety of cervical trauma collars: differences in immobilization, effect on jugular venous pressure and patient comfort. *Scandinavian Journal of Trauma, Resuscitation and Emergency Medicine*, 22, 37.

Klein, Y., Arieli, I., Sagiv, S., Peleg, K. and Ben-Galim, P., 2016. Cervical spine injuries in civilian victims of explosions: should cervical collars be used? *Journal of Trauma and Acute Care Surgery*, 80(6), 985–988.

Kodadek, L.M., Kieninger, A. and Haut, E.R., 2017. Penetrating trauma to the larynx and the cervical trachea. In *Penetrating trauma*. Berlin/Heidelberg: Springer, pp. 243–248.

Kreinest, M., Goller, S., Rauch, G., Frank, C., Gliwitzky, B., Wölfl, C.G., Matschke, S. and Münzberg, M., 2015. Application of cervical collars – an analysis of practical skills of professional emergency medical care providers, *PLOS ONE*, 10(11), e0143409.

Maissan, I.M., Ketelaars, R., Vlottes, B., Hoeks, S.E. and Stolker, R.J., 2017. Increase in intracranial pressure by application of a rigid cervical collar: a pilot study in healthy volunteers. *European Journal of Emergency Medicine*, 25(6), pp. e24–e28.

Mann, V., Spitzner, T., Schwandner, T., Mann, S.T.W., Müller, M., Ahlbrandt, J., Weigand, M.A. and Röhrig, R., 2012. The effect of a cervical collar on the seal pressure of the LMA Supreme™: a prospective, crossover trial. *Anaesthesia*, 67(11), 1260.

Mobbs, R.J., Stoodley, M.A. and Fuller, J., 2002. Effect of cervical hard collar on intracranial pressure after head injury. *ANZ Journal of Surgery*, 72(6), 389.

Moscote-Salazar, L.R., Godoy, D.A., Agrawal, A. and Rubiano, A.M., 2018. Effect of cervical collars on intracranial pressure in patients with head neurotrauma. *Journal of Emergency Practice and Trauma*, 4(1), 1–2.

Papadopoulos, M.C., Chakraborty, A., Waldron, G. and Bell, B.A., 1999. Exacerbating cervical spine injury by applying a hard collar. *BMJ*, 319(7203), 171–172.

Ramrattan, N.N., Öner, F.C., Boszczyk, B.M., Castelein, R.M. and Heini, P.F., 2012. Cervical spine injury in the young child. *European Spine Journal*, 21(11), 2205–2211.

Sridhar, S. and Hagberg, C.A., 2014. Airway management in cervical spine injured patients. In *Airway management*. Cham: Springer, pp. 157–175.

Sundstrøm, T., Asbjørnsen, H., Habiba, S., Sunde, G.A. and Wester, K., 2014. Prehospital use of cervical collars in trauma patients: a critical review. *Journal of Neurotrauma*, 31(6), 531–540.

Turnock, A.R., Carney, M.J., Fleischer, B.P., Jr, Mcswain, N.E. and Vanderlan, W.B., 2016. Cervical spine immobilization in penetrating cervical trauma is associated with an increased risk of indirect central neurological injury. *Trauma Emergency Care*, 2(1), 1–8.

Whitcroft, K.L., Massouh, L., Amirfeyz, R. and Bannister, G.C., 2011. A comparison of neck movement in the soft cervical collar and rigid cervical brace in healthy subjects. *Journal of Manipulative and Physiological Therapeutics*, 34(2), 119.

Chapter objectives

At the end of this chapter the reader will be able to:

1. Describe the rationale for applying a pelvic splint

2. Recognise when pelvic splint application is required

3. Demonstrate the method of applying a pelvic splint

Resources required for this assessment

- Simulated patient/mannequin
- Disposable gloves
- Towel
- Triangular bandages
- Sheet/pelvic splint
- Clinical waste bag
- Method of documenting the results

Skill matrix

This assessment requires:

- Infection control (CS 1.3)
- Communication (CS 1.5)
- Consent (CS 1.6)
- Trauma assessment (CS 5.1)

This assessment is a component of:

- Trauma (Chapter 5)

Introduction

The fractured pelvis is one of the few musculoskeletal injuries that can prove life threatening. It carries a high mortality rate, usually from the significant bleeding it can cause (Clamp and Moran, 2011; Ojodu et al., 2015; Stahel et al., 2005). Any strategy that can reduce this bleeding has the potential to reduce associated mortality. Applying a pelvic splint is one such strategy (Scott et al., 2013; Stahel et al., 2005).

Pelvic fractures are uncommon, representing 3–8% of fractures. Of these, only 2–4% are life-threatening, open book fractures, which are the target of pelvic splinting (Saxena et al., 2014). This chapter discusses the management of open book fractures using pelvic splinting.

Anatomy and physiology

The pelvis forms a major structural component of the human skeleton. It is ring-shaped when viewed from above. Either side of the posterior sacrum are the two large iliac bones connected by the strong sacroiliac joints. The anterior pelvis is comprised of smaller bones, including the ischium, acetabulum and pubic bone. The mid-anterior point is the cartilaginous symphysis pubis joint. Pelvic stability relies on intact internal ligaments.

Much of the body weight is borne by the pelvis. It forms the attachment point for the spine and the legs, making it pivotal for walking and standing.

A major function of the pelvis is to provide protection for the organs and blood vessels it encircles. The bladder, urethra and large intestine lie within the pelvis. Major blood vessels running to the legs pass near the pelvic bones, including iliac arteries and veins. The presacral venous plexus is near the sacroiliac joint, and is easily injured in open book fractures (Saxena et al., 2014; Tran et al., 2016).

Clinical rationale

The strong pelvis is not easily broken, and significant force is required to do so. High-impact mechanisms are usually involved, including road trauma (pedestrian/motorcycle/vehicle) and falls from height (Scott et al., 2013). The elderly are more vulnerable to pelvic fracture, with low-impact forces known to cause injury (Saxena et al., 2014; Verbeek et al., 2018). Fractures can be stable or, less commonly, unstable (Alwaal et al., 2015; Alton and Gee, 2014).

The direction of force is significant, and has three broad classifications. Lateral impact causes inward-side compression. Fractures resulting from this direction of force are most common and frequently stable. The fracture is not usually open book, although it can lead to internal organ and vascular injury. Pelvic binders are not necessarily helpful with these fractures (Scott et al., 2013; Tran et al., 2016), though there is no great evidence of them causing harm (Shackelford et al., 2017). Ilium fractures are usually stable and are not usually associated with open book injury.

A head-on direction is more concerning because of the result of anterior-posterior (AP) forces applied to the pelvis. The greater pelvis rotates externally, injuring the weaker central pubic region and creating an open book fracture. If the injury is largely contained in the pubis, the opening is minimal (<2.5 cm). However, if there is accompanying posterior sacroiliac injury, the widening can be greater (Alton and Gee, 2014). This mechanism leads to the open book fracture and is most associated with vascular injury and haemodynamic instability (Scott et al., 2013). The sacral venous plexus, hypogastric artery and soft tissue are all sources of haemorrhage, the injury being caused by nearby fractured bone (Lee and Porter, 2007).

The third direction is the vertical shear, where the force is transmitted up through the pelvis from below, typically via the femurs. It results from falling from height and landing on the legs. Fractures from this direction of force lead to severe pelvic disruptions, including to ligaments (Alton and Gee, 2014; Scott et al., 2013).

Assessment

Recognising pelvic fracture is not always easy. Determining the mechanism of injury is important, as is a physical examination. Patients are frequently unable to weight bear. Pain is typical and associated with widespread fracture of the pelvis, including the ilium, lower back and groin.

Bruising, swelling and deformity may be observable over the fractured site. Asymmetry of the lower limbs may be evident, including differing lengths or abnormal rotation. This must be differentiated from limb fracture. Urethral or rectal bleeding may suggest internal injury from fracture (Lee and Porter, 2007; Saxena et al., 2014; Shackelford et al., 2017).

Pelvic 'springing' (using the hands to apply direct force inwards and distract force over the iliac crests) is unreliable, often producing no result despite the presence of a fracture. It can also increase bleeding or injury. It is not usual to move a fractured bone to aid diagnosis (Lee and Porter, 2007; Scott et al., 2013; Shackelford et al., 2017), and assessing for pelvic fracture should be no different.

Pelvic binder (splint)

Significant bleeding does not pool in a damaged pelvis. Rather, bleeding escapes into the retroperitoneum and surrounds the bladder. The actual increase in pelvic volume is comparatively small, and the bleeding tamponade effect arising from closure of the fractured pelvic ring is a factor in haemorrhage control. While some low-pressure (including venous) bleeding can be controlled, major arterial bleeding may continue unabated. Bone end stabilisation reduces ongoing injury and improves the likelihood of clot formation (Clamp and Moran, 2011; Hsu et al., 2017; Lee and Porter, 2007; Saxena et al., 2014; Shackelford et al., 2017).

Since the aim of splinting is to reduce the pelvic diameter, closing the open pubis must occur. Bring the legs together by binding the (padded) knees and ankles before applying the splint (Fig. 5.7.1) (Morris et al., 2016). Pelvic splints are best applied over bare skin or, at most, undergarments, as they are less effective over clothing (Lee and Porter, 2007; Scott et al., 2013). If clothing is left on, ensure solid objects are removed from the pockets, as these can cause pain or injury if compressed.

The pelvic splint should be applied early, as part of major bleeding control (Halliwell et al., 2011; Saxena et al., 2014; Scott et al., 2013; Shackelford et al., 2017). It must be applied over the greater trochanters, since these are at the level of the opening of the pelvic ring (Fig. 5.7.1). Commonly, the splint is erroneously applied over the

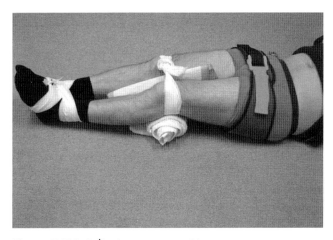

Figure 5.7.1 Splint in correct position

higher and more prominent iliac crests. If it is incorrectly applied in this way, there is no benefit from compression and additional pain may be caused. This can be avoided by applying the splint from beneath the thighs and then moving it up, rather than applying it under the lumbar arch and attempting to move it downwards (Shackelford et al., 2017).

Once applied, a pelvic binder should be left in place until definitive diagnosis and management can be applied. Distal circulation should be assessed after application (Saxena et al., 2014).

Log rolling patients with major pelvic fractures can disrupt clotting and worsen bleeding. It should be avoided where possible, or performed only partially (see Chapter 7.1) (Saxena et al., 2014; Scott et al., 2013; Shackelford et al., 2017).

Once the splint is applied, maintaining slight knee flexion with a pillow or rolled blanket may improve the patient's comfort, depending on limb injury.

Binder options

Several manufactured pelvic binder splints are available. Each operates by wrapping around the pelvis and providing compressive force when pulled tight (Shackelford et al., 2017). The SAM® pelvic binder is referred to for the purposes of this instruction. The application of other devices may differ slightly.

Alternatively, improvised options may be used. Of these, the best supported option is the pelvic sheet wrap. A folded sheet is placed beneath the patient's buttocks, extending an equal distance above and below the trochanters (Shackelford et al., 2017). As compression is applied, force will automatically contact the widest point first: the trochanters. It can be difficult to get the sheet in place beneath the patient and then ensure sufficient force is applied and maintained (Lee and Porter, 2007). The wrap can cover a larger area than manufactured splints do, impeding ongoing assessment and other procedures (Saxena et al., 2014).

The sheet wrap can be as effective as a manufactured option, depending on how much force is applied and how well it is secured (Shackelford et al., 2017). The most widely used method is the sheet knot method (Fig. 5.7.2) but the wrist roll alternative has proven effective (Fig. 5.7.3a and b).

Clinical skill assessment process

The following section outlines the clinical skill assessment tools that should be used to determine a student's ability to demonstrate effective pelvic splinting.

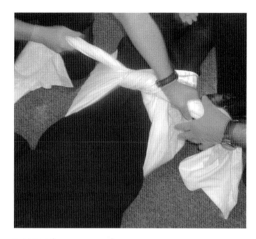

Figure 5.7.2 Sheet wrap knot

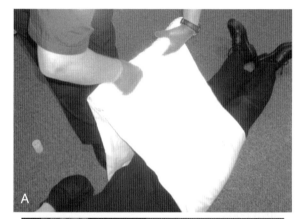

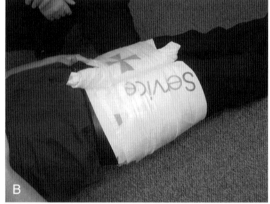

Figure 5.7.3 Sheet wrap wrist roll
(a) Applying the pelvic binder splint. (b) Fitted splint.

1. Clinical Skill Work Instruction
2. Formative Clinical Skill Assessment (F-CSAT)
3. Performance Improvement Plan (PIP)
4. Summative Clinical Skill Assessment (S-CSAT)
(5. Direct Observation of Procedural Skills (DOPS) – see Chapter 1.1)

Clinical Skill Work Instruction

Equipment and resources: Simulated patient/mannequin; pelvic splint/sheet; towel; triangular bandages; disposable gloves; clinical waste bag; method of documenting results

Associated Clinical Skills: Infection control; Communication; Consent; Trauma assessment

Pelvic splint application

Activity	Critical Action	Rationale
Personal protection	Don gloves.	Decreases infection risk.
Prepare patient	Discuss procedure. Obtain informed consent.	To reduce patient's stress and gain their cooperation.
	Expose pelvis and lower limbs. If clothing is left on, remove hard objects from pockets.	To visualise area and provide access.
	Assess for open book pelvic fracture.	These fractures benefit from pelvic splinting. Choose option to splint if unsure.
	Bring patient's legs together. Lightly pad bony ankle and knee prominences. Secure legs in place with broad-fold triangular bandage over knees and in figure of eight around ankles. Modify approach as required where limb injury is encountered.	To close pubis and avoid pressure areas.
Apply splint (SAM®)	Open pelvic splint and flatten out, ensuring inner side will be facing inwards towards the patient.	To avoid inverted application.
	Feed splint beneath thighs, buckle end first. Ensure sufficient buckle end appears to rest against patient's anterior thigh.	Applying from below assists in correct positioning.
	Gently sliding left and right, manipulate splint upwards until in place over trochanters. If necessary, gently lift patient's buttocks fractionally to assist. Palpate trochanters to confirm location.	Gentle handling minimises pain. Trochanter location ensures compression is applied correctly.
	The distal splint end has a small loop handle. Bring this end across and feed it into the buckle loop. Pull distal end back to original side again, trapping the buckle.	In preparation for compression.
	Ideally with a second operator holding the buckle loop handle and pulling in the opposite direction, pull the distal loop handle laterally away from patient. If there is only one operator, they can apply the opposing force by holding both handles.	The two opposing lateral forces apply the correct compression force.
	Continue force until a locking click is felt or heard. While maintaining tension, secure distal end using the Velcro® lining.	To lock compression in place.
Release splint tension	**The splint should be released only on medical examination.** When ready to do so, release distal end from Velcro® and move back towards the buckle side. The buckle will release.	Pelvic compression must be maintained to avoid pain and continuing haemorrhage.

Pelvic splint application continued

Activity	Critical Action	Rationale
Sheet wrap splint	If the alternative sheet wrap is used, assess and prepare patient similarly. Fold sheet along its width until it is approximately 30 cm wide. Extend sheet length perpendicular to the patient and feed it under the thighs as above. Pull it through, ensuring there are equal lengths on both sides and the trochanters are in the centre. Bring the two sheet ends together above patient's groin and roll the ends tightly until they contact the patient. Roll one end with one hand tightly then secure with a long length of broad adhesive tape. Repeat for the other roll end.	The sheet wrap is an alternative where no manufactured splint is available.
Assess patient	Assess distal circulation and pain. Lower limb injuries permitting, slight knee flexion maintained by a rolled blanket or pillow may improve the patient's comfort.	Splint may cause improvement or concerns.
Report	Accurately document/hand over assessment findings and procedure.	Accurate record kept and continuity of patient care.

Source: *Adapted from SAM® manufacturer's instructions.*

Formative Clinical Skill Assessment (F-CSAT)

Equipment and resources: Simulated patient/mannequin; pelvic splint/sheet; towel; triangular bandages; disposable gloves; clinical waste bag; method of documenting results

Associated Clinical Skills: Infection control; Communication; Consent; Trauma assessment

Staff/Student being assessed: _____

Pelvic splint application

Activity	Critical Action	Participant Performance				
Personal protection	Dons gloves.	0	1	2	3	4
Prepares patient	Discusses procedure. Obtains informed consent.	0	1	2	3	4
	Exposes pelvis and lower limbs. If clothing is left on, removes hard objects from pockets.	0	1	2	3	4
	Assesses for open book pelvic fracture.	0	1	2	3	4
	Brings patient's legs together. Lightly pads bony ankle and knee prominences. Secures legs in place with broad-fold triangular bandage over knees and in figure of eight around ankles. Modifies approach as required where limb injury is encountered.	0	1	2	3	4
Applies splint (SAM®)	Opens pelvic splint and flattens out, ensuring inner side faces inwards towards patient.	0	1	2	3	4
	Feeds splint beneath thighs, buckle end first. Ensures sufficient buckle end appears to rest against patient's anterior thigh.	0	1	2	3	4
	Gently sliding left and right, manipulates splint upwards until in place over trochanters. If necessary, gently lifts patient's buttocks fractionally to assist. Palpates trochanters to ensure location.	0	1	2	3	4
	Brings distal loop handle across and feeds into buckle loop. Pulls distal end back to the original side again, trapping the buckle.	0	1	2	3	4

Pelvic splint application continued

Activity	Critical Action	Participant Performance				
	With a second operator holding buckle loop handle and pulling in the opposite direction, pulls distal loop handle laterally to patient. If necessary, applies opposing force by holding both handles.	0	1	2	3	4
	Continues force until locking click is felt/heard. While maintaining tension, secures distal end using Velcro® lining.	0	1	2	3	4
Releases splint tension	**Releases only on medical examination.** When ready, releases distal end from Velcro® and moves back towards buckle side until it releases.	0	1	2	3	4
Sheet wrap splint	If alternative sheet wrap is used, assesses/prepares patient similarly. Folds sheet along its width until it is approximately 30 cm wide. Extends sheet length perpendicular to patient and feeds under thighs. Pulls through, ensuring there are equal lengths on both sides and the trochanters are in the centre. Brings the two sheet ends together above patient's groin and rolls them tightly together until they contact the patient. Rolls one end with one hand tightly, then secures with a long length of broad adhesive tape. Repeats for other roll end.	0	1	2	3	4
Assesses patient	Assesses distal circulation and pain. Lower limb injuries permitting, maintains slight knee flexion with a rolled blanket or pillow.	0	1	2	3	4
Reports	Accurately documents/hands over assessment findings and procedure.	0	1	2	3	4

Source: *Adapted from SAM® manufacturer's instructions.*

Standard Achieved: (please circle one)

Competent (C)   Not Yet Competent* (NYC)

Staff/Student Name: _____

Assessor (please print name)**:** _____

Signed (Assessor)**:** _____

Date of Assessment: _____

Comments:

*If Not Yet Competent (NYC) a PIP needs to be completed and a repeat of the F-CSAT

Formative Clinical Skill Assessment (F-CSAT) Key

Skill level	Standard of procedure	Quality of performance	Outcome	Level of assistance required
4 Safe for unsupervised practice	Safe Accurate Behaviour is appropriate to context	Confident Accurate Expedient	Achieved intended outcome	No supporting cues* required
3 Requires supervision	Safe Accurate Behaviour is appropriate to context	Confident Accurate Takes longer than required	Achieved intended outcome	Requires occasional supportive cues*

Skill level	Standard of procedure	Quality of performance	Outcome	Level of assistance required
2 Requires assistance	Safe Accurate Behaviour generally appropriate to context	Lacks certainty	Would not have achieved outcome without support	Requires frequent verbal and occasional physical directives in addition to supportive cues*
1 Requires direction	Safe only with guidance Not completely accurate	Unskilled Inefficient	Would not have achieved outcome without support	Requires continuous verbal and frequent physical directive cues*
0 Unsafe	Unsafe Unable to demonstrate behaviour Lack of insight into behaviour appropriate to context	Unskilled	Would not have achieved outcome	Requires continuous verbal and continuous physical directive cues*

*Refers to physical directives or verbal supportive cues

Performance Improvement Plan (PIP)

Please document the agreed education plan and completion timelines for areas assessed as less than 4.

This plan should be presented to assessor prior to commencement of summative assessment.

Where was supervisor support required?	Student summary of deficit. (Why was there a problem?)	Improvement Plan	Completed (Y/N)

Staff/Student Name: _____

Staff/Student Signature: _____

Educator Name: _____

Educator Signature: _____

Summative Clinical Skill Assessment (S-CSAT)

Equipment and resources: Simulated patient/mannequin; pelvic splint/sheet; towel; triangular bandages; disposable gloves; clinical waste bag; method of documenting results

Associated Clinical Skills: Infection control; Communication; Consent; Trauma assessment

Staff/Student being assessed: _____

- Completed Formative Clinical Skill Assessment (F-CSAT): **YES**   **NO**

- Completed Performance Improvement Plan (PIP): **YES**   **NO**   **N/A**

Pelvic splint application		Achieved Without Direction	
Activity	**Critical Action**		
Personal protection	Dons gloves.	NO	YES
Prepares patient	Discusses procedure. Obtains informed consent.	NO	YES
	Exposes pelvis and lower limbs. If clothing is left on, removes hard objects from pockets.	NO	YES
	Assesses for open book pelvic fracture.	NO	YES
	Brings patient's legs together. Lightly pads bony ankle and knee prominences. Secures legs in place with broad-fold triangular bandage over knees and in figure of eight around ankles. Modifies approach as required where limb fracture is encountered.	NO	YES
Applies splint (SAM®)	Opens pelvic splint and flattens out, ensuring inner side facing inwards towards patient.	NO	YES
	Feeds splint beneath thighs, buckle end first. Ensures sufficient buckle end appears to rest against patient's anterior thigh.	NO	YES
	Gently sliding left and right, manipulates splint upwards until in place over trochanters. If necessary, gently lifts buttocks fractionally to assist. Palpates trochanters to ensure location.	NO	YES
	Brings distal loop handle across and feeds into buckle loop. Pulls distal end back to the original side again, trapping the buckle.	NO	YES
	With a second operator holding buckle loop handle and pulling in the opposite direction, pulls distal loop handle laterally to the patient. If necessary, applies opposing force by holding both handles.	MO	YES
	Continues force until locking click is felt/heard. While maintaining tension, secures distal end using Velcro® lining.	NO	YES
Releases splint tension	**Releases only on medical examination.** When ready, releases distal end from Velcro® and moves back towards buckle side until it releases.	NO	YES
Sheet wrap splint	If alternative sheet wrap is used, assesses/prepares patient similarly. Folds sheet along its width until it is approximately 30 cm wide. Extends sheet length perpendicular to patient and feeds under thighs. Pulls through, ensuring there are equal lengths on both sides and the trochanters are in the centre. Brings the two sheet ends together above the patient's groin and rolls them tightly together until they contact the patient. Rolls one end with one hand tightly, then secures with a long length of broad adhesive tape. Repeats for other roll end.	NO	YES
Assesses patient	Assesses distal circulation and pain. Lower limb injuries permitting, maintains slight knee flexion with a rolled blanket or pillow.	NO	YES
Reports	Accurately documents/hands over assessment findings and procedure.	NO	YES

Source: *Adapted from SAM® manufacturer's instructions.*

Standard Achieved: (please circle one)

Competent (C)   Not Yet Competent* (NYC)

Staff/Student Name: _____

Assessor (please print name): _____

Signed (Assessor): _____

Date of Assessment: _____

Comments:

*If Not Yet Competent (NYC) a PIP needs to be completed and a repeat of the F-CSAT

Clinical findings

Uncertain assessment

It can be difficult to differentiate an uncomplicated fracture from an open book fracture, and a stable fracture from an unstable one, so it is critical to err on the side of pelvic splinting. Haemodynamic instability and shock should always prompt early pelvic splinting if injury is suspected (Shackelford et al., 2017).

Concurrent leg fractures

Given the large forces often involved, pelvic fracture is frequently accompanied by other forms of musculoskeletal trauma, including hip and femur fractures. Pelvic splinting should not worsen these injuries, though in some cases it may increase pain. Pelvic fractures must be prioritised, particularly if they are haemodynamically unstable. Limb splinting can then be considered, including simple anatomical immobilisation. If traction is considered necessary, this can be applied as long as the splint can be fitted over the pelvic splint. This may not be possible if a sheet wrap is used. It is possible for some unwanted force to be applied to the pelvis, so the need for traction must be considered absolutely necessary (Scott et al., 2013).

Obese adults

Manufactured pelvic binders do come in larger sizes. Where a patient is oversized for a splint, a sheet wrap option may be the only alternative.

Children

While pelvic fractures are far less common in children than in adults, they remain just as serious (Swaid et al., 2017). Manufactured binders also come in smaller sizes for paediatric patients. Where these are not available, sheet wrap methods are suitable.

PRACTICE TIP!

The management of open book pelvic fractures is not limited to applying a pelvic splint. It must be accompanied by leg closure and binding and possibly slight knee flexion. Other limb injuries must also be addressed.

PRACTICE TIP!

Correct positioning of the pelvic splint is critical. Fitting it from below the trochanters helps ensure it is not positioned too high. Palpate the trochanters to confirm placement before fitting the splint.

PRACTICE TIP!

Pelvic fractures are typically managed early, as part of the primary survey for controlling major haemorrhage. Multiple traumatic injuries and tasks (including analgesia) may distract from injury recognition. Consider pelvic fractures as a cause of shock early in the assessment.

TEST YOUR KNOWLEDGE QUESTIONS

1. **What are the two most common pelvic splint options?**
Manufactured purpose binder; pelvic sheet wrap.

2. **What are the most useful assessment clues to the presence of a pelvic fracture?**
The injury mechanism; pain, including in the ilium, lower back and groin; an inability to bear weight; bruising, swelling and deformity over the fractured site; lower limb asymmetry differentiated from limb fracture; urethral or rectal bleeding.

3. **What is the role of pelvic springing in assessment?**
It is unreliable, often producing no result despite the presence of a fracture. It can also increase bleeding and injury.

4. **Why is haemorrhage of such concern with open book pelvic fracture?**
Major vascular injury and haemodynamic instability including the iliac artery can occur. The sacral venous plexus, hypogastric artery and soft tissue are all sources of haemorrhage if injured by nearby fractured bone.

5. **How does pelvic fracture splinting help control haemorrhage?**
Pelvic compression can control some low-pressure bleeding; bone end stabilisation reduces ongoing injury and improves the likelihood of clot formation.

6. **When should a pelvic splint be applied?**
Early, as part of major haemorrhage control once an open book pelvic injury is suspected.

7. **Which is more effective: a pelvic binder splint or a sheet wrap?**
Both are equally effective if correctly applied.

8. **What is the most common error made when applying a pelvic binder splint?**
Applying the splint too high and above the correct greater trochanter point.

9. **Can pelvic splinting be applied to children?**
Yes, provided the splint is appropriately smaller sized. A sheet wrap is an alternative option.

10. **When is a pelvic binder removed?**
Only after definitive diagnosis and management can be applied.

References

Alton, T.B. and Gee, A.O., 2014. Classifications in brief: Young and Burgess classification of pelvic ring injuries. *Clinical Orthopaedics and Related Research*, 472(8), 2338–2342.

Alwaal, A., Zaid, U.B., Blaschko, S.D., Harris, C.R., Gaither, T.W., McAninch, J.W. and Breyer, B.N., 2015. The incidence, causes, mechanism, risk factors, classification, and diagnosis of pelvic fracture urethral injury. *Arab Journal of Urology*, 13(1), 2–6.

Clamp, J.A. and Moran, C.G., 2011. Haemorrhage control in pelvic trauma. *Trauma*, 13(4), 300–316.

Halliwell, D., Jones, P., Ryan, L. and Clark, R., 2011. The revision of the primary survey: a 2011 review. *Journal of Paramedic Practice*, 3(7), 366–374.

Hsu, S.D., Chen, C.J., Chou, Y.C., Wang, S.H. and Chan, D.C., 2017. Effect of early pelvic binder use in the emergency management of suspected pelvic trauma: a retrospective cohort study. *International Journal of Environmental Research and Public Health*, 14(10), 1217.

Lee, C. and Porter, K., 2007. The prehospital management of pelvic fractures. *Emergency Medicine Journal*, 24(2), 130–133.

Morris, R., Loftus, A., Lygas, A., Mahmood, R. and Pallister, I., 2016. Pelvic pressure changes after a fracture: a pilot cadaveric study assessing the effect of pelvic binders and limb bandaging. *Injury*, 47(2), 295.

Ojodu, I., Pohlemann, T., Hopp, S., Rollmann, M.F., Holstein, J.H. and Herath, S.C., 2015. Predictors of mortality for complex fractures of the pelvic ring in the elderly: a twelve-year review from a German level I trauma center. *Injury*, 46(10), 1996–1998.

Saxena, P., Sakale, H. and Agrawal, A.C., 2014. Introduction to pelvic injury and its acute management. *Journal of Orthopedics, Traumatology and Rehabilitation*, 7(1), 1.

Scott, I., Porter, K., Laird, C., Greaves, I. and Bloch, M., 2013. The prehospital management of pelvic fractures: initial consensus statement. *Emergency Medicine Journal*, 30(12), 1070–1072.

Shackelford, S., Hammesfahr, R., Morissette, D., Montgomery, H.R., Kerr, W., Broussard, M., Bennett, B.L., Dorlac, W.C., Bree, S. and Butler, F.K., 2017. The use of pelvic binders in tactical combat casualty care: TCCC guidelines change 1602 7 November 2016. *Journal of Special Operations Medicine*, 17(1), 135.

Stahel, P.F., Heyde, C.E. and Ertel, W., 2005. Current concepts of polytrauma management. *European Journal of Trauma*, 31, 200–211.

Swaid, F., Peleg, K., Alfici, R., Olsha, O., Givon, A. and Kessel, B., 2017. A comparison study of pelvic fractures and associated abdominal injuries between pediatric and adult blunt trauma patients. *Journal of Pediatric Surgery*, 52(3), 386–389.

Tran, T.L.N., Brasel, K.J., Karmy-Jones, R., Rowell, S., Schreiber, M.A., Shatz, D.V., Albrecht, R.M., Cohen, M.J., DeMoya, M.A., Biffl, W.L. and Moore, E.E., 2016. Western Trauma Association critical decisions in trauma: management of pelvic fracture with hemodynamic instability – 2016 updates. *Journal of Trauma and Acute Care Surgery*, 81(6), 1171–1174.

Verbeek, D.O., Ponsen, K.J., Fiocco, M., Amodio, S., Leenen, L.P. and Goslings, J.C., 2018. Pelvic fractures in the Netherlands: epidemiology, characteristics and risk factors for in-hospital mortality in the older and younger population. *European Journal of Orthopaedic Surgery & Traumatology*, 28(2), 197–205.

5.8 | Anterior shoulder dislocation reduction

Anna Pearce and Liam Langford

Chapter objectives

At the end of this chapter the reader will be able to:

1. Identify different types of shoulder dislocation.
2. State common anterior shoulder dislocation (ASD) injury mechanisms
3. Identify indications and contraindications for prehospital ASD reduction
4. Perform safe and effective ASD reduction based on the Stimson method and post care

Resources required for this assessment

- Standardised patient/mannequin capable of demonstrating joint dislocation
- Disposable gloves
- Hand decontamination agent
- Stretcher or flat horizontal surface for prone patient position with affected arm hanging over the side
- Approximately 5–7 kg weight (e.g. a small medical kit)
- Triangular bandage
- Method of documenting results

Skill matrix

This assessment requires:

- Infection control (CS 1.3)
- Communication (CS 1.5)
- Consent (CS 1.6)
- Pain assessment (CS 2.16)

This assessment is a component of:

- Trauma (Chapter 5)

Introduction

A shoulder dislocation is an injury where the humeral head is displaced from its normal position in the glenoid cavity (Tintinalli et al., 2011). Shoulder dislocations account for 50% of all major joint dislocations, and are divisible into four different types (Tintinalli et al., 2011). Anterior dislocation is the most common, accounting for approximately 95% of cases. Posterior dislocation accounts for about 1%, while inferior (luxatio erecta) and superior dislocations are very rare (Tintinalli et al., 2011).

This chapter focuses on the management of ASD, which, under certain strict conditions and in certain patient populations, can be safely reduced by paramedics (Helfen et al., 2016). While numerous reduction techniques are described in the literature (Alkaduhimi et al., 2016; Tintinalli et al., 2011), there is no clear evidence to support the superiority of one method over another (Sherman, 2016; Helfen et al., 2016).

The reduction technique presented here is the Stimson method. This technique is used in the Australasian prehospital environment (WFAS, 2019).

Anatomy and physiology

The shoulder (glenohumeral) joint (Fig. 5.8.1) is a ball-and-socket synovial joint. Articulation is between the glenoid fossa of the scapular and the head of the humerus (Sherman, 2016). The shoulder is known for its instability due to the structurally shallow socket of the glenoid fossa and the multiaxial movements of flexion, extension, abduction, adduction, internal and external rotation and circumduction (Sherman, 2016; Tintinalli et al., 2011). The shoulder socket is deepened by the fibrocartilaginous ring of the glenoid labrum. Further stability is provided by the tendinous attachments of the four rotator cuff muscles. The subscapularis muscle assists in preventing anterior dislocation. The supraspinatus, infraspinatus and teres minor pull the humerus head into the glenoid cavity (Sherman, 2016).

The axillary nerve is most commonly injured in shoulder dislocations (Sherman, 2016; Tintinalli et al., 2011). This nerve originates from the posterior cord of the brachial plexus and innervates the deltoid and teres minor muscles and the skin overlying the lateral shoulder, known as the 'shoulder badge' distribution (Sherman, 2016). The axillary nerve is usually damaged during fractures of the head of humerus, as this nerve path tracks inferiorly to the humeral head and wraps around the surgical head of humerus (Sherman, 2016).

Clinical rationale

ASDs are usually caused by force to an abducted, extended and externally rotated humerus, such as when the body rotates internally over a fixed outstretched arm (van der Brand and Kelly, 2015). It is common in young adults in contact sports (e.g. football, hockey) or sports with a high risk of falls (e.g. downhill skiing, volleyball, gymnastics). Other mechanisms include trauma (vehicle accidents) or falls from height onto an outstretched hand (Tintinalli et al., 2011).

Previous dislocations may result in stretched ligaments weakening the shoulder joint and increasing the risk of future dislocations. Increased shoulder joint laxity also occurs with age, predisposing the elderly to a higher risk of dislocation.

Shoulder dislocation results in inevitable stretching or tearing of the joint capsule, which may be associated with damage to the subscapularis muscle or the glenoid cavity (Tintinalli et al., 2011). ASDs are also associated with several fractures including Hills-Sachs deformity (impression fracture) of the humeral head, bony Bankart lesions (impaction fracture) to the bony glenoid margin and fractures of the greater tuberosity of humerus (Tintinalli et al., 2011). The most common complication associated with ASD is recurrence (Sherman, 2016). Other complications include rotator cuff injury, axillary nerve damage and, rarely, injury to the brachial plexus and axillary vessels (Tintinalli et al., 2011). Rotator cuff tears are more common in the elderly, as these muscles weaken with age (Sherman, 2016).

The clinical features of ASD include severe pain and shoulder deformity with a history of mechanical displacement (van der Brand and Kelly, 2015). On clinical examination, the affected arm will be slightly abducted and externally rotated (Sherman, 2016; van der Brand and Kelly, 2015). The shoulder appears 'squared off', lacking the normal rounded contour and with a palpable gap just under the acromion where the humeral head usually lies (van der Brand and Kelly, 2015) (Fig. 5.8.2). The humeral head may be palpable anteriorly in the hollow behind the pectoral muscles (van der Brand and Kelly, 2015).

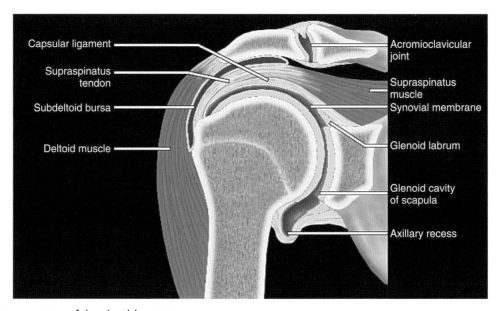

Figure 5.8.1 Cross-section of the shoulder joint

Source: *Woodward P. J., Griffith J. and Antonio G. et al., 2018,* Imaging anatomy: ultrasound, *2nd edn (Chapter: Shoulder, Figure 4), Elsevier Inc.*

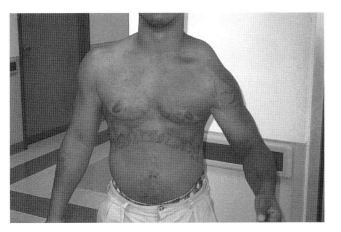

Figure 5.8.2 Anterior shoulder dislocation

Obvious left shoulder dislocation. This chronic dislocation occurred frequently with minimal trauma, and the patient was able to dislocate it at will, feign a new injury, and obtain narcotics from multiple emergency departments.

Source: *Thomsen, T.W., Custalow, C.B. and Roberts, J.R., 2019, Roberts and Hedges' clinical procedures in emergency medicine and acute care, 7th edn (Chapter 49, Figure 49.4), Elsevier.*

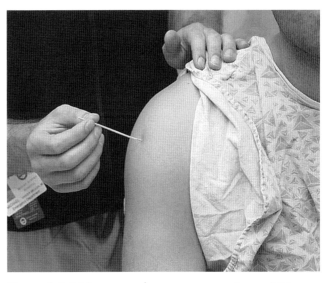

Figure 5.8.3 Neurovascular assessment prior to ASD reduction

Neurovascular evaluation of the upper extremity with a shoulder dislocation. Axillary (circumflex) nerve palsy is the most common neurologic complication. The axillary nerve has sensory and motor function. Test the integrity of the nerve by assessing sensation to pinprick in its distribution over the 'regimental badge' area. (The shoulder is usually too painful to allow assessment of deltoid activity with certainty.)

Source: *Thomsen, T.W., Custalow, C.B. and Roberts, J.R., 2019, Roberts and Hedges' clinical procedures in emergency medicine and acute care, 7th edn (Chapter 49, Figure 49.5), Elsevier.*

Range of motion is restricted, with the patient showing reluctance to move the shoulder and supporting the arm at the elbow or wrist (van der Brand and Kelly, 2015). The patient resists adduction and internal rotation, and is unable to touch the contralateral shoulder with the hand of the affected side (Sherman, 2016).

It is important to perform a comprehensive neurovascular examination both pre and post reduction, paying particular attention to the axillary and musculocutaneous nerves (Sherman, 2016; van der Brand and Kelly, 2015) (Fig. 5.8.3). The axillary nerve is most commonly injured and can be assessed by testing sensation over the skin of the deltoid muscle. Assess for posterior brachial plexus injury by testing the radial nerve; this is done by assessing the strength of the muscles used in wrist extension. Brachial and radial pulses should be assessed, as well as clinical signs of limb ischaemia (pallor, pulselessness, paraesthesia, poikilothermia, paralysis, pain) (van der Brand and Kelly, 2015). Limb ischaemia is a time-critical emergency (Sherman, 2016). There is significant pain associated with all types of shoulder dislocations, and appropriate analgesia is therefore important (van der Brand and Kelly, 2015).

A dislocated shoulder should be relocated at the earliest possible time to relieve pain and reduce further injury. Risk to nerves, blood vessels and ligaments increases with prolonged displacement (Sherman, 2016). In specific circumstances, ASD may be reduced in the prehospital field (Helfen et al., 2016).

The safe indications for ASD reduction are:
- clinically evident uncomplicated anterior shoulder dislocation *and*
- a history of multiple recurrent dislocations of the same joint *and*
- the joint dislocation is a result of minor force (e.g. sporting injury) only

- low risk or no evidence of concurrent humerus fracture or concomitant acromioclavicular joint dislocation.

Currently, there is little evidence to ascertain whether the risk outweighs the benefit of prehospital ASD reduction (Bath and Lord, 2009). Delaying reduction may lead to prolonged pain from muscle spasm, more difficult reduction requiring procedural sedation or surgical reduction and an increased likelihood of future dislocations. Successful reduction is more likely when performed by skilled clinicians (Helfen et al., 2016).

The Stimson method is discussed in this chapter, although alternative relocation methods include the Cunningham, Kocher, Hippocratic and scapular manipulation techniques (Sherman, 2016). Reduction techniques known to be successful without sedation and minimal analgesia include the Cunningham technique and the Stimson method (Amar et al., 2012; Cunningham, 2003).

The Stimson method achieves shoulder reduction using traction (Amar et al., 2012). The patient is placed prone on the stretcher, with the dislocated limb hanging freely over the side of the stretcher (Fig. 5.8.4) and a 5–10 kg weight attached to the wrist (Fig. 5.8.5). The patient's head is placed on a pillow in either direction for comfort. In the absence of a suitable weight, gentle manual downward traction can be used (Fig. 5.8.6) (Amar et al., 2012). Most importantly, complete muscle relaxation is required, which is achieved by providing reassurance and appropriate analgesia (Sherman, 2016). Gentle elbow flexion relaxes the biceps brachii, reducing muscular tension at the shoulder (Fig. 5.8.7) (Sherman, 2016).

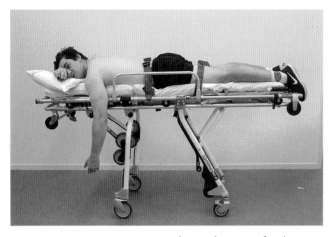

Figure 5.8.4 Prone position with arm hanging freely

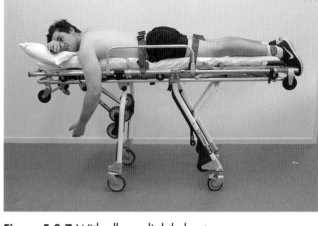

Figure 5.8.7 With elbow slightly bent

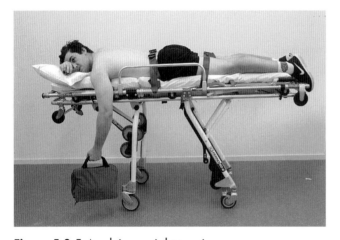

Figure 5.8.5 Applying weight traction

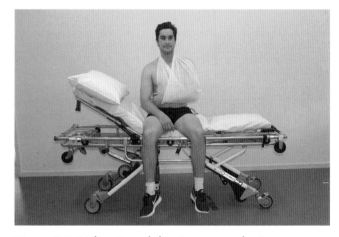

Figure 5.8.8 Sling immobilisation post reduction

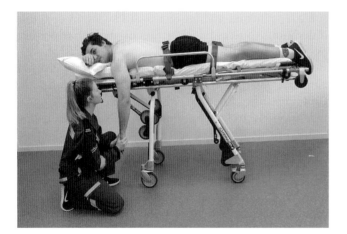

Figure 5.8.6 Applying manual traction

Short-duration procedural analgesia is ideal, as pain resolves quickly after relocation (Raftos and Locke, 2001). An audible 'clunk' may be heard as the humerus enters the glenoid cavity (van der Brand and Kelly, 2015). Using the Stimson method, reduction usually occurs within 30 minutes, after which the shoulder requires repeat neurovascular assessment, immobilisation (Fig. 5.8.8) and

transport to an appropriate receiving facility for follow-up care (Sherman, 2016).

Contraindications

ASD management should not precede the primary and secondary survey or the management of life-threatening injuries.

Elderly patients or those with metabolic bone disease, such as osteoporosis, are at risk of vascular injury and fractures during reduction attempts (van der Brand and Kelly, 2015), so prehospital reduction is contraindicated.

Prehospital relocation is not appropriate for patients with evidence of arm fracture, or where the mechanism of injury involves significant force and the risk of being associated with fractures. What constitutes 'significant force' is difficult to define and this must therefore be assessed case by case (van der Brand and Kelly, 2015).

Inferior, posterior and complicated anterior shoulder dislocations should only be reduced by experienced clinicians in the appropriate environment where radiology and procedural sedation are available. In hospital, radiographs are usually obtained before reduction to identify the type of dislocation and any coexisting fractures. There is currently no safe clinical decision tool to eliminate the need for pre-reduction radiographs. Where there is compromised perfusion or sensation distal to the dislocated shoulder, relocation is time critical. Shoulder dislocations with proximal humeral head fractures require operative repair. The prehospital treatment for these types of dislocations is to administer appropriate analgesia, splint the joint and transport the patient to an appropriate receiving facility (Sherman, 2016).

Reduction should not be attempted where there is no previous history of shoulder dislocations in the affected joint.

Clinical skill assessment process

The following section outlines the clinical skill assessment tools that should be used to determine a student's ability to demonstrate safe and accurate anterior shoulder dislocation reduction.
1. Clinical Skill Work Instruction
2. Formative Clinical Skill Assessment (F-CSAT)
3. Performance Improvement Plan (PIP)
4. Summative Clinical Skill Assessment (S-CSAT)
(5. Direct Observation of Procedural Skills (DOPS) – see Chapter 1.1)

Clinical Skill Work Instruction

Equipment and resources: Standardised patient/mannequin capable of demonstrating joint dislocation; disposable gloves; stretcher/flat horizontal surface for prone patient position with affected arm hanging over side; 5–10 kg weight (e.g. small medical kit); triangular bandage; method of documenting results

Associated Clinical Skills: Infection control; Communication; Consent; Pain assessment

Anterior shoulder dislocation reduction

Activity	Critical Action	Rationale
Assess patient	Determine mechanism of action, other injuries, pain level, history of dislocations/shoulder injuries and comorbidities.	To establish appropriate management and determine indications/contraindications for reduction.
	Cut or remove clothing to carefully expose injury.	To allow clinical examination and reduction.
	Assess for ASD by the principles of 'look, feel, move'. Conduct neurovascular assessment: sensory distribution of axillary nerve and distal vasculature of axillary artery, including brachial and radial pulses.	Axillary nerve injury is a complication of dislocation and reduction. Rarely, the axillary artery is injured. If this occurs, it is a surgical emergency to maintain limb viability.
Prepare patient	Inform patient that specific procedure risks are usually minimal/rare but may include fractures and injury to nerves or arteries.	Facilitates patient autonomy and empowers patient responsibility of their care.
	Administer procedural analgesia.	Facilitates musculature relaxation and provides pain management.
Position patient	Lay patient prone on raised stretcher with affected arm hanging freely over side (Fig. 5.8.4). Secure patient to the stretcher using stretcher straps. Wait 1–2 minutes, as reduction may occur with simple positioning.	Facilitates appropriate safe patient position.
Slightly bend elbow	Encourage patient to relax shoulder musculature and slightly bend the elbow (Fig. 5.8.7). Wait 1–2 minutes as reduction may occur with repositioning.	Facilitates appropriate patient position.
Apply traction	*Either:* Grasp patient's hand of affected arm and gently apply constant downward traction (Fig. 5.8.6); continue for 10–15 minutes or until evidence of successful reduction *or:* Hang approximately 5–10 kg of weight from the hand of the affected arm (e.g. small medical kit; Fig. 5.8.5); continue for 10–15 minutes or until evidence of successful reduction.	Use gentle traction with constant pressure only. Avoid jerky movements as this may cause further injury.

Anterior shoulder dislocation reduction continued

Activity	Critical Action	Rationale
Confirm reduction	Reduction may be confirmed by an audible clunk, immediate pain relief, resolution of normal shoulder contour and restoration of movement.	Reduction may take up to 30 minutes. Use traction for an appropriate time. If reduction is unsuccessful, transport to appropriate care.
Continuing care	Reassess neurovascular status of arm, apply sling, immobilise shoulder (Fig. 5.8.8), follow local pain management guidelines and transport to appropriate facility.	Stabilise joint and manage pain en route to hospital.
Report	Accurately document/hand over assessment findings and procedure.	Accurate record kept and continuity of patient care.

Source: *Adapted from Amar et al., 2012.*

Formative Clinical Skill Assessment (F-CSAT)

Equipment and resources: Standardised patient/mannequin capable of demonstrating joint dislocation; disposable gloves; stretcher/flat horizontal surface for prone patient position with affected arm hanging over side; 5–10 kg weight (e.g. small medical kit); triangular bandage; method of documenting results

Associated Clinical Skills: Infection control; Communication; Consent; Pain assessment

Staff/student being assessed: _____

Anterior shoulder dislocation reduction

Activity	Critical Action	Performance				
Assesses patient	Determines mechanism of action, other injuries, pain level, dislocations/ shoulder injury history and comorbidities.	0	1	2	3	4
	Cuts/removes clothing to carefully expose injury.	0	1	2	3	4
	Assesses for ASD using 'look, feel, move'. Conducts neurovascular assessment, including the axillary nerve and axillary artery.	0	1	2	3	4
Prepares patient	Informs patient of specific procedure risks.	0	1	2	3	4
	Administers procedural analgesia as needed.	0	1	2	3	4
Positions patient	Lays patient prone on raised stretcher with affected arm hanging freely over side. Secures patient to the stretcher using stretcher straps. Waits 1–2 minutes. Reassesses.	0	1	2	3	4
Slightly bends elbow	Encourages patient to relax the shoulder musculature and slightly bend the elbow. Waits 1–2 minutes. Reassesses.	0	1	2	3	4
Applies traction	*Either:* Grasps patient's hand of affected arm and gently applies constant downward traction; continues for 10–15 minutes or until evidence of successful reduction *or:* Hangs approximately 5–10 kg of weight from the hand of the affected arm (e.g. a small medical kit); continues for 10–15 minutes or until evidence of successful reduction.	0	1	2	3	4
Confirms reduction	Confirms reduction, checking for audible clunk, immediate pain relief, resolution of normal shoulder contour and restoration of movement.	0	1	2	3	4

Anterior shoulder dislocation reduction continued

Activity	Critical Action	Performance				
Continuing care	Reassesses arm neurovascular status, applies sling, immobilises shoulder, provides analgesia as necessary and transports to appropriate facility.	0	1	2	3	4
Reports	Accurately documents/hands over assessment findings and procedure.	0	1	2	3	4

Source: *Adapted from Amar et al., 2012.*

Standard Achieved: (please circle one)

Competent (C)   Not Yet Competent* (NYC)

Staff/Student Name: _____

Assessor (please print name): _____

Signed (Assessor): _____

Date of Assessment: _____

Comments:

*If Not Yet Competent (NYC) a PIP needs to be completed and a repeat of the F-CSAT

Formative Clinical Skill Assessment (F-CSAT) Key

Skill level	Standard of procedure	Quality of performance	Outcome	Level of assistance required
4 Safe for unsupervised practice	Safe Accurate Behaviour is appropriate to context	Confident Accurate Expedient	Achieved intended outcome	No supporting cues* required
3 Requires supervision	Safe Accurate Behaviour is appropriate to context	Confident Accurate Takes longer than required	Achieved intended outcome	Requires occasional supportive cues*
2 Requires assistance	Safe Accurate Behaviour generally appropriate to context	Lacks certainty	Would not have achieved outcome without support	Requires frequent verbal and occasional physical directives in addition to supportive cues*
1 Requires direction	Safe only with guidance Not completely accurate	Unskilled Inefficient	Would not have achieved outcome without support	Requires continuous verbal and frequent physical directive cues*
0 Unsafe	Unsafe Unable to demonstrate behaviour Lack of insight into behaviour appropriate to context	Unskilled	Would not have achieved outcome	Requires continuous verbal and continuous physical directive cues*

*Refers to physical directives or verbal supportive cues

Performance Improvement Plan (PIP)

Please document the agreed education plan and completion timelines for areas assessed as less than 4.

This plan should be presented to assessor prior to commencement of summative assessment.

Where was supervisor support required?	Student summary of deficit. (Why was there a problem?)	Improvement Plan	Completed (Y/N)

Staff/Student Name: _____

Staff/Student Signature: _____

Educator Name: _____

Educator Signature: _____

Summative Clinical Skill Assessment (S-CSAT)

Equipment and resources: Standardised patient/mannequin capable of demonstrating joint dislocation; disposable gloves; stretcher/flat horizontal surface for prone patient position with affected arm hanging over side; 5–10 kg weight (e.g. small medical kit); triangular bandage; method of documenting results

Associated Clinical Skills: Infection control; Communication; Consent; Pain assessment

Staff/student being assessed: _____

- Completed Formative Clinical Skill Assessment (F-CSAT):   **YES   NO**

- Completed Performance Improvement Plan (PIP):   **YES   NO   N/A**

Anterior shoulder dislocation reduction			
Activity	**Critical Action**	**Achieved Without Direction**	
Assesses patient	Determines mechanism of action, other injuries, pain level, dislocations/ shoulder injury history and comorbidities.	NO	YES
	Cuts/removes clothing to carefully expose injury.	NO	YES
	Assesses for ASD using 'look, feel, move'. Conducts neurovascular assessment, including the axillary nerve and axillary artery.	NO	YES
Prepares patient	Informs patient of specific procedure risks.	NO	YES
	Administers procedural analgesia if needed.	NO	YES
Positions patient	Lays patient prone on raised stretcher with affected arm hanging freely over side. Secures patient to the stretcher using stretcher straps. Waits 1–2 minutes. Reassesses.	NO	YES

Anterior shoulder dislocation reduction continued

Activity	Critical Action	Achieved Without Direction	
Slightly bends elbow	Encourages patient to relax the shoulder musculature and slightly bend the elbow. Waits 1–2 minutes. Reassesses.	NO	YES
Applies traction	*Either:* Grasps patient's hand on affected arm and gently applies constant downward traction; continues for 10–15 minutes or until evidence of successful reduction *or:* Hangs approximately 5–10 kg of weight from the hand of the affected arm (e.g. small medical kit); continues for 10–15 minutes or until evidence of successful reduction.	NO	YES
Confirms reduction	Confirms reduction, checking for audible clunk, immediate pain relief, resolution of normal shoulder contour and restoration of movement.	NO	YES
Continuing care	Reassesses arm neurovascular status, applies sling, immobilises shoulder, provides analgesia as necessary and transports to appropriate facility.	NO	YES
Reports	Accurately documents/hands over assessment findings and procedure.	NO	YES

Source: *Adapted from Amar et al., 2012.*

Standard Achieved: (please circle one)

Competent (C)   Not Yet Competent* (NYC)

Staff/Student Name: _____

Assessor (please print name)**:** _____

Signed (Assessor)**:** _____

Date of Assessment: _____

Comments:

*If Not Yet Competent (NYC) a PIP needs to be completed and a repeat of the F-CSAT

Clinical findings

Attempt limitations

No more than two attempts should be made using a single technique. If the shoulder does not relocate, support the arm in the most comfortable position, provide analgesia and transport the patient to an Emergency Department (Sherman, 2016). Post-reduction radiographs are required in all patients, for confirming shoulder relocation and screening for complications associated with relocation (Sherman, 2016).

PRACTICE TIP!

Complete shoulder muscle relaxation is fundamental to successful relocation. Gentle massage of the trapezius, deltoid and biceps can help relax the shoulder. Slightly flexing the elbow reduces bicep tension on the shoulder joint and can help relocation. Relax the patient using good communication skills.

PRACTICE TIP!

Given the procedure may take some time or, on occasion, even be ineffective, early analgesia should be considered according to local clinical guidelines. This can be continued according to patient need.

PRACTICE TIP!

Remember to reassess the patient's neurovascular status, paying attention to the axillary nerve. An injured axillary nerve results in the inability to contract the deltoid muscle and numbness over the insertion of the deltoid, also known as the 'badge area'.

PRACTICE TIP!

A detailed history and comprehensive examination helps ensure the patient meets the inclusion criteria and that shoulder relocation is not contraindicated. Relocation is contraindicated in patients who are elderly or those with metabolic bone disease, no previous history of shoulder dislocations in the affected joint, concomitant arm fracture or major trauma. Life-threatening injuries require prioritised treatment.

PRACTICE TIP!

Patients with reoccurring shoulder dislocations will know when the shoulder is relocated.

TEST YOUR KNOWLEDGE QUESTIONS

1. **Why is methoxyflurane an ideal medication to use for patients with ASD?**
There is rapid onset to effectiveness; it has good analgesic and sedative properties to enable reduction procedure; there is rapid offset after a successful reduction.

2. **Which nerve is most likely to be injured in ASD?**
The axillary nerve.

3. **What clinical features are likely with ASD?**
Severe pain; patient's reluctance/inability to move the shoulder; patient splinting their elbow/wrist, often in slight abduction; loss of normal round shoulder contour to a 'flattened-off' appearance; a palpable gap under the acromion; displaced humeral head; axillary nerve disruption, involving an inability to contract the deltoid or an abnormality in badge sensation.

4. **What are the potential complications of ASD?**
Reoccurring dislocations; rotator cuff injury; fractures such as Bankart lesions – bony (avulsion of the glenoid) and soft (injury to the glenoid labrum), Hill-Sachs deformity (impression fracture of humeral head) and humeral tuberosity head fractures; axillary nerve injury; vascular injury.

5. **What is the best clinical method to reduce ASD?**
There is no clear evidence to support the superiority of any one of the many methods used to reduce anterior shoulder dislocations.

6. **What are the indications for ASD reduction?**
Clinically evident ASD with a history of multiple recurrent dislocations of the same joint, and where the dislocation is a result of minor force (e.g. sporting injury) only.

7. **ASD is contraindicated in elderly patients (>70 years) or for those with known metabolic bone disorders (e.g. osteoporosis). Why?**
Because of the risk of vascular injury and fractures with reduction attempts.

8. **Shoulder muscle relaxation can increase successful relocation likelihood. What methods help facilitate this?**
Reassurance through good communication; analgesia; prone positioning with arm hanging; slightly bending arm at elbow; gently massaging the trapezius, deltoid and biceps.

9. **What signs and symptoms help confirm reduction?**
An audible clunk; immediate pain relief; resolution of normal shoulder contour; restoration of movement.

10. **If reduction has not occurred after 20–30 minutes of the Stimson method, outline your contingency management plan.**
Provide continued rest and reassurance; provide continued analgesia; position patient comfortably and practically; transport patient to an appropriate facility.

References

Alkaduhimi, H., van der Linde, J.A., Flipsen, M., van Deurzen, D.F.P. and van den Bekerom, M.P.J., 2016. A systematic and technical guide on how to reduce a shoulder dislocation. *Turkish Journal of Emergency Medicine*, 16, 155–168.

Amar, E., Maman, E., Khashan, M., Kauffman, E., Rath, E. and Chechik, O., 2012. Milch versus Stimson technique for nonsedated reduction of anterior shoulder dislocation: a prospective randomized trial and analysis of factors affecting success. *Journal of Shoulder and Elbow Surgery*, 21, 1443–1449.

Bath, T. and Lord, B., 2009. Risk and benefits of paramedic-initiated shoulder reduction. *Journal of Paramedic Practice*, 1, 235–240.

Cunningham, N., 2003. A new drug free technique for reducing anterior shoulder dislocations. *Emergency Medicine Australasia*, 15, 521–524.

Helfen, T., Ockert, B., Pozder, P., Regauer, M. and Haasters, F., 2016. Management of prehospital shoulder dislocation: feasibility and need of reduction. *European Journal of Trauma and Emergency Surgery*, 42, 357–362.

Raftos, J. and Locke, P., 2001. Orthopaedic principles – fractures and dislocations. In Fulde, G. and Fulde, S., Emergency medicine. *Current Therapeutics*, 42(8), 304–342.

Sherman, S.C., 2016. *Shoulder dislocation and reduction.* Retrieved from: www.uptodate.com

Tintinalli, J.E., Stapczynski, J.S., Ma, O.J., Yealy, D.M., Meckler, G.D. and Cline, D.M., 2011. *Emergency medicine: a comprehensive study guide.* New York: McGraw-Hill.

van der Brand, C. and Kelly, A., 2015. Section 4: Orthopaedic emergencies. In Cameron, P., Jelinek, G., Kelly, A.-M., Brown, A.F.T. and Little, M., *Textbook of adult emergency medicine*, 4th edn. Sydney: Churchill Livingstone/Elsevier.

WFAS (Wellington Free Ambulance Service), 2019. *Clinical procedures and guidelines: comprehensive edition 2019–2022.* Retrieved from: https://www.wfa.org.nz/assets/What-we-do/b8a3986cc7/WFA-CPG-Comprehensive-2019-2022.pdf

Dislocated patella relocation

John Suringa

Chapter objectives

At the end of this chapter the reader will be able to:

1. Describe the common mechanism and presentation for patella dislocation
2. Demonstrate the method for safe relocation of a closed dislocated patella

Resources required for this assessment

- Standard patient or mannequin suitable for practising patella relocation
- Disposable gloves
- Leg splint options, including triangular bandages
- Alcohol-based hand wash
- Clinical waste bag
- Method for documenting results

Skill matrix

This assessment requires:

- Infection control (CS 1.3)
- Communication (CS 1.5)
- Consent (CS 1.6)
- Assessment of motor and sensory nerve function (CS 2.13)
- Pain assessment (CS 2.16)
- Medication administration (Chapter 4)

This assessment is a component of:

- Trauma (Chapter 5)

Introduction

Patella dislocations are common sporting and dancing injuries, typically arising where the knee twists while the foot remains fixed to the ground (Longo et al., 2017; Smith et al., 2015). A previous similar injury is common (Jain et al., 2011; Longo et al., 2017), and dislocation is second only to anterior cruciate ligament tears in prevalence among knee injuries (Duthon, 2015; Longo et al., 2017; Vetrano et al., 2017). It is most common among adolescents (Sanders et al., 2017).

Dislocations occur when the patella slips out of the patellofemoral groove due to either a twisting motion of the knee or direct force applied to the patella (Frosch et al., 2011). This causes intense pain and swelling in the knee joint. The dislocation is usually obvious, as the patella is visibly displaced and the limb is typically held flexed (Duthon, 2015).

In most cases, surgical intervention is avoided unless there are fracture fragments or other damage to the ligaments (Smith et al., 2015). The patella generally dislocates laterally and, provided there are no fracture concerns, can be easily relocated.

This chapter discusses the safe relocation of a dislocated patella.

Anatomy and physiology

The patella is a small, roughly triangular-shaped bone that sits anterior to the knee joint. The knee is arguably the most complex joint, largely concealed beneath the patella. Superiorly, the patella is attached to the quadriceps femoris muscle via the quadriceps tendon. Distally, the patella is attached to the tibial head via the large patella ligament. This is essentially a continuation of the quadriceps tendon, and so it is also referred to as the patella tendon. Smaller ligaments attach to the medial (medial patellofemoral) and lateral patella. The patella normally sits and moves in a groove on the distal femur; it moves out of this groove when dislocated.

The purpose of the patella is to provide a stable attachment point for the quadriceps femoris muscle when the knee is flexed. It also provides some protection for the underlying knee joint.

The popliteal artery lies behind the knee, as does the tibial nerve. The common peroneal nerve lies laterally of the patella. All are potentially vulnerable during patella injury, with injuries including vascular occlusion or tearing and nerve impingement.

Clinical rationale

The most common form of patellar dislocation is lateral (Duthon, 2015; Longo et al., 2017) due to the natural pull of the quadriceps muscle (Fig. 5.9.1). Uncommonly, the patella can dislocate horizontally (turned on a horizontal axis) or vertically (turned on a vertical axis). This method of reduction applies to lateral dislocation, which is identifiable by the distinctive lateral position of the patella when found.

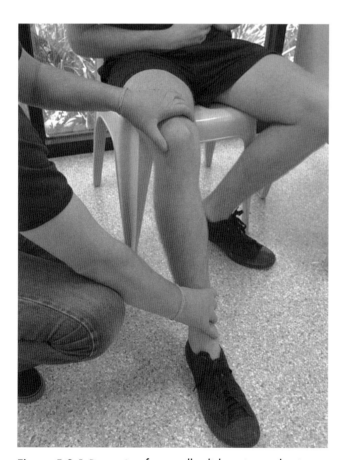

Figure 5.9.1 Preparing for patella dislocation reduction

Before commencing a patella reduction, exclude injuries that can be complicated by this procedure (see Table 5.9.1). Distal circulation and sensation are not usually compromised; where this occurs, consider knee dislocation as the more likely cause. If this is suspected, the tibia is likely to be out of alignment with the femur, which is not the case with patella dislocation.

Injuries to the quadriceps tendon or patella fracture can cause the patella to sit above its normal location instead of laterally. These injuries should be splinted in the position in which they are found. Fractures of the proximal tibia or distal femur are a contraindication for the procedure, given the potential to worsen injury and increase pain during any manipulation attempted.

In all cases, monitor distal circulation and sensation before and following the reduction procedure.

If there are no contraindications, a dislocated patella should be reduced as soon as practicable to avoid quadriceps muscle spasm and swelling. It may be necessary to provide procedural analgesia before doing so.

Attempt to manage the patient as found. If they are supine, flex the hip of the injured leg to relax the quadriceps muscle. If sitting, allow the leg to hang downwards. This position will naturally flex the hip.

Stand on the lateral side of the leg. Grasp the ankle with the nearest hand. The other hand is placed braced against the lateral thigh, with the arc between thumb and forefinger circling the displaced patella. The thumb should contact the lower edge of the patella (Fig. 5.9.1).

The ankle is then moved to extend the knee and straighten the leg. Simultaneous medial pressure is gently applied to the knee, pushing it back towards its correct position while the leg straightens (Duthon, 2015).

Clinical skill assessment process

The following section outlines the clinical skill assessment tools that should be used to determine a student's ability to demonstrate safe and accurate relocation of a dislocated patella.
1. Clinical Skill Work Instruction
2. Formative Clinical Skill Assessment (F-CSAT)
3. Performance Improvement Plan (PIP)
4. Summative Clinical Skill Assessment (S-CSAT)
(5. Direct Observation of Procedural Skills (DOPS) – see Chapter 1.1)

Table 5.9.1 Indications and contraindications for relocating a dislocated patella

Indications	Contraindications
Lateral patella dislocation	Fractures of the proximal tibia or distal femur Knee dislocation Other forms of patella dislocation

Clinical Skill Work Instruction

Equipment and resources: Standard patient or mannequin suitable for practising patella relocation; disposable gloves; leg splint options, including triangular bandages; alcohol-based hand wash; clinical waste bag; method for documenting results

Associated Clinical Skills: Infection control; Communication; Consent; Assessment of motor and sensory nerve function; Pain assessment; Medication administration

Dislocated patella relocation

Activity	Critical Action	Rationale
Assess patient	Confirm indication. Exclude contraindication. Assess distal circulation and sensation.	Procedure has the potential to cause injury if not correctly applied. Identifies urgency of injury.
Prepare patient	Gain consent. Explain procedure to patient. Patient can lie supine, semi-reclined or sitting.	Decreases anxiety and informs the patient of the procedure.
Universal precautions	Wash hands, don gloves.	To control the risk of infection.
Analgesia	Administer procedural analgesia as required.	Procedure may increase pain until patella is relocated.
Position paramedic	Stand beside and facing patient on lateral side of injured leg.	To perform procedure.
Grasp limb in readiness	Partly flex patient's hip if it is not already flexed. Hold patient's ankle with closest hand and support the lower leg. Place fingers of other hand against lower thigh, with forefinger against superior patella edge. Spread thumb away from forefinger and move hand so that the arc encircles lateral patella. Rest thumb against inferior patella edge.	Positioned ready to provide movements necessary to relocate patella.
Relocate patella	Slowly straighten limb/flex knee. Simultaneously press arc of hand medially, applying gentle constant pressure on the patella. Watch for snap of patella relocating.	To relocate patella.
Confirm relocation	Confirm visible relocation and a decrease in pain.	Ensures procedure has been successful.
Reassess limb	Reassess distal circulation and sensation.	Ensures there is no impingement of nerves or circulation.
Splint limb	Splint limb comfortably in correct alignment.	Prevents patella from displacing again, supports the knee and minimises risk of further injury.
Report	Document/hand over procedure and responses.	Accurate record kept and continuity of patient care.

Formative Clinical Skill Assessment (F-CSAT)

Equipment and resources: Standard patient or mannequin suitable for practising patella relocation; disposable gloves; leg splint options, including triangular bandages; alcohol-based hand wash; clinical waste bag; method for documenting results

Associated Clinical Skills: Infection; Communication; Consent; Assessment of motor and sensory nerve function; Pain assessment; Medication administration

Staff/Student being assessed: _____

Dislocated patella relocation

Activity	Critical Action	Performance				
Assesses patient	Confirms indication. Excludes contraindication. Assesses distal circulation and sensation.	0	1	2	3	4
Prepares patient	Gains consent. Explains procedure.	0	1	2	3	4
Universal precautions	Washes hands, dons gloves.	0	1	2	3	4
Analgesia	Administers procedural analgesia as required.	0	1	2	3	4
Positions paramedic	Stands beside and facing patient on lateral side of injured leg.	0	1	2	3	4
Grasps limb in readiness	Partly flexes patient's hip if not already flexed. Holds patient's ankle with closest hand. Supports lower leg. Places fingers of other hand against lower thigh, with forefinger against superior patella edge. Spreads thumb away from forefinger and moves hand so that the arc encircles lateral patella. Rests thumb against inferior patella edge.	0	1	2	3	4
Relocates patella	Slowly straightens limb/flexes knee. Simultaneously presses arc of hand medially, applying gentle constant pressure on the patella. Watches for snap of patella relocating.	0	1	2	3	4
Confirms relocation	Confirms visible relocation and decrease in pain.	0	1	2	3	4
Reassesses limb	Reassesses distal circulation and sensation.	0	1	2	3	4
Splints limb	Splints limb comfortably in correct alignment.	0	1	2	3	4
Reports	Documents/hands over procedure and responses.	0	1	2	3	4

Standard Achieved: (please circle one)

Competent (C) Not Yet Competent* (NYC)

Staff/Student Name: _____

Assessor (please print name)**:** _____

Signed (Assessor)**:** _____

Date of Assessment: _____

Comments:

*If Not Yet Competent (NYC) a PIP needs to be completed and a repeat of the F-CSAT

Formative Clinical Skill Assessment (F-CSAT) Key

Skill level	Standard of procedure	Quality of performance	Outcome	Level of assistance required
4 Safe for unsupervised practice	Safe Accurate Behaviour is appropriate to context	Confident Accurate Expedient	Achieved intended outcome	No supporting cues*required
3 Requires supervision	Safe Accurate Behaviour is appropriate to context	Confident Accurate Takes longer than required	Achieved intended outcome	Requires occasional supportive cues*
2 Requires assistance	Safe Accurate Behaviour generally appropriate to context	Lacks certainty	Would not have achieved outcome without support	Requires frequent verbal and occasional physical directives in addition to supportive cues*
1 Requires direction	Safe only with guidance Not completely accurate	Unskilled Inefficient	Would not have achieved outcome without support	Requires continuous verbal and frequent physical directive cues*
0 Unsafe	Unsafe Unable to demonstrate behaviour Lack of insight into behaviour appropriate to context	Unskilled	Would not have achieved outcome	Requires continuous verbal and continuous physical directive cues*

*Refers to physical directives or verbal supportive cues

Performance Improvement Plan (PIP)

Please document the agreed education plan and completion timelines for areas assessed as less than 4.

This plan should be presented to assessor prior to commencement of summative assessment.

Where was supervisor support required?	Student summary of deficit. (Why was there a problem?)	Improvement Plan	Completed (Y/N)

Staff/Student Name: _____

Staff/Student Signature: _____

Educator Name: _____

Educator Signature: _____

Summative Clinical Skill Assessment (S-CSAT)

Equipment and resources: Standard patient or mannequin suitable for practising patella relocation; disposable gloves; leg splint options, including triangular bandages; alcohol-based hand wash; clinical waste bag; method for documenting results

Associated Clinical Skills: Infection control; Communication; Consent; Assessment of motor and sensory nerve function; Pain assessment; Medication administration

Staff/Student being assessed: _____

- Completed Formative Clinical Skill Assessment (F-CSAT):   **YES**   **NO**
- Completed Performance Improvement Plan (PIP):   **YES**   **NO**   **N/A**

Dislocated patella relocation

Activity	Critical Action	Achieved Without Direction	
Assesses patient	Confirms indication. Excludes contraindication. Assesses distal circulation and sensation.	NO	YES
Prepares patient	Gains consent. Explains procedure.	NO	YES
Universal precautions	Washes hands, dons gloves.	NO	YES
Analgesia	Administers procedural analgesia as required.	NO	YES
Positions paramedic	Stands beside and facing patient on lateral side of injured leg.	NO	YES
Grasps limb in readiness	Partly flexes patient's hip if not already flexed. Holds patient's ankle with closest hand. Supports lower leg. Places fingers of other hand against lower thigh, with forefinger against superior patella edge. Spreads thumb away from forefinger and moves hand so that the arc encircles lateral patella. Rests thumb against inferior patella edge.	NO	YES
Relocates patella	Slowly straightens limb/flexes knee. Simultaneously presses arc of hand medially, applying gentle constant pressure on the patella. Watches for snap of patella relocating.	NO	YES
Confirms relocation	Confirms visible relocation and decrease in pain.	NO	YES
Reassesses limb	Reassesses distal circulation and sensation.	NO	YES
Splints limb	Splints limb comfortably in correct alignment.	NO	YES
Reports	Documents/hands over procedure and responses.	NO	YES

Standard Achieved: (please circle one)

Competent (C)   Not Yet Competent* (NYC)

Staff/Student Name: _____

Assessor (please print name): _____

Signed (Assessor): _____

Date of Assessment: _____

Comments:

*If Not Yet Competent (NYC) a PIP needs to be completed and a repeat of the F-CSAT

Clinical findings

Reduction success

Performed correctly, patella dislocation reduction should only take a few seconds once commenced. As the leg straightens, the knee will snap back into position with a sudden movement.

Typically, the patient feels an immediate improvement in pain but may still require further analgesia. Reassess the patient following the procedure and during care.

Once relocated, the leg can be held immobilised in this straightened position pending further assessment. Soft tissue injury may require further therapy or rehabilitation (Longo et al., 2017; Smith et al., 2015; Vetrano et al.,

2017), with the medial patellofemoral ligament commonly injured (Duthon, 2015; Frosch et al., 2011).

Reduction failure

Uncommonly, the patella will not reduce (Vetrano et al., 2017), likely due to a concurrent fracture or a physical impediment to the patella's return (Delagrammaticas and Cordes, 2016; Grewal et al., 2016). In such cases, continue analgesia as required and immobilise and support the leg in the position in which it is found.

PRACTICE TIP

As with many practical procedures, rehearsing the method of patella relocation assists with its effective performance.

PRACTICE TIP

Lateral patella dislocation typically results from lesser trauma mechanisms and has a distinctive appearance. It should not prove challenging to recognise the injury. Where the trauma mechanism is more significant or the injury is not distinctive, consider the contraindications to avoid worsening the pain or injury.

TEST YOUR KNOWLEDGE

1. **What is the most common form of patella dislocation?**
   Lateral.

2. **Why is this the most common form of dislocation?**
   The quadriceps muscle naturally pulls it that way.

3. **What is the most common mechanism for patella dislocation?**
   Sporting or dancing, where the foot is fixed and the knee twists.

4. **List three contraindications to lateral patella relocation.**
   Fractures of the proximal tibia or distal femur; knee dislocations; other forms of patella dislocation.

5. **What two motions occur simultaneously to reduce lateral patella dislocation?**
   Knee extension/straightening with medial patella pressure.

6. **What are the indications that a patella reduction has been successful?**
   The patella should snap back into place and pain may quickly reduce.

7. **What main tendons and ligaments attach to the patella?**
   Superiorly, the quadriceps femoris muscle attaches to the patella via the quadriceps tendon. Distally, the tibial head attaches to the patella via the large patella ligament. Smaller ligaments attach to the medial (medial patellofemoral) and lateral patella.

8. **Why might a lateral patella dislocation fail to reduce?**
   Due to concurrent fracture or physical impediment.

9. **If the patella cannot be reduced, what should you do?**
   Continue analgesia as required; splint the patella as found.

10. **What vascular/nerve risk exists with knee injuries?**
    The popliteal artery lies behind the knee, as does the tibial nerve. The common peroneal nerve lies laterally of the patella. Possible injuries include vascular occlusion or tearing and nerve impingement.

References

Delagrammaticas, D.E. and Cordes, S.D., 2016. A rare case of an irreducible patella dislocation. *Case Reports in Medicine*, doi: 10.1155/2016/3728425.

Duthon, V.B., 2015. Acute traumatic patellar dislocation. *Orthopaedics & Traumatology: Surgery & Research*, 101(1), S59–S67.

Frosch, S., Balcarek, P., Walde, T.A., Schüttrumpf, J.P., Wachowski, M.M., Ferleman, K.G., Stürmer, K.M. and Frosch, K.H., 2011. The treatment of patellar dislocation: a systematic review. *Zeitschrift für Orthopadie und Unfallchirurgie*, 149(6), 630–645.

Grewal, B., Elliott, D., Daniele, L. and Reidy, J., 2016. Irreducible lateral patellar dislocation: a case report and literature review. *Ochsner Journal*, 16(2), 180–184.

Jain, N.P., Khan, N. and Fithian, D.C., 2011. A treatment algorithm for primary patellar dislocations. *Sports Health*, 3(2), 170–174.

Longo, U.G., Ciuffreda, M., Locher, J., Berton, A., Salvatore, G. and Denaro, V., 2017. Treatment of primary acute patellar dislocation: systematic review and quantitative synthesis of the literature. *Clinical Journal of Sport Medicine*, 27(6), 511–523.

Sanders, T.L., Pareek, A., Hewett, T.E., Stuart, M.J., Dahm, D.L. and Krych, A.J., 2017. Incidence of first-time lateral patellar dislocation: a 21-year population-based study. *Sports Health*, 10(2), 146–151.

Smith, T.O., Donell, S., Song, F. and Hing, C.B., 2015. *Surgical versus non-surgical interventions for treating patellar dislocation*. Online: The Cochrane Library.

Vetrano, M., Oliva, F., Bisicchia, S., Bossa, M., De Carli, A., Di Lorenzo, L., Erroi, D., Forte, A., Foti, C., Frizziero, A. and Gasparre, G., 2017. IS Mu. LT first-time patellar dislocation guidelines. *Muscles, Ligaments and Tendons Journal*, 7(1), 1.

Bibliography

Craft, J., Gordon, C., Huether, S.E., McCance, K.L. and Brashers, V.L., 2015. *Understanding pathophysiology* (ANZ adaptation). Sydney: Elsevier.

McCance, K.L. and Huether, S.E., 2015. *Pathophysiology: the biologic basis for disease in adults and children*. Sydney: Elsevier.

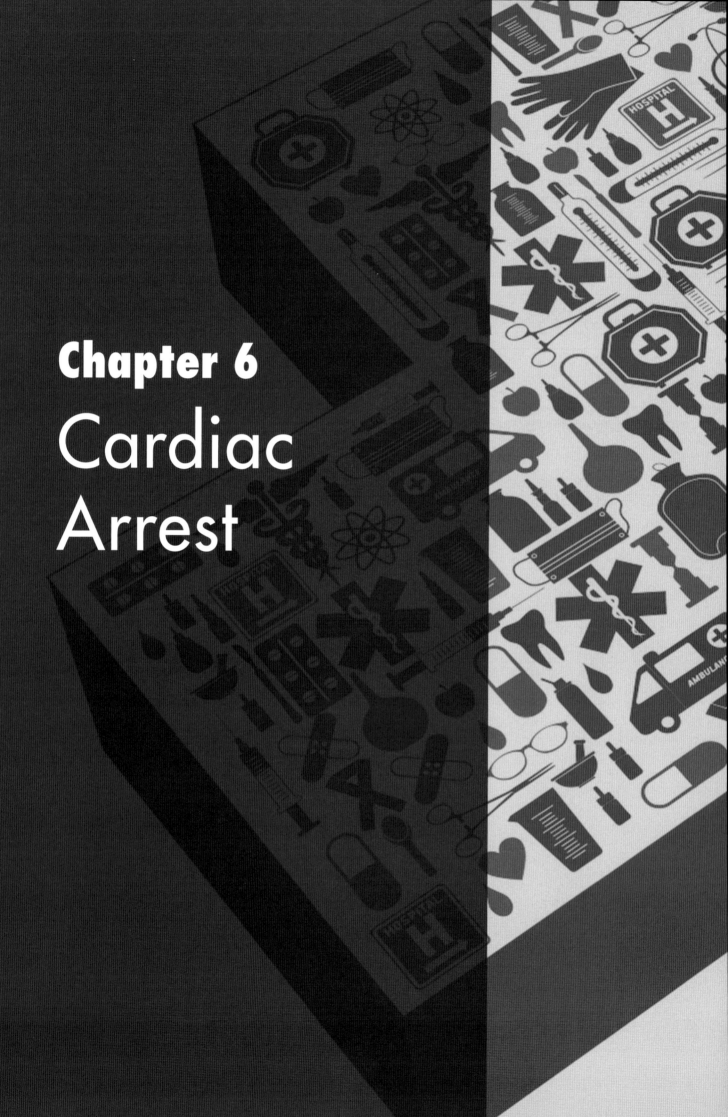

Chapter 6
Cardiac Arrest

6.1 | Chest compressions

Bre Jennings

Chapter objectives

At the end of this chapter the reader will be able to:

1. Understand the principles of providing effective cardiac compressions
2. Understand the pathophysiology behind cardiac compressions
3. Demonstrate effective cardiac compressions

Resources required for this assessment

- Mannequin for CPR training
- Hand decontamination agent
- Disposable gloves and eye protection
- Clinical waste bag
- Method of documenting results

Skill matrix

This assessment requires:
- Infection control (CS 1.3)
- Patient assessment skills (Chapter 2, CS 2.2, 2.3, 2.6, 2.7)

This assessment is a component of:
- Cardiac arrest (Chapter 6)

Introduction

Cardiac compressions provide perfusion to the heart, brain and other essential organs during cardiac arrest to minimise ischaemia and cell death while awaiting defibrillation or advanced care measures (Johnson et al., 2015). Compressions are paired with ventilations in resuscitation and together form cardiopulmonary resuscitation (CPR) (Kim et al., 2008). They must be initiated as early as possible, by any capable person, in the event a person is unresponsive with ineffective or absent breathing, where absence of pulse is suspected (ANZCOR, 2016).

This chapter describes the performance of effective cardiac compressions and discusses the difficulties and challenges in doing so. This skill is frequently performed by others on scene, who are described in this chapter as rescuers.

Anatomy and physiology

Performed correctly, the heart is compressed between the sternum and thoracic spine. The exact mechanism of how

blood is then moved through the heart and body is debated in the literature. The thoracic pump theory suggests that during compressions, intrathoracic pressure changes cause blood to move through the heart and around the body. The cardiac pump theory suggests that the left ventricle acts as a pump as it is directly compressed, pulling blood in and then ejecting it forwards into the aorta (John et al., 2017).

Regardless of which theory is more accurate, it is known that even, effective, uninterrupted compressions provide between 15% and 25% of normal cardiac output (Lurie et al., 2016). This highlights the importance of ensuring the quality of compressions is high in all resuscitation efforts.

Clinical rationale

Although compressions alone are rarely attributed to the survival of cardiac arrest patients, they are an essential component of resuscitation guidelines. In cardiac arrest, compressions are the only non-invasive method of maintaining cardiac output. When effective compressions

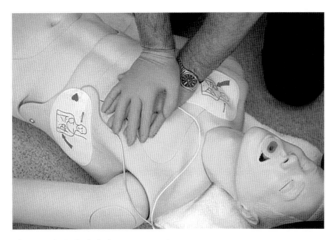

Figure 6.1.1 Adult compressions

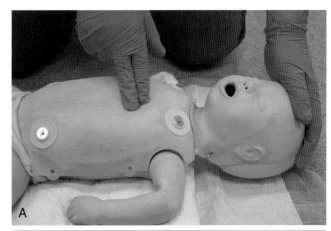

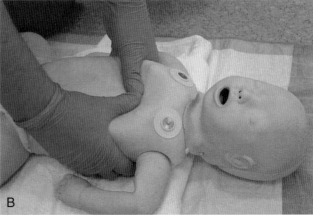

Figure 6.1.2 Alternatives for infant compression
(a) Two fingers placed over the lower half of the sternum. (b) Thumbs in the middle over the lower half of the sternum.

are implemented, other resuscitation methods, including defibrillation, airway management, ventilation and pharmacological interventions, can follow.

Effective compressions increase the likelihood of successful defibrillation and minimise major organ ischaemia. CPR is often referred to as 'buying time' (Kim et al., 2008). Regardless of whether other more advanced resuscitation interventions are used, poor compression quality is associated with reduced rates of survival.

Emphasis is placed on the following key principles.

Rescuer position

Ideally, the rescuer kneels beside the patient, who has been placed supine, facing their chest. This allows effective compressions as well as subsequent access to the airway, defibrillation and blood vessels. Where there is only a single rescuer, or if space is limited, it may be necessary to have one person positioned superior to the patient's head and leaning over their face while performing chest compressions (Perkins et al., 2015).

Hand position

For an adult patient, the two-hand technique is recommended (ANZCOR, 2016). The heel of one hand is placed in the middle of the lower half of the sternum, with the second hand placed on top (ANZCOR, 2016; Perkins et al., 2015) (Fig. 6.1.1). Interlacing fingers, or holding the top of the bottom hand or wrist, are acceptable options.

For infants, two fingers are placed over the lower half of the sternum (Fig. 6.1.2a). Alternatively, the hands can loosely circle either side of the chest with the thumbs meeting in the middle over the lower half of the sternum (Fig. 6.1.2b). For larger children, the heel of one hand is used, ensuring it remains at least one finger width above the xiphisternum.

The rescuer's body should be stable, with knees hip distance apart, shoulders over wrists and arms outstretched. In an even and appropriately paced rhythm, the rescuer depresses and releases the chest wall. If the patient is on a bed, the rescuer will need to stand on a stable platform to achieve the correct position.

Compression depth and recoil

Cardiac compressions should depress the chest wall approximately one-third anterior/posterior diameter by 50 mm but no more than 60 mm (Perkins et al., 2015; Stiell et al., 2014; Vadeboncoeur et al., 2014). For infants, this is approximately 40 mm and for older people approximately 50 mm (Maconochie et al., 2015).

Allow full recoil immediately after each compression without removing the hands from the patient's chest. Avoid leaning on the chest. This is important to maximise cardiac output and allow the ventricles to refill again.

Compression rate

A balance is required between moving sufficient blood for perfusion against allowing sufficient time for venous return and ventricular refilling. The recommended rate of cardiac compressions for an adult patient is 100–120 per minute (ANZCOR, 2016; Idris et al., 2015).

Minimising interruptions

During cardiac compressions, coronary perfusion pressure (CPP) increases. When compressions are interrupted, CPP drops, requiring 10–12 compressions to restore it (Curtis and Ramsden, 2016).

Minimising interruptions to compressions during resuscitation is therefore critical to survival (Brouwer et al., 2015). Pauses for ventilations, pulse checks or advanced airway interventions should be <10 seconds where possible (Nichol et al., 2015). Pauses for myocardial rhythm assessment and defibrillation should be minimal (see Chapter 6.2).

Hard surface
Compression force is lost if the patient is pressed downwards into a soft surface. It is therefore necessary to use a hard surface for compressions. If necessary, move the patient from a soft mattress or place a hard board beneath them (Perkins et al., 2015).

Rescuer rotation
Change rescuers every 2 minutes to avoid complications of fatigue. The logical time to change is during defibrillation attempts.

High performance CPR
The implementation of the numerous elements of CPR in the most effective manner is commonly referred to by ambulance services as high performance CPR (HP-CPR). It includes using a 'pit crew' approach, with a defined team leader and effective communication. Specific inclusions are:

- create a 360° view around the patient where possible, with strategic placement of equipment and personnel access/egress
- ensure the compression rate and depth are correct, allowing each time for full chest recoil
- rotate compression providers every 2 minutes, and have the replacement positioned in advance for rapid changeover
- keep the hands hovered over the chest, ready to resume compressions after ECG rhythm analysis or shock.

Clinical skill assessment process
The following section outlines the clinical skill assessment tools that should be used to determine a student's ability to demonstrate safe and accurate chest compressions.
1. Clinical Skill Work Instruction
2. Formative Clinical Skill Assessment (F-CSAT)
3. Performance Improvement Plan (PIP)
4. Summative Clinical Skill Assessment (S-CSAT)
(5. Direct Observation of Procedural Skills (DOPS) – see Chapter 1.1)

Clinical Skill Work Instruction

Equipment and resources: Mannequin for CPR training; hand decontamination agent; disposable gloves and eye protection; clinical waste bag; method of documenting the results

Associated Clinical Skills: Infection control; Patient assessment skills

Chest compressions

Activity	Critical Action	Rationale
Prepare rescuer	Apply personal protective equipment, including gloves and goggles.	Infectious risk can occur during compressions.
Prepare patient	Position patient supine with adequate space surrounding them. Expose patient's chest.	Access to the patient's chest and airway is essential for compressions and resuscitation.
Position rescuer	Position alongside patient, facing the chest. If on the floor, kneel, stack hips over knees and shoulders over wrists so that hands can be placed on the centre of the patient's chest.	Correct positioning increases the quality of compressions and reduces rescuer fatigue and injury risk.
Position hands	*Adults:* Place heel of one hand in the middle of the lower half of the sternum and the other hand on top of the first, with fingers interlacing. *Children:* As for adults, except use only one hand. *Infants:* Use two fingers or two thumbs over lower half of sternum.	Compression should occur directly over the heart.
Apply compressions	Compress the chest one-third anterior/posterior depth: • *adults and children* – 5 cm • *infants* – 4 cm.	This is the recommended depth of compression.

Chest compressions continued

Activity	Critical Action	Rationale
Compression recoil	Release each compression and allow full recoil before recompressing. Maintain hand contact with the chest without applying any pressure.	Full recoil is associated with greater cardiac output during compressions.
Compression rate	Continue compression and recoil at a rate of 100–120 per minute.	This is the recommended rate of compressions for an adult and child.
Alternate rescuers	Change rescuers every 2 minutes if possible.	Reduces fatigue and maintains compression quality.
Minimise interruptions	Minimise interruptions to compressions (<10 seconds when necessary).	Maintains coronary perfusion pressure.
Report	Document and hand over procedure and responses.	Accurate record kept and continuity of patient care.

Source: *Adapted from ANZCOR, 2016.*

Formative Clinical Skill Assessment (F-CSAT)

Equipment and resources: Mannequin for CPR training; hand decontamination agent; disposable gloves and eye protection; clinical waste bag; method of documenting the results

Associated Clinical Skills: Infection control; Patient assessment skills

Staff/Student being assessed: _____

Chest compressions

Activity	Critical Action	Performance				
Prepares rescuer	Applies personal protective equipment, including gloves and goggles.	0	1	2	3	4
Prepares patient	Positions patient supine with adequate space surrounding them. Exposes chest.	0	1	2	3	4
Positions rescuer	Positions alongside patient, facing the chest. If on the floor, kneels, stacks hips over knees and shoulders over wrists so that hands can be placed on the centre of the patient's chest.	0	1	2	3	4
Positions hands	*Adults:* Places heel of one hand in the middle of the lower half of the sternum and the other hand on top of the first, with fingers interlacing. *Children:* As for adults, except uses only one hand. *Infants:* Uses two fingers or two thumbs over lower half of sternum.	0	1	2	3	4
Applies compressions	Compresses the chest one-third anterior/posterior depth: • *adults and children* – 5 cm • *infants* – 4 cm.	0	1	2	3	4
Compression recoil	Releases each compression and allows full recoil before recompressing.	0	1	2	3	4
Compression rate	Continues compression and recoil at a rate of 100–120 per minute.	0	1	2	3	4
Rotates rescuer	Changes rescuer every 2 minutes if possible.	0	1	2	3	4

Chest compressions continued

Activity	Critical Action	Performance				
Minimises interruptions	Minimises interruptions to compressions (<10 seconds when necessary).	0	1	2	3	4
Reports	Documents and hands over procedure and responses.	0	1	2	3	4

Source: *Adapted from ANZCOR, 2016.*

Standard Achieved: (please circle one)

Competent (C)   Not Yet Competent* (NYC)

Staff/Student Name: _____

Assessor (please print name)**:** _____

Signed (Assessor)**:** _____

Date of Assessment: _____

Comments:

*If Not Yet Competent (NYC) a PIP needs to be completed and a repeat of the F-CSAT

Formative Clinical Skill Assessment (F-CSAT) Key

Skill level	Standard of procedure	Quality of performance	Outcome	Level of assistance required
4 Safe for unsupervised practice	Safe Accurate Behaviour is appropriate to context	Confident Accurate Expedient	Achieved intended outcome	No supporting cues* required
3 Requires supervision	Safe Accurate Behaviour is appropriate to context	Confident Accurate Takes longer than required	Achieved intended outcome	Requires occasional supportive cues*
2 Requires assistance	Safe Accurate Behaviour generally appropriate to context	Lacks certainty	Would not have achieved outcome without support	Requires frequent verbal and occasional physical directives in addition to supportive cues*
1 Requires direction	Safe only with guidance Not completely accurate	Unskilled Inefficient	Would not have achieved outcome without support	Requires continuous verbal and frequent physical directive cues*
0 Unsafe	Unsafe Unable to demonstrate behaviour Lack of insight into behaviour appropriate to context	Unskilled	Would not have achieved outcome	Requires continuous verbal and continuous physical directive cues*

*Refers to physical directives or verbal supportive cues

Performance Improvement Plan (PIP)

Please document the agreed education plan and completion timelines for areas assessed as less than 4.

This plan should be presented to assessor prior to commencement of summative assessment.

Where was supervisor support required?	Student summary of deficit. (Why was there a problem?)	Improvement Plan	Completed (Y/N)

Staff/Student Name: _____

Staff/Student Signature: _____

Educator Name: _____

Educator Signature: _____

Summative Clinical Skill Assessment (S-CSAT)

Equipment and resources: Mannequin for CPR training; hand decontamination agent; disposable gloves and eye protection; clinical waste bag; method of documenting the results

Associated Clinical Skills: Infection control; Patient assessment skills

Staff/student being assessed: _____

- Completed Formative Clinical Skill Assessment (F-CSAT):   **YES**   **NO**

- Completed Performance Improvement Plan (PIP):   **YES**   **NO**   **N/A**

Chest compressions

Activity	Critical Action	Achieved Without Direction	
Prepares rescuer	Applies personal protective equipment, including gloves and goggles.	NO	YES
Prepares patient	Positions patient supine with adequate space surrounding them. Exposes chest.	NO	YES
Positions rescuer	Positions alongside patient, facing the chest. If on the floor, kneels, stacks hips over knees and shoulders over wrists so that hands can be placed on the centre of the patient's chest.	NO	YES
Positions hands	*Adults:* Places heel of one hand in the middle of the lower half of the sternum and the other hand on top of the first, with fingers interlacing. *Children:* As for adults, except uses only one hand. *Infants:* Uses two fingers or two thumbs over lower half of sternum.	NO	YES
Applies compressions	Compresses the chest one-third anterior/posterior depth: • *adults and children* – 5 cm • *infants* – 4 cm.	NO	YES

Chest compressions continued

Activity	Critical Action	Achieved Without Direction	
Compression recoil	Releases each compression and allows full recoil before recompressing.	NO	YES
Compression rate	Continues compression and recoil at a rate of 100–120 per minute.	NO	YES
Rotates rescuer	Changes rescuer every 2 minutes if possible.	NO	YES
Minimises interruptions	Minimises interruptions to compressions (<10 seconds when necessary).	NO	YES
Reports	Documents and hands over procedure and responses.	NO	YES

Source: *Adapted from ANZCOR, 2016.*

Standard Achieved: (please circle one)

Competent (C)   Not Yet Competent* (NYC)

Staff/Student Name: _____

Assessor (please print name): _____

Signed (Assessor): _____

Date of Assessment: _____

Comments:

*If Not Yet Competent (NYC) a PIP needs to be completed and a repeat of the F-CSAT

Clinical findings

Injuries

Despite chest compressions being lifesaving, they are not without adverse risk. Patient injuries resulting from compressions include rib and sternum fractures and intrathoracic bleeding, though these are infrequent and unlikely to greatly affect patient outcomes. Injuries to the internal organs, including the stomach, spleen, heart and liver are uncommon but can also occur (Boland et al., 2015; Olds et al., 2015).

The risk of injury increases with a compression depth exceeding 60 mm and an increased rate above 120 per minute (Hellevuo et al., 2013).

Poor posture during compressions can cause back soreness in rescuers.

Capnography

Monitoring end tidal capnography during CPR can help guide the compression depth, rate and recoil quality (Murphy et al., 2016; Nassar and Kerber, 2017; Ruiz et al., 2016).

Feedback devices

Numerous novel devices for monitoring compression quality that incorporate both verbal and visual rescuer feedback are increasingly available (Cortegiani et al., 2017; Sarma et al., 2017; Wutzler et al., 2017).

PRACTICE TIP!

Measuring hand placement is no longer recommended. Simply place the hands in the centre of the chest over the lower half of the sternum and start compressing.

PRACTICE TIP!

While performing CPR may be considered a normal paramedic activity, for many others, including family and bystanders, it can be intensely traumatic and distressing. Ensure paramedic conversations and body language reflect this mismatch by moderating conversations and body language accordingly.

PRACTICE TIP!

Use your body weight to gain adequate compression depth rather than using your arms alone. Try stacking your body over your wrists and straightening your arms and back, to reduce fatigue and injury.

PRACTICE TIP!

Fatigue reduces the quality of cardiac compression. It is essential to rotate rescuers every 2 minutes to minimise fatigue. For prolonged resuscitation, utilise bystanders or other emergency service personnel, or request further paramedic assistance.

TEST YOUR KNOWLEDGE QUESTIONS

1. **What are the principles of effective cardiac compression?**
    Rescuer position; hand position; compression depth and recoil; rate; minimal interruptions; hard surface; rescuer rotation.

2. **What is the correct hand position for adult cardiac compressions?**
    The heel of one hand is placed in the middle of the lower half of the sternum and the other hand is placed on top, with the fingers interlocked.

3. **Why is it important to rotate compression providers every 2 minutes?**
    Performing cardiac compressions is fatiguing. This causes the compressions to become shallow and slower, reducing their effectiveness.

4. **Why is it important to wear personal protective equipment when performing cardiac compressions?**
    Paramedics change roles, exposing them to a variety of airway and body fluid risks.

5. **When should cardiac compressions be commenced?**
    They should be commenced immediately for persons assessed to be unconscious, without effective breathing and with a suspected absent pulse.

6. **How is the role of compression rescuer cycled during cardiac arrest?**
    A new or refreshed rescuer takes over each 2 minutes, during the rhythm and pulse check.

7. **What is the aim of cardiac compressions?**
    To depress the chest wall and produce sufficient cardiac output to provide cerebral and vital organ perfusion, 'buying time' until circulation can be restored.

8. **What cultural issues should be considered when performing cardiac compressions?**
    Different cultures, rituals, rules and behaviours at times of critical illness or death are varied. Exposure of the patient's chest may cause discomfort for others present. The patient's dignity and privacy should also be respected where possible.

9. **Why is full recoil of the chest wall required between compressions?**
    This is the phase when the ventricle refills, allowing for maximum blood flow.

10. **What are the parameters for compressions?**
    Rate of 100–120; depth; one-third of the chest wall diameter; compressing the middle of the lower half of the sternum with minimal interruptions; allowing full chest recoil.

References

ANZCOR (Australian and New Zealand Committee on Resuscitation), 2016. *ANZCOR Guideline 6: Compressions.* Retrieved from: https://resus.org.au/guidelines

Boland, L.L., Satterlee, P.A., Hokanson, J.S., Strauss, C.E. and Yost, D., 2015. Chest compression injuries detected via routine post-arrest care in patients who survive to admission after out-of-hospital cardiac arrest. *Prehospital Emergency Care*, 19(1), 23–30.

Brouwer, T.F., Walker, R.G., Chapman, F.W. and Koster, R.W., 2015. Association between chest compression interruptions and clinical outcomes of ventricular fibrillation out-of-hospital cardiac arrest. *Circulation*, 132(11), 1030–1037.

Cortegiani, A., Russotto, V., Baldi, E., Contri, E., Raineri, S.M. and Giarratano, A., 2017. Is it time to consider visual feedback systems the gold standard for chest compression skill acquisition? *Critical Care*, 21(1), 166.

Curtis, K. and Ramsden, C., 2016. *Emergency and trauma care for nurses and paramedics*, 2nd edn. Melbourne: Mosby.

Hellevuo, H., Sainio, M., Nevalainen, R., Huhtala, H., Olkkola, K.T., Tenhunen, J. and Hoppu, S., 2013. Deeper chest compression – more complications for cardiac arrest patients? *Resuscitation*, 84(6), 760–765.

Idris, A.H., Guffey, D., Pepe, P.E., Brown, S.P., Brooks, S.C., Callaway, C.W., Christenson, J., Davis, D.P., Daya, M.R., Gray, R. and Kudenchuk, P.J., 2015. Chest compression rates and survival following out-of-hospital cardiac arrest. *Critical Care Medicine*, 43(4), 840–848.

John, A.R., Manivannan, M. and Ramakrishnan, T.V., 2017. Computer-based CPR simulation towards validation of AHA/ERC guidelines. *Cardiovascular Engineering and Technology*, 8(2), 229–235.

Johnson, M., Boyd, L., Grantham, H. and Eastwood, K., 2015. *Paramedic principles and practice ANZ: a clinical reasoning approach.* Sydney: Elsevier.

Kim, H., Sung, O.H., Lee, C.C., Kang, H.L., Kim, J.Y., Yoo, B.S., Lee, S.H., Yoon, J.H., Kyung, H.C. and Singer, A.J., 2008. Direction of blood flow from the left ventricle during cardiopulmonary resuscitation in humans – its implications for mechanism of blood flow. *American Heart Journal*, 156(6), 1222.e1–1222.e7.

Lurie, K.G., Nemergut, E.C., Yannopoulos, D. and Sweeney, M., 2016. The physiology of cardiopulmonary resuscitation. *Anesthesia & Analgesia*, 122(3), 767–783.

Maconochie, I.K., Bingham, R., Eich, C., López-Herce, J., Rodríguez-Núñez, A., Rajka, T., van de Voorde, P., Zideman, D.A., Biarent, D., Monsieurs, K.G. and Nolan, J.P., 2015.

European Resuscitation Council Guidelines for Resuscitation 2015. *Resuscitation*, 95, 223–248.

Murphy, R.A., Bobrow, B.J., Spaite, D.W., Hu, C., McDannold, R. and Vadeboncoeur, T.F., 2016. Association between prehospital CPR quality and end-tidal carbon dioxide levels in out-of-hospital cardiac arrest. *Prehospital Emergency Care*, 20(3), 369–377.

Nassar, B.S. and Kerber, R., 2017. Improving CPR performance. *Chest*, 152(5), 1061–1069.

Nichol, G., Leroux, B., Wang, H., Callaway, C.W., Sopko, G., Weisfeldt, M., Stiell, I., Morrison, L.J., Aufderheide, T.P., Cheskes, S. and Christenson, J., 2015. Trial of continuous or interrupted chest compressions during CPR. *New England Journal of Medicine*, 373(23), 2203–2214.

Olds, K., Byard, R.W. and Langlois, N.E., 2015. Injuries associated with resuscitation – an overview. *Journal of Forensic and Legal Medicine*, 33, 39–43.

Perkins, G.D., Handley, A.J., Koster, R.W., Castrén, M., Smyth, M.A., Olasveengen, T., Monsieurs, K.G., Raffay, V., Gräsner, J.T., Wenzel, V. and Ristagno, G., 2015. European Resuscitation Council Guidelines for Resuscitation 2015. *Resuscitation*, 95, 81–99.

Ruiz, J.M., de Gauna, S.R., González-Otero, D.M., Daya, M., Russell, J.K., Gutiérrez, J.J. and Leturiondo, M., 2016. Relationship between EtCO2 and quality-parameters during cardiopulmonary resuscitation. In *Computing in Cardiology Conference (CinC), 2016.* New Jersey: IEEE, pp. 957–960.

Sarma, S., Bucuti, H., Chitnis, A., Klacman, A. and Dantu, R., 2017. Real-time mobile device–assisted chest compression during cardiopulmonary resuscitation. *American Journal of Cardiology*, 120(2), 196–200.

Stiell, I.G., Brown, S.P., Nichol, G., Cheskes, S., Vaillancourt, C., Callaway, C.W., Morrison, L.J., Christenson, J., Aufderheide, T.P., Davis, D.P. and Free, C., 2014. What is the optimal chest compression depth during out-of-hospital cardiac arrest resuscitation of adult patients? *Circulation*, 130(22), 1962–1970.

Vadeboncoeur, T., Stolz, U., Panchal, A., Silver, A., Venuti, M., Tobin, J., Smith, G., Nunez, M., Karamooz, M., Spaite, D. and Bobrow, B., 2014. Chest compression depth and survival in out-of-hospital cardiac arrest. *Resuscitation*, 85(2), 182–188.

Wutzler, A., von Ulmenstein, S., Bannehr, M., Völk, K., Förster, J., Storm, C. and Haverkamp, W., 2017. Improvement of lay rescuer chest compressions with a novel audiovisual feedback device. *Medizinische Klinik-Intensivmedizin und Notfallmedizin*, 1–7.

Bibliography

Cameron, P., Jelinek, G., Kelly, A., Brown, A. and Little, M., 2014. *Textbook of adult emergency medicine expert consult*, 4th edn. London: Elsevier.

6.2 | Safe defibrillation

Joe Karlek

Chapter objectives

At the end of this chapter the reader will be able to:

1. Understand the elements of safe defibrillation
2. Perform safe defibrillation

Resources required for this assessment

- Mannequin
- Disposable gloves and eyewear
- Manual defibrillator
- Defibrillation pads
- Cardiac rhythm generator
- Towel
- Shears/scissors
- Method of documenting results

Skill matrix

This assessment requires:

- Infection control (CS 1.3)
- Communication (CS 1.6)
- Consent (CS 1.6)
- Chest compressions (CS 6.1)

This assessment is a component of:

- Cardiac arrest (Chapter 6)

Introduction

Defibrillation is an integral component of basic and advanced life support algorithms and an adjunct to cardiopulmonary resuscitation (CPR). Successful defibrillation aims to return normal cardiac rhythm, spontaneous circulation and subsequent cerebral and other organ perfusion. International guidelines emphasise high quality CPR with minimal interruptions and early defibrillation. This chapter discusses effective manual defibrillation in the management of the patient in cardiac arrest.

Anatomy and physiology

The effectiveness of defibrillation and rates of survival correlate with the time taken from the onset of ventricular fibrillation or pulseless ventricular tachycardia (VF/pVT) to the delivery of the first shock. The Australian Resuscitation Council (ARC) shows for every minute defibrillation is delayed, the rate of survival to hospital discharge decreases by 10–12% (ANZCOR, 2016a). The result of this has been increasing numbers of publicly accessible defibrillators, which decrease the time between collapse and defibrillation.

The effectiveness of defibrillation and rate of survival are significantly reduced by even minimal interruptions to chest compressions (ANZCOR, 2016b). Chest compressions must be continuous, with all interventions that require a pause in compressions kept to an absolute minimum. This includes defibrillation.

Defibrillation aims to depolarise a critical mass of the myocardium by passing a direct current countershock, extinguishing ongoing uncontrolled activation or stimulation and allowing the sinoatrial node to re-establish pacing of the heart without initiating any further unwanted activation itself. Once this occurs and a pulse returns (return of spontaneous circulation), post-resuscitation care follows.

Clinical rationale

Pad positioning

Effective defibrillation must be delivered to bare, exposed skin, necessitating the removal of clothing beforehand. Defibrillation pads are routinely placed in the anterior-lateral position. The right pad is placed inferior to the collar bone of the anterior chest wall over the second intercostal space, just right of the sternum, and should not interfere with chest compressions (Fig. 6.2.1). The left is placed on the lateral chest wall in the mid-axillary line over the sixth intercostal space (ANZCOR, 2016b). The intent is for maximal current flow to pass through the affected area of the heart (Soar et al., 2015). Many defibrillation devices nominate one pad for sternum use and one for the lateral position, although, in practice, it does not matter if these are inadvertently reversed. The electrode wires should not be pulled on or interfere with resuscitation.

An alternative position for defibrillator pads is anterior-posterior placement. This option may be preferable when managing atrial arrhythmia. However, anterior-posterior placement is more difficult to achieve during CPR with the patient supine and means the posterior pad cannot be observed during use. Pads can be placed with one over the apex and the second on the right upper back or, alternatively, one over the left precordium and the other under the left scapula (Soar et al., 2015).

Pads should not be placed over permanent pacemakers and internal cardiac defibrillators (ICDs) to avoid damaging the device or resetting its functions. These devices are commonly in the left upper chest and are usually avoided with anterior-posterior pad placement. If necessary, place the pad 8 cm from any device (Soar et al., 2015). Avoid contact with any metal body piercing (such as nipple) in the same manner.

Large-breasted individuals may require the pad to be placed lateral to or underneath the breast. Medication patches and other jewellery should be removed from the area desired for pad placement. Underwire bras should be released and removed for safety, though inadvertent electrode contact is unlikely to be problematic (Di Maio et al., 2015).

Defibrillation safety

While there have been no reported incidents of harm to rescuers from defibrillation in wet environments (ANZCOR, 2016a), it remains a potential hazard. The patient's chest should be dried before applying the pad to assist adherence and the flow of the current. There have also been no reported incidents of fire when using self-adhesive pads (as opposed to paddles). For safety, move any free-flowing oxygen 1 m away during defibrillation. The ventilation bag can remain connected to the endotracheal tube or supraglottic airway device, as oxygen concentrations do not increase around the pads.

There may be rare occasions when defibrillation is contraindicated and must not be performed. Hazardous environments can include industrial and medical locations with areas of highly flammable materials, for example, or when on metal surfaces. Read the safety document related to the defibrillator for specific safety instructions. Defibrillation utilises electrical currents to achieve its desired outcome. For this reason, rescuers must not touch the patient or attached equipment while the shock is being delivered (ANZCOR, 2016b).

Selecting defibrillation energy

Current advanced life support recommendations (ANZCOR, 2016b; Soar et al., 2015) call for the initial energy level for biphasic adult patient defibrillation to be 200 joules for all shocks. Amounts less than 120 joules are not supported.

Typically, paediatric energy amounts are 4 joules/kg. Delivering lower levels of energy may not capture critical mass defibrillation. Where devices provide limited energy selection options, always round upwards to the nearest available amount. Up to 9 joules/kg has been safely administered to paediatric patients (Maconochie et al., 2015).

Transthoracic impedance

Electric current flows best through the path of least resistance. Bony patients with lean body mass have increased resistance, while obese patients have decreased resistance. Air-filled lungs increase resistance, so defibrillation is ideally administered at end expiration (Soar et al., 2015). Wet patient skin can decrease surface resistance, reducing the internal current.

Biphasic defibrillators typically do not have to be adjusted for variations in impedance. Most devices test impulse before delivering the shock to assess and allow for impedance. Roll the pads into position (see Fig. 6.2.1), avoiding the creation of air-filled spaces caused by skin rolls, incorrect adhesion or excess body hair. These all increase resistance and can cause burn injury. Hirsute individuals may require rapid removal of hair for adhesion

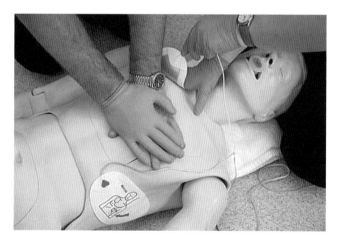

Figure 6.2.1 Placement of an anterior-lateral defibrillation pad

of the pad to successfully deliver the shock; however, this should not unreasonably delay defibrillation. If necessary, clip body hair, but avoid shaving as this can cause minor injury, predisposing the patient to burn injury or causing poor transmission of the current.

Reducing interruptions

The quality of chest compression performance is critical to patient outcome in cardiac arrest. When compressions are ceased to allow shock delivery, the pauses should not exceed 10 seconds (Deakin et al., 2015).

To reduce interruptions to chest compressions, rescuers should follow the COACHED method when assessing the rhythm:

Continue chest compressions
Oxygen away (if required)
All others stand clear
Charge defibrillator
Hands off (with confirmation rescuer is clear)
Evaluate rhythm
Deliver shock or disarm defibrillator.

This allows the defibrillator to be charged and ready to deliver a shock if required, minimising interruptions to chest compressions.

Pulselessness following even successful defibrillation is common and can last for up to 2 minutes. Chest compressions should be immediately recommenced, with pulse verification performed at the end of the current compression cycle (Pierce et al., 2015).

Paediatric defibrillation

Paediatric defibrillation is uncommon, as children typically succumb to bradycardia/asystole rather than shockable rhythms. Where it is required, the placement of pads is similar to that for adults. Many devices require use of specific, smaller paediatric electrode pads to suit the size of the patient. This lessens the ability of the device to dissipate the electrical energy. Lower discharge energy should be used to avoid causing injury.

If the pads prove large for infants, modify their placement as best as practicable, including extending the sternum pad onto the shoulder (but not the neck) and laterally around to the back (Fig. 6.2.2). Alternatively, adopt an anterior-posterior placement method (Maconochie et al., 2015).

Defibrillation principles in cardiac arrest

Defibrillation forms part of the management of cardiac arrest, along with high performance CPR. To deliver defibrillation in the most effective manner, the following principles should be followed:

- Charge the defibrillator during compressions, as each 2-minute cycle concludes with the operator verbally confirming no shock will be delivered by them until all persons have released contact with the patient.
- Analyse the presenting cardiac rhythm directly from the monitor screen in minimum time (ideally <5

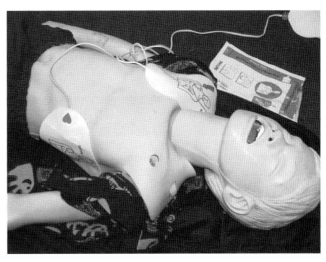

Figure 6.2.2 Modified placement of a large defibrillation pad on a child

seconds). This makes manual mode more effective than semi-automatic, as human interpretation is typically faster than device analysis algorithms.
- If in doubt about the presenting rhythm, where it could be a shockable rhythm and the patient is in cardiac arrest, deliver the shock.

Semi-automatic defibrillation

Members of the public or laypersons and, in some cases, medical responders can administer defibrillation using a semi-automatic device. The substantial difference between this method and manual defibrillation is that the device controls the decision to defibrillate rather than the operator. The operator must still recognise that the patient is in cardiac arrest (including unresponsiveness and absent or ineffective breathing with or without confirmation of pulselessness), apply the defibrillation pads (similarly to a manual device) and turn the defibrillator on.

Each automatic defibrillator contains an intrinsic algorithm for recognising shockable rhythms of ventricular tachycardia (above a minimum rate) and ventricular fibrillation. It does this by analysing multiple short sections of ECG. The device will then advise the operator to press a button to deliver the shock if it determines this is appropriate. It will not discharge without operator control. Alternatively, it will instruct the operator that no shock is advised and to immediately commence chest compressions. The device will typically then provide a 2-minute count with a metronome before repeating the cycle.

When using a semi-automatic defibrillator, the operator can neither override it to shock when the device chooses not to nor administer a shock sooner than the intrinsic 2-minute cycle allows.

Clinical skill assessment process

The following section outlines the clinical skill assessment tools that should be used to determine a student's ability to demonstrate safe and effective defibrillation.

1. Clinical Skill Work Instruction
2. Formative Clinical Skill Assessment (F-CSAT)
3. Performance Improvement Plan (PIP)

4. Summative Clinical Skill Assessment (S-CSAT)
(5. Direct Observation of Procedural Skills (DOPS) – see Chapter 1.1)

Clinical Skill Work Instruction

Equipment and resources: Mannequin; disposable gloves and eyewear; manual defibrillator; defibrillation pads; towel; shears/scissors; cardiac rhythm generator; method of documenting results

Associated Clinical Skills: Infection control; Communication; Consent; Chest compressions

Safe defibrillation

Activity	Critical Action	Rationale
Safety	Don PPE, including eyewear and gloves for universal precautions. Do not defibrillate in hazardous environments.	To provide electrical and biohazard protection for both rescuer and patient.
Prepare equipment	Position defibrillator to maximise operator view yet not interfere with resuscitation efforts. Ensure pad type is correct for the patient's age. Assess expiry date of pads, quality of gel and that wires/connections are undamaged.	More than one paramedic should be able to see the defibrillator. To ensure the safe transmission of electricity.
Prepare patient	Place the patient supine. If required: • remove or cut away sufficient clothing to expose chest • remove medication patches, jewellery or ECG electrodes • clip chest hair (if considered thick enough to interfere with electrode attachment) • dry the chest (with towel if available).	Allows effective pad contact for safe defibrillation.
Continue chest compressions	Continue chest compressions while the defibrillator operator continues preparation.	Minimises interruptions to chest compressions, increasing patient's chances of survival.
Position pads	Place pads in the anterior-lateral position (or anterior-posterior position if indicated). Avoid breast tissue, pacemakers and ICDs, placement over sternum and contact with patient's neck. Roll pads on to avoid air pockets. Ensure correct contact/adhesion.	Allows safe delivery of shock and increases efficacy of defibrillation. Pads will not reattach correctly if they are removed, so they are single-use only.
Move oxygen away	Move free-flowing oxygen 1 m away from the patient. Patients who are intubated or have a supraglottic airway can remain attached to oxygen.	Free-flowing oxygen can pose a risk of fire should sparks occur during shock delivery.
Move all others away	Rescuers not performing chest compressions should not touch the patient or attached equipment.	Prevents injury from electrical conduction.
Charge defibrillator	Charge defibrillator to recommended level.	Energy levels are dependent on local recommendations and those of the manufacturer.
Hands off	Rescuer performing compressions should move away and confirm they are safe.	The last person to contact the patient maintains chest compressions.
Evaluate rhythm	Rapidly evaluate the presenting rhythm to identify VF/pVT from non-shockable rhythms. Confirm with printed strip if available.	Only VF/pVT rhythms are indicated for defibrillation in cardiac arrest. Patient movement causes artifact, interfering with analysis.

Safe defibrillation continued

Activity	Critical Action	Rationale
Defibrillate/ disarm	If rhythm is VF/pVT, deliver shock if safe to do so. Confirm shock delivered on screen/printout. Disarm the defibrillator for non-shockable rhythms. Announce the shock has been delivered (or disarmed) and it is safe to touch the patient.	Ensures no one contacting the patient since instructed. Deliver shock or disarm defibrillator.
Continue resuscitation	Continue CPR or post-resuscitation care as indicated from the patient's presentation and rhythm analysis.	As per current resuscitation guidelines.
Report	Document/hand over details of presenting rhythm, shock(s), energy, pad placement and effectiveness.	Accurate record keeping and continuity of care.

Formative Clinical Skill Assessment (F-CSAT)

Equipment and resources: Mannequin; disposable gloves and eyewear; manual defibrillator; defibrillation pads; towel; shears/scissors; cardiac rhythm generator; method of documenting results

Associated Clinical Skills: Infection control; Communication; Consent; Chest compressions

Staff/Student being assessed: _____

Safe defibrillation

Activity	Critical Action	Performance				
Safety	Dons appropriate PPE. Does not defibrillate in hazardous environments.	0	1	2	3	4
Prepares equipment	Positions defibrillator optimally for situation. Ensures pad type is correct for patient's age. Assesses expiry date of pads, gel quality, undamaged wires/connections.	0	1	2	3	4
Prepares patient	Places patient supine. If required: • removes/cuts away sufficient clothing to expose chest • removes medication patches, jewellery, ECG electrodes • clips chest hair (if necessary) • dries chest (if necessary).	0	1	2	3	4
Continues chest compressions	Continues chest compressions while preparing for defibrillation.	0	1	2	3	4
Positions pads	Places pads in the anterior-lateral position (or anterior-posterior position if indicated). Avoids breast tissue, pacemakers, ICDs, placement over sternum and neck contact. Rolls pads on to avoid air pockets. Ensures correct contact/adhesion.	0	1	2	3	4
Moves oxygen away	Moves free-flowing oxygen 1 m away from the patient.	0	1	2	3	4
Moves all others away	Ensures rescuers not performing chest compressions are not touching the patient or attached equipment.	0	1	2	3	4
Charges defibrillator	Charges defibrillator to the recommended level.	0	1	2	3	4
Hands off	Ensures rescuer performing compressions moves away and confirms they are safe.	0	1	2	3	4

Safe defibrillation continued

Activity	Critical Action	Performance				
Evaluates rhythm	Rapidly evaluates presenting rhythm and identifies shockable rhythm.	0	1	2	3	4
Defibrillates/ disarms	Delivers shock to VF/pVT. Confirms shock delivered. Disarms defibrillator for non-shockable rhythms. Announces shock has been delivered (or disarmed) and it is safe to touch the patient.	0	1	2	3	4
Continues resuscitation	Continues CPR or post-resuscitation care as indicated from the patient's presentation and rhythm analysis.	0	1	2	3	4
Reports	Documents/hands over details of presenting rhythm, shock(s), energy, pad placement and effectiveness.	0	1	2	3	4

Standard Achieved: (please circle one)

Competent (C)   Not Yet Competent* (NYC)

Staff/Student Name: _____

Assessor (please print name): _____

Signed (Assessor): _____

Date of Assessment: _____

Comments:

*If Not Yet Competent (NYC) a PIP needs to be completed and a repeat of the F-CSAT

Formative Clinical Skill Assessment (F-CSAT) Key

Skill level	Standard of procedure	Quality of performance	Outcome	Level of assistance required
4 Safe for unsupervised practice	Safe Accurate Behaviour is appropriate to context	Confident Accurate Expedient	Achieved intended outcome	No supporting cues* required
3 Requires supervision	Safe Accurate Behaviour is appropriate to context	Confident Accurate Takes longer than required	Achieved intended outcome	Requires occasional supportive cues*
2 Requires assistance	Safe Accurate Behaviour generally appropriate to context	Lacks certainty	Would not have achieved outcome without support	Requires frequent verbal and occasional physical directives in addition to supportive cues*

Skill level	Standard of procedure	Quality of performance	Outcome	Level of assistance required
1 Requires direction	Safe only with guidance Not completely accurate	Unskilled Inefficient	Would not have achieved outcome without support	Requires continuous verbal and frequent physical directive cues*
0 Unsafe	Unsafe Unable to demonstrate behaviour Lack of insight into behaviour appropriate to context	Unskilled	Would not have achieved outcome	Requires continuous verbal and continuous physical directive cues*

*Refers to physical directives or verbal supportive cues

Performance Improvement Plan (PIP)

Please document the agreed education plan and completion timelines for areas assessed as less than 4.

This plan should be presented to assessor prior to commencement of summative assessment.

Where was supervisor support required?	Student summary of deficit. (Why was there a problem?)	Improvement Plan	Completed (Y/N)

Staff/Student Name: _____

Staff/Student Signature: _____

Educator Name: _____

Educator Signature: _____

Summative Clinical Skill Assessment (S-CSAT)

Equipment and resources: Mannequin; disposable gloves and eyewear; manual defibrillator; defibrillation pads; towel; shears/scissors; cardiac rhythm generator; method of documenting results

Associated Clinical Skills: Infection control; Communication; Consent; Chest compressions

Staff/Student being assessed: _____

- Completed Formative Clinical Skill Assessment (F-CSAT):   **YES**   **NO**

- Completed Performance Improvement Plan (PIP):   **YES**   **NO**   **N/A**

Safe defibrillation

Activity	Critical Action	Achieved Without Direction	
Safety	Dons appropriate PPE. Does not defibrillate in hazardous environments.	NO	YES
Prepares equipment	Positions defibrillator optimally for situation. Ensures pad type is correct for patient's age. Assesses expiry date of pads, gel quality, undamaged wires/connections.	NO	YES
Prepares patient	Places patient supine. If required: • removes/cuts away sufficient clothing to expose chest • removes medication patches, jewellery, ECG electrodes • clips chest hair (if necessary) • dries chest (if necessary).	NO	YES
Continues chest compressions	Continues chest compressions while preparing for defibrillation.	NO	YES
Positions pads	Places pads in the anterior-lateral position (or anterior-posterior position if indicated). Avoids breast tissue, pacemakers, ICDs, placement over sternum and neck contact. Rolls pads on to avoid air pockets. Ensures correct contact/adhesion.	NO	YES
Moves oxygen away	Moves free-flowing oxygen 1 m away from the patient.	NO	YES
Moves all others away	Ensures rescuers not performing chest compressions are not touching the patient or attached equipment.	NO	YES
Charges defibrillator	Charges defibrillator to the recommended level.	NO	YES
Hands off	Ensures rescuer performing compressions moves away and confirms they are safe.	NO	YES
Evaluates rhythm	Rapidly evaluates presenting rhythm and identifies shockable rhythm.	NO	YES
Defibrillates/disarms	Delivers shock to VF/pVT. Confirms shock delivered. Disarms defibrillator for non-shockable rhythms. Announces shock has been delivered (or disarmed) and it is safe to touch the patient.	NO	YES
Continues resuscitation	Continues CPR or post-resuscitation care as indicated from the patient's presentation and rhythm analysis.	NO	YES
Reports	Documents/hands over details of presenting rhythm, shock(s), energy, pad placement and effectiveness.	NO	YES

Standard Achieved: (please circle one)

Competent (C)   Not Yet Competent* (NYC)

Staff/Student Name: _____

Assessor (please print name)**:** _____

Signed (Assessor)**:** _____

Date of Assessment: _____

Comments:

*If Not Yet Competent (NYC) a PIP needs to be completed and a repeat of the F-CSAT

Clinical findings

Refractory shocks

Despite effective chest compressions and prompt defibrillation, some patients remain refractory to electrical therapy. Recent studies have examined the use of double sequential shock therapy using two defibrillators and two sets of strategically placed pads (Cortez et al., 2016; Ross et al., 2016; Stevenson, 2018) or repositioning the pads during resuscitation attempts to improve survival. These methods may receive future endorsement.

If the patient does not respond to the initial shock, it is reasonable to increase the energy levels for subsequent defibrillation. The safety of energy levels higher than 360 joules is unknown.

Patient contact during shock delivery

Inadvertent patient contact during defibrillation exposes the paramedic to risk of accidental electrocution and must be avoided. Minor nerve or burn injury are the worst outcomes reported by those feeling the shock. Most of the electrical current will still flow through the patient as planned. Nonetheless, rescuer safety is paramount and must not be compromised when trying to minimise the time between chest compressions (Deakin et al., 2015).

Arcing/burns

Electrodes in close contact with each other, or gel that is damaged, dried or in contact with other material, including metal jewellery or cardiac monitoring leads, can arc and cause burns. Pads must not be closer than 2.5 cm to each other and be of adequate quality before use. Quality inspection of pads includes assessing their expiry date and the quality of gel, and checking that wires/connections are undamaged. Avoid placing pads over wounds, nipples or other particularly sensitive or vulnerable skin.

Pad removal

To avoid injury, each pad should be removed after use by peeling it from the skin from one end back over itself, while the skin beneath is held taut.

PRACTICE TIP!

Paramedics should practise defibrillation and be familiar with placing defibrillator pads while chest compressions continue.

PRACTICE TIP!

The defibrillator operator must communicate clearly and effectively for the safety of all involved. This includes announcing the intention to shock, making eye contact with all nearby, confirming that everyone understands and calling 'Stand clear' before contacting the discharge button.

TEST YOUR KNOWLEDGE QUESTIONS

1. **What equipment inspections should occur before defibrillation?**
    Cables and wires are undamaged; pads are within expiry date; pads have sufficient gel.

2. **Where is the usual pad placement for patients in cardiac arrest?**
    Anterior-posterior: right pad to the right of sternum, inferior to the collar bone, over the second intercostal space. The left pad is placed on the lateral chest wall in the mid-axillary line over the sixth intercostal space.

3. **Why must the pad never be placed over the sternum?**
    Chest compressions over the pad could damage it.

4. **How are pacemakers or body piercings dealt with during defibrillation?**
    Do not place pads within 8 cm of them; relocate the pads to the nearest practicable position.

5. **What complications are posed by water on the patient?**
    Paramedic safety from electrical conduction; reduced effectiveness of defibrillation.

6. **What is the paediatric defibrillation energy and how is this delivered in practice?**
    4 joules/kg, rounded up to the nearest available setting.

7. **How is excessive body hair managed and why?**
    Body hair should be clipped, not shaved, to avoid causing minor cuts or injury leading to burns or the poor transmission of current.

8. **How is any nearby high-concentration oxygen hazard managed?**
    Move the source <1 m away from the defibrillator.

9. **Why must smaller paediatric defibrillation pads have less energy through them?**
    Their smaller size reduces the ability to dissipate electrical energy, leading to burns.

10. **Once a defibrillator is charged, what two options exist for using its energy?**
    Discharge; disarm.

References

ANZCOR (Australian and New Zealand Committee on Resuscitation), 2016a. *ANZCOR Guideline 7 – Automated external defibrillation in basic life support.* Retrieved from: https://resus.org.au/wpfb-file/anzcor-guideline-7-aed-jan16-pdf

ANZCOR (Australian and New Zealand Committee on Resuscitation), 2016b. *ANZCOR Guideline 11.4 – Electrical therapy for adult advanced life support.* Retrieved from: https://resus.org.au/download/section_11/anzcor-guideline-11-4-elect-jan16.pdf

Cortez, E., Krebs, W., Davis, J., Keseg, D.P. and Panchal, A.R., 2016. Use of double sequential external defibrillation for refractory ventricular fibrillation during out-of-hospital cardiac arrest. *Resuscitation*, 108, 82–86.

Deakin, C.D., Thomsen, J.E., Løfgren, B. and Petley, G.W., 2015. Achieving safe hands-on defibrillation using electrical safety gloves – a clinical evaluation. *Resuscitation*, 90, 163–167.

Di Maio, R., O'Hare, P., Crawford, P., McIntyre, A., McCanny, P., Torney, H. and Adgey, J., 2015. Self-adhesive electrodes do not cause burning, arcing or reduced shock efficacy when placed on metal items. *Resuscitation*, 96, 11.

Maconochie, I.K., Bingham, R., Eich, C., López-Herce, J., Rodríguez-Núnez, A., Rajka, T., van de Voorde, P., Zideman, D.A., Biarent, D., Monsieurs, K.G. and Nolan, J.P., 2015. European Resuscitation Council guidelines for resuscitation 2015, section 6: Paediatric life support. *Resuscitation*, 95, 223–248.

Pierce, A.E., Roppolo, L.P., Owens, P.C., Pepe, P.E. and Idris, A.H., 2015. The need to resume chest compressions immediately after defibrillation attempts: an analysis of post-shock rhythms and duration of pulselessness following out-of-hospital cardiac arrest. *Resuscitation*, 89, 162–168.

Ross, E.M., Redman, T.T., Harper, S.A., Mapp, J.G., Wampler, D.A. and Miramontes, D.A., 2016. Dual defibrillation in out-of-hospital cardiac arrest: a retrospective cohort analysis. *Resuscitation*, 106, 14–17.

Soar, J., Nolan, J.P., Böttiger, B.W., Perkins, G.D., Lott, C., Carli, P., Pellis, T., Sandroni, C., Skrifvars, M.B., Smith, G.B. and Sunde, K., 2015. European Resuscitation Council guidelines for resuscitation 2015, section 3: Adult advanced life support. *Resuscitation*, 95, 100–147.

Stevenson, L., 2018. Defibrillation: standard vs. double sequential in adult out-of-hospital cardiac arrest. *Journal of Paramedic Practice*, 10(2), 64–72.

Chapter 7
Manual Handling

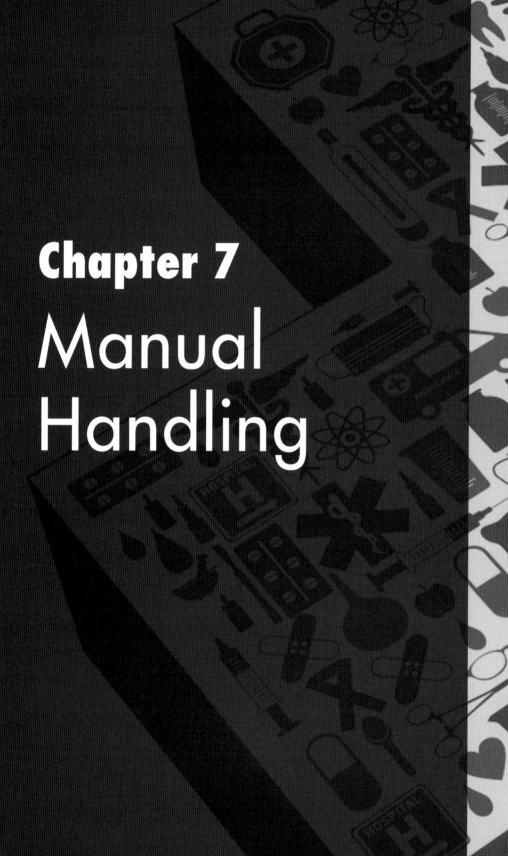

Chapter objectives

At the end of this chapter the reader will be able to:

1. Safely log roll a patient
2. Identify situations that interfere with safe patient log rolling and modify the process accordingly

Resources required for this assessment

- Patient or mannequin
- Gloves
- At least one and preferably three paramedic assistants

Skill matrix

This assessment requires:

- Infection control (CS 1.3)
- Communication (CS1.5)
- Consent (CS 1.6)
- Patient assessment skills (Chapter 2)
- Trauma asessment (CS 5.1)

This assessment is a component of:

- Manual handling (Chapter 7)

Introduction

Log rolling aims to move a patient who is lying supine onto their side as a single unit (or 'log'). This can be a component of transferring a patient, assessing their posterior aspect or removing things such as clothing from beneath them, or even adapted as part of the spinal immobilisation package. It can be used in conscious and unconscious patients.

This chapter will focus on the simple action of log rolling. The aim is to provide the principles of the task, which can be used in various specific situations. Despite log rolling being a commonly used skill, government agencies consider it 'High Risk: Very Likely to Cause Injury' to their employees utilising this method, because the shear forces produced exceed spinal capacity (Cohen et al., 2010; Workplace Health and Safety Queensland, 2001; Work Safe Victoria, 2009). Rigorous training in log rolling is required to ensure the safety of the patient and all those involved.

Anatomy and physiology

The two locations on the patient where the main force will be applied are the shoulder and hip. The advantages of these locations are that they are quite robust, well protected by bone, and generally not a sensitive place to handle (Marieb and Hoehn, 2007). These features allow the patient to be moved while minimising the possibility of injury and discomfort to the patient and paramedic.

Clinical rationale

The log roll is performed when a patient is unable to move themselves. This may be due to limitations in cognition or physical ability, injury or for medical reasons. Some patients may not be able to assist at all for various reasons; many will be able to provide at least some assistance (e.g. crossing their arms).

Log rolling may be required for numerous reasons, including:

- for assessment, where access to the patient's back is required
- for the patient's comfort, such as when removing wet or soiled clothing and bedding
- to allow the placement of a rigid spine board, pat slide and/or slide sheet under the patient
- as part of airway clearance, allowing the patient to be laterally positioned.

Log rolling therefore frequently forms part of a paramedic's day-to-day business. While appearing simple, the skill is often a small part of a larger goal, and practised in uncontrolled environments.

Assessing the need to log roll

Log rolling is a hazardous manual-handling activity, and should only be performed when required. Allow the patient to move with their own effort if appropriate.

Consider the patient's condition and injuries. Modify the log roll or choose an alternative method if necessary.

If log rolling/manual handling is necessary, seek sufficient human and equipment resources as early as practicable to maximise patient and paramedic safety.

Preparing the patient

Inform the patient of what will occur, and gain their cooperation where possible. Remove objects from the patient's pockets, especially the side they will be rolled onto.

Cross the patient's legs at the ankle, with the leg furthest from the paramedics on top. Allow the patient to do so themselves if able. Also cross the patient's arms over their chest, allowing them to do so themselves if they are able.

Instruct the patient to turn their head towards the paramedics who are performing the roll (Fig. 7.1.1) on the command of 'Roll', unless providing precautionary care for suspected spinal injury.

Preparing the team

Determine the log roll team leader. At least two paramedics, ideally no fewer than three, should be available to perform the roll. Consider requesting further assistance, depending on the size of both the patient and the paramedics.

Ensure that all those participating understand how the roll will be performed. A key part of the log roll is to move the patient simultaneously. Also ensure that the paramedics understand the commands and when the log roll will be executed. Using the command, 'Ready, set, roll' is recommended, as this avoids any confusion when to undertake the roll. Other commands are acceptable, provided all involved understand them clearly.

Paramedic positions

Paramedics should be positioned either kneeling or standing on the side towards which the patient will be rolled. Ensure proximity to the patient.

One paramedic places one cupped hand on the patient's shoulder and the second hand on the superior aspect of the hip to hold the torso (Fig. 7.1.2). Do not grab the patient's clothing to apply force. The second paramedic places one hand on the inferior aspect of hip and the other hand on the patient's leg. Where there are more paramedics available, consider having the second paramedic hold the pelvis or hip while a third holds the hip and legs and a fourth holds the lower legs only.

Where spinal injuries cannot be excluded, one paramedic should stand or kneel at the patient's head end, facing down the length of their body, and provide manual in-line neck stabilisation. To maintain neck alignment with body, the paramedic rests the forearms against the patient's head while grasping the clavicles with their fingers. The paramedic gently places inward pressure until they are lightly squeezing the patient's head between their forearms. This will move the head and body as one (Sahu and Lata, 2015). Holding the head alone allows separate movement of head/neck and torso, making this a difficult part of the log roll (Conrad et al., 2012; Del Rossi et al., 2003). As the patient is moved, this paramedic must rotate their arms with the patient to maintain head/neck/body alignment.

Performing the roll

The log roll team leader paramedic should be closest to the patient's head to control and command movement.

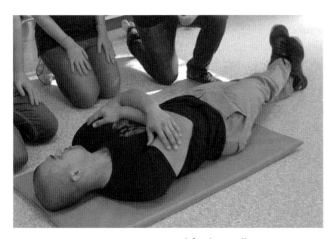

Figure 7.1.1 A patient prepared for log rolling

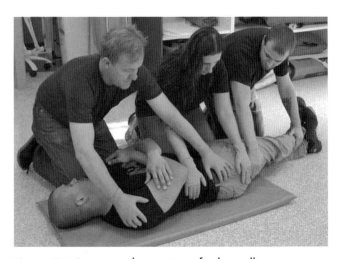

Figure 7.1.2 Paramedic positions for log rolling

The leader should loudly ask if everyone is ready. The roll must be performed as a team. Anyone who is not ready or who sees something unsafe must call 'Stop' loudly but calmly so the problem can be remedied.

The leader uses the command, 'Ready, set, roll'. On 'roll', both paramedics apply force, drawing the side of patient which is furthest from the paramedics upwards and creating a rolling action towards the paramedics. The patient is then rolled 90° onto their side.

As the roll is performed, the patient should turn their head looking towards the paramedics if they are able. If the patient is unable to do so, the team leader must stabilise their head in the neutral anatomical position with the spine held in alignment.

The paramedics then hold the patient in position to enable the task or procedure to occur. This should not place any strain on paramedics or cause patient adversity.

To lay the patient flat again, use the command, 'Ready, set, roll' and gently roll them back to a supine position in a continued controlled manner, avoiding letting them just drop back.

Clinical skill assessment process

The following section outlines the clinical skill assessment tools that should be used to determine a student's ability to demonstrate safe and effective log roll.
1. Clinical Skill Work Instruction
2. Formative Clinical Skill Assessment (F-CSAT)
3. Performance Improvement Plan (PIP)
4. Summative Clinical Skill Assessment (S-CSAT)
(5. Direct Observation of Procedural Skills (DOPS) – see Chapter 1.1)

Clinical Skill Work Instruction

Equipment and resources: Patient/mannequin; gloves; at least one and preferably three paramedic assistants

Associated Clinical Skills: Infection control; Communication; Consent; Patient asessment skills; Trauma assessment

Log roll

Activity	Critical Action	Rationale
Assess need for log roll	Consider whether a log roll needs to be performed.	The procedure involves a high risk of injury to paramedics, and should be avoided where possible.
	Consider the patient's condition and injuries.	Patient may not tolerate supine position due to respiratory compromise. Log rolling may cause further bleeding in pelvic injuries.
Prepare patient	Inform the patient and explain procedure.	To gain patient's cooperation, and assess whether they can assist.
	Don personal protection as required, including gloves.	To minimise the risk of infection.
	Remove objects from patient's pockets.	Avoids injury to patient.
	If able, patient to cross arms and legs, or otherwise paramedics to do this for them.	Crossing arms removes the need to roll on top of arm. Crossing the legs tilts the pelvis. Both actions reduce effort needed to roll.
Prepare team	Ensure suitable number of paramedics available to assist and are aware of how to perform log roll. Brief team on commands that will be used. Have all members don personal protection as required, including gloves.	Ensures log roll is performed as safely as possible.

Log roll continued

Activity	Critical Action	Rationale
Position paramedics	Either kneel or stand on the side the patient will be rolled towards. Ensure stand or kneel close to patient.	Ensures paramedics are at optimal height, avoiding bending their backs.
	First paramedic places one hand on shoulder and other hand on superior aspect of hip. Second paramedic places one hand on inferior aspect of hip and other hand on patient's leg. Where possible, use underneath sheet to apply pulling force.	Ensures patient will be rolled as a single unit.
	Paramedic closest to patient's head controls and commands the movement.	The head end of the patient is heaviest, and allows the control paramedic to best communicate with patient.
Perform roll	Command: 'Ready, set, roll'.	Avoids confusion of when to roll.
	On 'roll', both paramedics apply force, drawing side of patient which is furthest from paramedics upwards and creating a rolling action towards paramedics until patient is at 90° on their side. Take care not to grasp too tightly or pinch patient.	To apply teamwork in force application to move patient.
	At same time, patient turns head (if able) towards paramedics performing the roll, or otherwise paramedics do this for them.	Creates momentum and reduces effort required by paramedics.
Perform procedure	Hold patient steady while required procedure or task is completed.	This is the purpose of the log roll.
Return patient supine	On command of 'Read, set, roll', gently roll patient back to supine position.	Ensures patient moved as single unit. Reduces patient anxiety as they do not feel like they have been dropped.
Report	Accurately interpret, document and report on each patient movement and method used.	Accurate record kept and continuity of patient care.

Formative Clinical Skill Assessment (F-CSAT)

Equipment and resources: Patient/mannequin; gloves; at least one and preferably three paramedic assistants

Associated Clinical Skills: Infection control; Communication; Consent; Patient asessment skills; Trauma assessment

Staff/Student being assessed: _____

Log roll

Activity	Critical Action	Participant Performance				
Assesses need for log roll	Considers whether a log roll needs to be performed.	0	1	2	3	4
	Considers patient's condition and injuries.	0	1	2	3	4
Prepares patient	Informs patient and explains procedure.	0	1	2	3	4
	Checks/removes objects from patient's pockets.	0	1	2	3	4
	Instructs patient to cross arms and legs if able, or otherwise paramedics do this for them.	0	1	2	3	4

Log roll continued

Activity	Critical Action	Participant Performance				
Prepares team	Ensures suitable number of paramedics available to assist and are aware of how to perform log roll and the commands that will be used. All members don PPE as required.	0	1	2	3	4
Positions paramedics	Either kneels or stands on side the patient will be rolled towards, close to patient.	0	1	2	3	4
	First paramedic places one hand on shoulder and other hand on superior aspect of hip. Second paramedic places one hand on inferior aspect of hip and other hand on patient's leg.	0	1	2	3	4
	Paramedic closest to patient's head controls and commands movement.	0	1	2	3	4
Performs roll	Commands: 'Ready, set, roll'.	0	1	2	3	4
	On 'roll', both paramedics apply force, drawing side of patient which is furthest from paramedics upwards and creating a rolling action towards paramedics until patient is at 90° on their side.	0	1	2	3	4
	At same time, patient turns head (if able) towards paramedics performing roll, otherwise paramedics do this for them.	0	1	2	3	4
Performs procedure	Holds patient steady while required procedure or task is completed.	0	1	2	3	4
Returns patient supine	On command of 'Ready, set, roll', gently rolls patient back to supine position.	0	1	2	3	4
Reports	Accurately interprets, documents and reports on each patient movement and method used.	0	1	2	3	4

Standard Achieved: (please circle one)

Competent (C)   Not Yet Competent* (NYC)

Staff/Student Name: _____

Assessor (please print name): _____

Signed (Assessor): _____

Date of Assessment: _____

Comments:

*If Not Yet Competent (NYC) a PIP needs to be completed and a repeat of the F-CSAT

Formative Clinical Skill Assessment (F-CSAT) Key

Skill level	Standard of procedure	Quality of performance	Outcome	Level of assistance required
4 Safe for unsupervised practice	Safe Accurate Behaviour is appropriate to context	Confident Accurate Expedient	Achieved intended outcome	No supporting cues* required
3 Requires supervision	Safe Accurate Behaviour is appropriate to context	Confident Accurate Takes longer than required	Achieved intended outcome	Requires occasional supportive cues*
2 Requires assistance	Safe Accurate Behaviour generally appropriate to context	Lacks certainty	Would not have achieved outcome without support	Requires frequent verbal and occasional physical directives in addition to supportive cues*
1 Requires direction	Safe only with guidance Not completely accurate	Unskilled Inefficient	Would not have achieved outcome without support	Requires continuous verbal and frequent physical directive cues*
0 Unsafe	Unsafe Unable to demonstrate behaviour Lack of insight into behaviour appropriate to context	Unskilled	Would not have achieved outcome	Requires continuous verbal and continuous physical directive cues*

*Refers to physical directives or verbal supportive cues

Performance Improvement Plan (PIP)

Please document the agreed education plan and completion timelines for areas assessed as less than 4.

This plan should be presented to assessor prior to commencement of summative assessment.

Where was supervisor support required?	Student summary of deficit. (Why was there a problem?)	Improvement Plan	Completed (Y/N)

Staff/Student Name: _____

Staff/Student Signature: _____

Educator Name: _____

Educator Signature: _____

Summative Clinical Skill Assessment (S-CSAT)

Equipment and resources: Patient/mannequin; gloves; at least one and preferably three paramedic assistants

Associated Clinical Skills: Infection control; Communication; Consent; Patient asessment skills; Trauma assessment

Staff/Student being assessed: _____

• Completed Formative Clinical Skill Assessment (F-CSAT):	**YES**	**NO**	
• Completed Performance Improvement Plan (PIP):	**YES**	**NO**	**N/A**

Log roll

Activity	Critical Action	Achieved Without Direction	
Assesses need for log roll	Considers whether a log roll needs to be performed.	NO	YES
	Considers patient's condition and injuries.	NO	YES
Prepares patient	Informs patient and explains procedure.	NO	YES
	Checks/removes objects from patient's pockets.	NO	YES
	Instructs patient to cross arms and legs if able, otherwise paramedics do this for them.	NO	YES
Prepares team	Ensures suitable number of paramedics available to assist and are aware of how to perform log roll and the commands that will be used. All members don PPE as required.	NO	YES
Positions paramedics	Either kneels or stands on the side patient will be rolled towards, close to patient.	NO	YES
	First paramedic places one hand on shoulder and other hand on superior aspect of hip. Second paramedic places one hand on inferior aspect of hip and other hand on patient's leg.	NO	YES
	Paramedic closest to patient's head controls and commands movement.	NO	YES
Performs roll	Commands: 'Ready, set, roll'.	NO	YES
	On 'roll', both paramedics apply force, drawing side of patient which is furthest from paramedics upwards and creating a rolling action towards paramedics until patient is at 90° on their side.	NO	YES
	At same time, patient turns head (if able) towards paramedics performing roll, otherwise paramedics do this for them.	NO	YES
Performs procedure	Holds patient steady while required procedure or task is completed.	NO	YES
Returns patient supine	On command of 'Ready, set, roll', gently rolls patient back to supine position.	NO	YES
Reports	Accurately interprets, documents and reports on each patient movement and method used.	NO	YES

Standard Achieved: (please circle one)

Competent (C)   Not Yet Competent* (NYC)

Staff/Student Name: _____

Assessor (please print name): _____

Signed (Assessor): _____

Date of Assessment: _____

Comments:

*If Not Yet Competent (NYC) a PIP needs to be completed and a repeat of the F-CSAT

Clinical findings

Spinal cord injury

The log roll can cause significant motion in the patient's thoracolumbar spine (Conrad et al., 2012; Cornish and Jones, 2010; Prasarn et al., 2012), and it is difficult to maintain spinal alignment even when care is taken. To mitigate this risk, the team must move slowly and in a coordinated manner, particularly where spinal injury is not excluded. The benefit of log rolling where such injury exists has more recently been challenged (Rowell, 2014), though the likelihood of lateral rotation having any adverse impact on a vertebral injury is considered low (Hyldmo et al., 2015).

Pelvic fractures

Where possible, log rolling should be avoided where there is suspicion of pelvic fracture, due to its propensity to aggravate this potentially life-threatening injury (da Cunha Rodrigues, 2017; National Institute for Health and Care Excellence, 2016).

Musculoskeletal injuries

Patients should be rolled away from any obvious injuries, to avoid placing weight on and aggravating them. Consider splinting options and the need for analgesia before rolling.

PRACTICE TIP!

You need to perform a log roll of a patient with an injured shoulder or hip. Practise how you would modify hand positions, to avoid discomfort and any further injury to the patient.

PRACTICE TIP!

You have a patient who is unresponsive. Practise what changes might need to be made to log roll this patient effectively. *Hint:* The head will be unsupported in the unconscious patient.

Bariatric patients

Increased adipose tissue changes body size, which can adversely affect movement through log rolling. Men have greater propensity for abdominal adipose tissue while women tend more to hips and buttocks (Al-Benna, 2011; Sturman-Floyd, 2013). Rolling the patient may be more difficult, as their increased body mass is both more physically arduous to move and more resistant to reaching the intended position. Consider what outcomes are realistically achievable with the resources at hand and consider enlisting further paramedics to assist with log rolling if required.

Agitated behaviour

The proximity between paramedic and patient predisposes both of them to injury during log rolling. Agitated or aggressive behaviour increases the risk of injury. Consider using physical or chemical restraint before beginning the procedure if this is necessary for safe practice.

Non-paramedic assistance

Multiple or more challenging patients may necessitate the involvement of more than two people. In some cases, non-paramedics may need to assist. If so, ensure those involved take on the least difficult positions, such as the legs, and are well briefed before and during the procedure.

PRACTICE TIP!

Patients are often log rolled while on a bed or stretcher. Practise using a sheet to assist with the log roll. Your hands should grasp the sheet, roughly in line with where they would be placed on the patient.

PRACTICE TIP!

Sometimes patients will have multiple injuries, and despite best efforts may need to be moved towards an injured side. Practise log rolling a patient in a controlled manner, until the patient is at a lesser angle (say, 15°).

TEST YOUR KNOWLEDGE QUESTIONS

1. **When log rolling a patient, why are the shoulder and hip ideal locations to place your hands?**
   These locations are protected by bone and are generally not sensitive.

2. **If possible, why is it a good idea to have the patient turn their head towards you just as you roll them?**
   This creates momentum and reduces the effort required by paramedics.

3. **Why is log rolling a patient considered a high-risk manual-handling activity?**
   Through the shear forces produced, which exceed the spinal capacity to tolerate them.

4. **When rolling a patient back to supine, why is it important to do this in a controlled manner?**
   It ensures the patient is moved as single unit and reduces their anxiety, as they do not feel like they have been dropped.

5. **List at least three reasons a paramedic would perform a log roll.**
   For assessment, where access to the patient's back is required; for the patient's comfort, where removing wet or soiled clothing and bedding; to allow placement of a rigid spine board, pat slide and/or slide sheet under the patient; as part of airway clearance, allowing the patient to be laterally positioned.

6. **Why does log rolling a patient require training?**
   A key part of the log roll is to move the patient simultaneously. Training helps ensure that paramedics understand the commands and when the log roll will be executed.

7. **Why is it important that paramedics are positioned close to the patient when performing a log roll?**
   This ensures the paramedics are at the optimal height, avoiding bending their backs.

8. **Why should log rolling be avoided in patients with pelvic injuries?**
   Because this may aggravate this potentially life-threatening injury.

9. **Why should paramedics be familiar with the command used to coordinate a log roll?**
   It avoids confusion about when to roll the patient.

10. **A log roll is performed when a patient is unable to move themselves. What are some common reasons for this?**
    Limitations in cognition; limitations in physical ability; injury; medical reasons.

References

Al-Benna, S., 2011. Perioperative management of morbid obesity. *Journal of Perioperative Practice*, 21(7), 225.

Cohen, M.H., Faia, F., Nelson, G.G., Green, D.A. and Borden, C.M., 2010. *Patient handling and movement assessments* (white paper). Dallas: Facility Guidelines Institute.

Conrad, B.P., Del Rossi, G., Horodyski, M.B., Prasarn, M.L., Alemi, Y. and Rechtine, G.R., 2012. Eliminating log rolling as a spine trauma order. *Surgical Neurology International*, 3(Suppl 3), S188.

Cornish, J. and Jones, A., 2010. Factors affecting compliance with moving and handling policy: student nurses' views and experiences. *Nurse Education in Practice*, 10(2), 96–100.

da Cunha Rodrigues, I.F., 2017. To log-roll or not to log-roll – that is the question! A review of the use of log-roll on patients with pelvic fractures. *International Journal of Orthopaedic and Trauma Nursing*, 27, 36–40.

Del Rossi, G., Horodyski, M. and Powers, M.E., 2003. A comparison of spine-board transfer techniques and the effect of training on performance. *Journal of Athletic Training*, 38(3), 204.

Hyldmo, P.K., Vist, G.E., Feyling, A.C., Rognås, L., Magnusson, V., Sandberg, M. and Søreide, E., 2015. Does turning trauma patients with an unstable spinal injury from the supine to a lateral position increase the risk of neurological deterioration? A systematic review. *Scandinavian Journal of Trauma, Resuscitation and Emergency Medicine*, 23(1), 65.

Marieb, E.N. and Hoehn, K., 2007. *Human anatomy and physiology*, 7th edn. San Francisco: Pearson Benjamin Cummings.

National Institute for Health and Care Excellence, 2016. *Fractures (complex): assessment and management*. Retrieved from: https://www.nice.org.uk/guidance/ng37/chapter/Recommendations#pre-hospital-settings

Prasarn, M.L., Horodyski, M., Dubose, D., Small, J., Del Rossi, G., Zhou, H., Conrad, B.P. and Rechtine, G.R., 2012. Total motion generated in the unstable cervical spine during management of the typical trauma patient: a comparison of methods in a cadaver model. *Spine*, 37(11), 937–942.

Rowell, W., 2014. When emergency nurses should drop the log-rolling manoeuvre: William Rowell compares the potential outcomes of different ways to manipulate patients who have suspected spinal or pelvic injuries. *Emergency Nurse*, 22(4), 32–33.

Sahu, S. and Lata, I., 2015. Spine immobilization in trauma patient. *Manual of ICU procedures*. Delhi: Jaypee Brothers, p. 460.

Sturman-Floyd, M., 2013. Moving and handling: supporting bariatric residents. *Nursing & Residential Care*, 15(6), 432–437.

Workplace Health and Safety Queensland, 2001. *Manual tasks involving the handling of people: Code of Practice 2001*. Retrieved from: https://www.worksafe.qld.gov.au/__data/assets/pdf_file/0007/58174/manual-tasks-people-handling-cop-2001.pdf

Work Safe Victoria, 2009. *A handbook for workplaces, transferring people safely handling patients, residents and clients in health, aged care, rehabilitation and disability services*, 3rd edn. Retrieved from: https://content.api.worksafe.vic.gov.au/sites/default/files/2018-06/ISBN-Transferring-people-safely-handbook-2009-07.pdf

7.2 | Transfer: Supine to sitting position

Alex Vella and Shaun Wilkinson

Chapter objectives

At the end of this chapter the reader will be able to:

1. Identify anatomical landmarks to assist with patient movement
2. Assess patients' ability to stand safely
3. Demonstrate the ability to perform a risk assessment
4. Safely move the patient from supine to a sitting position

Resources required for this assessment

- Patient or mannequin
- Chair or other sturdy object
- Gloves
- At least one and preferably three paramedic assistants

Skill matrix

This assessment requires:

- Infection control (CS 1.3)
- Communication (CS1.5)
- Consent (CS 1.6)
- Patient assessment skills (Chapter 2)
- Trauma asessment (CS 5.1)
- Log roll (CS 7.1)

This assessment is a component of:

- Manual handling (Chapter 7)

Introduction

Paramedics are commonly called to patients who are lying supine and unable to get up from the ground. Purely lifting these patients poses an unacceptable risk of workplace injury, especially as a large cohort of these patients require minimal assistance to help themselves up. Healthcare workers are particularly susceptible to musculoskeletal injuries to the back, neck, shoulders, arms and knees when trying to help people who have fallen or need moving (Choi and Brings, 2016; Kim et al., 2012; Kurowski et al., 2017; Lapane et al., 2016; Ngan et al., 2010; Paul and Hoy, 2015). There is an increased risk of injury when such tasks are required to be performed by personnel who have not received adequate training (Cohen-Mansfield et al., 1996; Hogan et al., 2014). Safely changing patient posture from supine to sitting is discussed in this chapter.

Anatomy and physiology

The key anatomical locations for this patient movement are the acromion of the shoulder and the ilium on the pelvis (the greater trochanter can be substituted for the ilium if required). These are the two sturdy, anatomically significant points where the main force will be applied without likely detriment to the patient. They provide easily identifiable landmarks and solid skeletal points with little susceptibility to noxious stimuli of the nerve endings that can cause the patient pain (Marieb and Hoehn, 2007). These anatomical landmarks allow patient movement while minimising the risk of injury and discomfort for both patient and paramedic.

Clinical rationale

Wherever possible, encourage any patient needing postural change to contribute as much of the movement as they physically can. Sitting or standing from supine may be challenging, yet from a prone or kneeling position where the patient can use their own limbs it might be achievable. When moving a patient from supine, assistance might be required with part or all of the movement. A half log roll can help the patient to lift themselves by getting onto all fours and then pulling up to their feet.

Before undertaking any manual-handling task, formulate a plan, perform a risk assessment, identify hazards and manage those accordingly. This can be done informally as crew discussion on scene. Always have a back-up plan. Consider the possibility of:
• the patient reaching out and pulling the paramedic down, causing musculoskeletal injuries
• the patient falling on the paramedic
• supporting a patient who cannot sufficiently weight bear, placing excessive strain on the paramedic.

Next, perform a risk assessment. Risk assessment involves determining which factors may contribute to the risk of injury. Assess the hazards identified and plan to negate these. This should be done in consultation with all the paramedics involved in performing the task. Consider factors including:
• paramedic postures
• paramedic movements
• the forces and weight the paramedics will be exposed to
• the duration of the task
• the frequency of movements (is it an injurious, repetitive task?)
• situational considerations and the environmental conditions (Choi and Brings, 2016; Coenen et al., 2014; O'Keeffe et al., 2015; Villarroya et al., 2016; Worksafe Victoria, 2017).

Assessing the need to assist the patient

Perform an adequate clinical approach, including taking the patient's history, a survey of vital signs and a full secondary survey. Existing injuries or physiological compromise should be recognised before attempting to move any patient.

Rule out the need for full spinal immobilisation (see Clinical findings later in this chapter).

Log rolling is a hazardous manual-handling activity, and should only be performed when required (see Chapter 7.1). Allow the patient to move with their own effort if appropriate.

To test if the patient can bear weight, ask them to lift their buttocks off the bed with their back and heels flat on the floor, knees at 45° (known as 'bridging'; see Fig.

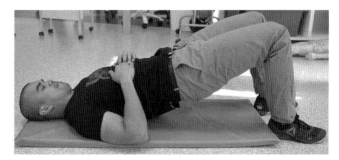

Figure 7.2.1 Patient bridging assessment

7.2.1). Have them hold the position for 5 seconds. Next, have them lift their legs in the air, one at a time, holding each up for 5 seconds while the other leg is bent with the heel firmly flat on the ground. If the patient cannot perform these tasks, an alternative manual-handling lifting device is necessary, as it is unlikely they will be able to stand (Doyle and McCutcheon, 2012).

If patient manual handling is necessary, seek sufficient human and equipment resources as early as practicable to maximise patient and paramedic safety.

Preparing the patient

Patients require precise instruction, time, coaching and encouragement to passively assist with bodily movement to reduce the workload of movement. Inform and engage the patient. Gain their cooperation where possible, to help ensure paramedics are not doing the bulk of lifting and shifting.

Remove objects from the patient's pockets so that they do not lie on them. Have the patient cross their legs at the ankle, with the leg furthest from paramedics on top, and get them to cross their arms over chest. Instruct the patient to turn head towards paramedics who are rolling, on the command of 'roll'.

Patients should be rolled away from any obvious injuries.

Preparing the team and equipment

The patient requires a stable object with a good edge to grip, large basal area and low centre of gravity to pull themselves up. A good example of a household object is a chair.

Ensure at least two paramedics perform the roll. Consider requesting further assistance, depending on the size and weight of the patient as well as the size and physical capabilities of the available paramedics.

Ensure the paramedics understand how to perform a roll, the commands that will be used and when the roll will be executed. The command, 'Ready, set, roll' is recommended to avoid any confusion.

Positioning the team

The initial movement is a patient log roll. This should be followed to the point where the patient is held steady and supported on their side (see Chapter 7.1).

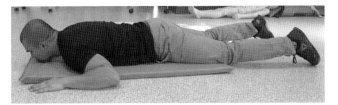

Figure 7.2.2 Patient in a prone, push-up position

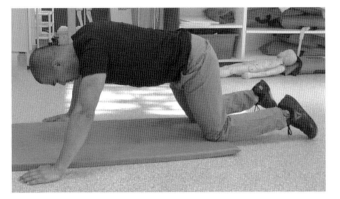

Figure 7.2.3 Patient on all fours

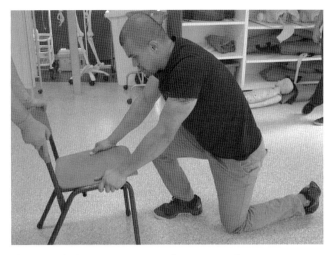

Figure 7.2.4 Patient using a chair to stand

To move patient into a prone position and then onto all fours, first instruct them to slowly outstretch their arms. Ensure the patient is stable, in a lateral position, supported by at least one arm. Instruct them to roll into prone position by continuing with the roll unaided. They will come to rest in a prone, push-up position (Fig. 7.2.2).

Instruct the patient to push up onto all fours (Fig. 7.2.3). The chair prepared earlier can now be placed in front or to the side of the patient, depending on their preference. The patient then grasps the edge of the chair and pulls themselves up slowly, first onto their knees and then into a crouch followed by a stand. Once standing or stooping upright, they can be guided to sit on the chair (Fig. 7.2.4).

Clinical skill assessment process

The following section outlines the clinical skill assessment tools that should be used to determine a student's ability to demonstrate safe transfer from supine to sitting position.
1. Clinical Skill Work Instruction
2. Formative Clinical Skill Assessment (F-CSAT)
3. Performance Improvement Plan (PIP)
4. Summative Clinical Skill Assessment (S-CSAT)
(5. Direct Observation of Procedural Skills (DOPS) – see Chapter 1.1)

Clinical Skill Work Instruction

Equipment and resources: Patient or mannequin; chair or other sturdy object; gloves; at least one and preferably three paramedic assistants

Associated Clinical Skills: Infection control; Communication; Consent; Patient assessment skills; Trauma assessment; Log roll

Transfer: Supine to sitting position

Activity	Critical Action	Rationale
Personal protection	Don gloves and PPE as required.	For infection risk management.
Assess need to assist	Assess patient for physiological status and injuries/illness. Ascertain patient's abilities for self-movement.	Unnecessary paramedic effort creates unwarranted risk.
Plan movement	Identify hazards and perform risk assessment. Develop a suitable plan for the situation. Ensure there are sufficient personnel for safe performance of the task. Brief all paramedics involved on their roles.	Cooperation ensures the patient assists and avoids unnecessary or incorrect paramedic involvement.

Transfer: Supine to sitting position continued

Activity	Critical Action	Rationale
Prepare patient	Gain consent and instruct patient on plan.	Preparation of patient to assess in task.
	Remove objects from patient's pockets. Prepare patient for log rolling.	To avoid causing discomfort or injury.
Prepare equipment	Ensure stable object is in readiness for patient to use, such as a solid chair. Place in useable position near patient's head or side, within easy reach but not obstructing log roll.	In readiness for standing effort. A solid, non-wheeled chair is suitable.
Log roll to prone	Log roll patient to stable lateral position (see Chapter 7.1).	In advance of completing rotation to prone.
Prone posture to all fours	Have patient stretch out their arms and then continue roll to prone unaided.	In readiness for standing.
	Instruct patient to push up onto all fours using stable object.	Part-way to upright position. Have patient move themselves as much as possible.
All fours to standing	Encourage patient to continue motion to standing.	Avoid unnecessary lifting.
Standing to sitting	Have patient move to a seated position.	Intended final position for patient.
Report	Document as required.	Accurate record kept and continuity of patient care.

Formative Clinical Skill Assessment (F-CSAT)

Equipment and resources: Patient or mannequin; chair or other sturdy object; gloves; at least one and preferably three paramedic assistants

Associated Clinical Skills: Infection control; Communication; Consent; Patient assessment skills; Trauma assessment; Log roll

Staff/Student being assessed: _____

Transfer: Supine to sitting position

Activity	Critical Action	Participant Performance				
Personal protection	Dons gloves and PPE as required.	0	1	2	3	4
Assesses need to assist	Assesses patient for physiological status and injuries/illness. Ascertains patient's abilities for self-movement.	0	1	2	3	4
Plans movement	Identifies hazards and performs risk assessment. Develops a suitable plan for situation. Ensures sufficient personnel for safe task performance. Briefs all paramedics involved on their roles.	0	1	2	3	4
Prepares patient	Gains consent and instructs patient on plan.	0	1	2	3	4
	Removes objects from patient's pockets. Prepares patient for log rolling.	0	1	2	3	4

Transfer: Supine to sitting position continued

Activity	Critical Action	Participant Performance				
Prepares equipment	Ensures stable object in is readiness for patient to use, such as a solid chair. Places in useable position near patient's head or side, within easy reach but not obstructing log roll.	0	1	2	3	4
Log roll to prone	Log rolls patient to stable lateral position.	0	1	2	3	4
Prone posture to all fours	Has patient stretch out their arms and then continue roll to prone unaided.	0	1	2	3	4
	Instructs patient to push up onto all fours using stable object.	0	1	2	3	4
All fours to standing	Encourages patient to continue motion to standing.	0	1	2	3	4
Standing to sitting	Has patient move to a seated position.	0	1	2	3	4
Reports	Documents as required.	0	1	2	3	4

Standard Achieved: (please circle one)

Competent (C)   Not Yet Competent* (NYC)

Staff/Student Name: _____

Assessor (please print name): _____

Signed (Assessor): _____

Date of Assessment: _____

Comments:

*If Not Yet Competent (NYC) a PIP needs to be completed and a repeat of the F-CSAT

Formative Clinical Skill Assessment (F-CSAT) Key

Skill level	Standard of procedure	Quality of performance	Outcome	Level of assistance required
4 Safe for unsupervised practice	Safe Accurate Behaviour is appropriate to context	Confident Accurate Expedient	Achieved intended outcome	No supporting cues* required
3 Requires supervision	Safe Accurate Behaviour is appropriate to context	Confident Accurate Takes longer than required	Achieved intended outcome	Requires occasional supportive cues*
2 Requires assistance	Safe Accurate Behaviour generally appropriate to context	Lacks certainty	Would not have achieved outcome without support	Requires frequent verbal and occasional physical directives in addition to supportive cues*

Skill level	Standard of procedure	Quality of performance	Outcome	Level of assistance required
1 Requires direction	Safe only with guidance Not completely accurate	Unskilled Inefficient	Would not have achieved outcome without support	Requires continuous verbal and frequent physical directive cues*
0 Unsafe	Unsafe Unable to demonstrate behaviour Lack of insight into behaviour appropriate to context	Unskilled	Would not have achieved outcome	Requires continuous verbal and continuous physical directive cues*

*Refers to physical directives or verbal supportive cues

Performance Improvement Plan (PIP)

Please document the agreed education plan and completion timelines for areas assessed as less than 4.

This plan should be presented to assessor prior to commencement of summative assessment.

Where was supervisor support required?	Student summary of deficit. (Why was there a problem?)	Improvement Plan	Completed (Y/N)

Staff/Student Name: _____

Staff/Student Signature: _____

Educator Name: _____

Educator Signature: _____

Summative Clinical Skill Assessment (S-CSAT)

Equipment and resources: Patient or mannequin; chair or other sturdy object; gloves; at least one and preferably three paramedic assistants

Associated Clinical Skills: Infection control; Communication; Consent; Patient assessment skills; Trauma assessment; Log roll

Staff/Student being assessed: _____

- Completed Formative Clinical Skill Assessment (F-CSAT): **YES**   **NO**
- Completed Performance Improvement Plan (PIP): **YES**   **NO**   **N/A**

Transfer: Supine to sitting position

Activity	Critical Action	Achieved Without Direction	
Personal protection	Dons gloves and PPE as required.	NO	YES
Assesses need to assist	Assesses patient for physiological status and injuries/illness. Ascertains patient's abilities for self-movement.	NO	YES
Plans movement	Identifies hazards and performs risk assessment. Develops a suitable plan for situation. Ensures there are sufficient personnel for safe task performance. Briefs all paramedics involved on their roles.	NO	YES
Prepares patient	Gains consent and instructs patient on plan.	NO	YES
	Removes objects from patient's pockets. Prepares patient for log rolling.	NO	YES
Prepares equipment	Ensures stable object is in readiness for patient to use, such as a solid chair. Places in useable position near patient's head or side within easy reach, but not obstructing log roll.	NO	YES
Log roll to prone	Log rolls patient to stable lateral position.	NO	YES
Prone posture to all fours	Has patient outstretch their arms then continues roll to prone unaided.	NO	YES
	Instructs patient to push up onto all fours using stable object.	NO	YES
All fours to standing	Encourages patient to continue motion to standing.	NO	YES
Standing to sitting	Has patient move to a seated position.	NO	YES
Reports	Documents as required.	NO	YES

Standard Achieved: (please circle one)

Competent (C)   Not Yet Competent* (NYC)

Staff/Student Name: _____

Assessor (please print name): _____

Signed (Assessor): _____

Date of Assessment: _____

Comments:

*If Not Yet Competent (NYC) a PIP needs to be completed and a repeat of the F-CSAT

Clinical findings

Patients who are unable to stand

Patients who are unable to stand unaided may have physiological reasons for this. Altered consciousness, respiratory difficulty or inadequate perfusion are all reasons why a patient may be unable to stand or why their condition may be worsened during the attempt.

A traumatic fall could cause musculoskeletal injuries that make the movement difficult if not impossible. This includes limb and potential spinal injuries. Spinal clearance should be performed routinely on all patients who have had a fall. Always immobilise the spine of patient who cannot be effectively cleared of spinal injury (Cox et al., 2017).

Delays to standing

Patients who have been supine and motionless on the ground for a prolonged period may experience symptoms of dizziness, feel faint or light-headed or have signs of orthostatic hypotension (Potter et al., 2010). Allow these patients time during this process for homeostasis to correct these imbalances.

PRACTICE TIP!

Everybody is slightly different in their anatomical makeup. Practise finding manual-handling landmarks on friends or family members.

PRACTICE TIP!

Perform the bridging exercise yourself so you can gain valuable insight into how you should instruct and coach the patient to do this effectively.

PRACTICE TIP!

In a group, practise rolling a person to get the feel of the amount of force required and the level of inertia involved. Roll the patient safely backwards and forwards a few times.

PRACTICE TIP!

Look around the home or workplace. Search for appropriate objects that would be suitable as safe options for the patient to use as a standing aid. Perform these actions yourself and assess whether these are adequate to mobilise a patient.

PRACTICE TIP!

Decide whether the task requires manual-handling equipment to assist. Suitable assist devices include lifting mattresses, lifting cushions, a hardboard patient slide, a slide sheet, the Kendrick Extrication Device and walk-assist belts.

TEST YOUR KNOWLEDGE QUESTIONS

1. **List six risk assessment factors for manual handling.**
    Paramedic postures and movements; forces and weight exposed to; task duration; frequency of movements; situational considerations; environmental conditions.

2. **Name two areas of paramedics' bodies that are particularly susceptible to manual-handling injury.**
    Back; neck; shoulders; arms; knees.

3. **Which anatomical place on the shoulder is rigid enough to assist patient movement?**
    The acromion.

4. **What are some signs/symptoms a patient may present with if they have been supine for a long period of time?**
    Dizziness; feeling faint or light-headed; orthostatic hypotension.

5. **What set of commands should you use with your partner when performing any supine patient movement?**
    Ready, set, roll.

6. **Name two inanimate household objects that could be used as support for a patient to help them to their knees or standing position.**
    Chair; table; four-wheel frame (with brakes **on**); firm sofa; stretcher (with brakes **on**); bedframe.

7. **What are two reasons a patient laying supine may not be able to stand?**
    For physiological reasons; due to the injuries they have incurred, including during a fall.

8. **Name at least two pieces of manual-handling equipment you should consider when performing the supine to sitting manual-handling task.**
    Lifting mattress; lifting cushion; hardboard patient slide; slide sheet; Kendrick Extrication Device; walk-assist belt.

9. **What is the safest way for a paramedic to get a patient up from the ground?**
    Coaching the patient to stand themselves.

10. **What should be considered before electing to manually transfer a patient from supine to sitting?**
    Sitting or standing from supine may be challenging, yet from a prone or kneeling position where the patient can use their own limbs it might be achievable. Can the patient complete some or all of the movement themselves? A half log roll can help the patient to lift themselves by getting onto all fours and then pulling up to their feet.

References

Choi, S.D. and Brings, K., 2016. Work-related musculoskeletal risks associated with nurses and nursing assistants handling overweight and obese patients: a literature review. *Work*, 53(2), 439–448.

Coenen, P., Gouttebarge, V., Van Der Burght, A.S., van Dieën, J.H., Frings-Dresen, M.H., van der Beek, A.J. and Burdorf, A., 2014. The effect of lifting during work on low back pain: a health impact assessment based on a meta-analysis. *Occupational and Environmental Medicine*, 71(12), 871–877.

Cohen-Mansfield, J., Culpepper, W.J. and Carter, P., 1996. Nursing staff back injuries. Prevalence and costs in long term care facilities. *American Association of Occupational Health Nurses Journal*, 44(1), 9–16.

Cox, S., Jennings, P., Middleton, J., Oteir, A., Smith, K., Sharwood, L. and Stoelwinder, J., 2017. Prehospital predictors of traumatic spinal cord injury in Victoria, Australia. *Prehospital Emergency Care*, 21(5).

Doyle, G. and McCutcheon, J., 2012. *Clinical procedures for safer patient care*. Victoria, BC: British Columbia Institute of Technology. Retrieved from: https://opentextbc.ca/clinicalskills

Marieb, E.N. and Hoehn, K., 2007. *Human anatomy and physiology*, 7th edn. San Francisco: Pearson Benjamin Cummings.

Hogan, D.A., Greiner, B.A. and O'Sullivan, L., 2014. The effect of manual handling training on achieving training transfer, employees' behaviour change and subsequent reduction of work-related musculoskeletal disorders: a systematic review. *Ergonomics*, 57(1), 93–107.

Kim, H., Dropkin, J., Spaeth, K., Smith, F. and Moline, J., 2012. Patient handling and musculoskeletal disorders among hospital workers: Analysis of 7 years of institutional workers' compensation claims data. *American Journal of Industrial Medicine*, 55(8), 683–690.

Kurowski, A., Gore, R., Roberts, Y., Kincaid, K.R. and Punnett, L., 2017. Injury rates before and after the implementation of a safe resident handling program in the long-term care sector. *Safety Science*, 92, 217–224.

Lapane, K., Dube, C. and Desdale, B., 2016. Worker injuries in nursing homes: Is safe patient handling legislation the solution? *Journal of Nursing Home Research Sciences*, 2, 110–117.

Ngan, K., Drebit, S., Siow, S., Yu, S., Keen, D. and Alamgir, H., 2010. Risks and causes of musculoskeletal injuries among health care workers. *Occupational Medicine*, 60(5), 389–394.

O'Keeffe, V.J., Tuckey, M.R. and Naweed, A., 2015. Whose safety? Flexible risk assessment boundaries balance nurse safety with patient care. *Safety Science*, 76, 111–120.

Paul, G. and Hoy, B., 2015. An exploratory ergonomic study of musculoskeletal disorder prevention in the Queensland Ambulance Service. *Journal of Health, Safety and Environment*, 31(3), 1–13.

Potter, P.A., Perry, A.G., Ross-Kerr, J.C. and Wood, M.J. (eds), 2010. *Canadian fundamentals of nursing*, 4th edn. Toronto: Elsevier.

Villarroya, A., Arezes, P., Díaz-Freijo, S. and Fraga, F., 2016. Comparison between five risk assessment methods of patient handling. *International Journal of Industrial Ergonomics*, 52, 100–108.

Worksafe Victoria, 2017. *Identify the risk*. Retrieved from: http://www.worksafe.vic.gov.au/pages/safety-and-prevention/health-and-safety-topics/manual-handling/identify-the-risk

7.3 | Transfer: Sitting to standing position

Alex Vella and Shaun Wilkinson

Chapter objectives

At the end of this chapter the reader will be able to:

1. Assess the risks to paramedic and patient in moving from sitting to standing
2. Formulate a plan to stand the sitting patient
3. Effectively communicate with the patient and paramedics when moving a patient from sitting to stand position unaided
4. Safely move a patient from sitting to standing position

Resources required for this assessment

- Patient
- Chair
- At least one and preferably three paramedic assistants
- Gloves

Skill matrix

This assessment requires:

- Infection control (CS 1.3)
- Communication (CS1.5)
- Consent (CS 1.6)
- Patient assessment skills (Chapter 2)
- Trauma asessment (CS 5.1)

This assessment is a component of:

- Manual handling (Chapter 7)

Introduction

Commonly, paramedics are called to attend patients who are found unwell while seated in a chair or sofa and unable to stand on their own. A variety of reasons could be implicated, including acute medical emergencies or the effects of chronic illness or degeneration. Lifting patients from sitting to standing poses a considerable risk of paramedic injury, which should always be avoided (Jäger et al., 2012; Jordan et al., 2011). This chapter discusses effective assessment and safe patient movement in this situation.

Anatomy and physiology

The anatomically significant sites for this exercise are the torso, the sacrum and the acromion of the shoulder. The torso is sturdy and offers support; the sacrum offers a point for gently pushing and assisting the patient to pivot while standing; and the shoulder is robust (Marieb and Hoehn, 2007). These strong points allow the patient to be guided in movement while minimising the chances of injury and discomfort.

Clinical rationale

High-risk patient-handling tasks are characterised by significant biomechanical and postural stressors imposed while moving loads. Examples include the patient's weight, the transfer distance, a confined workspace, unpredictable patient behaviour, awkward positions such as stooping or bending, and reaching out significantly (see Chapter 7.2). Isolated or together, these factors contribute to the risk of performing manual-handling tasks on patients.

One of the highest risk tasks when handling patients is transferring them from sitting to standing (Baptiste and Nelson, 2006; Burnfield et al., 2013). It is considered a task that can be biomechanically improved to lower the risk of injury through improved technique (Jäger et al., 2012; Jordan et al., 2011). Even small reductions in manual handling can provide long-term benefit against cumulative strain (Holmes et al., 2010).

Helping the patient move themselves from sitting to standing position is important for paramedic safety. It can also be a useful clinical tool to assess whether the patient is unable to weight bear due to injury or has physical deficits due to a medical condition.

Risk assessment

When performing any manual handling of the patient, a risk assessment must first be performed to identify and manage any hazards (see Chapter 7.2), including:

- awkward posturing such as bending or twisting, especially with failure to adopt a bent-knee, straight-leg position
- the patient's weight and subsequent difficulty to shift, lift and/or carry
- the patient's condition – altered consciousness or physical weakness could suggest a dead weight (how much support and assistance can the patient offer on their own?)
- unpredictable movements, such as grabbing onto the paramedic or sudden falls
- the hazards and risks posed by lifting a person (which can cause sprains, strains and other injuries; Worksafe Victoria, 2017).

Assessing the need to assist the patient

Wherever reasonable, encourage the patient to stand themselves. Gather clinical evidence to assess their capacity and analyse why they cannot stand. This includes previous observation or nursing/family advice.

This is a hazardous manual-handling activity, and should only be performed when required. Allow the patient to move with their own effort if appropriate, coaching and encouraging them as much as possible (Taylor, 2017). Time constraints can incorrectly prompt paramedics to turn to manual handling where mechanical options are available (Burnfield et al., 2013).

If patient manual handling is necessary, seek sufficient human and equipment resources as early as practicable to maximise patient and paramedic safety.

Preparing the patient

Inform and engage the patient. Give precise directions, detail the timing and provide coaching and encouragement throughout to passively assist them with body movement (Taylor, 2017).

Consider administering pain relief prior to movement if appropriate, if pain is a factor in limiting the patient's own movement.

Preparing the team and equipment

Place a sturdy object in front of the patient. Ensure it has a large basal area and low centre of gravity, such as a dining chair positioned with the backrest towards the patient. Encourage the patient to grip this and use it to apply force to stand and to remain steady once upright.

If necessary, have the stretcher or other mobile device nearby, ready to wheel in behind the patient for a quick and easy transfer if necessary. This can assist in the event the patient is unable to weight bear for long periods or walk without assistance.

Ensure at least two paramedics are available, briefed on the procedure as planned. Consider requesting further assistance or manual-handling equipment as a back-up plan.

Preparing for transfer to standing

Allocate a lead paramedic to control and command the movement.

Perform a verbal 'dry run' with your partner, discussing actions to ensure the safety and effectiveness of the plan. The command, 'Ready, set, stand' should be used.

Confirm the patient is ready.

One paramedic stands in a side-lunge position with legs slightly wider than shoulder width apart, the leg closest to the patient's back bent at the knee and the other leg straight. From here, this paramedic rocks their own position from one side to another in time with the patient as they stand (Fig. 7.3.1). It is essential to avoid

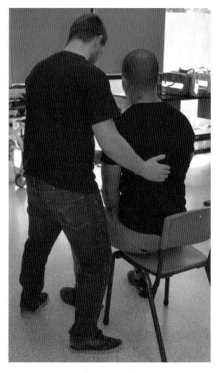

Figure 7.3.1 Preparing the seated patient to stand

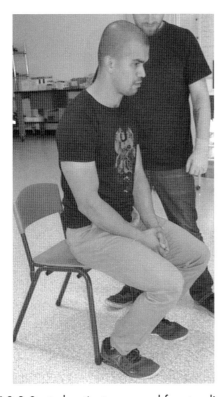

Figure 7.3.2 Seated patient prepared for standing attempt

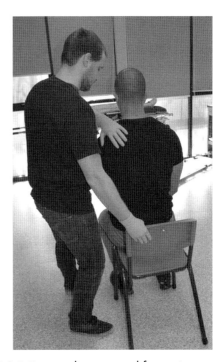

Figure 7.3.3 Paramedic prepared for patient standing attempt

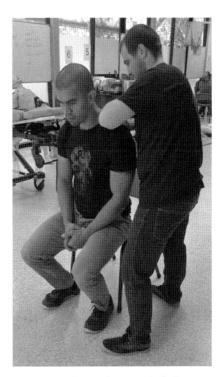

Figure 7.3.4 Paramedic rocking to shift the patient's posture

bending and twisting movements and using the limbs to apply force, as this can lead to injury (Theilmeier et al., 2010). The body should be kept in line with the necessary impetus for patient movement provided by the shifting of overall weight by the rocking motion.

Transferring the patient to standing position

Have the patient shuffle their buttocks forwards, close to the edge of their chair. Their weight should be leaning forwards in the direction they are to move, rather than leaning back in their chair and working in opposition to standing. Being seated further back in the chair increases the work and effort required to stand.

Place patient's feet as close to the base of the chair as possible. If space allows, the patient's heels can be slightly underneath the chair they are seated on but their feet must be firmly flat on the floor (Fig. 7.3.2).

The paramedic's hand closest to the patient is placed on the anterior acromion of the shoulder, with the other hand on the back of the chair the patient is seated on (see Fig. 7.3.3). The paramedic must maintain a straight-backed, non-twisting posture to ensure no strain is placed on their arms or lower back.

The paramedic assists the patient to lean forwards by straightening their bent knee, rocking to the other side, ensuring the straight knee now bends. They gently push against the patient's shoulder, leaning the torso forwards, to ensure the patient bends at the hips (Fig. 7.3.4).

Simultaneously, the patient is instructed to push down on their knees or the chair in front of them. If necessary, they can rock back and forth a few times to help generate

forwards momentum out of the chair. The paramedic's hand moves from the chair to now push forwards gently on the patient's sacrum, ensuring the hand on the shoulder is an open palm, facing the shoulder and gently pushing forwards (Fig. 7.3.5).

As the paramedic gently pushes forwards on the sacrum and shoulder, the patient stands themselves using their arms to increase upward force if they are able. The patient can either place both hands on the arms of the chair they are sitting in or one hand in advance on the chair they

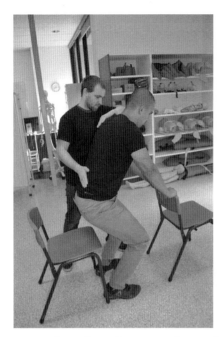

Figure 7.3.5 Gently pushing the patient forwards to stand

are to stand against to help steady them as they rise. They should not place both hands on the chair they are to stand against yet in case it shifts during the procedure as the patient moves.

Ideally, the paramedic stands on the side the patient is pushing up with their arm. This reduces the chance of the patient panicking and grabbing the paramedic with that arm.

Once standing, instruct the patient to hold the inanimate object in front of them for stabilisation.

If at any time the patient says they cannot weight bear, guide them to descend gently back into the seat they were sitting in.

Clinical skill assessment process

The following section outlines the clinical skill assessment tools that should be used to determine a student's ability to safely demonstrate a transfer from sitting to standing.
1. Clinical Skill Work Instruction
2. Formative Clinical Skill Assessment (F-CSAT)
3. Performance Improvement Plan (PIP)
4. Summative Clinical Skill Assessment (S-CSAT)
(5. Direct Observation of Procedural Skills (DOPS) – see Chapter 1.1)

Clinical Skill Work Instruction

Equipment and resources: Patient; chair; at least one and preferably three paramedic assistants; gloves

Associated Clinical Skills: Infection control; Communication; Consent; Patient assessment skills; Trauma assessment

Transfer: Sitting to standing position

Activity	Critical Action	Rationale
Personal protection	Don gloves and PPE as required.	For infection risk management.
Assess need to assist	Assess patient for physiological status and injuries/illness. Ascertain patient's abilities for self-movement.	Unnecessary paramedic effort creates unwarranted risk.
Plan movement	Identify hazards and perform a risk assessment. Develop a suitable plan for the situation. Ensure there are sufficient personnel for safe performance of the task. Brief all paramedics involved on their roles.	Cooperation ensures the patient assists and avoids unnecessary or incorrect paramedic involvement.
Prepare patient	Gain consent and instruct patient on the plan.	Prepares the patient to assist in task.
	Consider analgesia if needed to facilitate movement.	To avoid causing patient increased pain.
Prepare equipment	Place stable object in useable position in front of patient where they can lean forwards and easily reach it. If necessary, place alternative wheeled option ready to assist if patient proves unable.	In readiness for standing effort. A solid, non-wheeled chair is suitable.
Prepare to stand	Nominate lead paramedic for control. Rehearse procedure. Ensure all parties, including patient, are ready.	Brief team and ensure plan is safe and effective.

Transfer: Sitting to standing position continued

Activity	Critical Action	Rationale
Stand patient	Stand in a side-lunge position, legs slightly wider than shoulder length apart, with leg closest to patient's back bent at the knee and the other leg straight.	In readiness for patient standing.
	Shuffle patient's bottom close to edge of chair, leaning forwards. Place their feet, firmly flat, as close to chair base as possible.	Weight distribution to move patient forwards, not leaning back.
	Place hand nearest to patient's back on their shoulder, the further hand against their chair back.	Postured to help guide patient motion.
	Rock away from the chair back by bending straight knee and straightening bent knee while pushing gently against patient's shoulder.	Patient is providing effort, while paramedic is providing guide.
	Instruct patient to push down on their arms and knees to rise. At the same time, move hand from chair to now push gently on the patient's sacrum, with the other hand still on the shoulder.	To continue guiding patient effort to stand.
Patient standing	Encourage patient to continue motion to standing and grasp the inanimate object to help stabilise them.	To avoid unnecessary lifting.
Report	Document as required.	Accurate record keeping and continuity of care.

Formative Clinical Skill Assessment (F-CSAT)

Equipment and resources: Patient; chair; at least one and preferably three paramedic assistants; gloves

Associated Clinical Skills: Infection control; Communication; Consent; Patient assessment skills; Trauma assessment

Staff/Student being assessed: _____

Transfer: Sitting to standing position

Activity	Critical Action	Participant Performance				
Personal protection	Dons gloves and PPE as required.	0	1	2	3	4
Assesses need to assist	Assesses patient for physiological status and injuries/illness. Ascertains patient's abilities for self-movement.	0	1	2	3	4
Plans movement	Identifies hazards and performs risk assessment. Develops a suitable plan for situation. Ensures sufficient personnel for safe task performance. Briefs all paramedics involved on their roles.	0	1	2	3	4
Prepares patient	Gains consent and instructs patient on plan.	0	1	2	3	4
	Considers analgesia if needed to facilitate movement.	0	1	2	3	4
Prepares equipment	Places stable object in readiness for patient to use, such as a solid chair, in useable position in front within easy reach.	0	1	2	3	4
Prepares to stand	Nominates lead paramedic for control. Rehearses procedure. Ensures all parties, including patient, are ready.	0	1	2	3	4

Transfer: Sitting to standing position continued

Activity	Critical Action	Participant Performance				
Stands patient	Stands in a side-lunge position, legs slightly wider than shoulder length apart, with leg closest to patient's back bent at the knee and the other leg straight.	0	1	2	3	4
	Shuffles patient's bottom close to edge of chair, leaning forwards with feet placed firmly flat, as close to chair base as possible.	0	1	2	3	4
	Places hand nearest to patient on their shoulder, the further hand against their chair back.	0	1	2	3	4
	Rocks away from chair back by bending straight knee and straightening bent knee while pushing gently against patient's shoulder.	0	1	2	3	4
	Instructs patient to push down on their arms and knees to rise. At the same time, moves hand from chair to now push gently on the patient's sacrum, with the other hand still on the shoulder.	0	1	2	3	4
Patient standing	Encourages patient to continue motion to standing and grasp the inanimate object to help stabilise themselves.	0	1	2	3	4
Reports	Documents as required.	0	1	2	3	4

Standard Achieved: (please circle one)

Competent (C)   Not Yet Competent* (NYC)

Staff/Student Name: _____

Assessor (please print name): _____

Signed (Assessor): _____

Date of Assessment: _____

Comments:

*If Not Yet Competent (NYC) a PIP needs to be completed and a repeat of the F-CSAT

Formative Clinical Skill Assessment (F-CSAT) Key

Skill level	Standard of procedure	Quality of performance	Outcome	Level of assistance required
4 Safe for unsupervised practice	Safe Accurate Behaviour is appropriate to context	Confident Accurate Expedient	Achieved intended outcome	No supporting cues* required
3 Requires supervision	Safe Accurate Behaviour is appropriate to context	Confident Accurate Takes longer than required	Achieved intended outcome	Requires occasional supportive cues*
2 Requires assistance	Safe Accurate Behaviour generally appropriate to context	Lacks certainty	Would not have achieved outcome without support	Requires frequent verbal and occasional physical directives in addition to supportive cues*

Skill level	Standard of procedure	Quality of performance	Outcome	Level of assistance required
1 Requires direction	Safe only with guidance Not completely accurate	Unskilled Inefficient	Would not have achieved outcome without support	Requires continuous verbal and frequent physical directive cues*
0 Unsafe	Unsafe Unable to demonstrate behaviour Lack of insight into behaviour appropriate to context	Unskilled	Would not have achieved outcome	Requires continuous verbal and continuous physical directive cues*

Refers to physical directives or verbal supportive cues

Performance Improvement Plan (PIP)

Please document the agreed education plan and completion timelines for areas assessed as less than 4.

This plan should be presented to assessor prior to commencement of summative assessment.

Where was supervisor support required?	Student summary of deficit. (Why was there a problem?)	Improvement Plan	Completed (Y/N)

Staff/Student Name: _____

Staff/Student Signature: _____

Educator Name: _____

Educator Signature: _____

Summative Clinical Skill Assessment (S-CSAT)

Equipment and resources: Patient; chair; at least one and preferably three paramedic assistants; gloves

Associated Clinical Skills: Infection control; Communication; Consent; Patient assessment skills; Trauma assessment

Staff/Student being assessed: _____

- Completed Formative Clinical Skill Assessment (F-CSAT):   **YES**   **NO**

- Completed Performance Improvement Plan (PIP):   **YES**   **NO**   **N/A**

Transfer: Sitting to standing position

Activity	Critical Action	Achieved Without Direction	
Personal protection	Dons gloves and PPE as required.	NO	YES
Assesses need to assist	Assesses patient for physiological status and injuries/illness. Ascertains patient's abilities for self-movement.	NO	YES
Plans movement	Identifies hazards and performs risk assessment. Develops a suitable plan for situation. Ensures there are sufficient personnel for safe task performance. Briefs all paramedics involved on their roles.	NO	YES
Prepares patient	Gains consent and instructs patient on plan.	NO	YES
	Considers analgesia if needed to facilitate movement.	NO	YES
Prepares equipment	Places stable object in readiness for patient to use, such as solid chair, in useable position in front within easy reach.		
Stands patient	Stands in a side-lunge position, legs slightly wider than shoulder length apart, with leg closest to patient's back bent at the knee and the other leg straight.	NO	YES
	Shuffles patient's bottom close to edge of chair, leaning forwards with feet placed firmly flat, as close to chair base as possible.	NO	YES
	Places hand nearest to patient on their shoulder and the further hand against their chair back.	NO	YES
	Rocks away from chair back by bending straight knee and straightening bent knee while pushing gently against patient's shoulder.	NO	YES
	Instructs patient to push down on their arms and knees to rise. At the same time, moves hand from chair to now push gently on the patient's sacrum, with the other hand still on the shoulder.	NO	YES
Patient standing	Encourages patient to continue motion to standing and grasp the inanimate object to help stabilise themselves.	NO	YES
Reports	Documents as required.	NO	YES

Standard Achieved: (please circle one)

Competent (C)   Not Yet Competent* (NYC)

Staff/Student Name: _____

Assessor (please print name)**:** _____

Signed (Assessor)**:** _____

Date of Assessment: _____

Comments:

*If Not Yet Competent (NYC) a PIP needs to be completed and a repeat of the F-CSAT

Clinical finding

Patients who are unable to stand

Patients who are unable to stand may have interfering physiological reasons for this (see Chapter 7.2). Pre-existing injuries may reduce movement or cause pain, interfering with movement from a chair. Pre-existing illness, such as stroke or neuromuscular disorders, may similarly create difficulty with balance, strength and the patient's ability to stand themselves. If balance is an issue, a walk/lift belt secured to the patient's waist might help to steady them.

Sitting position modifications

The ability to move the patient to the edge of the chair and allow them to create their own forward momentum onto standing legs is pivotal to the success of this procedure. If the chair is able to be raised or tilted forwards, this can improve the chances of success.

Alternatively, it may be possible to assist pushing the patient forwards by using slide sheets folded and passed around the patient's waist, supported by paramedics holding either end, or by lifting cushions positioned behind their back.

PRACTICE TIP!

Perform a side lunge. Stand with feet slightly wider than shoulder width (approximately 1 m) and gently rock from side to side, facing forwards. At all times, one leg should be bent at the knee and the other leg straight.

PRACTICE TIP!

Ensure a back-up plan has been devised to remove the patient from the chair if they are unable to stand with instruction and minimal assistance. Lifting a patient from a chair is a dangerous exercise that poses an unacceptable risk to the health and safety of the paramedic.

PRACTICE TIP!

Practise placing one hand on your partner's shoulder and another on their sacrum. Push the two together in a firm, steady fashion while your partner stands up. You will see how this straightens the body and aids upright positioning while standing.

PRACTICE TIP!

Decide whether the task requires manual-handling equipment to assist the patient's own effort. Suitable assist devices include lifting mattresses, lifting cushions, a hardboard patient slide, a slide sheet, the Kendrick Extrication Device and walk-assist belts.

TEST YOUR KNOWLEDGE QUESTIONS

1. **What is the purpose of gently pushing in on the patient's sacrum and shoulder?**
   To straighten their back towards a standing posture.

2. **Why is a patient first shifted forwards in their seat with their feet flat on the floor before standing them?**
   To allow their body weight to lean forwards in the direction of intended movement.

3. **What should the patient do with their arms during the movement?**
   Push down into the chair arms to help them stand. One hand can be used to lean against the chair/object they are going to hold once they stand.

4. **When assisting the patient from sitting to standing using a side lunge, what anatomical landmarks should you identify?**
   Torso; sacrum; acromion of shoulder.

5. **What is the most appropriate way to assist the patient if, on standing, they find they are unable to weight bear or fully stand up?**
   Let the patient sit back down. Reassess and find another option.

6. **Name at least two causes of biomechanical and postural stressors on the paramedic when performing manual-handling tasks.**
   The patient's weight; transfer distance; confined workspace; unpredictable patient behaviour; awkward positions.

7. **Why is encouraging the patient to stand unaided safest for the paramedic?**
   This offers the least chance of injury or discomfort to both patient and paramedic.

8. **What therapeutic intervention can the paramedic administer prior to movement that may help the patient to stand by themselves?**
   Pain relief.

9. **Name at least two factors affecting the paramedic that should make up part of the risk assessment.**
   Posturing; movements; forces; duration; frequency of movements; situational considerations; environmental conditions.

10. **What methods can be used to identify whether a patient can stand?**
    Gather clinical evidence to assess their capacity and (if applicable) analyse why they cannot stand. This includes previous observation or nursing/family advice.

References

Baptiste, A. and Nelson, A., 2006. Evidence-based practices for safe patient handling and movement. *Orthopaedic Nursing*, 25(6), 366–379.

Burnfield, J.M., McCrory, B., Shu, Y., Buster, T.W., Taylor, A.P. and Goldman, A.J., 2013. Comparative kinematic and electromyographic assessment of clinician-and device-assisted sit-to-stand transfers in patients with stroke. *Physical Therapy*, 93(10), 1331–1341.

Marieb, E.N. and Hoehn, K., 2007. *Human anatomy and physiology*, 7th edn. San Francisco: Pearson Benjamin Cummings.

Holmes, M.W., Hodder, J.N. and Keir, P.J., 2010. Continuous assessment of low back loads in long-term care nurses. *Ergonomics*, 53(9), 1108–1116.

Jäger, M., Jordan, C., Theilmeier, A., Wortmann, N., Kuhn, S., Nienhaus, A. and Luttmann, A., 2012. Lumbar-load analysis of manual patient-handling activities for biomechanical overload prevention among healthcare workers. *Annals of Occupational Hygiene*, 57(4), 528–544.

Jordan, C., Luttmann, A., Theilmeier, A., Kuhn, S., Wortmann, N. and Jäger, M., 2011. Characteristic values of the lumbar load of manual patient handling for the application in workers' compensation procedures. *Journal of Occupational Medicine and Toxicology*, 6(1), 17.

Taylor, J., 2017. How to assist patients with sit-stand transfers. *Nursing Standard*, 31(37), 41–45.

Theilmeier, A., Jordan, C., Luttmann, A. and Jäger, M., 2010. Measurement of action forces and posture to determine the lumbar load of healthcare workers during care activities with patient transfers. *Annals of Occupational Hygiene*, 54(8), 923–933.

Worksafe Victoria, 2017. *Your health and safety guide to hazardous manual handling*. Retrieved from: https://www.worksafe.vic.gov.au/__data/assets/pdf_file/0003/211287/ISBN-Hazardous-manual-handling-guide-2017-06.pdf

7.4 | Transfer: Supine from bed to bed

Alex Vella and Shaun Wilkinson

Chapter objectives

At the end of this chapter the reader will be able to:

1. Safely move the supine patient from bed to bed
2. Identify situations that interfere with supine transfer from bed to bed and modify the process accordingly

Resources required for this assessment

- Patient or mannequin
- Two beds
- Pat slide
- Slide sheet
- Gloves

Skill matrix

This assessment requires:

- Infection control (CS 1.3)
- Communication (CS 1.5)
- Consent (CS 1.6)
- Patient assessment skills (Chapter 2)
- Trauma asessment (CS 5.1)
- Log roll (CS 7.1)

This assessment is a component of:

- Manual handling (Chapter 7)

Introduction

Transferring a supine patient from bed to bed is an essential part of any paramedic's role. Often this is the relatively controlled patient moving from ambulance stretcher to hospital bed. Bed-to-bed transfers are also utilised in moving the patient from their own bed to an ambulance stretcher, and between ambulance stretchers. These situations, especially moving the patient from bed to stretcher, present challenges. Despite this skill being frequently performed, it still presents paramedics with substantial injury risk from manual handling (Cohen et al., 2010; Workplace Health and Safety Queensland, 2001; Work Safe Victoria, 2009).

The skill of moving a supine patient from bed to bed utilises the log roll (see Chapter 7.1) and is discussed in this chapter.

Anatomy and physiology

When transferring a supine patient from bed to bed, it is important to note which areas of the body will create the most resistance to movement. Looking at the human body from a lateral view, the posterior shoulders and buttocks protrude the most (Marieb and Hoehn, 2007). When in the supine position, these are the two areas that will create the most resistance. It is therefore important that devices such as pat slides are placed in a way that ensures coverage of the shoulders and buttocks as a minimum. These areas will otherwise catch and create resistance during the transfer, increasing the risk of injury to paramedics.

Clinical rationale

The supine bed-to-bed transfer is a commonly used practice within the health industry around Australia. Ambulance services frequently use this method of loading and unloading patients from stretchers. However, like other manual transfers, it should be used only where patients cannot move themselves, for reasons including:

- cognitive impairment, where patients cannot understand instructions for effecting a transfer themselves
- a physical inability to move between beds
- injuries and/or medical conditions that may prevent movement or risk being exacerbated if the patient attempts to move themselves.

For clarity, the bed the patient commences on will be referred to as 'the ambulance stretcher' and the bed the patient is being transferred to will be referred to as 'the bed'. This skill can be used to transfer patients from stretcher to stretcher, bed to stretcher or any other combination.

Assessing the need for manual transfer

Supine bed-to-bed transfers are risky for paramedics. Where possible, the patient should effect their own transfer. This is safer for paramedics, and patients often feel more comfortable moving themselves.

If patient manual handling is necessary, seek sufficient human and equipment resources as early as practicable to maximise patient and paramedic safety.

Preparing the patient

Explain what will occur with the movement. Ensure the patient understands they will be moved between ambulance stretcher and bed. Emphasise the need to keep the arms crossed and not reach out during the transfer.

Lie the patient supine. If they are sitting or semi-reclined and you are using an ambulance stretcher with manual head lowering, have the patient sit forwards (if possible), release the catch and have the patient slowly lie back. Lower the head end of the bed until the patient is supine. If they are not able to do this, support the stretcher head as the catch is released and it is lowered, as it may jolt with the patient's weight on it.

Make further preparations as described in Chapter 7.1, Log roll.

Preparing the equipment

Lower the side rail of the ambulance stretcher and untuck ambulance stretcher sheets. Position the stretcher beside the bed the patient will be transferred to, ensuring the brakes are applied on both. Adjust the stretcher height, ideally so the patient is at the hip height of the shortest paramedic performing the transfer, with the bed slightly lower than the ambulance stretcher.

Place the pat slide (mini pat slides can be substituted) on the bed the patient will be transferred to. Position it in line with the patient to ensure the shoulders and hips/buttocks are covered.

Friction-reducing devices such as slide sheets should be used where available, and placed on top of the pat slide in preparation (Lloyd and Baptiste, 2006). Patients who are clothed will slide more easily than those whose skin contacts the surface of the slide, increasing friction.

Preparing the team

Ensure at least four paramedics are available to ensure equitable sharing of the manual load. More may be required depending on the size of the patient and the individual abilities of the paramedics.

Ensure all team members understand the method of performing the transfer and the commands to be used. The command, 'Ready, set, slide' is recommended, as this avoids confusion about when the transfer will occur. Other commands can be used as long as all paramedics understand when to perform the transfer.

Position the team. Two paramedics stand in line with the patient's shoulders, one at the side of the ambulance stretcher and one in the same position at the side of the bed. Position two paramedics in line with the patient's hips, again with one paramedic at the side of the ambulance stretcher and one at the side of the bed (Fig. 7.4.1).

Rolling the patient

Grasping the ambulance stretcher bedsheet, roll the patient as described in Chapter 7.1.

While the patient is at 90°, the paramedics at the side of bed place the pat slide and slide sheet onto the ambulance stretcher, just contacting the patient's back (Fig. 7.4.2).

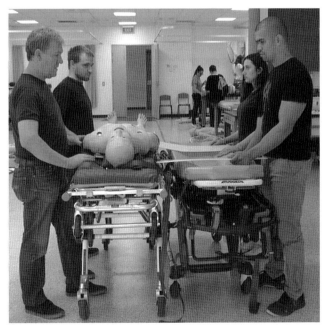

Figure 7.4.1 Paramedic positions for supine bed-to-bed transfer

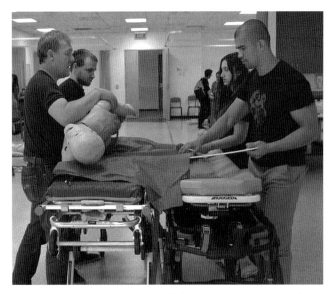

Figure 7.4.2 Placing the pat slide in position using a log roll

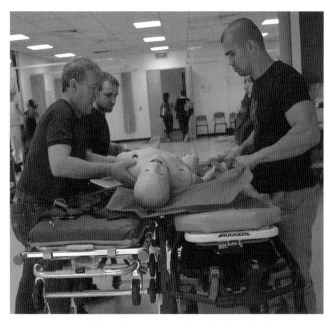

Figure 7.4.3 Sliding the patient from bed to bed

Ensure the pat slide is in a position that the patient will be lying on it when they are laid back to supine, and that the slide has coverage between the ambulance stretcher and bed.

Return the patient to supine as described in Chapter 7.1.

Sliding the patient

The paramedics at the side of the ambulance stretcher grasp the sheet closest to them. The paramedics beside the second bed reach and grasp the sheet. Providing ongoing manual in-line spinal support may not always be necessary. Where it is not, one paramedic on the pulling side of the patient should be the leader for movements.

Ensure all paramedics are ready.

Inform the patient that movement is about to begin. Surprise movement must be avoided to ensure the patient does not flail or resist. The patient must keep their arms crossed.

The team leader calls, 'Ready, set, slide'. In unison, the team members slide the patient in one smooth motion, shifting their weight from front leg to rear leg away from the patient and with their arms held straight to apply pulling force. Those on the side of the ambulance stretcher do not push the patient; they steady the patient's movement and stop the pat slide from moving with the patient (Fig. 7.4.3).

With the patient now on the bed, those on the ambulance stretcher side can slip the pat slide out laterally from under the patient towards themselves. If there is any resistance, stop the procedure. The paramedics on the bed side can then perform a slight roll of the patient towards them to free the pat slide, allowing it to slide out from under the patient. Store the pat slide when this is completed.

The side rails of the bed should be raised where fitted, and the ambulance stretcher can be removed. The patient should be positioned in a position of comfort and/or according to clinical need.

Clinical skill assessment process

The following section outlines the clinical skill assessment tools that should be used to determine a student's ability to demonstrate safe supine transfer from bed to bed.
1. Clinical Skill Work Instruction
2. Formative Clinical Skill Assessment (F-CSAT)
3. Performance Improvement Plan (PIP)
4. Summative Clinical Skill Assessment (S-CSAT)
(5. Direct Observation of Procedural Skills (DOPS) – see Chapter 1.1)

Clinical Skill Work Instruction

Equipment and resources: Patient or mannequin: two beds; pat slide; slide sheet; gloves

Associated Clinical Skills: Infection control; Communication; Consent; Patient assessment skills; Trauma assessment; Log roll

Transfer: Supine from bed to bed

Activity	Critical Action	Rationale
Assess need for transfer	Assess the need for manual transfer.	Manual patient transfer carries a risk for paramedics. Only perform it when necessary.
Prepare patient	Explain procedure.	Reduces patient anxiety and risk to paramedic.
	Slowly lie patient supine in a controlled manner.	Bed-to-bed transfer is most efficient when performed with the patient supine.
	Prepare patient for log roll (see Chapter 7.1).	Patient log roll is a key step within this skill.
Prepare equipment	Lower side rail of ambulance stretcher. Untuck ambulance stretcher sheets.	Need to lower side rail to allow access to sheet.
	Position ambulance stretcher beside bed patient will be transferred to.	Reduces the distance patient will be transferred.
	Ensure brakes are applied on both beds.	Reduces risk of beds moving during transfer.
	Adjust the bed height, ideally so patient is at hip height of the shortest paramedic involved in transfer, with ambulance stretcher slightly higher than bed.	While it is impossible for shorter paramedics to use correct technique when the bed is too high, taller paramedics can adjust to a lower bed. Provides gravity assistance during transfer.
	Place pat slide on bed, with slide sheet ready.	Pat slides and slide sheets reduce the force required for patient transfer.
Prepare team	Ensure at least four paramedics are available for the transfer.	This is the minimum number to undertake the transfer safely.
	Ensure all team members are competent and understand the commands to be used.	There is a risk of injury if paramedics not trained in this skill or are unfamiliar with commands to be used.
	Position team, either side of patient, in line with patient's shoulders and hips.	Ensures spread of effort.
Position pat slide	Grasping ambulance stretcher bedsheet, roll patient utilising log roll.	Using the stretcher bedsheet reduces risk of pinching the patient and avoids paramedics needing to reach awkwardly over the patient.
	Position pat slide so patient will lie on pat slide and slide sheet. Ensure pat slide has coverage to bridge between ambulance stretcher and bed. Log roll patient back onto board.	Ensures pat slide and slide sheet will assist optimally.

Transfer: Supine from bed to bed continued

Activity	Critical Action	Rationale
Perform slide	Paramedics either side of patient grasp ambulance stretcher bedsheet and take up slack.	Ensures a smooth slide across.
	One paramedic at head of patient commands the transfer and keeps the patient informed.	This is the easiest position in which to communicate with the patient.
	Instruct patient to keep arms crossed.	This position slightly raises the patient's shoulders, reducing friction, as well as preventing patient from grasping onto bed or paramedics.
	The command, 'Ready, set, slide' is called by either head support paramedic or leader on the pulling side.	Avoids confusion. Other commands can also be used if all paramedics are familiar with them.
	Slide patient in one smooth motion, using weight to shift front to back, with arms straight.	Maintains momentum of transfer.
	Paramedics at side of ambulance stretcher slide pat slide out from under patient.	Attempt should cease if excessive force is required.
	Raise side rails of patient bed and remove ambulance stretcher.	To ensure patient safety.
Report	Document as required.	Accurate record keeping and continuity of care.

Formative Clinical Skill Assessment (F-CSAT)

Equipment and resources: Patient or mannequin: two beds; pat slide; slide sheet; gloves

Associated Clinical Skills: Infection control; Communication; Consent; Patient assessment skills; Trauma assessment; Log roll

Staff/Student being assessed: _____

Transfer: Supine from bed to bed

Activity	Critical Action	Participant Performance				
Assesses transfer need	Assesses need for manual transfer.	0	1	2	3	4
Prepares patient	Explains procedure.	0	1	2	3	4
	Slowly lies patient supine in a controlled manner.	0	1	2	3	4
	Prepares patient for log roll (see Chapter 7.1).	0	1	2	3	4
Prepares equipment	Lowers side rail of ambulance stretcher. Untucks ambulance stretcher sheets.	0	1	2	3	4
	Positions ambulance stretcher beside bed patient will be transferred to.	0	1	2	3	4
	Ensures brakes are applied on both beds.	0	1	2	3	4
	Adjusts bed height, ideally so patient is at hip height of shortest paramedic involved in transfer and ambulance stretcher is slightly higher than bed.	0	1	2	3	4
	Places pat slide on bed, with slide sheet ready.	0	1	2	3	4

Transfer: Supine from bed to bed continued

Activity	Critical Action	Participant Performance				
Prepares team	Ensures at least four paramedics are available for transfer.	0	1	2	3	4
	Ensures all team members are competent and understand commands to be used.	0	1	2	3	4
	Positions team, either side of patient, in line with patient's shoulders and hips.	0	1	2	3	4
Positions pat slide	Grasping ambulance stretcher bedsheet, rolls patient utilising log roll.	0	1	2	3	4
	Positions pat slide so patient will lie on pat slide and slide sheet. Ensures pat slide has coverage to bridge between ambulance stretcher and bed. Log rolls patient back onto board.	0	1	2	3	4
Performs slide	Paramedics either side of patient grasp ambulance stretcher bedsheet, and take up slack.	0	1	2	3	4
	One paramedic at head end of patient commands transfer and keeps patient informed.	0	1	2	3	4
	Instructs patient to keep arms crossed.	0	1	2	3	4
	Uses command, 'Ready, set, slide'.	0	1	2	3	4
	Slides patient in one smooth motion.	0	1	2	3	4
	Paramedics at side of ambulance stretcher slide pat slide out from under patient.	0	1	2	3	4
	Raises side rails of bed and removes ambulance stretcher.	0	1	2	3	4
Reports	Documents as required.	0	1	2	3	4

Standard Achieved: (please circle one)

Competent (C)   Not Yet Competent* (NYC)

Staff/Student Name: _____

Assessor (please print name): _____

Signed (Assessor): _____

Date of Assessment: _____

Comments:

*If Not Yet Competent (NYC) a PIP needs to be completed and a repeat of the F-CSAT

Formative Clinical Skill Assessment (F-CSAT) Key

Skill level	Standard of procedure	Quality of performance	Outcome	Level of assistance required
4 Safe for unsupervised practice	Safe Accurate Behaviour is appropriate to context	Confident Accurate Expedient	Achieved intended outcome	No supporting cues* required
3 Requires supervision	Safe Accurate Behaviour is appropriate to context	Confident Accurate Takes longer than required	Achieved intended outcome	Requires occasional supportive cues*
2 Requires assistance	Safe Accurate Behaviour generally appropriate to context	Lacks certainty	Would not have achieved outcome without support	Requires frequent verbal and occasional physical directives in addition to supportive cues*
1 Requires direction	Safe only with guidance Not completely accurate	Unskilled Inefficient	Would not have achieved outcome without support	Requires continuous verbal and frequent physical directive cues*
0 Unsafe	Unsafe Unable to demonstrate behaviour Lack of insight into behaviour appropriate to context	Unskilled	Would not have achieved outcome	Requires continuous verbal and continuous physical directive cues*

*Refers to physical directives or verbal supportive cues

Performance Improvement Plan (PIP)

Please document the agreed education plan and completion timelines for areas assessed as less than 4.

This plan should be presented to assessor prior to commencement of summative assessment.

Where was supervisor support required?	Student summary of deficit. (Why was there a problem?)	Improvement Plan	Completed (Y/N)

Staff/Student Name: _____

Staff/Student Signature: _____

Educator Name: _____

Educator Signature: _____

Summative Clinical Skill Assessment (S-CSAT)

Equipment and resources: Patient or mannequin: two beds; pat slide; slide sheet; gloves

Associated Clinical Skills: Infection control; Communication; Consent; Patient assessment skills; Trauma assessment; Log roll

Staff/Student being assessed: _____

- Completed Formative Clinical Skill Assessment (F-CSAT): **YES** **NO**
- Completed Performance Improvement Plan (PIP): **YES** **NO** **N/A**

Transfer: Supine from bed to bed

Activity	Critical Action	Achieved Without Direction	
Assesses transfer need	Assesses the need for manual transfer.	NO	YES
Prepares patient	Explains procedure.	NO	YES
	Slowly lays patient supine in controlled manner.	NO	YES
	Prepares patient for log roll (see Chapter 7.1).	NO	YES
Prepares equipment	Lowers side rail of ambulance stretcher and untucks ambulance stretcher sheets.	NO	YES
	Positions ambulance stretcher beside bed patient will be transferred to.	NO	YES
	Ensures brakes are applied on both beds.	NO	YES
	Adjusts bed height, ideally so patient is at hip height of shortest paramedic involved in transfer and ambulance stretcher is slightly higher than bed.	NO	YES
	Places pat slide on bed, with slide sheet ready.	NO	YES
Prepares team	Ensures at least four paramedics are available for transfer.	NO	YES
	Ensures all team members are competent and understand commands to be used.	NO	YES
	Positions team either side of patient, in line with patient's shoulders and hips.	NO	YES
Positions pat slide	Grasping ambulance stretcher bedsheet, rolls patient utilising log roll.	NO	YES
	Positions pat slide so that patient will lie on pat slide and slide sheet. Ensures pat slide has coverage to bridge between ambulance stretcher and bed.	NO	YES
Performs slide	Paramedics either side of patient grasp ambulance stretcher bedsheet and take up slack.	NO	YES
	One paramedic at head of patient commands transfer and keeps patient informed.	NO	YES
	Instructs patient to keep arms crossed.	NO	YES
	Uses command, 'Ready, set, slide'.	NO	YES
	Slides patient in one smooth motion.	NO	YES
	Paramedics at side of ambulance stretcher slide pat slide out from under patient.	NO	YES
	Raises side rails of patient bed and removes ambulance stretcher.	NO	YES
Reports	Documents as required.	NO	YES

Standard Achieved: (please circle one)

Competent (C)   Not Yet Competent* (NYC)

Staff/Student Name: _____

Assessor (please print name)**:** _____

Signed (Assessor)**:** _____

Date of Assessment: _____

Comments:

*If Not Yet Competent (NYC) a PIP needs to be completed and a repeat of the F-CSAT

Clinical findings

Inability to fully log roll patient

Patients with injuries such as spinal, pelvic and musculoskeletal injuries can be adversely affected by the log rolling aspect of this procedure (see Chapter 7.1). This risk can be minimised by rolling the patient less than the 90° advocated where no physical examination will occur (Conrad et al., 2012; Del Rossi et al., 2008; Horodyski et al., 2011). The slide method may not be possible in patients who cannot be placed in a supine position (Del Rossi et al., 2003).

Inability to place patient supine

Unconsciousness reduces airway reflexes. Supine positioning of an unprotected airway is not supported, and lateral or upright positioning is preferred (Camacho et al., 2014; Hyldmo et al., 2015; Joosten et al., 2014). Similarly, full-term pregnant women are managed laterally to avoid aortocaval compression (Kinsella, 2003; Morris and Stacey, 2003; Palmer et al., 2017; Zelop et al., 2018). To facilitate bed-to-bed transfer, some patients may have to be briefly placed supine during transfer and then immediately returned to the preferred posture. If this is not possible, a modified slide transfer with the patient maintained laterally may be required.

Patients in respiratory distress frequently do not tolerate being positioned supine, as this increases both breathing difficulty and anxiety. Where such a patient refuses to tolerate supine positioning, a modified slide method, transferring the patient in a head-raised position, is required. Provided the slide mechanism is beneath the buttocks and legs, the raised upper body will have notably less friction. Both beds should have the head position raised equally. The paramedics at the head end must be tall enough to reach the patient pull points without stretching.

PRACTICE TIP!

If a patient does not tolerate lying supine (e.g. if they are in respiratory distress), modify the supine bed-to-bed transfer by placing the slide sheet under the bottom half of the patient only (buttocks and legs) while leaving the patient semi-recumbent.

PRACTICE TIP!

Many ambulance services have specialised manual-handling equipment available, such as hover mats that can be used to move the patient.

TEST YOUR KNOWLEDGE QUESTIONS

1. **Why do we use the ambulance stretcher bedsheet to assist with the transfer?**
   It reduces the risk of pinching the patient and avoids paramedics needing to reach awkwardly over patients.

2. **What action can be taken to ensure neither bed moves during patient transfer?**
   Engage the brakes.

3. **Why should a slide sheet be utilised?**
   Slide sheets significantly reduce friction and the effort needed to transfer the patient.

4. **What is the command used to initiate the patient slide transfer?**
   The command 'Ready, set, slide' is preferred.

5. **Why should the ambulance stretcher be slightly higher than the bed to which the patient is being transferred?**
   Having the ambulance stretcher slightly higher allows the use of gravity, which can offer slight assistance with the sliding motion.

6. **What modified strategies can be employed where a patient cannot be positioned supine ready for bed-to-bed sliding transfer?**
   Use a modified slide method, transferring the patient in a head-raised position. Provided the slide mechanism is beneath the buttocks and legs, the raised upper body will have notably less friction. Both beds should have the head position raised equally. The paramedics at the head end must be tall enough to reach the patient pull points without stretching.

7. **Why do we adjust the bed heights to the shortest paramedic?**
   Short paramedics cannot use an ergonomic position to transfer a patient who is situated too high. Tall paramedics can compensate for a patient who is too low, and still use an acceptable position.

8. **How many paramedics do you need as a minimum when performing a supine bed-to-bed transfer?**
   A minimum of four, but more may be required.

9. **Why do supine transfers from bed to bed require comprehensive training in the skill?**
   They are commonly used and present a high risk of injury to paramedics.

10. **Name at least three reasons why a patient may not be able to move themselves.**
    Cognition; physical ability; injury; medical conditions.

References

Camacho, M., Capasso, R. and Schendel, S., 2014. Airway changes in obstructive sleep apnoea patients associated with a supine versus an upright position examined using cone beam computed tomography. *Journal of Laryngology & Otology*, 128(9), 824–830.

Cohen, M.H., Faia, F., Nelson, G.G., Green, D.A. and Borden, C.M., 2010. *Patient handling and movement assessments* (white paper). Dallas, Texas: Facility Guidelines Institute.

Conrad, B.P., Del Rossi, G., Horodyski, M.B., Prasarn, M.L., Alemi, Y. and Rechtine, G.R., 2012. Eliminating log rolling as a spine trauma order. *Surgical Neurology International*, 3(Suppl 3), S188.

Del Rossi, G., Horodyski, M., Conrad, B.P., DiPaola, C.P., DiPaola, M.J. and Rechtine, G.R., 2008. Transferring patients with thoracolumbar spinal instability: are there alternatives to the log roll maneuver? *Spine*, 33(14), 1611–1615.

Del Rossi, G., Horodyski, M. and Powers, M.E., 2003. A comparison of spine-board transfer techniques and the effect of training on performance. *Journal of Athletic Training*, 38(3), 204.

Horodyski, M., Conrad, B.P., Del Rossi, G., DiPaola, C.P. and Rechtine, G.R., 2011. Removing a patient from the spine board: is the lift and slide safer than the log roll? *Journal of Trauma and Acute Care Surgery*, 70(5), 1282–1285.

Hyldmo, P.K., Vist, G.E., Feyling, A.C., Rognås, L., Magnusson, V., Sandberg, M. and Søreide, E., 2015. Is the supine position associated with loss of airway patency in unconscious trauma patients? A systematic review and meta-analysis. *Scandinavian Journal of Trauma, Resuscitation and Emergency Medicine*, 23(1), 50.

Joosten, S.A., O'Driscoll, D.M., Berger, P.J. and Hamilton, G.S., 2014. Supine position related obstructive sleep apnea in adults: pathogenesis and treatment. *Sleep Medicine Reviews*, 18(1), 7–17.

Kinsella, S.M., 2003. Lateral tilt for pregnant women: why 15 degrees? *Anaesthesia*, 58(9), 835–836.

Lloyd, J.D. and Baptiste, A., 2006. Friction-reducing devices for lateral patient transfers: a biomechanical evaluation. *AAOHN Journal*, 54(3), 113–119.

Marieb, E.N. and Hoehn, K., 2007. *Human anatomy and physiology*, 7th edn. San Francisco: Pearson Benjamin Cummings.

Morris, S. and Stacey, M., 2003. ABC of resuscitation: resuscitation in pregnancy. *BMJ*, 327(7426), 1277.

Palmer, J., Wallis, M. and Borhart, J., 2017. Cardiac arrest in the pregnant patient. In *Emergency Department management of obstetric complications*. Cham: Springer, pp. 117–127.

Workplace Health and Safety Queensland, 2001. *Manual tasks involving the handling of people: Code of Practice 2001*. Retrieved from: https://www.worksafe.qld.gov.au/__data/assets/pdf_file/0007/58174/manual-tasks-people-handling-cop-2001.pdf

Work Safe Victoria, 2009. *A handbook for workplaces, transferring people safely handling patients, residents and clients in health, aged care, rehabilitation and disability services*, 3rd edn. Retrieved from: https://content.api.worksafe.vic.gov.au/sites/default/files/2018-06/ISBN-Transferring-people-safely-handbook-2009-07.pdf

Zelop, C.M., Einav, S., Mhyre, J.M. and Martin, S., 2018. Cardiac arrest during pregnancy: ongoing clinical conundrum. *American Journal of Obstetrics and Gynecology*, 219(1), 52–61.

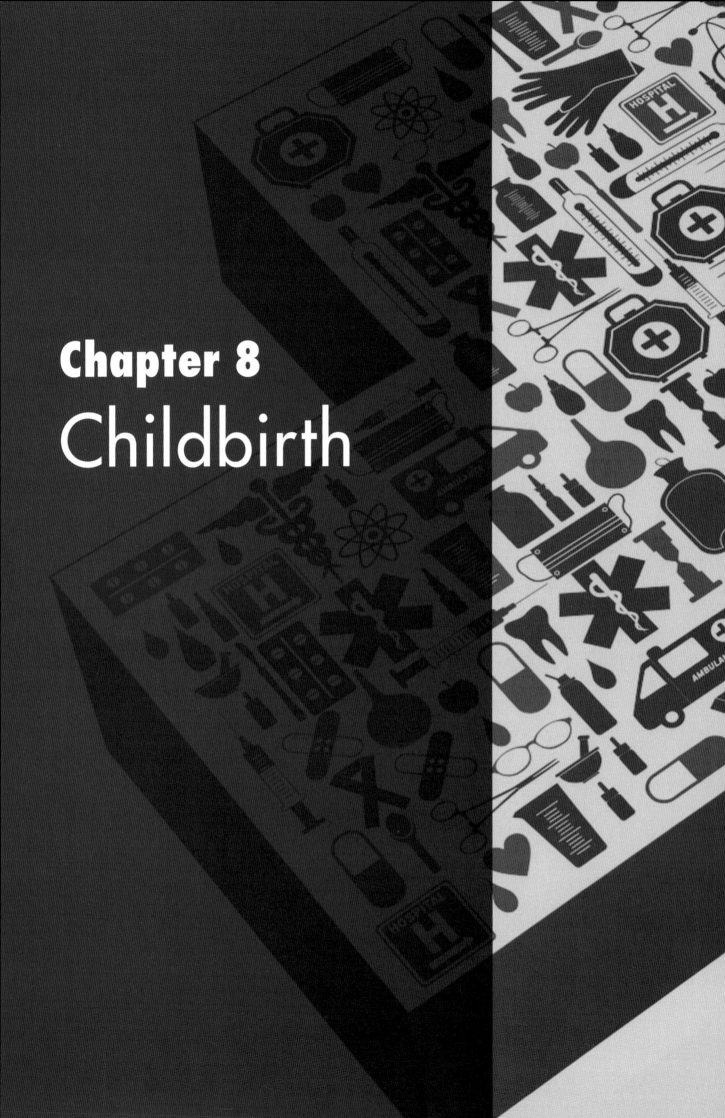

Chapter 8
Childbirth

8.1 | Normal birth

Christine Quinn

Chapter objectives

At the end of this chapter the reader will be able to:

1. Identify the four stages of normal labour and birth
2. Demonstrate how to assist with normal birth
3. Accurately document the event

Resources required for this assessment

- Mannequin capable of simulating vaginal birth
- Hand decontamination agent
- Clinical waste bag
- Ambulance obstetric kit (recommended contents: newborn blanket, newborn cap, maternity pads, gown, cord clamps, sterile scissors, large combine dressings, under-pads (Blueys), large zip lock bags for placenta or premature newborn management, bulb suction device)
- Disposable gloves and eyewear
- Towels and blankets
- Method of documenting results

Skill matrix

This assessment requires:

- Infection control (CS 1.3)
- Communication (CS 1.5)
- Consent (CS 1.6)
- Childbirth skills (Chapter 8, CS 8.2, 8.3, 8.4, 8.5)

This assessment is a component of:

- Childbirth (Chapter 8)

Introduction

In Australia and New Zealand, most women give birth just once or twice in their lives, and a few more often than this. It is an intensely emotional and physically challenging experience etched into a woman's memory and can have long-lasting impacts on relationships with those involved.

A birth requiring paramedic attendance is not part of any woman's birth plan. However, the woman will have considered birth preferences and these should be acknowledged where possible. The arrival of paramedics can occur at any stage of the childbirth process, necessitating consultation with the woman regarding her care and transition to a birthing facility.

This chapter discusses normal birth. Note that the term 'patient' is used in this chapter for consistency. However, normal birth is a natural event and neither mother nor baby are considered 'patients' in the first instance.

Anatomy and physiology

The pregnant uterus grows significantly from 60 g, 5–8 cm long and approximately 10 mL volume to

1.1 kg, 38 cm long and 5 L volume at term. Uterine blood supply increases to 800 mL/minute or around 15% of cardiac output, much of it supplying the placenta (Curtis and Ramsden, 2015). After birth, the uterus contracts and shrinks, and the placenta separates from the endometrium soon afterwards. The rich placental blood supply runs through a uterine muscle mesh. Blood supply to the attached placenta is stopped post birth by uterine contraction. This muscle contraction minimises any bleeding as the placenta detaches and is expelled (Burbank, 2009).

By the seventh week of pregnancy the embryo has become the fetus, enveloped in the amniotic sac and attached by the umbilical cord to the uterine wall. The fundus is the upper pole of the uterus rising from pelvic brim to umbilical level at 20 weeks' gestation to around the xiphoid process at term. The cervix lengthens and thickens during pregnancy, filling with a mucous plug (Curtis and Ramsden, 2015).

Clinical rationale

Patient history

Childbirth is a natural physiological event with numerous potential complications. It can be broken into four stages. Establishing the imminence of birth and identifying urgency includes quickly gathering relevant patient history.

The patient history is impacted by the woman's ability to communicate if she is in active labour. If you are unable to gather a comprehensive history, it is important to ask at least the key questions below. If you are able to take a more comprehensive history, include the remaining questions. Also determine a routine history/examination of health, medications and allergies.

Current pregnancy

The key questions:
- How many weeks pregnant is she?
- Is she expecting a singleton or is this a multiple pregnancy?
- Have her membranes ruptured? What colour was any amniotic fluid?
- Is she having contractions? (Assess frequency and duration)
- Does she have an urge to push?

The comprehensive history questions:
- Has she felt fetal movements? Less than usual or the same as normal?
- What, if any, hospital interventions have been performed?
- Does she anticipate any problems/complications (for baby or mother)?
- Has she had any antenatal care? Is there a physical record of this available?
- Have there been any problems noted?:
  - vaginal bleeding
  - high blood pressure

- pain other than contractions
- trauma
- any other issues.

Previous pregnancies

The key questions:
- Have there been any previous pregnancies? If so, how many?
- Has she had a previous caesarean section or interventions?
- Were there any complications or problems with previous pregnancies?
- What was the length of her previous labours?

Preparation

If birthing at home, select a suitable place that allows comfort and hygiene for the mother. Prepare the equipment required for birthing, newborn and maternal management, including analgesia and resuscitation. If any difficulty is anticipated, call for further paramedic support and consult for advice as soon as practicable, ideally before any emergency unfolds.

Stages of labour

First stage

The first stage of labour is from commencement of contractions to full cervical dilatation (10 cm). The average labour length for a primigravida is 10–12 hours and for a multigravida 6–8 hours.

Labour is often divided into two phases: latent and active. In the latent early phase, contractions are generally shorter in duration, lasting 20–60 seconds. They may be irregular, occurring approximately every 3–5 minutes. The mucous plug or operculum may be released from the cervix, resulting in a 'show'. This presents as vaginal mucoid discharge and is frequently blood-stained.

In the active phase, contractions build in intensity, strength and duration, becoming more painful and lasting longer (30–90 seconds).

Contractions begin in the uterine fundus and are palpated there. With each contraction, the smooth uterine muscles retract, becoming shorter, pulling the lower uterine segment up and resulting in cervical dilatation.

Towards the end of first stage the woman enters transition. Transition is poorly defined and lasts a varying amount of time. This phase is often associated with intensely painful contractions. Women in transition may panic, experience loss of control and feel they cannot continue with the labour.

Spontaneous rupture of the membranes (SROM) can occur at any time before or during labour. It most commonly occurs at commencement of the second stage. Note the time of SROM and the colour of the amniotic fluid, which is normally clear or pink. Brownish/green-stained fluid suggests meconium staining and may indicate fetal distress or a mature gut in a term baby. Heavily blood-stained liquor may indicate antepartum haemorrhage. Offensive-smelling and/or turgid liquor indicates infection. These abnormalities are associated with fetal compromise.

Second stage

The second stage of labour is from full cervical dilatation to newborn birth. Signs of second stage labour can prompt paramedics to remain on scene or stop the ambulance to assist birth if it is imminent. These include:

- shaking
- nausea and/or vomiting
- presence of bowel pressure and uncontrollable urge to push
- fresh, heavily blood-stained 'show'
- a purple or dark-red line seen to rise from the anal margin and extend between the buttocks just below the sacrococcygeal joint (Shepherd et al., 2010)
- contractions that may be slightly less frequent but more expulsive
- bulging and/or pouting of the vagina or anus.

The average length of second stage for a primigravida is 1–2 hours. For a multigravida this stage can be unpredictable, lasting from 1 hour to a few minutes.

The urge to push is initiated when the presenting part of the fetus (or bulging membranes if they have not yet ruptured) reaches the pelvic floor. Under normal circumstances, women should be encouraged to push with this urge.

If second stage is progressing fast and the head is emerging rapidly, it may be appropriate to instruct the woman to breathe instead of pushing as the head is born. Gentle counterpressure can be applied with fingers on the newborn's occiput to control the birth of the head. This may help avoid perineal trauma (Fig. 8.1.1).

After the birth of the head, assess for nuchal cord (see Clinical findings later in this chapter) and observe for restitution. This is when the newborn's head rotates towards the mother's thigh to align with its shoulders in the maternal pelvic anterior-posterior (AP) diameter.

The completion of the birth process is usually passive but may require assistance. Holding the newborn's head carefully (it will be slippery), gently press downwards to birth the anterior shoulder while the mother is pushing (Fig. 8.1.2) and then, if necessary, gently press upwards to birth the posterior shoulder.

Following birth, provide newborn and maternal care as needed, including clamping/cutting the umbilical cord. Delay cord clamping/cutting for at least 60 seconds or until it stops pulsating (McDonald et al., 2014). If postpartum haemorrhage (PPH) occurs, clamp/cut the cord immediately and administer uterotonics (see Chapter 8.2).

With the mother's consent, clamp the cord at approximately 10 cm, 15 cm and 20 cm allowing two clamps on the newborn's side and one on the mother's (Fig. 8.1.3).

The benefits of delayed cord clamping include increased blood volume, red cells and iron in the newborn

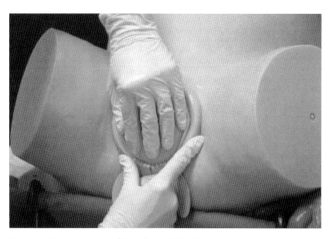

Figure 8.1.1 Controlling head birthing

As the crowning progresses, the vaginal opening becomes circular. This change results in the movement of the wings together. The posterior commissure is effectively locked between the tongue and the wings, and the device prevents the initiation of tearing when the head is maximally crowned. The device should be kept in place by the assistant during delivery of the shoulders. If an episiotomy is required, it can be performed laterally of the device. In the case of an instrumental delivery, the device can be used as described earlier. The assistant then holds the device in place to reduce the risk of tears, while the obstetrician performs the instrumental delivery by steering the head gently through the introitus. The device is preferably kept in place during the delivery of the shoulders.

Source: *Lavesson T., Griph I.D., Skärvad A. et al., 2014, A perineal protection device designed to protect the perineum during labor: a multicenter randomized controlled trial, European Journal of Obstetrics & Gynecology and Reproductive Biology, 181, Figure 2, 10–14.*

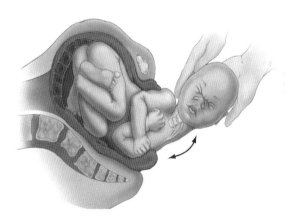

Figure 8.1.2 Birthing the anterior shoulder

The most common mechanism of brachial plexus injury during vertex delivery. Lateral flexion of the neck is applied to free the shoulder from the pubic arch.

Source: *Winn, R.H., 2017, Youmans & Winn neurological surgery, 7th edn (Chapter 228, Figure 228-1), Elsevier.*

(Committee on Obstetric Practice, 2017; Hubbard and Stanford, 2017; McDonald et al., 2014). Once newborn breathing is established, placental circulation is less beneficial (Hooper et al., 2016). If newborn resuscitation is required, this takes priority over delayed cord clamping (ANZCOR, 2017).

The newborn should not require any more care than being placed against the mother's chest for warmth, dried and covered with a blanket. Gently dry the newborn and, if preferred, wrap in a suitable clean sheet or blanket. Assess the newborn's APGAR score (see Table 8.1.1) at 1 and 5 minutes. APGAR assesses heart rate, work of

Table 8.1.1 APGAR score

Sign	0	1	2
Appearance/colour	Pale blue	Body pink, blue extremities	Completely pink
Pulse/heart rate	Absent	<100	>100
Grimace/response to stimulation	No response	Grimace	Vigorous crying
Activity/muscle tone	Flaccid/limp	Some flexion of extremities	Active motion
Respiratory effort	Absent	Slow/irregular	Good crying

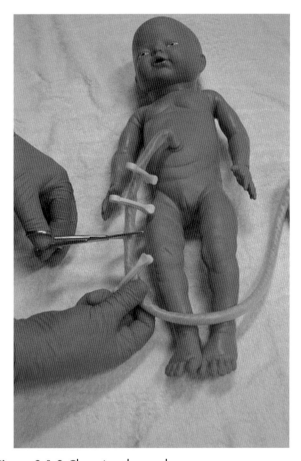

Figure 8.1.3 Clamping the cord

breathing, reflex irritability, muscle tone and colour. A rating of 2, 1 or 0 is given at 1 and 5 minutes. The 1 minute score focuses attention on the infant's condition immediately after delivery and the 5 minute score assesses the effectiveness of resuscitation (Finster and Wood, 2005). Generally, newborns scoring of 8, 9 or 10 are vigorous and usually breathe within seconds of delivery; scores of 5, 6 or 7 are mildly depressed; and scores of 4 or less are blue and limp, with respirations not established at 1 minute.

The acronym APGAR (Appearance, Pulse, Grimace, Activity and Respiration) was created in 1962 to facilitate teaching (Finster and Wood, 2005).

The APGAR score is never used as a guide or prompt for newborn resuscitation. A newborn who at birth is not breathing, has poor tone and a heart rate <100 requires *immediate* stimulation and/or ventilation (see Chapter 8.3).

Third stage

The third stage of labour is from the birth of the newborn to the birth of the placenta and membranes (see Chapter 8.2). The physiological third stage of labour can take from a few minutes to 1 hour.

Fourth stage

The fourth stage of labour extends from the birth of the placenta to the next 1–2 hours where uterine tone is established and post-birth recovery begins. This may include 'crampy' (after birth) pains caused by uterine contractions. Continue vigilance for PPH (see Chapter 8.2), which is indicated by excessive vaginal bleeding, pain, poor uterine fundal tone and haemodynamic instability.

Clinical skill assessment process

The following section outlines the clinical skill assessment tools that should be used to determine a student's ability to demonstrate the procedure of birth.
1. Clinical Skill Work Instruction
2. Formative Clinical Skill Assessment (F-CSAT)
3. Performance Improvement Plan (PIP)
4. Summative Clinical Skill Assessment (S-CSAT)
(5. Direct Observation of Procedural Skills (DOPS) – see Chapter 1.1)

Clinical Skill Work Instruction

Equipment and resources: Mannequin capable of simulating vaginal birth; hand decontamination agent; clinical waste bag; ambulance obstetric kit; disposable gloves and eyewear; towels and blankets; method of documenting results

Associated Clinical Skills: Infection control; Communication; Consent; Childbirth skills

Normal birth		
Activity	**Critical Action**	**Rationale**
Personal protection	Don PPE – eye protection, gown, gloves.	To prevent/minimise infection.
Patient assessment	Obtain obstetric and antenatal history. Identify signs of second stage labour and imminent birth, including blood-stained show, vulva/anal pouting, perineum distension, crowning, defecation. Ask if there is urge to push. Ascertain membrane rupture and liquor colour/consistency.	Assesses complication risks. Identifies imminent birth and descent of presenting part. Clear/pink liquor is normal. Heavily blood-stained or meconium-stained liquor may indicate a compromised newborn requiring resuscitation.
Prepare environment	Prepare environment, including privacy and temperature. Prevent draughts. Maintain hygienic environment.	To help prevent newborn hypothermia or infection.
Prepare equipment	Open maternity kit and lay out near to the mother. Ensure all equipment is present.	In preparation for birth.
Prepare patient	Allow mother to find a comfortable position; adapt to suit her. If birth is imminent during transport, stop vehicle. Positioning mother on all fours or lateral may be appropriate on a narrow stretcher. Clean faecal matter where appropriate.	Position patient allowing perineum vision and access. Prevent newborn faecal contamination. The descending presenting part flattens the rectum against sacral curve, causing possible defecation.
Monitor for imminent birth	If signs of advancing presenting part, monitor perineum. Encourage mother to push with contractions.	Birth may occur rapidly and forcefully, presenting risk of fetal injury from falling.
Deliver baby's head	Encourage mother to breathe rather than push as head is born. Apply gentle counterpressure to head to control delivery speed if required. If membranes have not yet ruptured, they may do so on the birth of the head. This may require membrane removal from the newborn's face after birth. Note time of head birth.	To help prevent explosive birth and reduce perineal damage.
Inspect for cord	With head birthed, check if cord is around the neck. If it is present and loose, slip it over newborn's head. If unable to do so, continue to birth through the cord and then unravel it. If cord is tight, preventing birthing, utilise somersault manoeuvre.	Minimal nuchal cord handling prevents cord vasoconstriction and tearing.

Normal birth continued

Activity	Critical Action	Rationale
Deliver baby's shoulders and body	Observe fetal head restitute and signs of external rotation.	The fetal head turns to one side (restitution). As the shoulders move into the pelvis in the AP diameter the head restitutes to align with the plane of the fetal body.
	If the woman is not actively pushing, wait for next contraction. Apply gentle traction on fetal head with one hand either side, posteriorly away from the symphysis pubis. Apply gentle traction on the fetal head in the opposite, anterior direction.	Posterior pressure births anterior shoulder. Anterior pressure births posterior shoulder.
	Deliver body/limbs anteriorly. Place the newborn on the mother's chest/abdomen (bare skin preferable). Dry and stimulate the newborn with a dry towel or blanket. Note the time.	Direction follows birth canal curve. Skin-to-skin contact is desired to provide newborn warmth and emotional contact. Drying stimulates breathing.
Exclude further unborn	Gently palpate uterine fundus to exclude presence of any other fetus.	Undiagnosed twins are rare but can occur, especially if there has been no antenatal care.
Assess newborn	Assess newborn respiratory effort, tone and heart rate. Measure newborn APGAR at 1 and 5 minutes.	A newborn who is not breathing, has poor tone and a heart rate <100 requires immediate stimulation and/or ventilation (see Chapter 8.3). The APGAR score is conducted at 1 and 5 minutes to assess extra-uterine life transition.
Cut cord	Delay cord clamping/cutting for at least 60 seconds or until pulsing stops. With mother's consent, clamp cord at approximately 10 cm, 15 cm and 20 cm from newborn. Cut between 15 cm and 20 cm (two clamps on newborn side, one on maternal).	Benefits to the newborn of delayed cord clamping include increased blood volume, red blood, stem and immune cells. Newborn cord length provides umbilical vein access if required.
Postpartum care	Change mother's bedding and remove wet/soiled linen/clothing. Make mother comfortable. Observe as indicated by clinical condition. Include fundal tone/height and ongoing blood loss assessment. Transport newborn skin to skin on the mother's chest if possible, provided mother and newborn are stable. Consider third stage labour (see Chapter 8.2). *Note:* Keeping soiled items may assist with blood loss estimation.	Promotes bonding and helps prevent neonatal hypothermia.
Report	Document time of birth, birthing details and newborn observations/APGAR.	Accurate record kept and continuity of patient care.

Formative Clinical Skill Assessment (F-CSAT)

Equipment and resources: Mannequin capable of simulating vaginal birth; hand decontamination agent; clinical waste bag; ambulance obstetric kit; disposable gloves and eyewear; towels and blankets; method of documenting results

Associated Clinical Skills: Infection control; Communication; Consent; Childbirth skills

Staff/Student being assessed: _____

Normal birth

Activity	Critical Action	Participant Performance				
Personal protection	Dons PPE.	0	1	2	3	4
Patient assessment	Obtains obstetric and antenatal history. Identifies signs of second stage labour. Ascertains membrane rupture and liquor colour/consistency.	0	1	2	3	4
Prepares environment	Prepares environment, including for privacy and temperature.	0	1	2	3	4
Prepares equipment	Prepares maternity equipment.	0	1	2	3	4
Prepares patient	Positions mother comfortably, usually semi-recumbent or on all fours.	0	1	2	3	4
Monitors for imminent birth	If there are signs of advancing presenting part, monitors perineum. Encourages mother to push with each contraction.	0	1	2	3	4
Delivers baby's head	Encourages mother to breathe rather than push as the head is born. Controls head birth as required. Documents time.	0	1	2	3	4
	Checks for nuchal cord. Manages as appropriate.	0	1	2	3	4
Delivers baby's shoulders and body	Observes fetal head restitute and signs of external rotation.	0	1	2	3	4
	Waits for next contraction. Applies gentle traction on the fetal head with one hand either side, posteriorly away from the symphysis pubis.	0	1	2	3	4
	Applies gentle traction on the fetal head in the opposite direction.	0	1	2	3	4
	Delivers body and limbs anteriorly and places newborn on mother's chest/abdomen (preferably bare skin). Dries newborn.	0	1	2	3	4
	Documents time of birth.	0	1	2	3	4
Excludes further unborn	Palpates uterine fundus to exclude any other fetus.	0	1	2	3	4
Assesses newborn	Appropriately assesses newborn. Measures APGAR. Documents.	0	1	2	3	4
Cuts cord	Clamps/cuts umbilical cord after 60 seconds or when pulsating stops. Documents time.	0	1	2	3	4
Postpartum care	Provides postpartum care, including maternal comfort, newborn care, ongoing assessment. Considers third stage labour.	0	1	2	3	4
Reports	Documents time of birth, birthing details and newborn observations/APGAR.	0	1	2	3	4

Standard Achieved: (please circle one)

Competent (C)   Not Yet Competent* (NYC)

Staff/Student Name: _____

Assessor (please print name): _____

Signed (Assessor): _____

Date of Assessment: _____

Comments:

*If Not Yet Competent (NYC) a PIP needs to be completed and a repeat of the F-CSAT

Formative Clinical Skill Assessment (F-CSAT) Key

Skill level	Standard of procedure	Quality of performance	Outcome	Level of assistance required
4 Safe for unsupervised practice	Safe Accurate Behaviour is appropriate to context	Confident Accurate Expedient	Achieved intended outcome	No supporting cues* required
3 Requires supervision	Safe Accurate Behaviour is appropriate to context	Confident Accurate Takes longer than required	Achieved intended outcome	Requires occasional supportive cues*
2 Requires assistance	Safe Accurate Behaviour generally appropriate to context	Lacks certainty	Would not have achieved outcome without support	Requires frequent verbal and occasional physical directives in addition to supportive cues*
1 Requires direction	Safe only with guidance Not completely accurate	Unskilled Inefficient	Would not have achieved outcome without support	Requires continuous verbal and frequent physical directive cues*
0 Unsafe	Unsafe Unable to demonstrate behaviour Lack of insight into behaviour appropriate to context	Unskilled	Would not have achieved outcome	Requires continuous verbal and continuous physical directive cues*

*Refers to physical directives or verbal supportive cues

Performance Improvement Plan (PIP)

Please document the agreed education plan and completion timelines for areas assessed as less than 4.

This plan should be presented to assessor prior to commencement of summative assessment.

Where was supervisor support required?	Student summary of deficit. (Why was there a problem?)	Improvement Plan	Completed (Y/N)

Staff/Student Name: _____

Staff/Student Signature: _____

Educator Name: _____

Educator Signature: _____

Summative Clinical Skill Assessment (S-CSAT)

Equipment and resources: Mannequin capable of simulating vaginal birth; hand decontamination agent; clinical waste bag; ambulance obstetric kit; disposable gloves and eyewear; towels and blankets; method of documenting results

Associated Clinical Skills: Infection control; Communication; Consent; Childbirth skills

Staff/Student being assessed: _____

- Completed Formative Clinical Skill Assessment (F-CSAT): **YES   NO**
- Completed Performance Improvement Plan (PIP): **YES   NO   N/A**

Normal birth

Activity	Critical Action	Achieved Without Direction	
Personal protection	Dons PPE.	NO	YES
Patient assessment	Obtains obstetric and antenatal history. Identifies signs of second stage labour. Ascertains membrane rupture and liquor colour/consistency.	NO	YES
Prepares environment	Prepares environment, including for privacy and temperature.	NO	YES
Prepares equipment	Prepares maternity equipment.	NO	YES
Prepares patient	Positions mother comfortably, usually semi-recumbent or on all fours.	NO	YES

Normal birth continued

Activity	Critical Action	Achieved Without Direction	
Monitors for imminent birth	If there are signs of advancing presenting part, monitors perineum. Has mother push with each contraction.	NO	YES
Delivers baby's head	Encourages mother to breathe rather than push as the head is born. Controls head birth as required. Documents time.	NO	YES
	Checks for nuchal cord. Manages as appropriate.	NO	YES
Delivers baby's shoulders and body	Observes fetal head restitute and for signs of external rotation.	NO	YES
	Waits for next contraction. Applies gentle traction on the fetal head with one hand either side, away from the symphysis pubis.	NO	YES
	Delivers body and limbs in an upward direction and places newborn on the mother's chest/abdomen (preferably bare skin). Dries newborn.	NO	YES
	Documents time of birth.	NO	YES
Excludes further unborn	Palpates uterine fundus to exclude any other fetus.	NO	YES
Assesses newborn	Appropriately assesses newborn and measures APGAR. Documents.	NO	YES
Cuts cord	Clamps/cuts umbilical cord after 60 seconds or when it stops pulsating. Documents time.	NO	YES
Postpartum care	Provides postpartum care including maternal comfort, newborn care, ongoing assessment. Considers third stage labour.	NO	YES
Reports	Documents time of birth, birthing details and newborn observations/APGAR.	NO	YES

Standard Achieved: (please circle one)

Competent (C)   Not Yet Competent* (NYC)

Staff/Student Name: _____

Assessor (please print name)**:** _____

Signed (Assessor)**:** _____

Date of Assessment: _____

Comments:

*If Not Yet Competent (NYC) a PIP needs to be completed and a repeat of the F-CSAT

Clinical findings

Nuchal cord

A nuchal cord is where the umbilical cord is wrapped around the fetus's neck. This is common and in most cases the cord loop can be slipped over the head after the birth (Hubbard and Stanford, 2017). It is not routinely problematic (Clapp et al., 2003; Cohain, 2010; Reed et al., 2009) even if the cord is tight (Henry et al., 2013).

A nuchal cord can cause hypoxia by compromising or occluding umbilical blood supply. It can prevent descent and delay birth (Sheiner et al., 2006). Avoid clamping and cutting the cord to relieve nuchal cord before birth of the body but consider doing so if there is no alternative (Hubbard and Stanford, 2017; Mercer et al., 2005; Reed et al., 2009). Cutting severs the blood supply, which can be problematic if there is a delay between the birth of the head and the body.

If the cord is too tight to loop over the head, the somersault manoeuvre may be used to effect birth (David, 2013; Hanson, 2017; Mercer et al., 2005). The somersault manoeuvre is where the fetal head is flexed sideways to the maternal thigh or towards the pubic bone after the birth of the shoulders (Fig. 8.1.4). In effect, the fetal head is kept as close as possible to the mother to avoid further pulling on the cord. This allows the baby to 'somersault' out and the nuchal cord is then removed after birth, restoring the blood supply.

Breech birth

Breech birth is where a body part other than the fetal head is observed first during second stage labour. Breech birth should be managed as described in Chapter 8.4.

Shoulder dystocia

Following the appearance of the head, birthing may not progress. This could represent shoulder dystocia (see Chapter 8.5).

Premature birth

Labour may commence before full term. Premature birth can be problematic and requires management as described in Chapter 8.3.

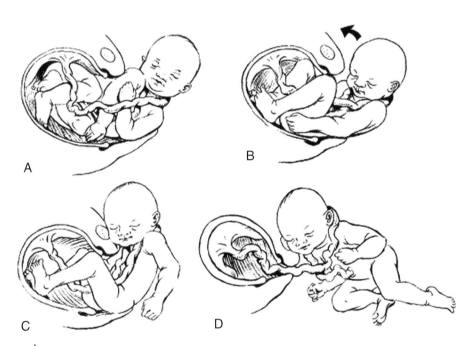

Figure 8.1.4 Somersault manoeuvre

The somersault manoeuvre involves holding the infant's head flexed and guiding it upwards or sideways towards the pubic bone or thigh, so the baby does a 'somersault', ending with the infant's feet towards the mother's knees and the head still at the perineum. (a) Once the nuchal cord is discovered, the anterior and posterior shoulders are slowly delivered under control without manipulating the cord. (b) As the shoulders are delivered, the head is flexed so that the face of the baby is pushed towards the maternal thigh. (c) The baby's head is kept next to the perineum while the body is delivered and 'somersaults' out. (d) The umbilical cord is then unwrapped, and the usual management ensues.

Source: Mercer, J.S., Erickson-Owens, D.A., Graves, G. and Mumford Haley, M., 2007, Evidence-based practices for the fetal to newborn transition, Journal of Midwifery & Women's Health, 52(3), Figure 1, 262–272.

PRACTICE TIP!

Women cannot be 'talked out of' pushing. If a woman is bearing down or saying she needs to push, then prepare for birth. Asking her to breathe through her contractions and ignore the urge to push is pointless, as it is impossible for her to do so. Instead, tell her to do what her body is saying and follow her instincts.

PRACTICE TIP!

Despite childbirth not being considered a medical emergency, unplanned out-of-hospital childbirth can have high-risk complications that develop quickly and without warning. Planning for emergencies as early as practicable is essential, including early expert obstetric consultation as necessary.

PRACTICE TIP!

The newborn can be slippery and easily dropped if the woman is kneeling or standing. Holding a towel beneath the mother or having her lower herself closer to the ground can help. Ensure there is a soft place for the newborn to land in the event of an expulsive birth. If the woman is sitting on the toilet, place a towel across the seat to stop the newborn falling into the bowl. The toilet can be comfortable for some women, as they often feel the need to open their bowels.

PRACTICE TIP!

It is essential to wear appropriate PPE with universal precautions when managing imminent birth, due to the potential for contact with bodily fluids (amniotic fluid, urine, blood and faeces).

PRACTICE TIP!

While paramedics cannot be aware of all religious and cultural beliefs, it is appropriate to acknowledge specific childbirth rituals and support women's preferences.

TEST YOUR KNOWLEDGE QUESTIONS

1. **What are three key questions to ask when taking antenatal history?**
    How many weeks' gestation? Is this a single or multiple pregnancy? Have there been any previous pregnancies?

2. **What marks the change from latent to active first stage labour?**
    Contractions build in intensity and strength, and duration increases to 30–90 seconds.

3. **What is the average duration for second stage labour for a primigravida and a multigravida?**
    Primigravida: 1–2 hours; multigravida: from 1 hour to minutes.

4. **What reasons support the decision to remain on scene for the birth?**
    Signs of second stage labour.

5. **What physical signs help establish that birth is imminent?**
    The presence of bowel pressure and/or urge to push.

6. **How is nuchal cord managed?**
    If the cord is loose, slip it over the baby's head. If it is too tight, use the somersault manoeuvre. Clamp and cut only as a last resort.

7. **What time is allowed for delayed cord clamping?**
    At least 60 seconds or until the cord stops pulsating.

8. **What is the best time to call for support during an obstetric emergency?**
    As soon as practicable once a difficulty is anticipated or identified.

9. **What two maternal observations are particularly important post birth?**
    Fundal tone/height; ongoing vaginal blood loss.

10. **Newborns are often hypothermic when admitted to hospital after unplanned out-of-hospital birth. What should paramedics do to maintain newborn normothermia?**
    Skin-to-skin care on the mother's chest, with the abdomen covered in sheet/blanket within a warm environment.

References

ANZCOR (Australian and New Zealand Committee on Resuscitation), 2017. *Guideline 13.1: Introduction to resuscitation of the newborn infant*. Retrieved from: https://resus.org.au/guidelines

Burbank, F., 2009. Hemodynamic changes in the uterus and its blood vessels in pregnancy. In *Fibroids, menstruation, childbirth, and evolution: the fascinating story of uterine blood vessels*. Tucson: Wheatmark, pp. 177–182.

Clapp, J.F., Stepanchak, W., Hashimoto, K., Ehrenberg, H. and Lopez, B., 2003. The natural history of antenatal nuchal cords. *American Journal of Obstetrics & Gynecology*, 189(2), 488–493.

Cohain, J.S., 2010. Nuchal cords are necklaces, not nooses. *Midwifery Today with International Midwife*, (93), 46–48.

Committee on Obstetric Practice, 2017. Committee Opinion No. 684: Delayed umbilical cord clamping after birth. *Obstetrics and Gynecology*, 129(1), e5.

Curtis, K. and Ramsden, C., 2015. *Emergency and trauma care for nurses and paramedics*. Sydney: Elsevier.

David, J.R., 2013. Management of the nuchal cord at birth. *Journal of Midwifery and Reproductive Health*, 1(1), 4–6.

Finster, M. and Wood, M., 2005. The Apgar score has survived the test of time. *Anesthesiology*, 102(4), 855–857.

Hanson, L., 2017. Low-technology clinical interventions to promote labor progress. In Simson, P., Hanson, L. and Ancheta, R. (eds), *The labor progress handbook: early interventions to prevent and treat dystocia*, 4th edn. New Jersey: Wiley, p. 231.

Henry, E., Andres, R.L. and Christensen, R.D., 2013. Neonatal outcomes following a tight nuchal cord. *Journal of Perinatology*, 33(3), 231.

Hooper, S.B., Binder-Heschl, C., Polglase, G.R., Gill, A.W., Kluckow, M., Wallace, E.M., Blank, D. and te Pas, A.B., 2016. The timing of umbilical cord clamping at birth: physiological considerations. *Maternal Health, Neonatology and Perinatology*, 2(1), 4.

Hubbard, L.J. and Stanford, D.A., 2017. The umbilical cord lifeline. *Journal of Emergency Nursing*, 43(6), 593–595.

McDonald, S.J., Middleton, P., Dowswell, T. and Morris, P.S., 2014. Effect of timing of umbilical cord clamping of term infants on maternal and neonatal outcomes. *Evidence-Based Child Health*, 9(2), 303–397.

Mercer, J.S., Skovgaard, R.L., Peareara-Eaves, J. and Bowman, T.A., 2005. Nuchal cord management and nurse-midwifery practice. *Journal of Midwifery & Women's Health*, 50(5), 373–379.

Reed, R., Barnes, M. and Allan, J., 2009. Nuchal cords: sharing the evidence with parents. *British Journal of Midwifery*, 17(2), 106–109.

Sheiner, E., Abramowicz, J.S., Levy, A., Silberstein, T., Mazor, M. and Hershkovitz, R., 2006. Nuchal cord is not associated with adverse perinatal outcome. *Archives of Gynecology and Obstetrics*, 274(2), 81–83.

Shepherd, A., Cheyne, H., Kennedy, S., McIntosh, C., Styles, M. and Niven, C., 2010. The purple line as a measure of labour progress: a longitudinal study. *BMC Pregnancy and Childbirth*, 10(1), 54.

Bibliography

Coad, J. and Dunstall, M., 2011. *Anatomy and physiology for midwives*. London: Elsevier Churchill Livingston.

Pairman, S., Tracy, S.K., Thorogood, C. and Pincombe, J., 2010. *Midwifery: preparation for practice*. Sydney: Elsevier.

Managing third stage labour

Christine Quinn

Chapter objectives

At the end of this chapter the reader will be able to:

1. Describe the signs of placental separation
2. Manage third stage labour delivery with active or physiological methods
3. Describe emergency measures for managing postpartum haemorrhage (PPH)

Resources required for this assessment

- Mannequin capable of simulating vaginal birth
- Hand decontamination agent
- Ambulance obstetric kit
- Disposable gloves and eyewear
- Towels and blankets
- Clinical waste bag
- Method of documenting results

Skill matrix

This assessment requires:
- Infection control (CS 1.3)
- Communication (CS 1.5)
- Consent (CS 1.6)
- Childbirth skills (Chapter 8, CS 8.1, 8.3, 8.4)

This assessment is a component of:
- Childbirth (Chapter 8)

Introduction

The third stage of labour is from newborn birth to expulsion of the placenta and membranes (Begley et al., 2015). In third stage there are two patients, mother and newborn, both of whom are in vulnerable physiological states. Most women who are birthing naturally deliver the placenta and membranes physiologically. There is no rushed cord clamping, allowing the placenta and membranes to be birthed by maternal effort.

Physiological third stage is a holistic approach where postpartum haemorrhage is minimised by promoting skin-to-skin contact, breastfeeding and an upright position for placental delivery (Saxton et al., 2014).

This chapter discusses methods of normal third stage delivery and the emergency management of postpartum haemorrhage (PPH).

Note that the term 'patient' is used in this chapter for consistency. Normal birth is a natural event and neither mother nor baby are considered 'patients' in the first instance.

Anatomy and physiology

During labour, uterine muscles shorten with each contraction. As the newborn progresses down the birth canal in the second stage of labour, the size of the uterus, including its interior surface area, reduces. The placenta is unable to reduce its surface area. After fetal expulsion, placental separation occurs, leaving a raw placental bed on the uterine wall that is up to the size of a dinner plate. Uterine muscle fibres are arranged in an interlacing fashion around the arterioles that supply the placenta, and constrict around these vessels to control bleeding. These fibres are known as 'living ligatures' (Fig. 8.2.1).

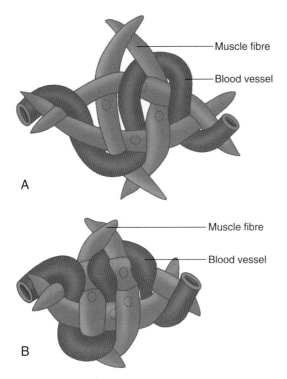

- Muscle fibre
- Blood vessel

A

- Muscle fibre
- Blood vessel

B

Figure 8.2.1 Living ligatures
How the blood vessels run between the interlacing muscle fibres of the uterus. (a) Muscle fibres relaxed and blood vessels not compressed. (b) Muscle fibres contracted, blood vessels compressed and bleeding arrested.
Source: Johnson, G. and Macdonald, S., 2017, Mayes' midwifery, 15th edn (Chapter 39, Figure 39.4), Elsevier.

Physiological third stage can take up to 60 minutes. If uterotonics are available, active third stage management can be undertaken, shortening the third stage to 30 minutes or less and minimising the risk of maternal haemorrhage (Fathima and Rao, 2017).

As the placenta separates, a retroplacental clot often forms. Signs of placental separation include:
- vaginal bleeding (a 30–60 mL gush of fresh blood)
- cord lengthening as the placenta descends through the birth canal
- an urge to push
- bulging at or appearance of the placenta at the vaginal introitus.

The third stage of labour may be accompanied by 'crampy' pelvic pains.

On palpation, the uterine fundus should feel firm and contracted (like a hard ball) at about the level of the umbilicus. This indicates placenta separation from the uterine wall. Massaging the fundus prior to placental separation is inappropriate, as it can cause postpartum haemorrhage.

Clinical rationale

The management of physiological (expectant) third stage delivery is passive and relies on support measures only. Minimal intervention is usually required, apart from waiting for the signs of placental separation before encouraging maternal pushing for delivery.

Management of modified active third stage labour involves a three-part strategy to reduce bleeding. It includes administration of uterotonics, delayed cord clamping (see Chapter 8.1) where appropriate and delivery of the placenta/membranes with controlled cord traction (CCT) *after* signs of placental separation. Uterotonics can be administered just after cord cutting (Begley et al., 2015). Pushing the fundus upwards with one hand while applying CCT with the other involves risks but unclear benefits and is **best omitted if unskilled** (Gülmezoglu et al., 2012). Placing a hand just above the symphysis pubis to stabilise the uterus and apply counterpressure while applying CCT is recommended (Lalonde et al., 2006). Active management is frequently not an option for paramedics.

Placental delivery

Before the placenta and membranes are delivered, mother and newborn are separated by clamping and cutting the umbilical cord, which is delayed for >60 seconds or until the cord stops pulsating (McDonald et al., 2014) (see Chapter 8.1). If PPH occurs, clamp and cut the cord immediately and administer uterotonics.

Skin-to-skin contact and initiating breastfeeding increases the natural release of oxytocin, helping placental separation by promoting contraction of the uterus. The mother frequently feels pelvic pain, pressure or an urge to push when the placenta reaches the pelvic floor. Encourage her to push as she desires. The placenta often emerges unaided, but if there is a delay in expulsion when the placenta is more than half delivered, use both hands to support it and complete the delivery.

If the woman is not bleeding and there are no signs of third stage labour, transport her with the placenta in situ.

Postpartum haemorrhage

Understanding normal blood loss during birth and third stage labour is key to early identification of abnormal bleeding and PPH. Normal blood loss is <500 mL (WHO, 2012). Bleeding can be occult and occur in an empty or near empty uterine cavity. This is best detected by palpating the abdomen to determine increasing uterine fundal height and diminishing uterine tone. Pregnant and postnatal women compensate for large blood loss as they have increased blood volume during pregnancy and labour. Most will not show signs of circulatory compromise until about 1000 mL of blood loss.

Blood loss is easily concealed under the mother's buttocks. Check thoroughly when observing for vaginal loss.

There are four causes of PPH, often referred to as the '4 Ts':
1. *Tone* – poor uterine tone following birth, where the living ligatures are not compressing placental site arterioles
2. *Tissue* – all or part of the placenta and membranes in the uterine cavity are preventing the uterus contracting properly; the living ligatures are not compressing placental site arterioles

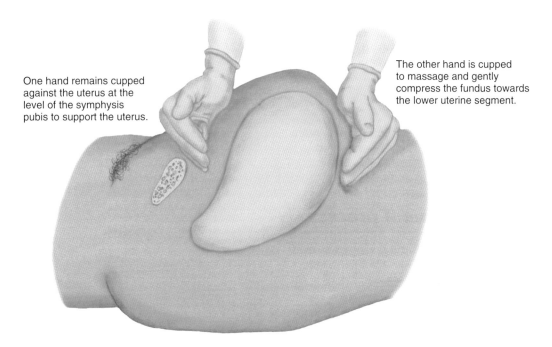

One hand remains cupped against the uterus at the level of the symphysis pubis to support the uterus.

The other hand is cupped to massage and gently compress the fundus towards the lower uterine segment.

Figure 8.2.2 Fundal massage
Source: Weiler Ashwill, J., Smith Murray, S., Slone McKinney, E., Nelson, K.A. and Rowen James, S., 2013, Maternal-child nursing, 4th edn (Chapter 28, Figure 28-2), Elsevier.

3. *Trauma* – lacerations of the birth canal or perineum
4. *Thrombin* – consumption of clotting factors, usually secondary to haemorrhage.

Why is this important? Because you need to manage the cause to stop the bleeding.

Most PPHs are caused by lack of uterine tone. Management depends on whether the placenta is in or out.

If the placenta is in but signs of separation are evident, massage the uterus to expel clots, blood or tissue that may collect and prevent it from contracting. Seek urgent advice. Uterotonics are typically used, particularly intramuscular syntocinon. (Note that ergometrine and syntometrine should not be used in this case as these cause tonic uterine contractions and may delay expulsion of the placenta.) Large-gauge intravenous access and resuscitation are likely to be necessary.

If the placenta is out, massage the uterus (Fig. 8.2.2) (Hofmeyr et al., 2013). If you have access to uterotonics, administer these intramuscularly to aid uterine contraction.

Massaging the uterus stimulates and maintains contraction (Saccone et al., 2017). Place one hand at the base of the uterus just above the pubic symphysis to prevent prolapse. The upper hand at the top of the uterus, just below the umbilicus, rotates until the fundus becomes firm.

Always assess the perineum and lower genital tract for evidence of bleeding from birth trauma. Apply pressure if there is any sign of external bleeding. PPH may have more than one cause.

In extreme circumstances where haemorrhage is torrential due to uterine atony, external aortic compression or bimanual compression may be required.

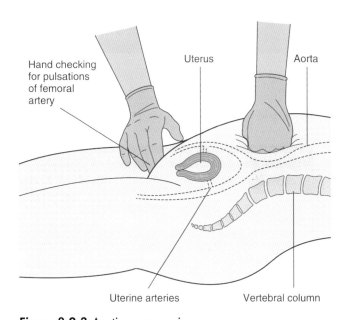

Hand checking for pulsations of femoral artery

Uterus

Aorta

Uterine arteries

Vertebral column

Figure 8.2.3 Aortic compression

External aortic compression

This is a painful procedure achieved by applying downward pressure with a closed fist above and slightly to the left of the umbilicus while feeling for the femoral pulse with the other hand (Fig. 8.2.3). If pressure is adequate, no femoral pulse should be palpable. If bleeding does not stop, proceed to bimanual compression.

Bimanual compression

Another painful procedure, bimanual compression, is achieved by inserting the whole fist into the vagina and pressing up against the posterior uterus wall while the other hand presses externally against the uterus (Fig. 8.2.4). This position must be maintained until the patient reaches hospital and the paramedic is instructed to release it.

Risk factors

There are many risk factors for PPH, including:
- rapid birth
- grand multiparity (four or more previous births), often resulting in rapid birth
- multiple pregnancy
- obesity.

Clinical skill assessment process

The following section outlines the clinical skill assessment tools that should be used to determine a student's ability to demonstrate the safety and management of third stage labour.
1. Clinical Skill Work Instruction
2. Formative Clinical Skill Assessment (F-CSAT)
3. Performance Improvement Plan (PIP)
4. Summative Clinical Skill Assessment (S-CSAT)
(5. Direct Observation of Procedural Skills (DOPS) – see Chapter 1.1)

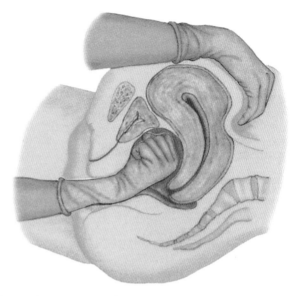

Figure 8.2.4 Bimanual compression
One hand is inserted in the vagina, and the other compresses the uterus through the abdominal wall.
Source: Murray, S., McKinney, E., Shaw Holub, K. and Jones, R., 2019, Foundations of maternal-newborn and women's health nursing, 7th edn (Chapter 18, Figure 18.3), Elsevier.

Clinical Skill Work Instruction

Equipment and resources: Mannequin capable of simulating vaginal birth; hand decontamination agent; ambulance obstetric kit; disposable gloves and eyewear; towels and blankets; clinical waste bag; method of documenting results

Associated Clinical Skills: Infection control; Communication; Consent; Childbirth skills

Managing third stage labour

Activity	Critical Action	Rationale
Personal protection	Don PPE – eye protection, gown, gloves.	To prevent/minimise infection.
Prepare environment	Prepare environment, including for privacy and temperature.	For comfort and dignity and to protect the newborn.
PPH monitoring	Monitor patient throughout for vaginal blood loss/PPH.	Can be life threatening and occur any time.
	If PPH is detected, assess for cause and manage accordingly. Manage uterine atony using uterine massage, uterotonics where available and direct pressure methods, including to perineal bleeding.	Prompt response to PPH can be lifesaving.
Initial management	Assist mother into comfortable position, usually semi-recumbent (modified active) or upright (physiological).	For maternal comfort.
	Delay cord clamping unless there is abnormal bleeding/PPH.	Delayed clamping offers benefit to the newborn.
	Determine active or physiological management.	Depends on skill set of paramedic and options available.
	Gently palpate uterus to exclude any other fetus.	Must be excluded before uterotonic administration.

Managing third stage labour continued

Activity	Critical Action	Rationale
For (expectant) physiological third stage	Encourage newborn breastfeeding and skin-to-skin contact.	Aids placental detachment and descent.
	Encourage mother to push when she feels the urge.	To expel placenta.
	Allow placenta to emerge unaided with maternal effort if appropriate.	Allows complete detachment.
For modified active third stage management	Administer uterotonic in accordance with recommended practice after cord clamping and maternal consent.	To initiate active third stage management.
	After signs of separation are observed, apply controlled cord traction to deliver placenta.	To determine placental separation.
	Cease controlled cord traction if resistance is met and await further descent. Encourage maternal effort if there is an urge to push.	To avoid uterine inversion if placenta is not ready.
Placenta and membrane delivery	If there is delay in complete expulsion, gently grasp placenta in both hands and ease out. Ease trailing membranes out if resistance met. Note expulsion time.	Gentle handling of placenta and membranes helps ensure they are delivered completely, reducing PPH and neurogenic shock risk.
Placenta storage	Place placenta and membranes in a plastic bag/container and transport with mother and newborn.	Allows inspection of placenta and membranes.
Report	Document/hand over placenta, delivery time, estimated blood loss.	Accurate record kept and continuity of patient care.

Formative Clinical Skill Assessment (F-CSAT)

Equipment and resources: Mannequin capable of simulating vaginal birth; hand decontamination agent; ambulance obstetric kit; disposable gloves and eyewear; towels and blankets; clinical waste bag; method of documenting results

Associated Clinical Skills: Infection control; Communication; Consent; Childbirth skills

Staff/Student being assessed: _____

Managing third stage labour

Activity	Critical Action	Participant Performance				
Personal protection	Dons PPE.	0	1	2	3	4
Prepares environment	Prepares environment, including for privacy and temperature.	0	1	2	3	4
PPH monitoring	Monitors for PPH throughout.	0	1	2	3	4
	Manages PPH if detected, according to cause. Manages atony if present, using uterine massage, uterotonics and direct pressure methods.	0	1	2	3	4
Initial management	Assists mother into a comfortable position.	0	1	2	3	4
	Provides delayed cord clamping unless PPH is present.	0	1	2	3	4
	Chooses active or physiological management.	0	1	2	3	4
	Excludes any other fetus present.	0	1	2	3	4

Managing third stage labour continued

Activity	Critical Action	Participant Performance				
For physiological third stage	Encourages newborn breastfeeding and skin-to-skin contact.	0	1	2	3	4
	Has mother push when she feels the urge to do so.	0	1	2	3	4
	Allows placenta and membranes to deliver unaided.	0	1	2	3	4
For modified active management	Gains maternal consent. Administers uterotonic after cord clamping if available.	0	1	2	3	4
	Applies controlled cord traction following signs of separation.	0	1	2	3	4
	Ceases if resistance is met. Awaits further descent. Has mother push if she feels the urge.	0	1	2	3	4
Placenta and membrane delivery	If expulsion is delayed, grasps placenta with both hands and gently eases it out, including trailing membranes. Notes time.	0	1	2	3	4
Placenta storage	Places placenta and membranes in plastic bag/container for transport.	0	1	2	3	4
Reports	Documents/hands over placenta, delivery time, estimated blood loss.	0	1	2	3	4

Standard Achieved: (please circle one)

Competent (C)   Not Yet Competent* (NYC)

Staff/Student Name: _____

Assessor (please print name): _____

Signed (Assessor): _____

Date of Assessment: _____

Comments:

*If Not Yet Competent (NYC) a PIP needs to be completed and a repeat of the F-CSAT

Formative Clinical Skill Assessment (F-CSAT) Key

Skill level	Standard of procedure	Quality of performance	Outcome	Level of assistance required
4 Safe for unsupervised practice	Safe Accurate Behaviour is appropriate to context	Confident Accurate Expedient	Achieved intended outcome	No supporting cues* required
3 Requires supervision	Safe Accurate Behaviour is appropriate to context	Confident Accurate Takes longer than required	Achieved intended outcome	Requires occasional supportive cues*

Skill level	Standard of procedure	Quality of performance	Outcome	Level of assistance required
2 Requires assistance	Safe Accurate Behaviour generally appropriate to context	Lacks certainty	Would not have achieved outcome without support	Requires frequent verbal and occasional physical directives in addition to supportive cues*
1 Requires direction	Safe only with guidance Not completely accurate	Unskilled Inefficient	Would not have achieved outcome without support	Requires continuous verbal and frequent physical directive cues*
0 Unsafe	Unsafe Unable to demonstrate behaviour Lack of insight into behaviour appropriate to context	Unskilled	Would not have achieved outcome	Requires continuous verbal and continuous physical directive cues*

*Refers to physical directives or verbal supportive cues

Performance Improvement Plan (PIP)

Please document the agreed education plan and completion timelines for areas assessed as less than 4.

This plan should be presented to assessor prior to commencement of summative assessment.

Where was supervisor support required?	Student summary of deficit. (Why was there a problem?)	Improvement Plan	Completed (Y/N)

Staff/Student Name: _____

Staff/Student Signature: _____

Educator Name: _____

Educator Signature: _____

Summative Clinical Skill Assessment (S-CSAT)

Equipment and resources: Mannequin capable of simulating vaginal birth; hand decontamination agent; ambulance obstetric kit; disposable gloves and eyewear; towels and blankets; clinical waste bag; method of documenting results

Associated Clinical Skills: Infection control; Communication; Consent; Childbirth skills

Staff/Student being assessed: _____

- Completed Formative Clinical Skill Assessment (F-CSAT):   **YES**   **NO**

- Completed Performance Improvement Plan (PIP):   **YES**   **NO**   **N/A**

Managing third stage labour

Activity	Critical Action	Achieved Without Direction	
Personal protection	Dons PPE as appropriate.	NO	YES
Prepares environment	Prepares environment, including for privacy and temperature.	NO	YES
PPH monitoring	Monitors for PPH throughout.	NO	YES
	Manages PPH if detected, according to cause. Manages atony if present using uterine massage, uterotonics and direct pressure methods.	NO	YES
Initial management	Assists mother into a comfortable position.	NO	YES
	Provides delayed cord clamping unless PPH is present.	NO	YES
	Chooses active or physiological management.	NO	YES
	Excludes any other fetus present.	NO	
For physiological third stage	Encourages newborn breastfeeding and skin-to-skin contact.	NO	YES
	Has mother push when she feels the urge to do so.	NO	YES
	Allows placenta and membranes to deliver unaided.	NO	YES
For modified active management	Gains maternal consent. Administers uterotonic after cord clamping if available.	NO	YES
	Applies controlled cord traction following separation signs.	NO	YES
	Ceases if resistance met. Awaits further descent. Has mother push if she feels the urge.	NO	YES
Placenta and membrane delivery	If expulsion is delayed, grasps placenta with both hands and gently eases it out, including trailing membranes. Notes time.	NO	YES
Placenta storage	Places placenta and membranes in plastic bag/container for transport.	NO	YES
Reports	Documents/hands over placenta, delivery time, estimated blood loss.	NO	YES

Standard Achieved: (please circle one)

Competent (C)   Not Yet Competent* (NYC)

Staff/Student Name: _____

Assessor (please print name): _____

Signed (Assessor): _____

Date of Assessment: _____

Comments:

*If Not Yet Competent (NYC) a PIP needs to be completed and a repeat of the F-CSAT

Clinical findings

Bladder

Uterine blood flow can be up to 500 mL/minute. An uncontracted uterus could bleed up to 2500 mL in 5 minutes. A full bladder can displace the uterus, preventing effective contraction. Allow the mother to (safely) void her bladder if needed, even with the placenta in.

Membranes

Membranes trail the placenta as it is delivered; resistance may be encountered with their delivery. Do not exert undue pressure to remove them; gently ease them out so they remain intact. Membrane fragments remaining in the uterine cavity or cervical canal can interfere with uterine contraction or cause neurogenic (cervical) shock. The delivered placenta and membranes should be transported to the hospital in a plastic bag or container with the mother and newborn, for inspection.

PRACTICE TIP!

Practise estimating blood loss. Measure coloured or stained water (e.g. coffee) and note how much is used when soaking different items – pads, towels, undersheets – inside a toilet bowl.

PRACTICE TIP!

Third stage labour now has two patients, each of whom require care, shared between paramedics or further support as needed. The most likely maternal problem is PPH while the most likely newborn problem is hypothermia, although more extensive resuscitation may be required. Continually reassess each patient and manage any problems accordingly.

PRACTICE TIP!

If the mother is showing no signs of imminent placenta delivery and there is no evidence of abnormal bleeding, leave well alone and transport the mother with placenta in situ.

PRACTICE TIP!

Enjoy the moment. Births can be one of the happiest events you will attend in your career and they are not commonly encountered in the prehospital setting. You are privileged to be involved in such a special 'rite of passage' with this family. Consider how important this is to everyone present. Congratulate yourself.

TEST YOUR KNOWLEDGE QUESTIONS

1. **Define the third stage of labour.**
    From birth of the baby to expulsion of the placenta and membranes.

2. **Describe the management of modified active and physiological third stage labour.**
    Modified active: uterotonic administration, delayed cord clamping and placenta/membrane delivery with controlled cord traction after signs of placental separation. Physiological: passive, reliant on support measures only waiting for placental separation signs before maternal pushing.

3. **What are the common signs of placental separation?**
    Gush of fresh blood; umbilical cord lengthening.

4. **How do breastfeeding and skin-to-skin contact promote placental separation?**
    They increase the release of natural oxytocin, helping placental separation by promoting uterine contraction.

5. **Why is it important that the placenta and membranes are delivered complete?**
    Membrane fragments remaining in the uterine cavity or cervical canal can interfere with uterine contraction.

6. **When is it safe to transport the mother with the placenta in situ?**
    If the woman is not bleeding and there are no signs of third stage.

7. **How do we define PPH?**
    >500 mL blood loss post birth.

8. **What are the four causes of PPH?**
    Tone; tissue; trauma; thrombin.

9. **List four common PPH risk factors.**
    Rapid birth; grand multiparity (four or more previous births), often resulting in rapid birth; multiple pregnancy; obesity.

10. **How much blood loss can occur from an uncontracted uterus?**
    Up to 2500 mL in 5 minutes.

References

Begley, C.M., Gyte, G.M., Devane, D., McGuire, W. and Weeks, A., 2015. *Active versus expectant management for women in the third stage of labour*. Online: The Cochrane Library.

Gülmezoglu, A.M., Lumbiganon, P., Landoulsi, S., Widmer, M., Abdel-Aleem, H., Festin, M., Carroli, G., Qureshi, Z., Souza, J.P., Bergel, E. and Piaggio, G., 2012. Active management of the third stage of labour with and without controlled cord traction: a randomised, controlled, non-inferiority trial. *Lancet*, 379(9827), 1721–1727.

Hofmeyr, G.J., Abdel-Aleem, H. and Abdel-Aleem, M.A., 2013. *Uterine massage for preventing postpartum haemorrhage*. Online: The Cochrane Library.

Fathima, N. and Rao, M.R., 2017. An evaluation of the practice of active management of third stage of labour in a teaching hospital. *International Journal of Reproduction, Contraception, Obstetrics and Gynecology*, 5(6), 1705–1708.

Lalonde, A., Daviss, B.A., Acosta, A. and Herschderfer, K., 2006. Postpartum hemorrhage today: ICM/FIGO initiative 2004–2006. *International Journal of Gynecology & Obstetrics*, 94(3), 243–253.

McDonald, S.J., Middleton, P., Dowswell, T. and Morris, P.S., 2014. Effect of timing of umbilical cord clamping of term infants on maternal and neonatal outcomes. *Evidence-Based Child Health*, 9(2), 303–397.

Saccone, G., Caissutti, C., Ciardulli, A., Abdel-Aleem, H., Hofmeyr, G.J. and Berghella, V., 2017. Uterine massage as part of active management of the third stage of labour for preventing postpartum haemorrhage during vaginal delivery: a systematic review and meta-analysis of randomised trials. *BJOG: An International Journal of Obstetrics & Gynaecology*, 125, 778–781.

Saxton, A., Fahy, K. and Hastie, C., 2014. Effects of skin-to-skin contact and breastfeeding at birth on the incidence of PPH: a physiologically based theory. *Women and Birth*, 27(4), 250–253.

WHO (World Health Organization), 2012. *Recommendations for the prevention and treatment of postpartum haemorrhage*. Retrieved from: http://apps.who.int/iris/bitstream/10665/75411/1/9789241548502_eng.pdf

Bibliography

Queensland Ambulance Service, 2019. *Clinical Practice Procedures: Obstetrics/External aortic compression and bimanual compression*. Retrieved from: https://www.ambulance.qld.gov.au/docs/clinical/cpp/CPP_External%20aortic%20and%20bimanual%20compression.pdf

Queensland Ambulance Service, 2020. *Clinical Practice Guidelines: Obstetrics/Physiological cephalic birth*. Retrieved from: https://ambulance.qld.gov.au/docs/clinical/cpp/CPP_Physiological%20cephalic%20birth.pdf

McLelland, G., 2014. Imminent birth. In Johnson, M., Boyd, L., Grantham, H. and Eastwood, K. (eds), *Paramedic principles and practice ANZ: a clinical reasoning approach*. Sydney: Elsevier, pp. 917–948.

Winter, C., Crofts, J., Draycott, T. and Muchatuta, N. (eds), 2017. *PROMPT course manual*. Cambridge: Cambridge University Press.

8.3 | Premature birth

Christine Quinn

Chapter objectives

At the end of this chapter the reader will be able to:

1. Recognise and respond to complications presented by premature birth
2. Identify and anticipate the special needs of premature newborns
3. Manage immediate post-birth care of the premature newborn

Resources required for this assessment

- Mannequin capable of simulating vaginal birth
- Newborn mannequin
- Ambulance obstetric kit
- Bag/mask/valve resuscitator
- Newborn suction
- Food-grade polyethylene bag
- Baby cap
- Newborn blanket
- Hand decontamination agent
- Disposable gloves, protective eyewear
- Ambulance obstetric kit
- Clinical waste bag
- Method of documenting results

Skill matrix

This assessment requires:

- Infection control (CS 1.3)
- Communication (CS 1.5)
- Consent (CS 1.6)
- Intermittent positive pressure ventilation (CS 3.11)
- Chest compressions (CS 6.1)
- Childbirth skills (Chapter 8, CS 8.1, 8.2, 8.4)

This assessment is a component of:

- Childbirth (Chapter 8)

Introduction

Premature birth is defined as birth occurring before 37 weeks' gestation.

The newborn support required is generally related to the degree of prematurity. The incidence of breech presentation (see Chapter 8.4) is higher (up to 20% at 28 weeks) in premature births, and multiple pregnancy is also often associated with premature birth. This chapter discusses premature delivery, the physiological differences between the premature and the full term newborn and appropriate paramedic management.

Anatomy and physiology

All premature newborns have an immature physiology proportionate to their gestation. The main immediate concerns are providing respiratory support as required and preventing heat loss. Unlike term newborns, premature newborns are less able to maintain body temperature using gluconeogenesis. In this process, glucose stores are mobilised to provide energy for heat production, increasing metabolic rate and therefore oxygen consumption. In the newborn, this can result in hypoglycaemia and further complicate respiratory function through increased oxygen demand. Preventing heat loss is vital to prevent this sequelae of events.

Premature babies are more vulnerable to heat loss as they have:

- less brown fat from which to draw glucose energy
- reduced white fat to insulate the body from heat loss
- a larger surface area relative to their size
- a variable ability to adopt a position of flexion in order to effectively reduce surface area.

The optimal body temperature in a newborn is 36.5 °C to 37.4 °C (Castrodale and Rinehart, 2014).

Lung development and respiratory function are related to gestational age at birth with most development in the third trimester (Islam et al., 2015). The key factor is surfactant. Premature newborns have less surfactant than those born at term. Surfactant is first produced by the fetus between 24 and 28 weeks' gestation and is primarily composed of lipids. It reduces fluid surface tension and prevents the alveoli from collapsing after each inflation (Veldhuizen and Haagsman, 2000). The fetus produces enough surfactant to adequately support independent respiratory function at about 35 weeks. Without sufficient surfactant, the newborn's airways collapse after each breath, requiring higher inflation pressures to reopen them. This represents enormous effort for the very preterm newborn, who will tire quickly and become hypoxic.

Newborn transition from placental-dependent to air breathing requires alveolar ventilation to reduce pulmonary vascular resistance, increase pulmonary circulation and force essential post-birth cardiovascular changes.

Clinical rationale

Delivery of the premature newborn is essentially the same as for the baby born at term. The birthing process may be more rapid as the fetus is smaller. Complications of preterm delivery largely revolve around the newborn. The shorter the gestation, the smaller the fetus and the increased likelihood of breech or cord presentation. A maternal age of <20 or >40 years and multiple pregnancy are all associated with increased prematurity rates (Oliveira et al., 2016).

The first key step is to identify imminent premature delivery. Where delivery is not thought imminent, alternative interventions, such as tocolytics and neuroprotective medication, may be possible. Delaying delivery creates a time opportunity, even if only small, that permits the administration of medication to promote and support fetus development and transfer of the mother to a higher level birthing facility.

As prematurity problems are inversely proportional to gestational age at birth, newborn management must be related to gestation. Premature newborns are divided into two categories for immediate management:

1. Those born at 28 weeks' gestation or less
2. Those born greater than 28 weeks' gestation.

Preventing heat loss

Babies born at 28 weeks' gestation onwards
Drying the late preterm newborn minimises heat loss from evaporation. Placing the newborn on the mother's bare skin and covering them together is the best way to maintain warmth, provided the newborn's condition permits this (Nimbalkar et al., 2014; Vilinsky and Sheridan, 2014; Wyckoff et al., 2015). This also depends on the mother's condition post birth and on her wishes.

Alternatively, drying and wrapping the newborn, ensuring the head (not face) is covered with a cap or bedclothing to prevent heat loss, may be more appropriate. The relatively large head size accounts for proportionately greater heat loss and should not be ignored. Remember that this newborn must be closely observed, which may be difficult when the baby is well wrapped.

Babies born at less than 28 weeks' gestation
Newborns of less than 28 weeks' gestation should not be dried at birth. Careful handling is required as they are at greater risk of damage to the skin and internal organs (ANZCOR, 2016b). The newborn should immediately be placed wet into a food-grade polyethylene bag of an appropriate size. This creates a warm, humid environment, permitting heat entry while minimising evaporative heat loss (Castrodale and Rinehart, 2014; Oatley et al., 2016; Pinheiro et al., 2014; Wyckoff, 2014). To achieve this, a hole is made in the bottom of the bag to allow placement over the newborn's head, with the opening at the foot end. This bag remains in place for transfer. The newborn's head should be covered with an appropriately sized cap (Fig. 8.3.1). If a polyethylene bag is unavailable, a soft plastic sheet or cling wrap may be used.

Respiratory support
Most very preterm babies require respiratory support immediately after birth (ANZCOR, 2016b). At birth, assess for vigorous breathing or crying. If these are present and the newborn has good muscle tone and a heart rate of >100 per minute, only basic care is required. If breathing is inadequate or absent, basic stimulation can precipitate breathing where body tone and heart rate are present. If there is no response, body tone is poor and the heart rate is <60 per minute, positive pressure ventilation in air is required (Wyllie et al., 2015). If the heart rate remains ≤60 after 30 seconds of adequate ventilation, then commence chest compressions using a 3 : 1 ratio (see Chapter 6.1). If chest compressions are required, ventilation should then take place in 100% oxygen.

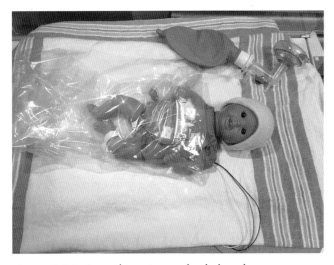

Figure 8.3.1 A newborn in a polyethylene bag

Source: *Gupta, A.G. and Adler, M.D., 2016, Management of an unexpected delivery in the Emergency Department, Clinical Pediatric Emergency Medicine, 17(2), 89–98.*

The technique for providing bag/mask ventilation is the same for preterm babies as for term babies, taking care not to over-inflate the lungs (see Chapter 3.11).

The preterm inflatable bag has a 240 mL reservoir. Each inflation should be 4–6 mL/kg of air. The extent of chest wall rise and fall and a heart rate rising to >100 guide ventilation. Premature newborns are at increased risk of barotrauma from bag/mask ventilation (Ganga-Zandzouet al., 1996).

Use of an appropriately sized ventilation mask is essential. The mask should cover the nose and mouth but not the eyes, nor should it overlap the chin. Small masks of 35 mm are suitable for premature babies of less than 29 weeks' gestation (O'Shea et al., 2015).

Clinical skill assessment process

The following section outlines the clinical skill assessment tools that should be used to determine a student's ability to demonstrate the safe management of premature birth.
1. Clinical Skill Work Instruction
2. Formative Clinical Skill Assessment (F-CSAT)
3. Performance Improvement Plan (PIP)
4. Summative Clinical Skill Assessment (S-CSAT)
(5. Direct Observation of Procedural Skills (DOPS) – see Chapter 1.1)

Clinical Skill Work Instruction

Equipment and resources: Mannequin capable of simulating vaginal birth; newborn mannequin; ambulance obstetric kit; bag/valve/mask resuscitator; newborn suction; food-grade polyethylene bag; baby cap; newborn blanket; hand decontamination agent; disposable gloves and protective eyewear; clinical waste bag; method of documenting the results

Associated Clinical Skills: Infection control; Communication; Consent; IPPV; Chest compressions; Childbirth skills

Premature birth

Activity	Critical Action	Rationale
Personal protection	Don PPE – eye protection, gown, gloves.	Decreases infection risk.
Patient assessment	Obtain mother's obstetric and antenatal history. Establish premature gestation. Observe for signs of second stage and imminent birth. Consider calling for back up or advice. Ascertain membrane rupture/fluid colour. Ask if there is an urge to push (see Chapter 8.1).	Clear or pink liquor is normal. Heavily blood- or meconium-stained liquor may indicate a compromised newborn requiring resuscitation. A prolapsed cord is more common in preterm labour. An urge to push is typically an uncontrollable sign of imminent birth.
Preparation	Prepare environment and equipment (see Chapter 8.1).	To minimise hypothermia and prepare for difficult outcomes.
Prepare patient	Allow mother to find a comfortable position, usually semi-recumbent or on all fours (see Chapter 8.1).	Aim for good access and vision of perineum.

Premature birth continued

Activity	Critical Action	Rationale
Birth imminent	If there are signs of the advancing presenting part, maintain perineum observation (see Chapter 8.1). Assess for prolapsed cord or breech presentation (see Chapter 8.4). Encourage mother to breathe rather than push as the head is born.	Smaller fetal size and prematurity increases the chance of cord or breech presentation.
Fetal delivery	Birth head, inspect/manage nuchal cord, observe restitution and birth body as described in Chapter 8.1.	The fetal head normally turns into the AP pelvis diameter. If the newborn is very premature, this may not occur and birth can be very rapid.
Newborn birth	*For late premature babies:* Dry and place the newborn on mother's bare chest and cover both mother and newborn. Place an appropriately sized cap on the newborn.	To prevent hypothermia. Drying can provide stimulation for breathing.
	For earlier premature babies: Do not dry the newborn. Place wet newborn in a food-grade plastic bag, leaving the head protruding. Place an appropriately sized cap on newborn's head. Place against mother for warmth unless resuscitation is required.	This provides a humidified, warm environment as the skin is very fragile.
Cord clamping and cutting	Allow at least 1 minute post birth before delayed cutting unless resuscitation demands otherwise. Double-clamp umbilical cord and cut between clamps (leave at least 10 cm of cord at the newborn end).	Cord length provides emergency umbilical vein access.
Newborn resuscitation	If the newborn has not established breathing following tactile stimulation, provide positive pressure ventilation in air using an appropriately sized face mask (see Chapter 3.11). Ventilate at 40–60 per minute, reassess every 30 seconds. Monitor newborn heart rate (ECG/auscultation). Commence cardiac compressions (see Chapter 6.1) if newborn heart rate is ≤60 after 30 seconds of adequate ventilation. CPR ratio is 3 compressions to 1 ventilation. Increase oxygen to 100%.	Lung inflation with air is critical for transition from placental to extra-uterine life and cardiovascular transition. CPR ratio differs from that for other ages, as ventilation remains priority.
Newborn APGAR	Assess APGAR score at 1 and 5 minutes after birth.	Newborn APGAR *does not* guide the resuscitation efforts required.
Maternal care	Monitor/reassess mother. Provide post-birth care as required (see Chapter 8.1).	Mother will be concerned for the newborn but may have maternal complications herself.
Report	Document time of birth, birthing details, newborn observations/ APGAR and any resuscitation required.	Accurate record kept and continuity of patient care.

Source: *Adapted from ANZCOR, 2016b.*

Formative Clinical Skill Assessment (F-CSAT)

Equipment and resources: Mannequin capable of simulating vaginal birth; newborn mannequin; ambulance obstetric kit; bag/valve/mask resuscitator; newborn suction; food-grade polyethylene bag; baby cap; newborn blanket; hand decontamination agent; disposable gloves and protective eyewear; clinical waste bag; method of documenting the results

Associated Clinical Skills: Infection control; Communication; Consent; IPPV; Chest compressions; Childbirth skills

Staff/Student being assessed: _____

Premature birth

Activity	Critical Action	Participant Performance				
Personal protection	Dons PPE.	0	1	2	3	4
Patient assessment	Obtains mother's obstetric and antenatal history. Establishes premature gestation. Observes for signs of second stage and imminent birth. Ascertains membrane rupture/fluid colour. Asks if there is an urge to push.	0	1	2	3	4
Preparation	Prepares environment and equipment as necessary. Considers calling for back up or advice.	0	1	2	3	4
Prepares patient	Positions patient with good perineum access, usually semi-recumbent or on all fours.	0	1	2	3	4
Birth imminent	If signs of birth are imminent, assesses for cord prolapse and breech presentation.	0	1	2	3	4
Fetal delivery	Births head, inspects/manages nuchal cord if present, observes restitution and births body.	0	1	2	3	4
Newborn birth	*For late premature babies:* Dries and places on mother's bare chest and covers both mother and newborn. Places appropriately sized cap on newborn.	0	1	2	3	4
	For earlier premature babies: Does not dry newborn. Places wet newborn in a food-grade plastic bag leaving head protruding. Places appropriately sized hat on newborn's head. Places against mother for warmth unless resuscitation is required.	0	1	2	3	4
Cord clamping and cutting	Allows >1 minute post birth before delayed cutting unless resuscitation demands otherwise. Double-clamps umbilical cord and cuts between clamps (leaving >10 cm of cord at the newborn end).	0	1	2	3	4
Newborn resuscitation	If newborn breathing has not been established following tactile stimulation, provides positive pressure ventilation in air at 40–60/minute. Reassesses every 30 seconds. Monitors newborn heart rate. Commences cardiac compressions if newborn heart rate is ≤60 after 30 seconds of adequate ventilation, using 3:1 ratio. Increases oxygen to 100%.	0	1	2	3	4
Newborn APGAR	Performs APGAR score at 1 and 5 minutes after birth.	0	1	2	3	4
Maternal care	Monitors/reassesses mother. Provides post-birth care as required.	0	1	2	3	4
Reports	Documents time of birth, birthing details, newborn observations/APGAR and any resuscitation required.	0	1	2	3	4

Source: *Adapted from ANZCOR, 2016b.*

Standard Achieved: (please circle one)

Competent (C)   Not Yet Competent* (NYC)

Staff/Student Name: _____

Assessor (please print name)**:** _____

Signed (Assessor)**:** _____

Date of Assessment: _____

Comments:

*If Not Yet Competent (NYC) a PIP needs to be completed and a repeat of the F-CSAT

Formative Clinical Skill Assessment (F-CSAT) Key

Skill level	Standard of procedure	Quality of performance	Outcome	Level of assistance required
4 Safe for unsupervised practice	Safe Accurate Behaviour is appropriate to context	Confident Accurate Expedient	Achieved intended outcome	No supporting cues* required
3 Requires supervision	Safe Accurate Behaviour is appropriate to context	Confident Accurate Takes longer than required	Achieved intended outcome	Requires occasional supportive cues*
2 Requires assistance	Safe Accurate Behaviour generally appropriate to context	Lacks certainty	Would not have achieved outcome without support	Requires frequent verbal and occasional physical directives in addition to supportive cues*
1 Requires direction	Safe only with guidance Not completely accurate	Unskilled Inefficient	Would not have achieved outcome without support	Requires continuous verbal and frequent physical directive cues*
0 Unsafe	Unsafe Unable to demonstrate behaviour Lack of insight into behaviour appropriate to context	Unskilled	Would not have achieved outcome	Requires continuous verbal and continuous physical directive cues*

*Refers to physical directives or verbal supportive cues

Performance Improvement Plan (PIP)

Please document the agreed education plan and completion timelines for areas assessed as less than 4.

This plan should be presented to assessor prior to commencement of summative assessment.

Where was supervisor support required?	Student summary of deficit. (Why was there a problem?)	Improvement Plan	Completed (Y/N)

Staff/Student Name: _____

Staff/Student Signature: _____

Educator Name: _____

Educator Signature: _____

Summative Clinical Skill Assessment (S-CSAT)

Equipment and resources: Mannequin capable of simulating vaginal birth; newborn mannequin; ambulance obstetric kit; bag/valve/mask resuscitator; newborn suction; food-grade polyethylene bag; baby cap; newborn blanket; hand decontamination agent; disposable gloves and protective eyewear; clinical waste bag; method of documenting the results

Associated Clinical Skills: Infection control; Communication; Consent; IPPV; Chest compressions; Childbirth skills

Staff/Student being assessed: _____

- Completed Formative Clinical Skill Assessment (F-CSAT):   **YES   NO**

- Completed Performance Improvement Plan (PIP):   **YES   NO   N/A**

Premature birth			
Activity	**Critical Action**	**Achieved Without Direction**	
Personal protection	Dons PPE.	NO	YES
Patient assessment	Obtains mother's obstetric and antenatal history. Establishes premature gestation. Observes for signs of second stage and imminent birth. Ascertains membrane rupture/fluid colour. Asks if there is an urge to push.	NO	YES
Preparation	Prepares environment and equipment as necessary. Considers calling for back up or advice.	NO	YES
Prepares patient	Positions patient with good perineum access, usually semi-recumbent or on all fours.	NO	YES
Birth imminent	If signs of birth are imminent, assesses for cord prolapse and breech presentation.	NO	YES

Premature birth continued

Activity	Critical Action	Achieved Without Direction	
Fetal delivery	Births head, inspects/manages nuchal cord if present, observes restitution and births body.	NO	YES
Newborn birth	*For late premature babies:* Dries and places on mother's bare chest and covers both mother and newborn. Places appropriately sized hat on the newborn.	NO	YES
	For earlier premature babies: Does not dry newborn. Places wet newborn in a food-grade plastic bag, leaving head protruding. Places appropriately sized hat on newborn's head. Places against mother for warmth unless resuscitation is required.	NO	YES
Cord clamping and cutting	Allows >1 minute post birth before delayed cutting unless resuscitation demands otherwise. Double-clamps umbilical cord and cuts between cord clamps (leaving >10 cm of cord at newborn end).	NO	YES
Newborn resuscitation	If newborn breathing has not been established following tactile stimulation, provides positive pressure ventilation in air at 40–60/minute. Reassesses every 30 seconds. Monitors newborn heart rate. Commences cardiac compressions if newborn heart rate is ≤60 after 30 seconds of adequate ventilation, using 3 : 1 ratio. Increases oxygen to 100%.	NO	YES
Newborn APGAR	Performs APGAR score at 1 and 5 minutes after birth.	NO	YES
Maternal care	Monitors and reassesses mother. Provides post-birth care as required.		
Reports	Documents time of birth, birthing details, newborn observations/APGAR and any resuscitation required.	NO	YES

Source: *Adapted from ANZCOR, 2016b.*

Standard Achieved: (please circle one)

Competent (C)   Not Yet Competent* (NYC)

Staff/Student Name: _____

Assessor (please print name)**:** _____

Signed (Assessor)**:** _____

Date of Assessment: _____

Comments:

*If Not Yet Competent (NYC) a PIP needs to be completed and a repeat of the F-CSAT

Clinical findings

Airway suctioning

The newborn airway does not normally require suctioning unless thick meconium liquor is noted and airway obstruction is found. Gently suctioning the mouth and *then* the nose allows for nasal breathing and the possibility of gasping. Unnecessary suctioning can cause bradycardia and reduced oxygenation (Willie et al., 2015; Wyckoff et al., 2015).

Supplemental oxygen

ANZCOR does not recommend routine resuscitation with oxygen for newborns. Premature newborns are more vulnerable to hyperoxia effects, which include lung damage (bronchopulmonary dysplasia), intraventricular haemorrhage and eye damage (retinopathy of prematurity). The lowest supplemental oxygen flow rate possible is advised to maintain suitable pulse oximetry, even during resuscitation (Saugstad et al., 2014; Willie et al., 2015; Wyckoff et al., 2015). If supplemental oxygen is administered, the target oxygen saturation of a newborn should not exceed 90% (ANZCOR, 2016a).

If chest compressions are required, resuscitation includes increased supplemental oxygen.

Positive end expiratory pressure

To help overcome alveolar collapse, the addition of 5 cm H_2O positive end expiratory pressure (PEEP) is advocated during assisted ventilation (Willie et al., 2015; Wyckoff et al., 2015).

Cord cutting

The umbilical cord is typically not cut until at least 1 minute after birth to increase blood volume and improve pulmonary blood flow (Wyllie et al., 2015). The cord may have to be cut earlier to allow effective resuscitation away from the mother. Lung ventilation increases pulmonary venous return, replacing umbilical venous return. Umbilical cord cutting can safely occur after effective breathing has been established (Hooper et al., 2016).

PRACTICE TIP

Always prepare for resuscitation for every birth. In particular, have a 'nesting' blanket and a plastic bag or cling wrap ready to protect the newborn. It is important to place the newborn skin to skin on the mother, if this is appropriate.

PRACTICE TIP

Premature labours can birth rapidly. Be ready. Anticipate risks such as breech, twins, prolapsed cord during delivery, hypothermia, respiratory compromise (newborn) and PPH (mother). Consult for clinical support.

PRACTICE TIP

Unlike in the resuscitation of all other age groups, ventilation is the critical determinant for the newborn. Early, rapid ventilation following tactile stimulation is the primary focus. Fetal circulation requires pulmonary pressure changes to progress the extra-uterine cardiovascular changes.

PRACTICE TIP

Babies can be born unexpectedly small. If a newborn is small enough to put into the plastic bag regardless of gestation, put it in the plastic bag.

PRACTICE TIP

Both mother and newborn are at risk of complications in a premature birth. The largest maternal risk is PPH, while the largest newborn risks are hypothermia and respiratory compromise.

PRACTICE TIP

The decision to resuscitate or not is a complex one in cases where the newborn may not be viable. When unsure, or parents express the wish for resuscitation to commence, commence resuscitation until further advice.

PRACTICE TIP

Expert obstetric consultation may prove critical. The parents will need explanation and reassurance throughout.

TEST YOUR KNOWLEDGE QUESTIONS

1. **Define premature birth.**
    A newborn born <37 weeks' gestation.

2. **Which delivery complications are associated with premature birth?**
    Multiple pregnancy; cord prolapse; breech delivery.

3. **What are the most *immediate* concerns for the premature newborn?**
    Respiratory distress; hypothermia.

4. **What is the optimum method for heat loss prevention in the stable premature baby born at 32 weeks' gestation?**
    Drying and placing the newborn skin to skin on the mother's chest.

5. **What is the best way of assessing ventilation adequacy in the premature newborn?**
    Observing the normal rise and fall of the chest with each ventilation and a heart rate rising to 100 and above.

6. **When should supplemental oxygen be administered to the premature newborn?**
    When cardiac compressions are required.

7. **What is the role of pulmonary surfactant?**
    To prevent alveolar collapse at the end of expiration.

8. **List three reasons why premature newborns are at greater risk of heat loss.**
    They have a greater surface area in relation to size, less brown fat from which to draw glucose energy and reduced white fat to insulate the body from heat loss.

9. **What is the role of gluconeogenesis in the newborn?**
    It assists the newborn in maintaining normal body temperature.

10. **What is the recommended guide for the administration of oxygen to all premature newborns?**
    Premature newborns are more vulnerable to hyperoxia effects, including lung and eye damage. Routine use of oxygen for newborns is not recommended. The lowest supplemental oxygen flow rate possible to maintain suitable pulse oximetry (up to 90%) should be used, even during resuscitation.

References

ANZCOR, 2016a. *Guideline 13.4 – Airway management and mask ventilation of the newborn infant.* Retrieved from: https://resus.org.au/wpfb-file/anzcor-guideline-13-4-jan16-pdf

ANZCOR, 2016b. *Guideline 13.8 – The resuscitation of the newborn infant in special circumstances.* Retrieved from: https://resus.org.au/wpfb-file/anzcor-guideline-13-8-jan16-pdf

Castrodale, V. and Rinehart, S., 2014. The golden hour: improving the stabilization of the very low birth-weight infant. *Advances in Neonatal Care*, 14(1), 9–14.

Ganga-Zandzou, P.S., Diependaele, J.F., Storme, L., Riou, Y., Klosowski, S., Rakza, T., Logier, R. and Lequien, P., 1996. Is Ambu ventilation of newborn infants a simple question of finger-touch? *Archives de Pediatrie*, 3(12), 1270–1272.

Hooper, S.B., Binder-Heschl, C., Polglase, G.R., Gill, A.W., Kluckow, M., Wallace, E.M., Blank, D. and te Pas, A.B., 2016. The timing of umbilical cord clamping at birth: physiological considerations. *Maternal Health, Neonatology and Perinatology*, 2(1), 4.

Islam, J.Y., Keller, R.L., Aschner, J.L., Hartert, T.V. and Moore, P.E., 2015. Understanding the short-and long-term respiratory outcomes of prematurity and bronchopulmonary dysplasia. *American Journal of Respiratory and Critical Care Medicine*, 192(2), 134–156.

Nimbalkar, S.M., Patel, V.K., Patel, D.V., Nimbalkar, A.S., Sethi, A. and Phatak, A., 2014. Effect of early skin-to-skin contact following normal delivery on incidence of hypothermia in neonates more than 1800 g: randomized control trial. *Journal of Perinatology*, 34(5), 364.

Oatley, H.K., Blencowe, H. and Lawn, J.E., 2016. The effect of coverings, including plastic bags and wraps, on mortality and morbidity in preterm and full-term neonates. *Journal of Perinatology*, 36(S1), S83.

Oliveira, L.L.D., Gonçalves, A.D.C., Costa, J.S.D.D. and Bonilha, A.L.D.L., 2016. Maternal and neonatal factors related to prematurity. *Revista da Escola de Enfermagem da USP*, 50(3), 382–389.

O'Shea, J.E., Thio, M., Owen, L.S., Wong, C., Dawson, J.A. and Davis, P.G., 2015. Measurements from preterm infants to guide face mask size. *Archives of Disease in Childhood – Fetal and Neonatal Edition*, F1–F5.

Pinheiro, J.M., Furdon, S.A., Boynton, S., Dugan, R., Reu-Donlon, C. and Jensen, S., 2014. Decreasing hypothermia during delivery room stabilization of preterm neonates. *Pediatrics*, 133(1), e218–e226.

Saugstad, O.D., Aune, D., Aguar, M., Kapadia, V., Finer, N. and Vento, M., 2014. Systematic review and meta-analysis of optimal initial fraction of oxygen levels in the delivery room at ≤32 weeks. *Acta Paediatrica*, 103(7), 744–751.

Veldhuizen, E.J. and Haagsman, H.P., 2000. Role of pulmonary surfactant components in surface film formation and dynamics. *Biochimica et Biophysica Acta –Biomembranes*, 1467(2), 255–270.

Vilinsky, A. and Sheridan, A., 2014. Hypothermia in the newborn: an exploration of its cause, effect and prevention. *British Journal of Midwifery*, 22(8), 557–562.

Wyckoff, M.H., 2014. Initial resuscitation and stabilization of the periviable neonate: the Golden-Hour approach. In *Seminars in Perinatology*, 38(1), 12–16.

Wyckoff, M.H., Aziz, K., Escobedo, M.B., Kapadia, V.S., Kattwinkel, J., Perlman, J.M., Simon, W.M., Weiner, G.M. and Zaichkin, J.G., 2015. Part 13: Neonatal resuscitation. *Circulation*, 132(18, Suppl 2), S543–S560.

Wyllie, J., Perlman, J.M., Kattwinkel, J., Wyckoff, M.H., Aziz, K., Guinsburg, R., Kim, H.S., Liley, H.G., Mildenhall, L., Simon, W.M. and Szyld, E., 2015. Part 7: Neonatal resuscitation: 2015 international consensus on cardiopulmonary resuscitation and emergency cardiovascular care science with treatment recommendations. *Resuscitation*, 95, e169–e201.

Bibliography

neoResus – The Victorian Newborn Resuscitation Project. *Breathing.* Retrieved from: https://www.neoresus.org.au/learning-resources/key-concepts/first-response/breathing

8.4 | Vaginal breech birth

Christine Quinn

Chapter objectives

At the end of this chapter the reader will be able to:

1. Describe the anatomy and physiology of vaginal breech birth
2. Identify vaginal breech presentation
3. Demonstrate manoeuvres that may be required to assist vaginal breech birth
4. Identify pathologies associated with vaginal breech birth

Resources required for this assessment

- Mannequin capable of simulating vaginal birth
- Hand decontamination agent
- Ambulance obstetric kit
- Disposable gloves, eyewear
- Towels and blankets
- Clinical waste bag
- Method of documenting results

Skill matrix

This assessment requires:

- Infection control (CS 1.3)
- Communication (CS 1.5)
- Consent (CS 1.6)
- Childbirth skills (Chapter 8, CS 8.1, 8.2, 8.3)

This assessment is a component of:

- Childbirth (Chapter 8)

Introduction

Breech presentation is where the fetus is presenting with the buttocks or feet. It accounts for only 3–4% of term presentations but up to 20% of premature presentations (Bergenhenegouwen et al., 2015). Breech presentation may not have been diagnosed antenatally, so the mother may be equally surprised when the fetal buttocks or feet emerge first.

There is increased risk of fetal birth injury and asphyxia from cord compression during vaginal breech birth (Berhan and Haileamlak, 2016; Bin et al., 2016; Bjellmo et al., 2017; Ekéus et al., 2017). Some newborns birth spontaneously (particularly those who are premature) but some will require assistance. Be prepared for a compromised baby that may require resuscitation.

This chapter discusses vaginal breech birth.

Anatomy and physiology

There are three types of breech presentations (Fig. 8.4.1): complete breech (both legs flexed at the hips and knees), incomplete or footling breech (one or both feet tucked under the buttocks) and frank breech (legs extended at the knees). Frank breech presentations account for 65% of breech presentations (Pairman et al., 2010).

The major concerns with vaginal breech birth are:

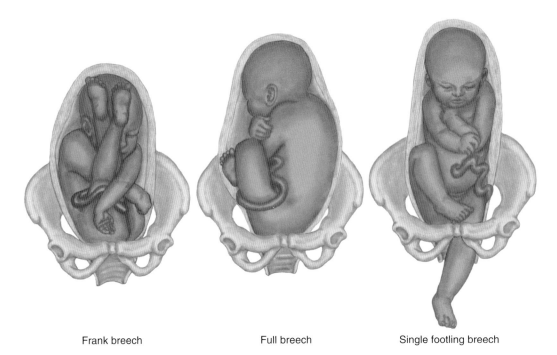

Frank breech   Full breech   Single footling breech

Figure 8.4.1 Breech presentations

Three variations of a breech presentation. Frank breech is the most common variation. Footling breeches may be single or double.

Source: Murray, S., McKinney, E., Shaw Holub, K. and Jones, R. (eds), 2019, Foundations of maternal-newborn and women's health nursing, 7th edn (Chapter 12, Figure 12.9), Elsevier.

- the largest part of the fetus (the head) is presenting last and has not had the opportunity to mould, so it may not fit
- the umbilical cord is compressed as the fetal head enters the pelvis, increasing the risk of hypoxia.

Clinical rationale

A breech birth is an obstetric emergency due to the increased risk to mother and newborn. Recognised manoeuvres may be needed to effect birth. Call for assistance or advice.

A 'hands off approach' is recommended for vaginal breech birth, assisting only when recognised manoeuvres are indicated. Even when required, it is important to keep these manoeuvres to a minimum. Trying to accelerate the birth can have serious consequences, resulting in the fetus becoming stuck or causing it unnecessary trauma.

Note: A breech birth is often associated with fresh meconium caused by mechanical compression of the lower part of the fetus body during birthing. It does not necessarily indicate meconium-stained liquor or fetal distress.

Spontaneous vaginal breech birth

Most spontaneous breech births occur very preterm (Bergenhenegouwen et al., 2015). Their birth is best accomplished in the standing, squatting or all-fours position, as this encourages optimum pelvic diameter (Louwen et al., 2017; Pairman et al., 2010; Reitter et al., 2014). If breech birth is progressing rapidly when you arrive, the maternal position should be led by the mother. Interference may result in a deflexed fetal head, delay the

birthing process and increase the need for assisted breech manoeuvres.

If the maternal position for birth is upright or on all fours, ensure the safety of the emerging fetus with gentle support so the newborn does not fall at birth.

Assisted vaginal breech manoeuvres

As for any birth that requires assistance, access is vital. Position the woman to enable maximum vaginal access; this may be on the edge of a bed or bench. A lithotomy or semi-recumbent position is preferred for assisted breech birth (Reitter et al., 2014). In the lithotomy position, the patient is supine with legs apart, flexed and held raised in stirrups (which are not usually found in ambulances) or supported by others in lieu of stirrups. This position requires two assistants to help, with one on each side and asking the mother to pull both her legs back towards her chest if she is able.

As the woman feels the urge to push with contractions, this should be encouraged.

The breech, legs and abdomen should birth spontaneously to the umbilicus level. Once the legs have birthed, you can gently palpate the umbilical cord to ascertain the fetal heart rate. Avoid unnecessary cord handling, as this may cause the vessels to spasm and compromise fetal blood supply. Cord prolapse is more likely in preterm and breech delivery (Kaymak et al., 2015).

If there is a delay and the legs do not release, apply pressure to the popliteal fossae to release them.

Once the legs have emerged, allow the fetus to hang and gravity to assist the birthing process. This should continue until the scapulae tips can be seen. Gentle support may be needed, depending on the woman's position, to prevent the newborn from falling should the birth proceed rapidly.

Wrapping a warm towel around the fetal trunk may assist in preventing hypothermia, although care must be taken not to obscure hand placement. **Poor hand placement can cause injury to underlying soft tissue and organs.**

The shoulders should present in the anterior-posterior (AP) plane and birth one at a time, followed by the arms. Once the shoulders are visible, the fetal head enters the maternal pelvis. The baby must be born within 6 minutes of this occurring (Pairman et al., 2010).

Lovset's manoeuvre

If the arms do not birth spontaneously, use Lovset's manoeuvre to assist (Fig. 8.4.2). **Do not pull on the trunk as this can cause a nuchal (upward raised) or trapped arm.**

Hold the baby over the bony part of the pelvis. Gently apply downward traction while rotating the body until one arm is uppermost. Using an index finger, follow the arm

down to the antecubital fossa; applying gentle pressure here will release the arm downwards for delivery.

Rotate the baby 180°, **keeping the back uppermost**, and deliver the other arm the same way. Failure to keep the back uppermost will result in the fetal head being trapped.

Allow the baby to 'hang' at the perineum until the nape of the neck is visible. Head descent into the pelvis uses the newborn's own weight to encourage flexion (Winter et al., 2017). Consider support if indicated.

Suprapubic pressure may be applied to assist the birth of the head.

Mauriceau-Smellie-Viet manoeuvre

If Lovset's manoeuvre is insufficient, the Mauriceau-Smellie-Viet manoeuvre should be used. This manoeuvre aims to maintain fetal head flexion to promote delivery.

Place the first and second (or third) fingers on the cheekbones, allowing the fetal body to straddle the forearm. **Do not insert a finger into the fetal mouth, as this is associated with injury.**

With the other hand, apply occipital pressure with the middle finger while placing the other fingers on the shoulders to promote flexion. Gently ease the newborn out in an upward motion (Fig. 8.4.3).

Provide post-birth care to the newborn and mother as required (see Chapters 8.1 and 8.2).

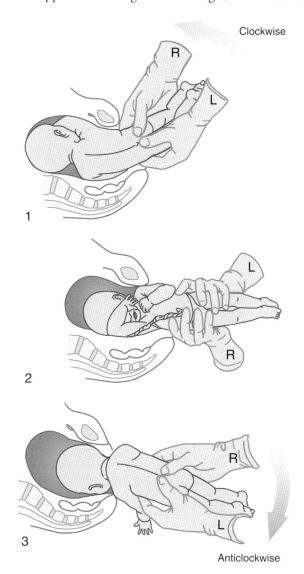

Figure 8.4.2 Lovset's manoeuvre
Source: Macdonald, S. and Johnson, G. (eds), 2017, Mayes' midwifery, 15th edn (Chapter 62, Figure 62.13), Elsevier.

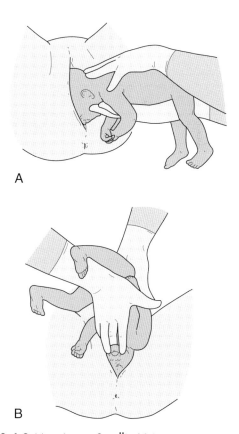

Figure 8.4.3 Mauriceau-Smellie-Veit manoeuvre
The Mauriceau-Smellie-Veit manoeuvre for delivering the after-coming head of breech presentation. (a) The hands are in position before the body is lifted. (b) Extraction of the head.
Source: Pairman, S., Pincombe, J., Thorogood, C. and Tracy, S., 2015, Midwifery: preparation for practice, 3rd edn (Chapter 38, Figure 38-7), Churchill Livingstone Australia.

Clinical skill assessment process

The following section outlines the clinical skill assessment tools that should be used to determine a student's ability to demonstrate management of vaginal breech delivery.

1. Clinical Skill Work Instruction
2. Formative Clinical Skill Assessment (F-CSAT)
3. Performance Improvement Plan (PIP)
4. Summative Clinical Skill Assessment (S-CSAT)
(5. Direct Observation of Procedural Skills (DOPS) – see Chapter 1.1)

Clinical Skill Work Instruction

Equipment and resources: Mannequin capable of simulating vaginal birth; hand decontamination agent; ambulance obstetric kit; disposable gloves and eyewear; towels and blankets; clinical waste bag; method of documenting results

Associated Clinical Skills: Infection control; Communication; Consent; Childbirth skills

Vaginal breech birth

Activity	Critical Action	Rationale
Personal protection	Don PPE – eye protection, gown, gloves.	To prevent/minimise infection.
Identify emergency	Confirm shoulder breech presentation on perineal view. Note time of fetal buttock birth.	The fetal buttocks may be birthed but the head trapped. The lapse in time can help identify if this is the case.
Preparation	Call for support/advice.	Clinical advice and extra personnel is valuable.
	Prepare for childbirth and newborn resuscitation.	Cord compression is more likely during birthing.
Position patient	Assist mother into semi-recumbent or lithotomy position.	Improves vaginal access. Recommended for breech birth.
Birth of trunk/legs	Allow the breech to descend with maternal pushing.	Spontaneous delivery of legs is preferable.
	If there is a delay, with legs not delivering spontaneously, release them using popliteal pressure.	Assistance is necessary to continue.
	Ensure the fetal back remains uppermost. Allow the fetus to hang until the scapulae are visible.	Fetal head may become trapped if allowed to deflex and move into posterior position.
	Note time of body/leg birth.	Newborn delivery is required within 6 minutes from shoulder appearance to minimise cord compression hypoxia.
	Consider wrapping a warm towel around fetal trunk.	To prevent hypothermia.

Vaginal breech birth continued

Activity	Critical Action	Rationale
Birth of shoulders/arms: Lovset's manoeuvre	If shoulders and arms do not birth spontaneously with maternal effort, hold fetus over body prominences of hips/sacrum with both hands.	Careful hand placement over bony prominences avoids fetal injury.
	Rotate baby using gentle downward traction until one arm is uppermost.	Allows arm release.
	If arm does not release spontaneously, release uppermost arm using index finger placed over fetal shoulder, following the arm to the antecubital fossa and flexing it to release.	The upward pointing arm is compressed against the pelvis and will not be able to be delivered otherwise.
	Rotate fetus 180°, keeping the back uppermost.	To present other arm and avoid fetal head entrapment.
	Repeat Lovset's manoeuvre to deliver second arm.	Arm also requires release assistance.
	Allow fetus to hang until nape of neck is visible. Support only if necessary. Check time.	Allows gravity to help pelvic head descent.
Birth of head: Mauriceau-Smellie-Viet manoeuvre	If spontaneous head birth does not follow, have an assistant apply suprapubic pressure. Encourage mother to push.	To promote fetal head flexion and facilitate birth.
	If head birth does not follow, use forearm to support the fetal body.	To support the fetus while pressing occiput away from pelvis and rotating free using natural occipital curve.
	Place first and second/third finger on either fetal cheek, avoiding the mouth.	
	Apply pressure using middle finger of other hand to the occiput, with other fingers on fetal shoulders.	
	Encourage mother to push. Gently use both hands to ease fetal head outwards in a rotating upward motion.	
	Note time.	To estimate the likelihood of complications.
Post delivery	Reassess mother and newborn. Provide care as required.	To provide normal care and respond to complications.
Report	Document/hand over presentation, times and interventions.	Accurate record keeping and continuity of care.

Source: *Adapted from RCOG, 2006.*

Formative Clinical Skill Assessment (F-CSAT)

Equipment and resources: Mannequin capable of simulating vaginal birth; hand decontamination agent; ambulance obstetric kit; disposable gloves and eyewear; towels and blankets; clinical waste bag; method of documenting results

Associated Clinical Skills: Infection control; Communication; Consent; Childbirth skills

Staff/Student being assessed: _____

Vaginal breech birth

Activity	Critical Action	Participant Performance				
Personal protection	Dons PPE.	0	1	2	3	4
Identifies emergency	Confirms breech presentation. Notes time of fetal buttock birth.	0	1	2	3	4
Preparation	Calls for support/advice. Prepares for childbirth and newborn resuscitation.	0	1	2	3	4
Positions patient	Assists mother into semi-recumbent or lithotomy position.	0	1	2	3	4
Birth of trunk/ legs	Allows breech to descend with maternal pushing. Identifies delay in birthing legs and releases them using popliteal pressure. Allows fetus to hang back uppermost until scapulae are visible. Notes time. Is aware of need to complete within 6 minutes from now. Applies warm towels to trunk if necessary.	0	1	2	3	4
Birth of shoulders/ arms (Lovset's manoeuvre)	If there is delay in birth of shoulders/arms, holds fetus over hip/sacrum prominences with both hands. Rotates fetus until one arm is uppermost. If arm does not spontaneously release, releases arm using finger over fetal shoulder, finding antecubital fossa. Rotates fetus 180°, keeping back uppermost. Releases the second arm, using same method. Notes time.	0	1	2	3	4
Birth of head (Mauriceau-Smellie-Viet manoeuvre)	If spontaneous birth does not follow, has assistant apply suprapubic pressure to assist birthing the head. Encourages mother to push. If head birth does not follow, uses forearm to support fetal body. Places first and second/third finger of hand onto cheekbones. Applies occipital pressure with second hand, with other fingers over shoulders. Encourages mother to push while using both hands to complete delivery in an upward motion. Notes time.	0	1	2	3	4
Post delivery	Reassesses mother and newborn. Provides care as required.	0	1	2	3	4
Reports	Documents/hands over required information.	0	1	2	3	4

Source: Adapted from RCOG, 2006.

Standard Achieved: (please circle one)

Competent (C)   Not Yet Competent* (NYC)

Staff/Student Name: _____

Assessor (please print name)**:** _____

Signed (Assessor)**:** _____

Date of Assessment: _____

Comments:

*If Not Yet Competent (NYC) a PIP needs to be completed and a repeat of the F-CSAT

Formative Clinical Skill Assessment (F-CSAT) key

Skill level	Standard of procedure	Quality of performance	Outcome	Level of assistance required
4 Safe for unsupervised practice	Safe Accurate Behaviour is appropriate to context	Confident Accurate Expedient	Achieved intended outcome	No supporting cues* required
3 Requires supervision	Safe Accurate Behaviour is appropriate to context	Confident Accurate Takes longer than required	Achieved intended outcome	Requires occasional supportive cues*
2 Requires assistance	Safe Accurate Behaviour generally appropriate to context	Lacks certainty	Would not have achieved outcome without support	Requires frequent verbal and occasional physical directives in addition to supportive cues*
1 Requires direction	Safe only with guidance Not completely accurate	Unskilled Inefficient	Would not have achieved outcome without support	Requires continuous verbal and frequent physical directive cues*
0 Unsafe	Unsafe Unable to demonstrate behaviour Lack of insight into behaviour appropriate to context	Unskilled	Would not have achieved outcome	Requires continuous verbal and continuous physical directive cues*

*Refers to physical directives or verbal supportive cues

Performance Improvement Plan

Please document the agreed education plan and completion timelines for areas assessed as less than 4.

This plan should be presented to assessor prior to commencement of summative assessment.

Where was supervisor support required?	Student summary of deficit. (Why was there a problem?)	Improvement Plan	Completed (Y/N)

Staff/Student Name: _____

Staff/Student Signature: _____

Educator Name: _____

Educator Signature: _____

Summative Clinical Skill Assessment (S-CSAT)

Equipment and resources: Mannequin capable of simulating vaginal birth; hand decontamination agent; ambulance obstetric kit; disposable gloves and eyewear; towels and blankets; clinical waste bag; method of documenting results

Associated Clinical Skills: Infection control; Communication; Consent; Childbirth skills

Staff/Student being assessed: _____

- Completed Formative Clinical Skill Assessment (F-CSAT):   **YES   NO**
- Completed Performance Improvement Plan (PIP):   **YES   NO   N/A**

Vaginal breech birth

Activity	Critical Action	Achieved Without Direction	
Personal protection	Dons PPE.	NO	YES
Identifies emergency	Confirms breech presentation. Notes time of fetal buttock birth.	NO	YES
Preparation	Calls for support/advice. Prepares for childbirth and newborn resuscitation.	NO	YES
Positions patient	Assists mother into semi-recumbent or lithotomy position.	NO	YES
Birth of trunk/legs	Allows breech to descend with maternal pushing. Identifies delay in birthing legs and releases them using popliteal pressure. Allows fetus to hang back uppermost until scapulae are visible. Notes time. Is aware of need to complete within 6 minutes from now. Applies warm towel to trunk if necessary.	NO	YES
Birth of shoulders/arms (Lovset's manoeuvre)	If there is delay in shoulders/arms birth, holds fetus over hip/sacrum prominences with both hands. Rotates fetus until one arm is uppermost. If arm does not spontaneously release, releases arm using finger over fetal shoulder, finding antecubital fossa. Rotates fetus 180°, keeping back uppermost. Releases the second arm using same method. Notes time.	NO	YES
Birth of head (Mauriceau-Smellie-Viet manoeuvre)	If spontaneous birth does not follow, has assistant apply suprapubic pressure to assist birthing the head. Encourages mother to push. If head birth does not follow, uses forearm to support fetal body. Places first and second/third finger of hand onto cheekbones. Applies occipital pressure with second hand, with other fingers over shoulders. Encourages mother to push while using both hands to complete delivery in an upward motion. Notes time.	NO	YES
Post delivery	Reassesses mother and newborn. Provides care as required.	NO	YES
Reports	Documents/hands over required information.	NO	YES

Source: *Adapted from RCOG, 2006.*

Standard Achieved: (please circle one)

Competent (C)   Not Yet Competent* (NYC)

Staff/Student Name: _____

Assessor (please print name): _____

Signed (Assessor): _____

Date of Assessment: _____

Comments:

*If Not Yet Competent (NYC) a PIP needs to be completed and a repeat of the F-CSAT

Clinical findings

Fetal head entrapment

Fetal head entrapment is a rare and serious complication that occurs when the trunk of the small preterm (particularly at <28 weeks) slips through an incompletely dilated cervix and the proportionately larger head remains trapped behind the cervix (Kayem et al., 2008).

This condition is identified if the head is not born quickly following the body. *The extremely preterm newborn is very small.* Fetal head entrapment is associated with very high perinatal morbidity and mortality if it occurs outside the controlled hospital environment.

Transport the mother and newborn in this partially delivered state (Robertson et al., 2015).

Tell the mother not to push. Consult for advice.

Monitor closely, as cervical dilation may occur at any time and the newborn may be delivered. Be prepared for newborn resuscitation.

Obstetric management of this condition may involve digitally pushing the cervix over the fetal head, or the use of tocolytic drugs or cervical incisions – all of which are outside the paramedic's usual scope.

PRACTICE TIP!

Hands off the breech. Allow the breech to birth until the scapula is visible and allow the limbs and trunk to birth unaided if possible.

PRACTICE TIP!

Avoid overhandling the umbilical cord, as this may cause vasospasm and further compromise blood supply to the fetus.

PRACTICE TIP!

Ensure the fetal back remains uppermost. Failure to do this may result in the head becoming trapped.

PRACTICE TIP!

Never pull on the fetal trunk, as this may cause the arms to become trapped.

PRACTICE TIP!

Handle the fetus over the bony prominences only, to avoid damage to soft tissue and the underlying organs.

PRACTICE TIP!

Breech birth is an obstetric emergency that poses a high risk to mother and fetus. The paramedic will almost certainly be inexperienced in managing breech delivery. Call for expert obstetric advice early and prepare for newborn resuscitation.

PRACTICE TIP!

Use Lovset's manoeuvre to release the shoulders and arms if they do not release spontaneously.

TEST YOUR KNOWLEDGE QUESTIONS

1. **Define breech presentation.**
   Where the fetus is presenting with the buttocks or the feet.

2. **If a breech birth is occurring and rapidly progressing on arrival, what should you do?**
   Call for clinical assistance/advice; prepare for birth and newborn resuscitation; allow the mother to determine the birth position unless delay is evident; provide physical support for the emerging fetus if necessary.

3. **Which baby population is more likely to present breech?**
   Early premature gestations.

4. **List two main concerns associated with vaginal breech birth for the baby.**
   Increased risk to the fetus from asphyxia due to cord compression; birth injury.

5. **What are the risks of unnecessarily interfering in this birthing process?**
   Entrapment of the fetal head or shoulders, causing delay in the birthing process and the need for further intervention.

6. **What are the recommended positions for an assisted breech birth?**
   Semi-recumbent or lithotomy.

7. **Why should you avoid overhandling the umbilical cord?**
   This may cause the vessels in the cord to spasm and further occlude fetal blood supply.

8. **Why is it important to always keep the fetal back uppermost?**
   To prevent the fetal head deflexing in the posterior position, causing fetal head entrapment.

9. **Where are the hands placed on the fetus to assist with birth of the shoulders and arms?**
   Over the bony prominences, to avoid organ and soft tissue injury.

10. **Once the shoulders appear, how long should it take for birth to be completed?**
    Once the shoulders are visible, the fetal head enters the maternal pelvis. The newborn must be born within 6 minutes of this occurring.

References

Bergenhenegouwen, L., Vlemmix, F., Ensing, S., Schaaf, J., van der Post, J., Abu-Hanna, A., Ravelli, A.C., Mol, B.W. and Kok, M., 2015. Preterm breech presentation: a comparison of intended vaginal and intended cesarean delivery. *Obstetrics & Gynecology*, 126(6), 1223–1230.

Berhan, Y. and Haileamlak, A., 2016. The risks of planned vaginal breech delivery versus planned caesarean section for term breech birth: a meta-analysis including observational studies. *BJOG*, 123(1), 49–57.

Bin, Y.S., Roberts, C.L., Ford, J.B. and Nicholl, M.C., 2016. Outcomes of breech birth by mode of delivery: a population linkage study. *Australian and New Zealand Journal of Obstetrics and Gynaecology*, 56(5), 453–459.

Bjellmo, S., Andersen, G.L., Martinussen, M.P., Romundstad, P.R., Hjelle, S., Moster, D. and Vik, T., 2017. Is vaginal breech delivery associated with higher risk for perinatal death and cerebral palsy compared with vaginal cephalic birth? Registry-based cohort study in Norway. *BMJ Open*, 7(4), e014979.

Ekéus, C., Norman, M., Åberg, K., Winberg, S., Stolt, K. and Aronsson, A., 2017. Vaginal breech delivery at term and neonatal morbidity and mortality – a population-based cohort study in Sweden. *Journal of Maternal-Fetal & Neonatal Medicine*, 1–6.

Kayem, G., Baumann, R., Goffinet, F., El Abiad, S., Ville, Y., Cabrol, D. and Haddad, B., 2008. Early preterm breech delivery: is a policy of planned vaginal delivery associated with increased risk of neonatal death? *American Journal of Obstetrics & Gynecology*, 198(3), 289–e1.

Kaymak, O., Iskender, C., Ibanoglu, M., Cavkaytar, S., Uygur, D. and Danisman, N., 2015. Retrospective evaluation of risk factors and perinatal outcome of umbilical cord prolapse during labor. *European Review for Medical and Pharmacological Sciences*, 19(13), 2336–2339.

Louwen, F., Daviss, B.A., Johnson, K.C. and Reitter, A., 2017. Does breech delivery in an upright position instead of on the back improve outcomes and avoid cesareans? *International Journal of Gynecology & Obstetrics*, 136(2), 151–161.

Pairman, S., Tracy, S.K., Thorogood, C. and Pincombe, J., 2010. *Midwifery: preparation for practice*. Sydney: Elsevier.

RCOG (Royal College of Obstetricians and Gynaecologists), 2006. *Management of breech presentation*. Green-top Guideline no. 20. London: RCOG.

Reitter, A., Daviss, B.A., Bisits, A., Schollenberger, A., Vogl, T., Herrmann, E., Louwen, F. and Zangos, S., 2014. Does pregnancy and/or shifting positions create more room in a woman's pelvis? *American Journal of Obstetrics & Gynecology*, 211(6), 662–e1.

Robertson, J.F., Braude, D.A., Stonehocker, J. and Moreno, J., 2015. Prehospital breech delivery with fetal head entrapment – a case report and review. *Prehospital Emergency Care*, 19(3), 451–456.

Winter, C., Crofts, J., Laxton, C., Barnfield, S. and Draycott, T.J. (eds), 2017. *PROMPT: Trainer's manual*. Cambridge: Cambridge University Press.

Bibliography

Kotaska, A., Menticoglou, S., Gagnon, R., Farine, D., Basso, M., Bos, H., Delisle, M.F., Grabowska, K., Hudon, L., Mundle, W. and Murphy-Kaulbeck, L., 2009. Vaginal delivery of breech presentation. *Journal of Obstetrics and Gynaecology Canada*, 31(6), 557–566.

Shoulder dystocia

Christine Quinn

Chapter objectives

At the end of this chapter the reader will be able to:

1. Describe the anatomy of shoulder dystocia
2. Identify shoulder dystocia
3. Demonstrate manoeuvres to relieve shoulder dystocia
4. Identify complications of newborn with shoulder dystocia

Resources required for this assessment

- Mannequin capable of simulating vaginal birth
- Hand decontamination agent
- Ambulance obstetric kit
- Towels and blankets
- Disposable gloves and eyewear
- Clinical waste bag
- Method of documenting results

Skill matrix

This assessment requires:

- Infection control (CS 1.3)
- Communication (CS 1.5)
- Consent (CS 1.6)
- Childbirth skills (Chapter 8, CS 8.1, 8.2, 8.3)

This assessment is a component of:

- Childbirth (Chapter 8)

Introduction

The most common cause of shoulder dystocia is impaction of the anterior fetal shoulder against the maternal symphysis pubis, preventing birth of the fetal body. It requires obstetric manoeuvres to complete the birth after routine traction fails to release the shoulders following birth of the head (Hansen and Chauhan, 2014; Resnik, 1980). As this is a pelvic problem, pulling on the fetus causes injury and increases impaction.

This is a rare complication that often has no recognisable risk factors. Though it is difficult to predict, shoulder dystocia is associated with maternal diabetes and larger birth weight (Dodd et al., 2012; Gupta et al., 2010; Mehta and Sokol, 2014; Revicky et al., 2012; Volpe et al., 2016).

This chapter discusses the recognition and emergency management of shoulder dystocia.

Anatomy and physiology

Shoulder dystocia most commonly occurs when the bisacromial fetal shoulder diameter (width) is bigger than the pelvic outlet in the presenting anterior-posterior (AP) plane. Manoeuvres to relieve shoulder dystocia aim to either reduce fetal shoulder width or increase pelvic outlet size.

The oblique or transverse planes of the pelvic outlet are larger than the AP plane (Fig. 8.5.1).

Shoulder dystocia occurs where the fetal head emerges slowly from the perineum and appears to slip back, presenting with the chin tucked back into the perineum;

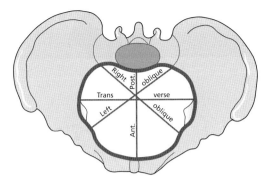

Figure 8.5.1 Pelvic inlet diameters
Source: Catling, C. and Raynor, M., 2017, Myles survival guide to midwifery, 3rd edn (Chapter 1, Figure 1.3), Elsevier.

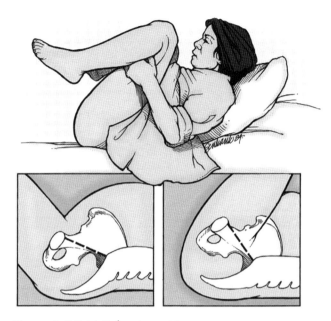

Figure 8.5.3 McRobert's position
Source: Lew, G.H. and Pulia, M.S., 2013, Emergency childbirth, in Roberts, J. (ed.), Roberts Hedges clinical procedures in emergency medicine, Elsevier, p. 1170.

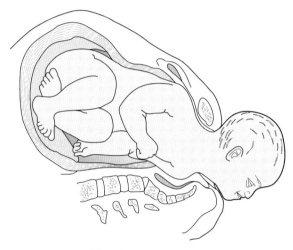

Figure 8.5.2 Shoulder dystocia
Source: Cooper, M.A. and Fraser, D.M., 2018, A–Z midwifery (Figure 31), Elsevier.

this is called the 'turtleneck sign' or 'turtling'. This fetal head often fails to restitute. There is difficulty birthing the face and chin, as the head is tightly applied to the vulva (Fig. 8.5.2). The anterior shoulder fails to release with maternal pushing or routine head traction (Winter et al., 2017).

Clinical rationale

Early recognition of shoulder dystocia is vital for prompt management. A fetus in this position is unable to initiate breathing, and cord compression and hypoxia require urgent relief. There is no safe time limit within which birth must take place, as it is entirely dependent on the condition of the fetus, which is unknown. Expect a compromised newborn requiring resuscitation, especially in the presence of meconium-stained liquor.

A series of steps is followed to relieve shoulder dystocia, including simple, external manoeuvres followed by more complicated, internal manoeuvres. Performed correctly, external manoeuvres relieve >90% shoulder dystocia (RCOG, 2012).

Immediately shoulder dystocia is suspected, ask the mother to stop pushing, as this only increases impaction. Remember:

- Time equals fetal hypoxia. Do not waste time on any manoeuvre that is not working (30–60 seconds maximum).
- Work from easy, external manoeuvres progressing to more complicated and invasive internal manoeuvres if needed.
- The anterior shoulder of the fetus corresponds to the mother's anterior. Changing the mother's position does not change which fetal shoulder is anterior, only which one is uppermost.

External manoeuvres

The external manoeuvres are McRobert's position, suprapubic pressure and the all fours position.

McRobert's position

This is the first manoeuvre to try; it has a success rate of up to 90% (Fig. 8.5.3) (RCOG, 2012). This position increases AP pelvic diameter by flattening the sacral curve.

Lay the mother flat, removing any excess pillows from behind her. Move her into a position that offers best access to the vagina, such as on the edge of the bed, bench or stretcher.

Two assistants are needed; the woman's partner may be able to assist. Having one assistant either side helps the mother hyperflex her legs, pointing her knees straight back towards her nipples. From this position, ask her to push and reattempt delivery of the fetal head, **applying normal axial traction**. Normal axial traction refers to the level of traction applied for normal delivery in the fetal spine and head axis. This keeps the fetus in alignment, preventing

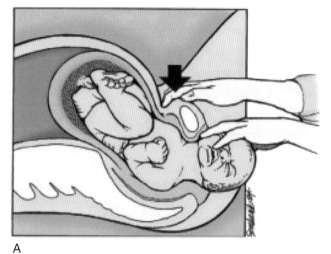

A

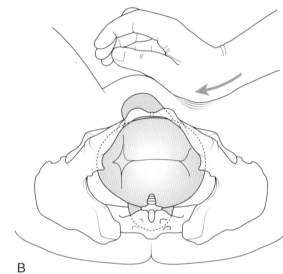

B

Figure 8.5.4 Suprapubic pressure

Source: (a) Lew, G.H. and Pulia, M.S., 2013, Emergency childbirth, in Roberts, J. (ed.), Roberts Hedges clinical procedures in emergency medicine, Elsevier, p. 1170; (b) Cooper, M.A. and Fraser, D.M., 2018, A–Z midwifery (Figure 32), Elsevier.

lateral head and neck flexion and nerve damage. It is repeated throughout with each additional manoeuvre.

If McRobert's position fails to relieve shoulder dystocia, the second manoeuvre is suprapubic pressure.

Suprapubic pressure

Keep the mother in McRobert's position.

Suprapubic pressure (Fig. 8.5.4) reduces fetal shoulder width in two ways:
1. Moving the fetal shoulders into the wider transverse or oblique diameter of the mother's pelvis
2. Adducting the fetal shoulders (if pressure is applied from the side of the fetal back).

Before beginning the manoeuvre, warn the mother that it will be uncomfortable and her cooperation is needed.

Identify the side of the fetal back if possible (do not waste time if unsure). Apply slow pressure from above the mother in a lateral downward direction just above her symphysis pubis (appears like performing CPR). With the

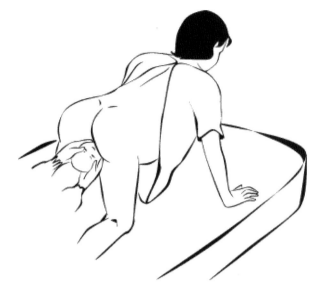

Figure 8.5.5 All fours position

Source: Kovavisarach, E., 2006, The 'all-fours' maneuver for the management of shoulder dystocia, International Journal of Gynaecology and Obstetrics, 95(2), 153–154.

mother in this position, ask her to push and reattempt delivery of the fetal head, **applying normal axial traction**.

Time is critical. If this does not relieve the problem after 30–60 seconds you can try applying pressure from the opposite side or move to the next step.

All fours position

Helping the mother into the all fours position (Fig. 8.5.5) has high success at releasing the trapped shoulder through the movement alone (Bruner et al., 1998). Its advantage is that the posterior shoulder (the one not trapped) is now uppermost.

With the mother in position, ask her to push and reattempt delivery of the fetal head, **applying normal axial traction**.

Episiotomy

If external manoeuvres fail to deliver the fetal shoulder, internal manoeuvres are required. It is unlikely paramedics will be trained in or perform any internal manoeuvre or episiotomy without guidance or consultation.

Cutting an episiotomy can improve access to the vagina before attempting internal manoeuvres, though it is not essential (Gurewitsch et al., 2004; Paris et al., 2011).

The safest incision is the mediolateral episiotomy (Fig. 8.5.6). With shoulder dystocia, cutting an episiotomy is more difficult than usual as the head has been incompletely delivered.

Internal manoeuvres

The internal manoeuvres are posterior arm delivery and rotational manoeuvres. No internal manoeuvre is superior to another: the choice is driven by which part of the fetal anatomy is felt when entering the vagina. If you locate the fetal back first, then try rotational manoeuvres. If the fetal chest is located first and the arms are flexed in front, try releasing the posterior arm.

These manoeuvres can be attempted in a supine or all fours position. If you are unable to relieve the dystocia in one position, try the other.

Internal manoeuvres require entering the vagina with your *whole hand*. You will only achieve this from the posterior vaginal wall, as the shoulder is firmly wedged in the anterior, preventing access.

Posterior arm delivery

Posterior arm delivery (Fig. 8.5.7) reduces the shoulder width by the breadth of an arm.

Inside the vagina, feel across the fetal chest. Most babies will present with both arms flexed across the chest. If this is the case, grasp the posterior arm by the wrist and draw it out in a straight line.

Ask the mother to push and reattempt delivery of the fetal head, **applying normal axial traction**.

If this manoeuvre fails or the fetal arm is not flexed across the chest, attempt rotational manoeuvres instead.

Internal rotation manoeuvres

Apply pressure to either the anterior or posterior aspect of the posterior fetal shoulder and push it into the oblique or transverse diameter of the maternal pelvis (Figs 8.5.8 and 8.5.9). Posterior aspect pressure also helps adduct

the shoulders, reducing the shoulder width. Suprapubic pressure applied by an assistant in the direction of rotation can assist.

Ask the mother to push and reattempt delivery of the fetal head, **applying normal axial traction**.

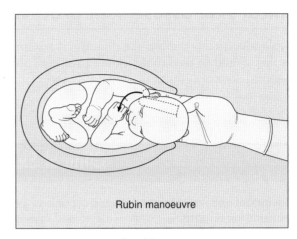

Rubin manoeuvre

Figure 8.5.8 Posterior shoulder rotation
Source: *Oats, J. and Abraham, S., 2010*, Llewellyn-Jones fundamentals of obstetrics and gynaecology, *9th edn (Chapter 22, Figure 22.5)*, Elsevier.

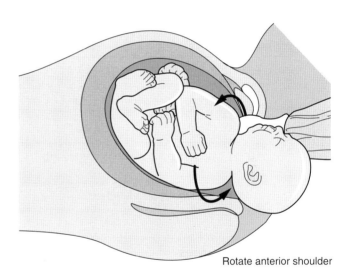

Rotate anterior shoulder

Figure 8.5.9 Anterior shoulder rotation

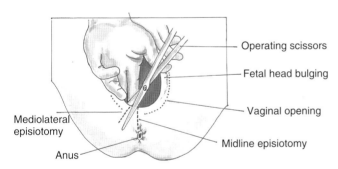

Operating scissors

Fetal head bulging

Vaginal opening

Mediolateral episiotomy

Midline episiotomy

Anus

Figure 8.5.6 Episiotomy
Source: *Kumari, U., 2019*, Textbook of obstetrics *(Chapter 14, Figure 14.11)*, RELX India.

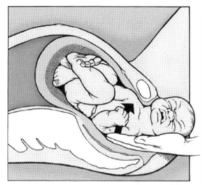
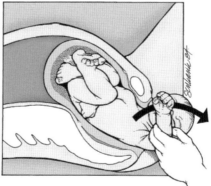

Figure 8.5.7 Posterior arm delivery
Source: *Lew, G.H. and Pulia, M.S., 2013, Emergency childbirth, in Roberts, J. (ed.)*, Roberts Hedges clinical procedures in emergency medicine, Elsevier, p. 1170.

If rotation in one direction fails, swap hands and try the other.

Rotating the anterior fetal shoulder is more difficult and will require working your fingers up around the fetal back to push the anterior shoulder forwards.

Clinical skill assessment process

The following section outlines the clinical skill assessment tools that should be used to determine a student's ability to demonstrate management of shoulder dystocia.

1. Clinical Skill Work Instruction
2. Formative Clinical Skill Assessment (F-CSAT)
3. Performance Improvement Plan (PIP)
4. Summative Clinical Skill Assessment (S-CSAT)
(5. Direct Observation of Procedural Skills (DOPS) – see Chapter 1.1)

Clinical Skill Work Instruction

Equipment and resources: Mannequin capable of simulating vaginal birth; hand decontamination agent; ambulance obstetric kit; disposable gloves and eyewear; towels and blankets; clinical waste bag; method of documenting results

Associated Clinical Skills: Infection control; Communication; Consent; Childbirth skills

Shoulder dystocia

Activity	Critical Action	Rationale
Personal protection	Don PPE as required.	To minimise the risk of infection.
Prepare patient	Confirm shoulder dystocia. Request partner assistance. Call for further support. Prepare for newborn resuscitation. Call for back up or advice.	To ensure maximum focus and assistance on emergency. The newborn will likely require resuscitation post cord compression hypoxia.
	Discourage the mother from pushing.	To avoid further shoulder impaction.
	Note time of fetal head birth.	The body should birth soon after. Timely recognition and intervention is critical from this point.

External manoeuvres

Activity	Critical Action	Rationale
McRobert's manoeuvre	Assist the woman to: • lie flat (one pillow only behind the head) • move into a position that maximises access (e.g. bed/bench edge).	In readiness for McRobert's manoeuvre.
	Bring mother's legs to 'knees-to-nipple' position, using assistant where available.	To increase AP diameter of maternal pelvis.
	Ask the mother to push and apply routine fetal head axial traction to effect delivery. Note the time. Allow 30–60 seconds maximum for the manoeuvre.	Excessive or downward traction will not relieve bony impaction and causes fetal nerve injury.

Shoulder dystocia continued

Activity	Critical Action	Rationale
Suprapubic pressure	Maintain McRobert's position.	This is an adjunct to the manoeuvre.
	Try to identify which side the fetal back is on. Do not waste time if this is not apparent.	Guides best direction to push from.
	Have assistant apply downward and lateral suprapubic pressure just above the maternal symphysis pubis in a continuous motion (from the side of fetal back if known).	To move the fetal shoulder into the wider, oblique maternal pelvis diameter.
	Apply routine fetal head axial traction head. Encourage mother to push.	To attempt delivery.
	If delivery is unsuccessful with routine axial traction, suprapubic pressure may be applied from mother's opposite side.	Important where position of fetal back is unclear.
	Note time taken. Allow 30–60 seconds maximum for the manoeuvre.	If unsuccessful, another option is required. Fetal cord compression remains.
All fours	Help the mother roll into the all fours position.	Position change can dislodge dystocia by placing free shoulder uppermost.
	Apply routine fetal head axial traction head. Encourage mother to push.	To attempt delivery.
	Note time taken. Allow 30–60 seconds maximum for the manoeuvre.	Failure dictates another option.

Internal manoeuvres

Activity	Critical Action	Rationale
Posterior arm removal	Instruct mother to stop pushing.	To avoid compounding impaction.
	All internal manoeuvres can be attempted in all fours or supine position.	Choose the quickest and most suitable position.
	Insert entire hand posteriorly into the sacral hollow.	Anterior access is difficult as this is where impaction is.
	Locate fetal hand and forearm across fetal chest.	Fetus is usually positioned with arms flexed across chest.
	Grasp the wrist and gently remove it in a straight line.	Removing posterior shoulder reduces fetal bisacromial diameter.
	Apply routine axial traction to fetal head. Encourage mother to push.	To attempt delivery.
	Note time taken. Allow 30–60 seconds maximum for the manoeuvre.	Failure dictates trying another option.

Shoulder dystocia continued

Activity	Critical Action	Rationale
Rotational manoeuvres	If unsuccessful or unable to locate posterior arm across chest, attempt rotational manoeuvre. Instruct mother to stop pushing.	To avoid compounding impaction.
	Insert entire hand posteriorly into sacral hollow. Apply pressure to anterior or posterior aspect of fetal posterior shoulder with fingers moving the fetus into the oblique pelvic plane.	Achieves posterior access. Push shoulder into wider oblique diameter of maternal pelvis.
	Apply routine axial traction to fetal head. Encourage mother to push.	To attempt delivery.
	If unsuccessful, have an assistant apply suprapubic pressure in the direction of rotation.	To dislodge shoulder.
	If still unsuccessful, swap hands and apply pressure to anterior fetal shoulder from the side of the fetal back. Suprapubic pressure in the direction of rotation can be applied to assist.	Substitutes anterior for posterior shoulder.
Outcome	If successful, provide newborn (see Chapter 8.3) and maternal care as required. If unsuccessful, continue efforts in the alternative maternal position.	Resuscitation/reassurance is likely necessary.
Report	Document/hand over times for head birth and procedural times/results as provided.	Accurate record keeping and continuity of care.

Source: *Adapted from RCOG, 2012.*

Formative Clinical Skill Assessment (F-CSAT)

Equipment and resources: Mannequin capable of simulating vaginal birth; hand decontamination agent; ambulance obstetric kit; disposable gloves and eyewear; towels and blankets; clinical waste bag; method of documenting results

Associated Clinical Skills: Infection control; Communication; Consent; Childbirth skills

Staff/Student being assessed: _____

Shoulder dystocia

Activity	Critical Action	Participant Performance				
Personal protection	Dons PPE.	0	1	2	3	4
Prepare patient	Confirms and states shoulder dystocia. Calls for support/advice. Prepares for newborn resuscitation. Discourages mother from pushing. Notes time of fetal head birth.	0	1	2	3	4
McRobert's manoeuvre	Assists mother to lie flat in a position that maximises access. Brings legs into knees-to-nipple position with assistance. Asks mother to push and attempts delivery using normal axial traction. Notes time taken – maximum 30–60 seconds.	0	1	2	3	4
Suprapubic pressure	Identifies which side fetal back is on if possible. Has assistant apply suprapubic pressure continuously from the side of the fetal back. Attempts delivery with mother pushing. Notes time taken – maximum 30–60 seconds.	0	1	2	3	4

Shoulder dystocia continued

Activity	Critical Action	Participant Performance				
Posterior arm removal	Instructs mother to stop pushing. Inserts entire hand posteriorly into the sacral hollow. Locates fetal hand and forearm across fetal chest. Grasps wrist and gently removes in straight line. Attempts delivery with mother pushing. Notes time taken – maximum 30–60 seconds.	0	1	2	3	4
Rotational manoeuvres	If still unsuccessful, instructs mother to stop pushing. Inserts hand into sacral hollow. Applies pressure to anterior or posterior aspect of posterior fetal shoulder with fingers, moving the fetus into the oblique pelvic plane. If unsuccessful, has assistant apply suprapubic pressure in the direction of rotation. If still unsuccessful, swaps hands and applies pressure to anterior fetal shoulder from the side of the fetal back. Suprapubic pressure in the direction of rotation can be applied to assist. Attempts delivery with mother pushing between each technique change.	0	1	2	3	4
Outcome	If successful, provides newborn (Chapter 8.3) and maternal care. If unsuccessful, continues efforts in the alternative maternal position.	0	1	2	3	4
Report	Accurately documents/hands over details of events.	0	1	2	3	4

Source: Adapted from RCOG, 2012.

Standard Achieved: (please circle one)

Competent (C)   Not Yet Competent* (NYC)

Staff/Student Name: _____

Assessor (please print name): _____

Signed (Assessor): _____

Date of Assessment: _____

Comments:

*If Not Yet Competent (NYC) a PIP needs to be completed and a repeat of the F-CSAT

Formative Clinical Skill Assessment (F-CSAT) Key

Skill level	Standard of procedure	Quality of skill delivery	Outcome	Level of assistance required
4 Safe for unsupervised practice	Safe Accurate Behaviour is appropriate to context	Confident Accurate Expedient	Achieved intended outcome	No supporting cues required
3 Requires supervision	Safe Accurate Behaviour is appropriate to context	Confident Accurate Takes longer than required	Achieved intended outcome	Requires occasional supportive cues

Skill level	Standard of procedure	Quality of skill delivery	Outcome	Level of assistance required
2 Requires assistance	Safe Accurate Behaviour generally appropriate to context	Lacks certainty	Would not have achieved outcome without support	Requires frequent verbal and occasional physical directives in addition to supportive cues
1 Requires direction	Safe only with guidance Not completely accurate	Unskilled Inefficient	Would not have achieved outcome without support	Requires continuous verbal and frequent physical directive cues
0 Unsafe	Unsafe Unable to demonstrate behaviour Lack of insight into behaviour appropriate to context	Unskilled	Would not have achieved outcome	Requires continuous verbal and continuous physical directive cues

Performance Improvement Plan (PIP)

Please document the agreed education plan and completion timelines for areas assessed as less than 4.

This plan should be presented to assessor prior to commencement of summative assessment.

Where was supervisor support required?	Student summary of deficit. (Why was there a problem?)	Improvement Plan	Completed (Y/N)

Staff/Student Name: _____

Staff/Student Signature: _____

Educator Name: _____

Educator Signature: _____

Summative Clinical Skill Assessment (S-CSAT)

Equipment and resources: Mannequin capable of simulating vaginal birth; hand decontamination agent; ambulance obstetric kit; disposable gloves and eyewear; towels and blankets; clinical waste bag; method of documenting results

Associated Clinical Skills: Infection control; Communication; Consent; Childbirth skills

Staff/Student being assessed: _____

- Completed Formative Clinical Skill Assessment (F-CSAT):   **YES**   **NO**

- Completed Performance Improvement Plan (PIP):   **YES**   **NO**   **N/A**

Shoulder dystocia			
Activity	**Critical Action**	**Achieved Without Direction**	
Personal protection	Dons PPE.	NO	YES
Prepares patient	Confirms and states shoulder dystocia. Calls for support/advice. Prepares for newborn resuscitation. Discourages mother from pushing. Notes time of fetal head birth.	NO	YES
McRobert's manoeuvre	Assists mother to lie flat in a position that maximises access. Brings legs into knees-to-nipple position with assistance. Asks mother to push and attempts delivery using normal axial traction. Notes time taken – maximum 30–60 seconds.	NO	YES
Suprapubic pressure	Identifies which side fetal back is on if possible. Has assistant apply suprapubic pressure continuously from the side of the fetal back. Attempts delivery with mother pushing. Notes time taken – maximum 30–60 seconds.	NO	YES
Posterior arm removal	Instructs mother to stop pushing. Inserts entire hand posteriorly into the sacral hollow. Locates fetal hand and forearm across fetal chest. Grasps wrist and gently removes in straight line. Attempts delivery with mother pushing. Notes time taken – maximum 30–60 seconds.	NO	YES
Rotational manoeuvres	If still unsuccessful, instructs mother to stop pushing. Inserts hand into sacral hollow. Applies pressure to anterior or posterior aspect of posterior fetal shoulder with fingers, moving the fetus into the oblique pelvic plane. If unsuccessful, has assistant apply suprapubic pressure in the direction of rotation. If still unsuccessful, swaps hands and applies pressure to anterior fetal shoulder from the side of the fetal back. Suprapubic pressure in the direction of rotation can be applied to assist. Attempts delivery with mother pushing between each technique change.	NO	YES
Outcome	If successful, provides newborn (Chapter 8.3) and maternal care. If unsuccessful, continues efforts in the alternative maternal position.	NO	YES
Reports	Accurately documents/hands over details of events.	NO	YES

Source: *Adapted from RCOG, 2012.*

Standard Achieved: (please circle one)

Competent (C)   Not Yet Competent* (NYC)

Staff/Student Name: _____

Assessor (please print name)**:** _____

Signed (Assessor)**:** _____

Date of Assessment: _____

Comments:

*If Not Yet Competent (NYC) a PIP needs to be completed and a repeat of the F-CSAT

Clinical findings

Newborn outcomes

The primary concern for the newborn is hypoxia from cord compression and birth injury. Newborn resuscitation is commonly required following prolonged entrapment (>5 minutes) that causes hypoxia. Fetal death is uncommon but it does occur (Dajani and Magann, 2014). Prepare for this in all events, particularly if initial manoeuvres are not successful.

Newborn injuries during the manoeuvres used for shoulder dystocia include brachial plexus palsy from forceful lateral pulling or traction on the head (Dajani and Magann, 2014; Leung et al., 2011; Thatte and Mehta, 2011) and clavicular or humeral fracture from suprapubic pressure (Dajani and Magann, 2014; Leung et al., 2011; Hoffman et al., 2011).

PRACTICE TIP!

Expect a compromised newborn that will need resuscitation. Seek help early.

PRACTICE TIP!

Never apply excessive and/or downward pressure to the fetal head – this will cause nerve damage.

PRACTICE TIP!

Always try the simple external manoeuvres first, alternating quickly until successful. Do not waste time on a manoeuvre that is not working – time equals fetal hypoxia.

TEST YOUR KNOWLEDGE QUESTIONS

1. **Describe shoulder dystocia.**
   The fetal anterior shoulder impacts against the maternal symphysis pubis, preventing birth of the fetal body.

2. **How does shoulder dystocia present?**
   The fetal head emerges slowly from the perineum and appears to slip back, presenting with chin tucked back into the perineum.

3. **When you identify shoulder dystocia, what immediate preparations should you make?**
   Instruct the mother to stop pushing; call for clinical support; prepare for newborn resuscitation.

4. **List the external manoeuvres to relieve shoulder dystocia in the order they are performed.**
   McRobert's position; suprapubic pressure; all fours position.

5. **List the two internal manoeuvres that may be required to effect delivery.**
   Posterior arm delivery; rotational manoeuvres.

6. **Which external manoeuvre can assist internal rotation manoeuvres?**
   Suprapubic pressure.

7. **What is the maximum time that should be spent on each manoeuvre?**
   30–60 seconds.

8. **Why is patient consent important?**
   Consent is enshrined in legal, ethical and moral healthcare.

9. **Why is it important not to apply excessive downward pressure on the fetal head?**
   This causes fetal nerve damage and increases bony impaction.

10. **If these manoeuvres fail, what could you try?**
    Repeat the manoeuvres with the woman in the opposite position (i.e. dorsal or all fours).

References

Bruner, J.P., Drummond, S.B., Meenan, A.L. and Gaskin, I.M.,1998. All-fours maneuver for reducing shoulder dystocia during labor. *Journal of Reproductive Medicine*, 43(5), 439–443.

Dajani, N.K. and Magann, E.F., 2014. Complications of shoulder dystocia. *Seminars in Perinatology,* 38(4), 201–204.

Dodd, J.M., Catcheside, B. and Scheil, W., 2012. Can shoulder dystocia be reliably predicted? *Australian and New Zealand Journal of Obstetrics and Gynaecology*, 52(3), 248–252.

Gupta, M., Hockley, C., Quigley, M.A., Yeh, P. and Impey, L., 2010. Antenatal and intrapartum prediction of shoulder dystocia. *European Journal of Obstetrics and Gynecology and Reproductive Biology*, 151(2), 134–139.

Gurewitsch, E.D., Donithan, M., Stallings, S.P., Moore, P.L., Agarwal, S., Allen, L.M. and Allen, R.H., 2004. Episiotomy versus fetal manipulation in managing severe shoulder dystocia: a comparison of outcomes. *American Journal of Obstetrics & Gynecology*, 191(3), 911–916.

Hansen, A. and Chauhan, S.P., 2014. Shoulder dystocia: definitions and incidence. *Seminars in Perinatology*, 38(4), 184–188.

Hoffman, M.K., Bailit, J.L., Branch, D.W., Burkman, R.T., Van Veldhusien, P., Lu, L., Kominiarek, M.A., Hibbard, J.U., Landy, H.J., Haberman, S. and Wilkins, I., 2011. A comparison of obstetric maneuvers for the acute management of shoulder dystocia. *Obstetrics and Gynecology*, 117(6), 1272.

Leung, T.Y., Stuart, O., Suen, S.S.H., Sahota, D.S., Lau, T.K. and Lao, T.T., 2011. Comparison of perinatal outcomes of shoulder dystocia alleviated by different type and sequence of manoeuvres: a retrospective review. *BJOG*, 118(8), 985–990.

Mehta, S.H. and Sokol, R.J., 2014. Shoulder dystocia: risk factors, predictability, and preventability. *Seminars in Perinatology*, 38(4), 189–193.

Paris, A.E., Greenberg, J.A., Ecker, J.L. and McElrath, T.F., 2011. Is an episiotomy necessary with a shoulder dystocia? *American Journal of Obstetrics & Gynecology*, 205(3), 217–e1.

RCOG (Royal College of Obstetricians & Gynaecologists), 2012. *Shoulder dystocia*, Green-top Guideline No. 42, 2nd edn. Retrieved from: https://www.rcog.org.uk/globalassets/documents/guidelines/gtg_42.pdf

Resnik, R., 1980. Management of shoulder girdle dystocia. *Clinical Obstetrics and Gynecology*, 23(2), 559–564.

Revicky, V., Mukhopadhyay, S., Morris, E.P. and Nieto, J.J., 2012. Can we predict shoulder dystocia? *Archives of Gynecology and Obstetrics*, 285(2), 291–295.

Thatte, M.R. and Mehta, R., 2011. Obstetric brachial plexus injury. *Indian Journal of Plastic Surgery*, 44(3), 380.

Volpe, K.A., Snowden, J.M., Cheng, Y.W. and Caughey, A.B., 2016. Risk factors for brachial plexus injury in a large cohort with shoulder dystocia. *Archives of Gynecology and Obstetrics*, 294(5), 925–929.

Winter, C., Crofts, J., Laxton, C., Barnfield, S. and Draycott, T.J. (eds), 2017. *PROMPT: Trainer's manual*. Cambridge: Cambridge University Press.

Bibliography

Johnson, R. and Taylor, W., 2016. *Skills for midwifery practice*. Sydney: Elsevier.

Pairman, S., Tracy, S.K., Thorogood, C. and Pincombe, J., 2010. *Midwifery: preparation for practice*. Sydney: Elsevier.

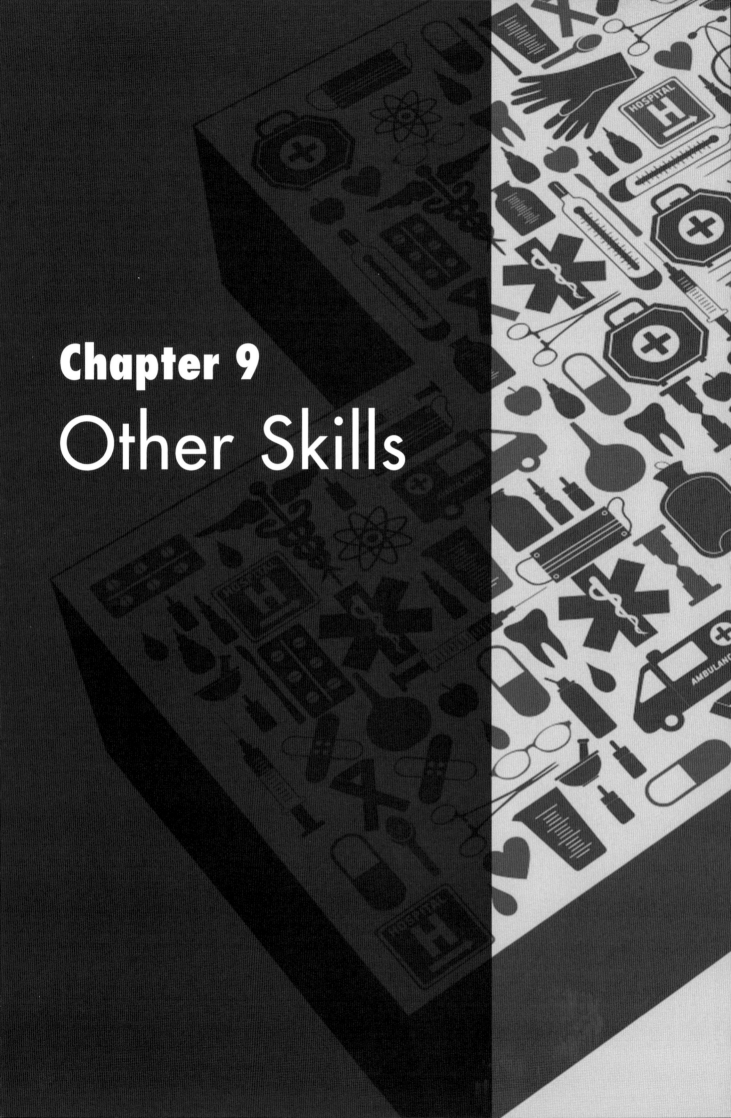

Chapter 9
Other Skills

9.1 | Urinary catheter insertion
John Suringa

Chapter objectives

At the end of this chapter the reader will be able to:

1. Describe the rationale for urinary catheter insertion
2. Safely insert a urinary catheter into a patient
3. Problem solve difficulties with insertion or failure of a catheter to drain

Resources required for this assessment

- Hand decontamination agent
- Disposable gloves
- Sterile urinary catheters
- Adult mannequin for urinary catheter insertion (ideally male and female)
- Urinary drainage bag
- Syringe and normal saline
- Clinical waste bag
- Method of documenting the results

Skill matrix

This assessment requires:
- Infection control (CS 1.3)
- Communication (CS 1.5)
- Consent (CS 1.6)

This assessment is a component of:
- Other skills (Chapter 9)

Introduction

Home care in Australia and New Zealand is increasingly commonplace, including use of devices for gastric feeding and urine retention. Also increasing are emergency calls for ambulance services where these devices have been blocked, are leaking or have even been removed altogether by the patient. In some ambulance services, extended care paramedics are utilised to manage these devices.

Urinary catheters becoming blocked is a common problem, and managing it has traditionally been the responsibility of nursing staff or community care organisations. Prehospital management not only resolves patient difficulties but also decreases the resources required to transport patients for further care. Management of urinary catheters is discussed in this chapter.

Anatomy and physiology

The urinary system has roles in eliminating metabolic waste from the body and maintaining homeostasis. It does this chiefly by filtering blood in the kidney to produce urine. Excreting toxins, acid base regulation, mineral conservation and balancing fluid regulation within the body are all essential urinary system functions.

The urinary system involves the:
- left and right kidneys
- ureters, one from each kidney, both draining into the bladder
- bladder for urine collection
- prostate (in males), which encircles the urethra immediately inferior to the bladder, providing fluid for semen during ejaculation

- urethra, the single outflow tube from the bladder for urine discharge; it has a voluntary and involuntary sphincter to control urine release.

Clinical rationale

The rationale for urinary catheter placement is relief of pain and the adverse effects of urine retention caused by outflow obstruction. The causes of such obstruction include:

- urinary tract infections among all age groups, caused by various bacteria; the urinary system is prone to infection due to the short external urethral opening, particularly females
- enlargement of the male prostate, typically with age
- obstructions such as strictures of the urethra or tumours, blood clots and calculi
- trauma
- abnormalities of the urinary system, such polycystic kidneys or spina bifida
- surgery
- renal failure (chronic or acute).

The aim of inserting a urinary catheter is to allow free drainage from the bladder. The catheter can be temporarily or permanently placed. A variety of catheters are available, the choice of which depends on their intended use.

Indications

The indications for a urinary catheter are:

- to relieve urinary retention (acute or chronic)
- to empty the bladder before surgery or investigations
- to instil medication
- to determine residual volume in the absence of ultrasound equipment
- to irrigate the bladder
- to keep the perineal area dry in order to assist healing
- to determine accurate fluid balance
- to collect a sterile specimen of urine
- for investigations of the lower urinary tract
- for management of intractable incontinence
- to allow healing following surgery on the lower urinary tract
- for the comfort of the terminally ill (Feneley et al., 2015; Meddings et al., 2013).

Urinary drainage systems include the following:

- urodomes, which fit over the penis
- surgical catheters, such as suprapubic catheters
- indwelling catheters, which are introduced through the urethral meatus.

This chapter discusses the latter method.

Urinary catheters come in a range of sizes, which are defined by the French gauge (Fg) scale. The size chosen should fit comfortably into the urethral opening without urine leakage around it. Adults most commonly require a 16–18 Fg catheter. A slightly larger catheter is required for urine that is more viscous or mixed with blood. The silicon type is most commonly used due to its resistance to chemical attack and temperature changes, the lower incidence of encrustation and the prevalence of latex allergies in some patients.

The standard Foley catheter has a straight tip at one end and an open drainage end at the other. There is a small inflatable balloon on some catheters near the distal tip to assist holding it in place after insertion. An inflation connection is found at the proximal drainage end. Saline or sterile water is used to inflate the balloon, typically 5–10 mL; this is printed on the device for reference (Feneley et al., 2015).

Insertion method

The patient should be placed supine in the 'frog leg' position with legs drawn up, knees bent and rotated outwards to either side.

The procedure should be aseptic, with sterile gloves worn and a sterile field created around the patient using drapes from a prepared catheter kit (Barbadoro et al., 2015).

Apply lubricant gel along the catheter distal tip. Ensure the urine drainage bag is connected to the catheter. Pour sterile saline into tray for use.

For males, hold the penis with the non-dominant hand and retract the foreskin if this is present. For females, separate the labia and locate the urethral opening. This hand is now non-sterile and should not perform any other role.

With the sterile hand, clean the urethral area using saline soaked cotton swabs, repeated several times with clean swab each time. Always move the swab away from the urethra, never towards it. For males, swab in a circular fashion; for females, swab downwards, away from the urethra.

Lidocaine 2% local anaesthesia gel can be administered into the urethra using a syringe. Allow several minutes for it to take effect.

For males, hold the penis stretched upright and gently introduce the catheter into the urethra. Advance the catheter slowly until the Y-ports are near the meatus. For females, hold the urethral opening steady and advance in a 30° upward direction. Observe for urine escape from the catheter as confirmation that it is positioned in the bladder, and progress several more centimetres to ensure the inflatable balloon is well clear of the sphincter.

Inflate the balloon with fluid to the specified volume. Gently pull back on the catheter until resistance is felt as the balloon occludes the urethra. Pain on inflation suggests the balloon is within the urethra. It is important to avoid this happening as injury to the urethra can occur (Ghaffary et al., 2013; Willette and Coffield, 2012). If this happens, deflate the balloon, push the catheter in further and reinflate.

Secure the drainage bag to the patient's thigh below the bladder, allowing it to drain.

Contraindications

A urinary catheter should not be inserted if there is traumatic injury to the urinary tract. This is betrayed by blood at the urethra opening or perineal bruising.

Clinical skill assessment process

The following section outlines the clinical skill assessment tools that should be used to determine a student's ability to demonstrate the safe and accurate insertion of a urinary catheter.

1. Clinical Skill Work Instruction
2. Formative Clinical Skill Assessment (F-CSAT)
3. Performance Improvement Plan (PIP)
4. Summative Clinical Skill Assessment (S-CSAT)
(5. Direct Observation of Procedural Skills (DOPS) – see Chapter 1.1)

Clinical Skill Work Instruction

Equipment and resources: Hand decontamination agent; disposable gloves; sterile urinary catheters; adult mannequin for urinary catheter insertion (ideally male and female); urinary drainage bag; syringe and normal saline; clinical waste bag; method of documenting the results

Associated Clinical Skills: Infection control; Communication; Consent

Urinary catheter insertion

Activity	Critical Action	Rationale
Prepare patient	Explain procedure and gain informed consent.	This is an invasive procedure requiring permission and cooperation.
Prepare equipment	Obtain catheterisation pack and drapes. Ensure catheter is the correct size.	Gather all equipment before commencing sterile procedure.
Position patient	Ensure patient privacy. Remove lower garments and place patient supine, with knees drawn up. Place a clean, absorbent towel beneath patient's buttocks.	To allow urethral access and absorb any urine leakage.
Unpack catheter kit	Wash hands with warm water and soap. Unfold pack on surface near to patient. Pour saline into catheterisation pack. Remove catheter from external package and drop on sterile field without touching it.	For ease of use and to maintain sterility.
Hand hygiene	Don sterile gloves.	This is an aseptic procedure.
Prepare equipment	Lay out sterile drapes around insertion area.	To maintain sterile field and asepsis.
Lubricate catheter	Expose insertion end of catheter and lubricate with gel. Maintain sterility. Ensure drainage bag is attached.	To maintain asepsis. Decreases pain and for ease of insertion.
Locate urethral opening	Using non-dominant hand only: • *males:* hold penis upright with non-dominant hand and fold back foreskin • *females:* fold back labia and hold with fingers to expose urethra above the vagina.	Locates urethral opening for insertion.
Clean area	Using forceps and saline moistened cotton, wipe urethral opening. Repeat several times with clean swab each time, moving away from urethra.	Infection prevention.
Insert catheter	Using dominant hand, push catheter tip into urethral opening: • *males:* straight 90° angle • *females:* 30° upward angle. Continue insertion without using force almost until Y junction. Note urine escape.	Ensures correct catheter placement and catheter balloon is inserted beyond urethral sphincter.
Inflate cuff	Using manufacturer's guidelines, inflate the cuff with normal saline. **Stop if pain is felt.** Do not inflate cuff until free flow of urine is observed.	Pain may indicate improper placement or bladder spasm.

Urinary catheter insertion continued		
Activity	**Critical Action**	**Rationale**
Drainage bag	Ensure there are no kinks in the catheter and that urine is flowing freely. Secure drainage tube and bag to leg at a level lower than the bladder.	To ensure effective drainage occurs and reduce risk of inadvertent removal.
Clean up	Discard all used and unused materials and gloves as clinical waste.	To reduce risk of cross-contamination.
Report	Accurately document procedure.	Accurate record kept and continuity of patient care.

Urinary catheter unblocking (non-assessable skill)

Equipment and resources: Sterile water for irrigation solution; 50 mL syringe with catheter tip; antiseptic swabs; waterproof sheet; drainage bag; pair sterile gloves; sterile catheter pack; personal protective equipment

Associated Clinical Skills: Infection control; Communication; Consent

Urinary catheter blockage care		
Activity	**Clinical Action**	**Rationale**
Prepare patient	Explain procedure.	To gain cooperation.
Position patient	Position patient supine. Ensure privacy.	Allows access to catheter.
Hand hygiene	Wash hands with warm water and soap. Don clean gloves.	For infection control.
Prepare equipment	Gather sterile dressing pack or catheter pack with sterile saline, sterile sheet and gloves, and alcohol wipes. Open and lay out equipment, maintaining asepsis.	To maintain aseptic technique.
Prepare syringe	Fill 50 mL catheter tip syringe with sterile saline solution.	For flushing.
Prepare catheter opening	Clean catheter and bag connection with antiseptic, and place waterproof sterile sheet beneath catheter opening. Disconnect drainage bag, ensuring catheter opening remains aseptic.	Prevents infection transmission of bacteria. Keeps patient dry and clean.
Flush catheter	Insert syringe tip into catheter using a twisting motion. Gently flush approximately 30 mL saline into the bladder. At no time use force.	To unblock catheter without trauma.
Withdraw the saline	Draw back the syringe to remove fluid and any foreign particles that have caused the blockage.	Reduces trauma and allows the urine to flow freely.
Repeat procedure	Repeat procedure if necessary. If still unsuccessful, consider changing the catheter.	Until urine flows freely and foreign particles are removed.
Clean up	Discard all used and unused materials and gloves as clinical waste.	To reduce risk of cross-contamination.
Report	Accurately document procedure.	Accurate record kept and continuity of patient care.

Formative Clinical Skill Assessment (F-CSAT)

Equipment and resources: Hand decontamination agent; disposable gloves; sterile urinary catheters; adult mannequin for urinary catheter insertion (ideally male and female); urinary drainage bag; syringe and normal saline; clinical waste bag; method of documenting the results

Associated Clinical Skills: Infection control; Communication; Consent

Staff/Student being assessed: _____

Urinary catheter insertion

Activity	Critical Action	Performance				
Prepares patient	Explains procedure and gains informed consent.	0	1	2	3	4
Prepares equipment	Obtains catheterisation pack and drapes. Ensures catheter is correct size.	0	1	2	3	4
Positions patient	Ensures patient privacy. Removes lower garments and places patient supine with knees drawn up. Places a clean, absorbent towel beneath patient's buttocks.	0	1	2	3	4
Unpacks catheter kit	Washes hands with warm water and soap. Unfolds pack on surface near to patient. Pours saline into catheterisation pack. Removes catheter from external package and drops on sterile field without touching it.	0	1	2	3	4
Hand hygiene	Dons sterile gloves.	0	1	2	3	4
Prepares equipment	Pours saline into catheterisation pack. Lays out sterile drapes around insertion area.	0	1	2	3	4
Lubricates catheter	Removes catheter from pack and lubricates with gel.	0	1	2	3	4
Locates urethral opening	Using non-dominant hand only: • *males:* holds penis upright and folds back foreskin • *females:* folds back labia and holds with fingers to expose urethra above the vagina.	0	1	2	3	4
Cleans area	Using forceps and saline moistened cotton, wipes urethral opening. Repeats several times, with clean swab each time, moving away from urethra.					
Inserts catheter	Using dominant hand, pushes catheter tip into urethral opening: • *males:* straight 90° angle • *females:* 30° upward angle. Continues insertion without using force almost until Y junction. Notes urine escape.	0	1	2	3	4
Inflates cuff	Using manufacturer's guidelines, inflates the cuff with normal saline or sterile water. **Stops if pain is felt.** Does not inflate cuff until free flow of urine is observed.	0	1	2	3	4
Drainage bag	Ensures there are no kinks in the catheter and urine is flowing freely. Secures drainage tube and bag to leg at a level lower than the bladder.	0	1	2	3	4
Cleans up	Discards all used and unused materials and gloves as clinical waste.	0	1	2	3	4
Reports	Accurately documents procedure.	0	1	2	3	4

Note: *Documentation of time and date of catheter change should follow the change of all catheters.*

Standard Achieved: (please circle one)

Competent (C)   Not Yet Competent* (NYC)

Staff/Student Name: _____

Assessor (please print name): _____

Signed (Assessor): _____

Date of Assessment: _____

Comments:

*If Not Yet Competent (NYC) a PIP needs to be completed and a repeat of the F-CSAT

Formative Clinical Skill Assessment (F-CSAT) Key

Skill level	Standard of procedure	Quality of performance	Outcome	Level of assistance required
4 Safe for unsupervised practice	Safe Accurate Behaviour is appropriate to context	Confident Accurate Expedient	Achieved intended outcome	No supporting cues* required
3 Requires supervision	Safe Accurate Behaviour is appropriate to context	Confident Accurate Takes longer than required	Achieved intended outcome	Requires occasional supportive cues*
2 Requires assistance	Safe Accurate Behaviour generally appropriate to context	Lacks certainty	Would not have achieved outcome without support	Requires frequent verbal and occasional physical directives in addition to supportive cues*
1 Requires direction	Safe only with guidance Not completely accurate	Unskilled Inefficient	Would not have achieved outcome without support	Requires continuous verbal and frequent physical directive cues*
0 Unsafe	Unsafe Unable to demonstrate behaviour Lack of insight into behaviour appropriate to context	Unskilled	Would not have achieved outcome	Requires continuous verbal and continuous physical directive cues*

*Refers to physical directives or verbal supportive cues

Performance Improvement Plan (PIP)

Please document the agreed education plan and completion timelines for areas assessed as less than 4.

This plan should be presented to assessor prior to commencement of summative assessment.

Where was supervisor support required?	Student summary of deficit. (Why was there a problem?)	Improvement Plan	Completed (Y/N)

Staff/Student Name: _____

Staff/Student Signature: _____

Educator Name: _____

Educator Signature: _____

Summative Clinical Skill Assessment (S-CSAT)

Equipment and resources: Hand decontamination agent; disposable gloves; sterile urinary catheters; adult mannequin for urinary catheter insertion (ideally male and female); urinary drainage bag; syringe and normal saline; clinical waste bag; method of documenting the results

Associated Clinical Skills: Infection control; Communication; Consent

Staff/Student being assessed: _____

• Completed Formative Clinical Skill Assessment (F-CSAT):   **YES   NO**

• Completed Performance Improvement Plan (PIP):   **YES   NO   N/A**

Urinary catheter insertion			
Activity	**Critical Action**	**Achieved Without Direction**	
Prepares patient	Explains procedure and gains informed consent.	NO	YES
Prepares equipment	Obtains catheterisation pack and drapes. Ensures catheter is correct size.	NO	YES
Positions patient	Ensures patient privacy. Removes lower garments and places patient supine, with knees drawn up. Places a clean, absorbent towel beneath patient's buttocks.	NO	YES
Unpacks catheter kit	Washes hands with warm water and soap. Unfolds pack on surface near to patient.	NO	YES
Hand hygiene	Dons sterile gloves.	NO	YES
Prepares equipment	Pours saline into catheterisation pack. Lays out sterile drapes around insertion area.	NO	YES

Urinary catheter insertion continued

Activity	Critical Action	Achieved Without Direction	
Lubricates catheter	Removes catheter from pack and lubricates with gel.	NO	YES
Locates urethral opening	Using non-dominant hand only: • *males:* holds penis upright and folds back foreskin • *females:* folds back labia and holds with fingers to expose urethra above the vagina.	NO	YES
Cleans area	Using forceps and saline moistened cotton, wipes urethral opening. Repeats several times, with a clean swab each time, moving away from urethra.	NO	YES
Inserts catheter	Using dominant hand, pushes catheter tip into urethral opening: • *males:* straight 90° angle • *females:* 30° upward angle. Continues insertion without using force almost until Y junction. Notes urine escape.	NO	YES
Inflates cuff	Using manufacturer's guidelines, inflates the cuff with normal saline or sterile water. **Stops if pain is felt.** Does not inflate cuff until free flow of urine is observed.	NO	YES
Drainage bag	Ensures there are no kinks in the catheter and urine is flowing freely. Secures drainage tube and bag to leg at a level lower than the bladder.	NO	YES
Cleans up	Discards all used and unused materials and gloves as clinical waste.	NO	YES
Reports	Accurately documents procedure.	NO	YES

Standard Achieved: (please circle one)

Competent (C)   Not Yet Competent* (NYC)

Staff/Student Name: _____

Assessor (please print name): _____

Signed (Assessor): _____

Date of Assessment: _____

Comments:

*If Not Yet Competent (NYC) a PIP needs to be completed and a repeat of the F-CSAT

Clinical findings

Unable to insert catheter

It can be difficult to insert catheters into some patients, particularly men. If the catheter will only proceed a short distance (<16 cm in adults), this may be due to spasm of the urethral meatus or stricture of the urethra. Consider reattempting the procedure with a smaller diameter catheter or having the patient take a few deep breaths to relax the voluntary sphincter. If the blockage is further along, prostatic obstruction is more likely the problem.

Flush a smaller catheter with saline as it is advanced. If still unsuccessful, the attempt may have to be abandoned (Gardi et al., 2013; Harkin et al., 1998; Villanueva and Hemstreet, 2008).

Catheter not draining after insertion

If the catheter is not draining, it may not be inserted far enough, it may be blocked by sediment or blood clots or there may be a kink in it. Ensure the insertion depth is correct and adjust it if necessary. If a blockage is suspected, attempt gentle flushing. Occasionally, bladder spasm may occur; this is betrayed by pain and a sudden urge to urinate, which usually settles without medication. The bladder may be empty of urine.

Drainage bags

There are different types of drainage bag that can be fitted, including smaller leg bags or larger hooked bags for attaching to a bed. They all must hang lower than the bladder for drainage. Urine quality and volume can be assessed from these bags. They should be kept clean and periodically emptied, making note of the drained volume. When transporting patients in ambulances, empty the drainage bag before commencing the trip and protect it from damage and contamination.

Catheter care

Catheter insertion is the most common source of infection acquired in a healthcare facility, and the risk of infection increases with the duration of catheter placement. Asepsis on insertion and during ongoing care and limiting the duration of placement are key to minimising infection (Nicolle, 2014; Chenoweth et al., 2014; Meddings et al., 2013).

Catheters interfere with the normal cycle of bladder filling and emptying. This leads to urine pooling, inadequate urethral flushing and biofilm development along the catheter lining, where infection grows (Feneley et al., 2015; Stickler, 2014).

To minimise the risk of infection:

- cleanse the urethral opening and the catheter itself
- disconnect the drainage bag from the catheter only with clean hands
- disconnect the drainage bag as seldom as possible
- keep the drainage bag connector clean
- use a thin catheter where possible to reduce the risk of harm to the urethra during insertion
- encourage the patient to drink sufficient liquid to produce at least 2 litres of urine daily.

PRACTICE TIP!

If you encounter any difficulty during urinary catheter insertion, consider an algorithm to respond. Is there sufficient lubricant? Is the insertion immediately blocked, necessitating a smaller catheter size? Might a saline flush during advancement help?

If the attempt at insertion is still unsuccessful, it may have to be abandoned.

PRACTICE TIP!

The decision to replace or clear a blockage of a urinary catheter involves several factors:

- the ease with which the blockage can be cleared
- the paramedic's skill in the procedure
- the catheterisation equipment available
- patient compliance.

PRACTICE TIP!

This procedure can be emotionally distressing for patients. Ensure explanation, reassurance, privacy and respect are all at the forefront. Consider the possibility of using clinicians who are the same sex as the patient if this is requested.

PRACTICE TIP!

Insertion of an indwelling catheter is a sterile procedure. All non-sterile support actions can be provided by an assistant away from the sterile field or prepared in advance.

TEST YOUR KNOWLEDGE QUESTIONS

1. **Why are urinary catheters a primary source of urinary tract infections?**
   Urine pooling; inadequate urethral flushing; development of catheter biofilm.

2. **List three common reasons for urinary catheter insertion.**
   To: relieve urinary retention; empty the bladder before surgery or investigations; instil medication; determine residual volume; irrigate the bladder; keep the perineal area dry in order to assist healing; determine accurate fluid balance; collect a urine specimen; investigate the lower urinary tract; relieve intractable incontinence; allow healing following lower urinary tract surgery; provide comfort for the terminally ill (Feneley et al., 2015; Meddings et al., 2013).

3. **List three types of urinary drainage system.**
   Urodome; suprapubic; indwelling.

4. **What is the contraindication for urinary catheter insertion?**
   Traumatic urinary tract injury, betrayed by blood at the urethral opening or perineal bruising.

5. **What are four possible reasons for a urinary catheter not draining after insertion?**
   The catheter is not inserted in far enough; it is blocked by sediment/blood clots; bladder spasm; there is no urine in the bladder.

6. **What are the two ports at the proximal urinary catheter end for?**
   One is for urine drainage, the other for cuff inflation.

7. **What finding suggests the balloon is incorrectly placed in the urethra?**
   Pain on inflation.

8. **List three reasons for difficulty inserting a urinary catheter.**
   Urethral meatus spasm; urethral stricture; prostatic obstruction.

9. **How is the urinary catheter cuff filled?**
   Using 5–10 mL sterile water or normal saline.

10. **List three options to assist difficulty inserting urinary catheters.**
    Using a smaller diameter catheter; having the patient take a few deep breaths to relax the voluntary sphincter; flushing the catheter with saline as it is advanced.

References

Barbadoro, P., Labricciosa, F.M., Recanatini, C., Gori, G., Tirabassi, F., Martini, E., Gioia, M.G., D'errico, M.M. and Prospero, E., 2015. Catheter-associated urinary tract infection: Role of the setting of catheter insertion. *American Journal of Infection Control*, 43(7), 707–710.

Chenoweth, C.E., Gould, C.V. and Saint, S., 2014. Diagnosis, management, and prevention of catheter-associated urinary tract infections. *Infectious Disease Clinics*, 28(1), 105–119.

Feneley, R.C., Hopley, I.B. and Wells, P.N., 2015. Urinary catheters: history, current status, adverse events and research agenda. *Journal of Medical Engineering & Technology*, 39(8), 459–470.

Gardi, M., Balta, G.M., Repele, M., Zanovello, N., Betto, G., Fracalanza, S., Battenello, W., Santoni, B., Secco, S., Agostini, A. and dal Bianco, M., 2013. The challenge of difficult catheterisation in men: a novel technique and review of the literature. *UroToday International Journal*, 6(4).

Ghaffary, C., Yohannes, A., Villanueva, C. and Leslie, S.W., 2013. A practical approach to difficult urinary catheterizations. *Current Urology Reports*, 14(6), 565–579.

Harkin, D.W., Hawe, M. and Pyper, P., 1998. A novel technique for difficult male urethral catheterization. *British Journal of Urology*, 82, 752–753.

Meddings, J., Rogers, M.A., Krein, S.L., Fakih, M.G., Olmsted, R.N. and Saint, S., 2013. Reducing unnecessary urinary catheter use and other strategies to prevent catheter-associated urinary tract infection: an integrative review. *BMJ Quality & Safety*, 23(4), 277–289.

Nicolle, L.E., 2014. Catheter associated urinary tract infections. *Antimicrobial Resistance and Infection Control*, 3(1), 23.

Stickler, D.J., 2014. Clinical complications of urinary catheters caused by crystalline biofilms: something needs to be done. *Journal of Internal Medicine*, 276(2), 120–129.

Villanueva, C. and Hemstreet III, G.P., 2008. Difficult male urethral catheterization: a review of different approaches. *International Brazilian Journal of Urology*, 34(4), 401–412.

Willette, P.A. and Coffield, S., 2012. Current trends in the management of difficult urinary catheterizations. *Western Journal of Emergency Medicine*, 13(6), 472.

Chapter objectives

At the end of this chapter the reader will be able to:

1. Describe the clinical rationale for applying pressure bandaging and immobilisation (PBI)
2. Identify the indications and contraindications for PBI application
3. Demonstrate the safe and effective application of PBI

Resources required for this assessment

- Standardised patient or mannequin (simulated bite/sting marks optional)
- Hand decontamination agent
- Broad elasticised compression bandages (approximately 15 cm wide)
- Equipment to immobilise limb (e.g. cardboard/formable splint, triangular bandages) or to immobilise patient (e.g. vacuum mattress)
- Tape
- Pen or marker
- Method of documenting results

Skill matrix

This assessment requires:

- Infection control (CS 1.3)
- Communication (CS 1.5)
- Consent (CS 1.6)

This assessment is a component of:

- Other skills (Chapter 9)

Introduction

Australian toxicologist Professor Struan Sutherland and colleagues proposed pressure bandaging and immobilisation as treatment for Australian venomous snakebite in 1979 (Sutherland et al., 1979). The principle is that toxins and other substances in venom can be slowed or stopped from reaching the circulation by application of pressure bandaging to the affected limb and immobilisation (PBI) of the patient (Dart and White, 2015). Some of the toxic substances can be inactivated in situ in the tissues, and others can be delayed from having systemic effects until the patient's arrival at an appropriate facility where resuscitation and antivenom can be administered if

required (White, 2013). PBI is not definitive treatment, but it can 'buy time' to reach definitive care.

While there is currently no high-grade evidence supporting the use of PBI, it remains considered best practice and is taught and used widely in Australia (Currie et al., 2008). However, it is not standard practice in many international medical systems (Bowers and Mustain, 2011; Warrell, 2010), in part due to the differing mechanisms of action of venoms (such as local tissue necrosis and molecular weight) of different types of snake (Seifert et al., 2011).

Venomous Australian snakes belong to the Elapidae family. This includes the brown snake, tiger snake, black snake, death adder, taipan and sea snake venom groups (White, 2013). While there are no snakes of medical importance native to New Zealand (Isbister, 2015), Australian snakes do make their way to New Zealand shores in shipping containers, and this is becoming an increasing problem for local authorities (Chapple et al., 2016). PBI should be applied to all suspected or confirmed Australian native snakebites to limbs (ARC, 2011a). Though this chapter refers predominantly to snakebite, the use of PBI is also recommended by expert consensus opinion for funnel-web spider bites (and bites from related species – check local information) (ARC, 2014), blue-ringed octopus bites and cone shell stings (ARC, 2011b). The Poisons Information Centre can be consulted on 13 11 26 in Australia or 0800 764 766 in New Zealand for advice on bites and stings from other creatures, including exotic snake species, that may benefit from PBI.

As this chapter is designed for paramedic professionals, aspects of the PBI described may vary from that taught in first aid courses to laypersons. In this context, PBI consists of two essential components:
1. pressure bandaging of the entire affected limb
2. immobilisation of the affected limb and immobilisation of the whole patient (if possible).

Anatomy and physiology

Australian snake venom consists of various toxins of different molecular weights. Once injected, most of these toxins are absorbed by the lymphatic system and travel towards the central circulation in the low-pressure lymphatic vessels. Application of a pressure bandage compresses these lymphatic vessels and superficial veins, retarding the movement of toxins (White, 2013). Immobilisation of the affected limb and the entire patient further reduces lymphatic drainage, slowing or stopping the spread of venom (CSL, 2005).

Clinical rationale

The majority of snakebites are 'dry bites', where no venom is injected (Isbister et al., 2013) or the venom injected is of insufficient quantity to have significant effects (White, 2013). The bite site may appear as a single or pair of puncture marks, a scratch or a bleeding wound (White, 2013).

Do not attempt to catch or kill the snake or other animal. If possible, record a description of the creature and its exact location and provide this to the receiving facility to assist species determination. For a suspected snakebite, a venom detection kit (VDK) can be used to identify the venom if required (White, 2013). If the animal has already been killed, take a photograph of the dead snake from a safe distance and show it to the hospital staff as it may aid in the overall identification of the snake genus.

Reassure and calm the patient. Explain the importance of them keeping any bitten limbs immobile as well as keeping themselves as still as practicable to reduce anxiety and movement, which increases cardiac output and venom circulation.

Immediately immobilise the patient in a comfortable position and do not allow them to walk (Queensland Ambulance Service, 2016), as even small amounts of walking have been shown to increase venom movement towards the central circulation (Howarth, 1994). Skeletal muscle movement promotes lymphatic drainage by way of mechanical pumping action of the muscles. Ensure the whole patient is immobilised, not just the affected limb (Currie et al., 2008; Isbister et al., 2013). A vacuum mattress can assist in immobilising the whole patient (if available).

Where possible, the site of the bite or sting should be kept below the level of the heart to minimise movement of venom with gravity towards the central circulation. A semi-recumbent position on a stretcher in an immobilising vacuum mattress is ideal.

Do not wash, cut or suction the wound. Do not apply ice or heat to the wound, or apply an arterial tourniquet. There is no evidence to support using any of these techniques. They may cause further harm by delaying identification of the venom, creating further tissue destruction at the site or causing tissue ischaemia (Avau et al., 2016).

Perform hand hygiene and follow standard precautions for all patients (WHO, 2006).

Remove any jewellery worn on the affected limb. There is a risk of oedema developing after PB application, which could cause digit ischaemia.

Removing the patient's clothing can increase muscle movement and lymphatic flow. Instead, cut off the clothing without moving the patient. If doing so is difficult and likely to result in significant limb movement, apply bandages over the top of the clothing instead.

Select a broad, elasticised compression bandage, preferably 15 cm wide (Vlad and Guthrie, 2016). Elasticised bandages maintain required compression more effectively than non-elasticised crepe bandages, especially during transport (Canale et al., 2009). Apply the bandage over the entire affected limb. Commence distally and work proximally as this improves patient comfort and does not increase the movement of venom. Ensure the tips of the digits are left exposed (Fig. 9.2.1). Use tape to firmly secure the bandage (Brinton and Fenton, 2016).

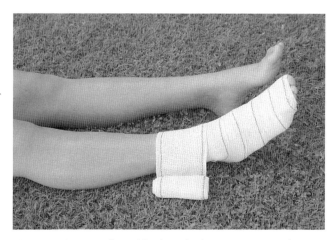

Figure 9.2.1 Bandaged limb with digit tips exposed

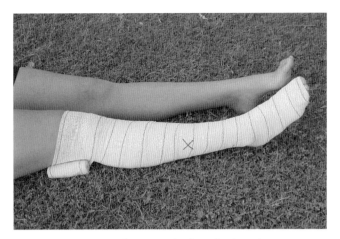

Figure 9.2.2 Wound site marked on the bandage

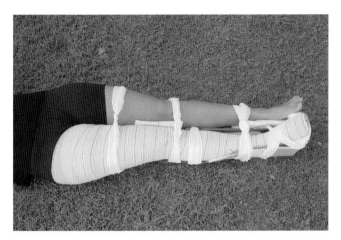

Figure 9.2.4 Limb immobilised using an appropriate splint

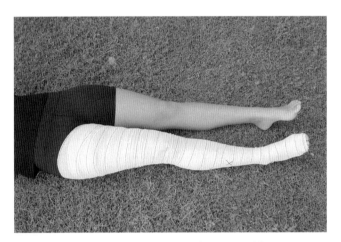

Figure 9.2.3 Limb covered as much as possible to groin or axilla

Identify the wound site on the top layer of bandaging, using a pen or marker (Fig. 9.2.2). This is helpful for the receiving facility to locate the wound and identify the type of venom by swab for VDK use (Stewart, 2003).

Cover as much of the affected limb as possible (St John Ambulance Australia, 2014) (Fig. 9.2.3). You should not easily be able to slide a finger underneath the bandage. The bandage should be applied firmly enough to reduce lymphatic drainage but still allow arterial circulation. Aim for the firmness of a bandage for a sprained ankle (NSW Ambulance, 2016).

Perform neurovascular observations regularly on the exposed digits. If the patient complains of severe pain, the limb may be becoming ischaemic. Removing the pressure bandage could result in rapid release of the toxin. Where possible, use non-opiate-based analgesia initially to avoid potentiating respiratory depression that can result from neurotoxic venoms.

Use an appropriate (e.g. cardboard) splint to completely immobilise the affected limb (Fig. 9.2.4). If the wound is on a lower limb, immobilise the lower limbs together. If the wound is on an upper limb, the bandaged arm may be held straight and splinted to the patient's body using triangular bandages (or kept inside a vacuum mattress if available). An arm sling is not indicated during transport

as this can cause skeletal muscle contraction and elevates the wound above the heart. It can also create a tourniquet effect at the elbow.

The patient may require extrication equipment and techniques, such as a rescue stretcher, to maintain immobilisation. Application of PBI is time-critical and takes precedence over patient extrication (Currie et al., 2008).

After the application of PBI, all potential snakebite victims should be transported promptly to a receiving facility that has antivenom available (Weber and Johnson, 2015). The PBI should only be removed after medical review and antivenom has been administered, where appropriate, or where there are no signs of envenomation (Isbister, 2006). This may take up to 12 hours to become fully apparent (Ireland et al., 2010; Isbister et al., 2013).

Indications for PBI

PBI must only be used on a limb for:
- Australian native terrestrial and marine snakebites
- funnel-web spider bites (and bites from related species – check local information)
- blue-ringed octopus bites
- cone shell stings (ARC, 2011b).

Contraindications for PBI

PBI must not be used for:
- other spider bites (e.g. redback spider)
- jellyfish stings
- any other stings or bites from marine or terrestrial animals (unless recommended by a Poisons Information Centre)
- non-Australian elapid snakes unless specifically approved.

In each case, local complications or non-neurotoxic venom makes PBI unlikely to be effective (ARC, 2011b).

Clinical skill assessment process

The following section outlines the clinical skill assessment tools that should be used to determine a student's ability to demonstrate safe and accurate pressure bandaging and immobilisation.

1. Clinical Skill Work Instruction
2. Formative Clinical Skill Assessment (F-CSAT)
3. Performance Improvement Plan (PIP)
4. Summative Clinical Skill Assessment (S-CSAT)
(5. Direct Observation of Procedural Skills (DOPS) – see Chapter 1.1)

Clinical Skill Work Instruction

Equipment and resources: Standardised patient or mannequin (simulated bite/sting marks optional); hand decontamination agent; broad elasticised compression bandages (approximately 15 cm wide); equipment to immobilise limb (e.g. splint, triangular bandages) or to immobilise patient (e.g. vacuum mattress); tape; pen or marker; method of documenting results

Associated Clinical Skills: Infection control; Communication; Consent

Pressure bandaging and immobilisation

Activity	Critical Action	Rationale
Immobilise patient	Immobilise patient in a semi-recumbent position. Do not allow them to walk.	Reduces skeletal muscle movement and retards lymphatic drainage. Semi-recumbent posture may help attenuate nausea and overstimulation of sympathetic nervous system.
Reassurance	Reassure and calm patient.	Reduces sympathetic activation and circulation pressures.
Assess for wound	Assess area where the patient reports being bitten or stung.	To locate possible wound.
Remove jewellery	Carefully remove any jewellery from affected limb.	Swelling may result from the compression bandage or a reaction to the bite/sting.
Apply pressure bandage	Cut off clothing.	Removing it may increase movement.
	Apply a firm, broad pressure spiralling bandage over entire limb. Commence distally and work proximally, leaving digit tips exposed.	Limb compression may slow toxin movement.
	Identify wound using pen/marker.	For later VDK swabbing.
Apply splint	Use an appropriate splint to immobilise limb (or vacuum mattress to immobilise whole patient if available).	Limb/patient immobilisation may slow movement of the toxin.
Assess distal circulation	Assess the exposed digits regularly for adequate circulation.	Bandaging should be firm enough to restrict lymphatic flow but still allow arterial circulation.
Report	Document/hand over details of type, time and site of bite/sting.	Accurate record kept and continuity of patient care.

Source: *Adapted from ARC, 2011a.*

Formative Clinical Skill Assessment (F-CSAT)

Equipment and resources: Standardised patient or mannequin (simulated bite/sting marks optional); hand decontamination agent; broad elasticised compression bandages (approximately 15 cm wide); equipment to immobilise limb (e.g. splint, triangular bandages) or to immobilise patient (e.g. vacuum mattress); tape; pen or marker; method of documenting results

Associated Clinical Skills: Infection control; Communication; Consent

Staff/Student being assessed: _____

Pressure bandaging and immobilisation

Activity	Critical Action	Performance				
Immobilises patient	Immobilises patient in a semi-recumbent position. Does not allow them to walk.	0	1	2	3	4
Reassurance	Reassures and calms patient.	0	1	2	3	4
Assesses for wound	Performs thorough assessment of area where the patient reports being bitten or stung.	0	1	2	3	4
Removes jewellery	Carefully removes any jewellery from the affected limb.	0	1	2	3	4
Applies pressure bandage	Cuts off clothing. Applies firm broad pressure spiralling bandage over entire limb. Commences distally and works proximally, leaving digit tips exposed. Identifies wound using pen/marker.	0	1	2	3	4
Applies splint	Uses an appropriate splint to immobilise the limb (or vacuum mattress to immobilise whole patient).	0	1	2	3	4
Assesses distal circulation	Assesses exposed digits regularly for adequate circulation.	0	1	2	3	4
Reports	Documents/hands over details of type, time and site of bite/sting.	0	1	2	3	4

Source: *Adapted from ARC, 2011a.*

Standard Achieved: (please circle one)

Competent (C)   Not Yet Competent* (NYC)

Staff/Student Name: _____

Assessor (please print name): _____

Signed (Assessor): _____

Date of Assessment: _____

Comments:

*If Not Yet Competent (NYC) a PIP needs to be completed and a repeat of the F-CSAT

Formative Clinical Skill Assessment (F-CSAT) Key

Skill level	Standard of procedure	Quality of performance	Outcome	Level of assistance required
4 Safe for unsupervised practice	Safe Accurate Behaviour is appropriate to context	Confident Accurate Expedient	Achieved intended outcome	No supporting cues* required
3 Requires supervision	Safe Accurate Behaviour is appropriate to context	Confident Accurate Takes longer than required	Achieved intended outcome	Requires occasional supportive cues*
2 Requires assistance	Safe Accurate Behaviour generally appropriate to context	Lacks certainty	Would not have achieved outcome without support	Requires frequent verbal and occasional physical directives in addition to supportive cues*
1 Requires direction	Safe only with guidance Not completely accurate	Unskilled Inefficient	Would not have achieved outcome without support	Requires continuous verbal and frequent physical directive cues*
0 Unsafe	Unsafe Unable to demonstrate behaviour Lack of insight into behaviour appropriate to context	Unskilled	Would not have achieved outcome	Requires continuous verbal and continuous physical directive cues*

*Refers to physical directives or verbal supportive cues

Performance Improvement Plan (PIP)

Please document the agreed education plan and completion timelines for areas assessed as less than 4.

This plan should be presented to assessor prior to commencement of summative assessment.

Where was supervisor support required?	Student summary of deficit. (Why was there a problem?)	Improvement Plan	Completed (Y/N)

Staff/Student Name: _____

Staff/Student Signature: _____

Educator Name: _____

Educator Signature: _____

Summative Clinical Skill Assessment (S-CSAT)

Equipment and resources: Standardised patient or mannequin (simulated bite/sting marks optional); hand decontamination agent; broad elasticised compression bandages (approximately 15 cm wide); equipment to immobilise limb (e.g. splint, triangular bandages) or to immobilise patient (e.g. vacuum mattress); tape; pen or marker; method of documenting results

Associated Clinical Skills: Infection control; Communication; Consent

Staff/Student being assessed: _____

- Completed Formative Clinical Skill Assessment (F-CSAT):   **YES**   **NO**

- Completed Performance Improvement Plan (PIP):   **YES**   **NO**   **N/A**

Pressure bandaging and immobilisation

Activity	Critical Action	Achieved Without Direction	
Immobilises patient	Immobilises patient in a semi-recumbent position. Does not allow the patient to walk.	NO	YES
Reassurance	Reassures and calms patient.	NO	YES
Assesses for wound	Performs thorough assessment of the area where the patient reports being bitten or stung.	NO	YES
Removes jewellery	Carefully removes any jewellery from the affected limb.	NO	YES
Applies pressure bandage	Cuts off clothing. Applies firm broad pressure spiralling bandage over entire limb. Commences distally and works proximally, leaving digit tips exposed. Identifies wound using pen/marker.	NO	YES
Applies splint	Uses appropriate splint to immobilise limb (or vacuum mattress to immobilise whole patient).	NO	YES
Assesses distal circulation	Assesses exposed digits regularly for adequate circulation.	NO	YES
Reports	Document/hands over details of type, time and site of bite/sting.	NO	YES

Source: *Adapted from ARC, 2011a.*

Standard Achieved: (please circle one)

Competent (C)   Not Yet Competent* (NYC)

Staff/Student Name: _____

Assessor (please print name)**:** _____

Signed (Assessor)**:** _____

Date of Assessment: _____

Comments:

*If Not Yet Competent (NYC) a PIP needs to be completed and a repeat of the F-CSAT

Clinical findings

If the PBI method is applied correctly, the patient should not subsequently develop any signs and symptoms before arriving at hospital. A pressure bandage applied more than 4 hours after the bite or sting occurs is unlikely to be effective (Isbister et al., 2013).

Non-limb bites and stings

Bites and stings on areas of the body other than limbs require varied management. The patient should be kept immobile. Pressure may be applied directly over the site but this may not be effective. If practical, consider keeping the bitten/stung areas lower than, or at least no higher than, the heart in order to retard venom movement towards the central circulation.

Patient deterioration

If applied correctly, PBI should ensure there is no further deterioration in the patient's condition or onset of any new clinical signs. Where this is not the case, consider whether the bandage has been applied firmly enough. Do not remove the bandage to retighten it; instead, apply a firmer pressure bandage over the top. Failure to apply a bandage with sufficient firmness is commonly observed (Avau et al., 2016).

Anaphylaxis

Severe allergic reaction can uncommonly occur due to the nature of protein-based venom and to the antivenom itself. This may be difficult to differentiate from venom toxicity. It is treated with adrenaline in a similar way to any other anaphylaxis (Isbister et al., 2013). The PBI method should not be changed despite this.

PRACTICE TIP!

If a patient reports, 'It was only a little snake that bit me', don't treat the bite as any less dangerous or venomous. Juvenile or hatchling snakebites may be no less dangerous than bites from mature snakes.

PRACTICE TIP!

More is missed by not looking than not knowing! Consider envenomation and conduct a thorough head-to-toe assessment on any patient showing unexplained signs consistent with neurotoxicity or coagulopathy, or general systemic signs of envenomation. Snakebites have occurred in unusual places without a patient realising they have been bitten!

PRACTICE TIP!

PBI is recommended for all Australian native snakebites, but may cause harm if used for bites by exotic, non-native snake species. Exotic snakes are often kept as pets in home vivariums. If you are unsure whether PBI is indicated, call the Poisons Information Centre on 13 11 26 in Australia or 0800 764 766 in New Zealand.

PRACTICE TIP!

One of the first specific clinical signs of snake envenomation may be ptosis (drooping eyelids), where neurotoxic-acting venom is involved. Be aware of this sign and be alert for other signs of evolving paralysis, usually beginning in the cranial nerves and descending, often resulting in the loss of airway reflexes. A patient may require ventilation for an extended period.

PRACTICE TIP!

Coagulopathy causing sudden cardiac arrest from transient coronary thrombosis is thought to be a leading cause of Australian deaths from snakebite. Cardiac monitoring is an essential adjunct for management of a suspected snakebite victim.

TEST YOUR KNOWLEDGE QUESTIONS

1. **What is the preferred minimum width of a bandage to be used for pressure bandaging?**
   The preferred minimum width is 10 cm, but ideally 15 cm wide.

2. **How tight should a pressure bandage be applied?**
   Firm enough to reduce lymphatic drainage but still allow arterial circulation. Aim for the firmness of a bandage for a sprained ankle. Once applied, you should not easily be able to slide a finger underneath the bandage.

3. **A farmer has been bitten on the calf muscle by a snake. He then killed the animal. His leg has been pressure bandaged and he is immobilised on a stretcher in the ambulance. His wife wishes to follow in the family car to the hospital. What should be done with the dead snake?**
   Leave the dead snake alone. Take a photograph of it from a safe distance and show this to the hospital staff, as it may aid in identifying the snake.

4. **A patient in the Blue Mountains of New South Wales reports being bitten by a large black spider on the finger approximately 15 minutes ago. The patient is conscious but now complaining of nausea and headache and is vomiting. They have no first aid established. What is your initial first aid management?**
   Immobilise and reassure the patient. Remove any jewellery from the limb, apply a pressure bandage and immobilise the limb (and the entire patient if possible). Transport the patient to an appropriate facility urgently for ongoing care.

5. **A tourniquet has been applied by a well-meaning first-aider just below a patient's knee after a snakebite. What action should you take?**
   Initially leave the tourniquet in situ as sudden release may worsen the patient's condition. Contact your usual medical control or the Poisons Information Centre for advice on further management.

6. **A patient offers to get up from the ground to walk a very short distance to the stretcher after a suspected snakebite to the foot. What advice should you give them?**
   Explain it is vital they stay still and not move, as even small movements can promote the distribution of venom. Paramedics will arrange to move them to the stretcher instead.

7. **A patient reports being bitten by a hatchling brown snake on the wrist 30 minutes ago. They feel fine and do not want to go to hospital. How should you respond?**
   Hatchling snakebites are just as dangerous as those from mature snakes and the onset of symptoms may take hours. PBI and appropriate hospital assessment is strongly advised.

8. **How is the venom of most Australian snakes thought to be transported around the body?**
   Venom is mostly absorbed into and then transported around the body via the lymphatic system. Lymphatic flow is reliant on muscle movement.

9. **A bandage has been applied by a first-aider to a patient's arm following suspected snakebite. It is clearly loose and does not cover the entire arm length. What should you do?**
   Do not remove the existing bandage. Apply a new pressure bandage in the normal method over the top of the existing bandage.

10. **You are bandaging a patient's leg following a suspected blue-ringed octopus bite. You run out of bandage just above the patient's knee. What should you do?**
    Continue with a new bandage from where the previous bandage finished and continue it all the way up to the groin.

References

ARC (Australian Resuscitation Council), 2011a. *Guideline 9.4.1: Envenomation – Australian snake bite*. Retrieved from: https://resus.org.au/download/9_4_envenomation/guideline_9-4-1-july11.pdf

ARC (Australian Resuscitation Council), 2011b. *Guideline 9.4.8: Envenomation – pressure immobilisation technique*. Retrieved from: https://resus.org.au/download/9_4_envenomation/guideline-9-4-8-aug11.pdf

ARC (Australian Resuscitation Council), 2014. *Guideline 9.4.2: Envenomation – spider bite*. Retrieved from: https://resus.org.au/download/9_4_envenomation/guideline-9-4-2-july-2014.pdf

Avau, B., Borra, V., Vandekerckhove, P. and de Buck, E., 2016. The treatment of snake bites in a first aid setting: a systematic review. *PLoS Neglected Tropical Diseases*, 10(10), 1–20.

Bowers, R.C. and Mustain, M.V., 2011. Disorders due to physical & environmental agents. In Stone, C. and Humphries, R. (eds), *Current diagnosis & treatment: emergency medicine*, 7th edn (Volume 30). New York: McGraw-Hill.

Brinton, J. and Fenton, W., 2016. Clinical skills. In Curtis, K. and Ramsden, C. (eds), *Emergency and trauma care for nurses and paramedics*, 2nd edn. Sydney: Elsevier.

Canale, E., Isbister, G.K. and Currie, B.J., 2009. Investigating pressure bandaging for snakebite in a simulated setting: bandage type, training and the effect of transport. *Emergency Medicine Australasia*, 21(3), 184–190.

Chapple, D.G., Knegtmans, J., Kikillus, H. and Van Winkel, D., 2016. Biosecurity of exotic reptiles and amphibians in New Zealand: building upon Tony Whitaker's legacy. *Journal of the Royal Society of New Zealand*, 46(1), 66–84.

CSL, 2005. Principles of first aid for snakebite. *In CSL antivenom handbook*. Retrieved from: http://www.toxinology.com/generic_static_files/cslavh_first_aid.html

Currie, B.J., Canale, E. and Isbister, G.K., 2008. Effectiveness of pressure-immobilization first aid for snakebite requires further study. *Emergency Medicine Australasia*, 20(3), 267–270.

Dart, R.C. and White, J., 2015. Reptile bites. In Cline, D.M., Ma, O.J., Meckler, G., Tintinalli, J., Stapczynski, J. and Yealy, D. (eds), *Tintinalli's emergency medicine: a comprehensive study guide*, 8th edn. New York: McGraw-Hill.

Howarth, D., Southee, A. and Whyte, I., 1994. Lymphatic flow rates and first-aid in simulated peripheral snake or spider envenomation. *Medical Journal of Australia*, 161, 695–700.

Ireland, G., Brown, S.G., Buckley, N.A., Stormer, J., Currie, B.J., White, J., Spain, D. and Isbister, G.K., 2010. Changes in serial laboratory test results in snakebite patients: when can we safely exclude envenoming? *Medical Journal of Australia*, 193(5), 285–290.

Isbister, G., 2006. Snake bite: a current approach to management. *Australian Prescriber*, 29(5), 125–129.

Isbister, G., 2015. Snakebite. In Cameron, P., Jelinek, G., Kelly, A., Bronw, A. and Little, M. (eds), *Textbook of adult emergency medicine*, 4th edn. London: Churchill Livingstone.

Isbister, G.K., Brown, S.G.A., Page, C.B., McCoubrie, D.L., Greene, S.L. and Buckley, N.A., 2013. Snakebite in Australia: a practical approach to diagnosis and treatment. *Medical Journal of Australia*, 199(11), 763–768.

NSW Ambulance, 2016. *Bandaging – compression bandage*. Retrieved from: http://www.ambulance.nsw.gov.au/media/docs/Snake%20bites%202016-534b9e15-595b-45c0-afde-6abfadb23a78-0.pdf

Queensland Ambulance Service, 2016. *Toxicology and toxinology/snake bite*. Retrieved from: https://www.ambulance.qld.gov.au/docs/clinical/cpg/CPG_Snakebite.pdf

Seifert, S.A., White, J. and Currie, B.J., 2011. Commentary: pressure bandaging for North American snake bite? No! *Journal of Medical Toxicology*, 7(4), 324–326.

St John Ambulance Australia, 2014. *Snake bite*. Retrieved from: http://stjohn.org.au/assets/uploads/factsheets/english/FS_snakebite.pdf

Stewart, C.J., 2003. Snake bite in Australia: first aid and envenomation management. *Accident and Emergency Nursing*, 11(2), 106–111.

Sutherland, S., Coulter, A. and Harris, R., 1979. Rationalisation of first-aid measures for elapid snakebite. *Lancet*, 1(8109), 183–186.

Vlad, I. and Guthrie, K., 2016. Envenomation. In Curtis, K. and Ramsden, C. (eds), *Emergency and trauma care for nurses and paramedics*, 2nd edn. Sydney: Elsevier.

Warrell, D.A., 2010. Snake bite. *Lancet*, 375(9708), 77–88.

Weber, A. and Johnson, M., 2015. Snake bites. In Johnson, M., Boyd, L., Grantham, H. and Eastwood, K. (eds), *Paramedic principles and practice ANZ*. Sydney: Elsevier.

White, J., 2013. *A clinician's guide to Australian venomous bites and stings: incorporating the updated CSL antivenom handbook*. CSL (Australia). Retrieved from: http://www.toxinology.com/generic_static_files/A%20Clinician's%20Guide%20to%20Venomous%20Bites%20&%20Stings%202013.pdf

WHO (World Health Organization), 2006. *Your 5 moments for hand hygiene*. Retrieved from: http://who.int/gpsc/tools/5momentsHandHygiene_A3-2.pdf?ua=1

Index

Page numers followed by 'b refer to boxes, by 'f' refer to figures and by 't' refer to tables.

A

abdomen 206–207
  quadrants 206–207, 207f
  regions 206–207, 207f
abdominal assessment 206–215
  anatomy and physiology in 206–207, 207f
  clinical findings in 214
  clinical rationale in 207–209
    auscultation 208
    history 207–208
    inspection 208
    palpation 208–209, 208f, 209f
    percussion 209
    position for 207, 207f
  clinical skill assessment process for 209
abdominal cavity 206
abdominal thrusts, for choking 251
abducens nerves. see VI (abducens) nerves
acceptability 2
access
  intraosseous 448–459
    anatomy and physiology of 448
    clinical findings of 457
    clinical rationale of 449–452
    clinical skill assessment process for 452–457
    device options 449, 449f
    embolism 457
    extravasation 457
    growth plate injury 457
    infection 457
    injection pain 457
    method of insertion and use 451, 451f
    practice tip 458
    sites and needle size 450
    specific site contraindications 451
    test your knowledge questions 459
  intravenous 435–446
    anatomy and physiology of 435–436
    arterial injection 445
    cannulation 437–439, 437f, 438f, 439f
    clinical findings of 444–445
    clinical rationale of 436–437, 436f
    clinical skill assessment process for 439–444
    difficult insertion 444–445
    embolism 445
    infection and inflammation 445
    infiltration/extravasation 445
    injection sites and cannula size 436, 436t, 437f
    nerve injection 445
    pain 445
    skill matrix 435
    test your knowledge questions 446
accessory nerves. see XI (accessory) nerves
action, right, before administering any medication 374
active vomiting, continuous positive airway pressure and 481
activities of daily living, in functional capacity assessment 183
acute coronary syndrome, oxygen therapy and 470
acute foreign body airway obstruction, stages of 250
adenosine triphosphate (ATP) 461
administration of medications
  buccal 373–374, 375
  enteral 373
  intranasal 382–390
    anatomy and physiology of 382, 383f
    clinical findings of 389

    clinical rationale of 383–384, 383f
    clinical skill assessment process for 384–388
    contraindications of 389
    indications for 384, 384f
    precautions of 389
  oral 373–380
    anatomy and physiology of 373–374
    clinical findings of 379
    clinical rationale of 374–375
    clinical skill assessment process for 375–379
    nine factors for patient safety 374–375
    solid and liquid 373
  rectal 374
  right form 374
  subcutaneous 403–404
  sublingual 373–374, 375
  venous 403–404
adolescent, respiratory rate 90
advance care directives 35–36
advanced social activities 183
AEIOU TIPS mnemonic 173
affect, mental status assessment 174
age, paramedic patient and 10–11
agitated behaviour, log roll and 612
agitation
  continuous positive airway pressure and 481
  speech and 125
agonal breathing 95
airborne infection protection 16–17
airway
  laryngeal mask 325–336
    airway preparation of 327
    anatomy and physiology in 325–326
    cardiovascular effects and 334
    children and 334
    clinical findings of 334–335
    clinical rationale of 326–328
    clinical skill assessment process for 328–334
    contraindications of 328
    cuff inflation 327–328, 327f
    device measurement of 327
    insertion method of 328, 328f
    intubation and 334
    patient positioning in 326–327
    pharyngeal injury and 334
    removal of 334
    return of airway reflexes and 334
  nasopharyngeal 290–298
    airway preparation of 291
    anatomy and physiology in 290
    aspiration and 297
    basal skull fracture and 297
    cardiovascular effects and 297
    children and 297
    clinical findings of 297
    clinical rationale of 290–292
    clinical skill assessment process for 292–296
    cough/gag reflex stimulated 297
    device measurement of 291, 291f
    facial injury and 297
    insertion method of 291–292, 291f, 292f
    patient positioning of 291
    remains non-patent 297
    resistance 297
    soft tissue injury and 297

C

posterior chest
   anatomy and physiology of 108, 108f
   auscultation of 110, 110f
posterior shoulder rotation 699f
postpartum haemorrhage (PPH) 664–665, 665f
   four causes of 664–665
   risk factors for 666
PPH. *see* postpartum haemorrhage
precordial limb leads, for 12-lead electrocardiogram, recording 79–80
pregnancy, in abdominal assessment 214
premature birth 659, 674–683
   anatomy and physiology for 674–675
   clinical findings for 682
   clinical rationale for 675–676
   clinical skill assessment process for 676–681
preparation, injection
   anatomy and physiology of 403–404
   clinical findings of 410
      diluting medication 410
      quantity of medication 410
   clinical rationale of 404–406
      clearing syringe of air bubbles 405
      documentation and handover 405–406
      hygiene 404
      labelling 405
      medication check 404
      medication inspection 404
      preparing ampoule 405, 405f
      preparing vial 404–405, 404f
   clinical skill assessment process for 406–410
pre-school, respiratory rate 90
pressure bandaging and immobilisation (PBI) 722–730
   anaphylaxis and 729
   anatomy and physiology in 723
   clinical findings in 729
   clinical rationale of 723–724, 723f, 724f
   clinical skill assessment process for 724–728
   contraindications for 724
   indications for 724
   for non-limb bites 729
   for non-limb stings 729
   patient deterioration and 729
pressurised metered dose inhaler (pMDI) 392, 393f
   complications of 400
   usage 393–394, 394f
primary school, respiratory rate 90
prolonged expiratory phase 95
proximal tibia 450, 450f
psychogenic pain 193
pulmonary barotrauma 368
pulse
   brachial, assessing 59–66
      absence/presence of 64
      anatomy and physiology for 59–60
      clinical findings for 64
      clinical rationale for 60
      clinical skill assessment process for 60
      palpation of 60f
      rate of 64
      rhythm of 64
      strength of 64–65
   oximetry 128–137
      anatomy and physiology in 128
      clinical findings for 135
      clinical rationale for 128–129, 129f, 130f
      clinical skill assessment process for 129
   radial, assessing 59–66
      absence/presence of 64
      anatomy and physiology for 59–60
      clinical findings for 64
      clinical rationale for 60
      clinical skill assessment process for 60

palpation of 60f
   rate of 64
   rhythm of 64
   strength of 64–65
pupils
   in assessment of cranial nerve function 156–157
   direction of, cranial nerve function and 157
pursed lip expiration 100f

Q

quality, of speech 121
quantity, of speech 121

R

race, paramedic patient and 11–12
radial pulse, assessing 59–66
   absence/presence of 64
   anatomy and physiology for 59–60
   clinical findings for 64
   clinical rationale for 60
   clinical skill assessment process for 60
   palpation of 60f
   rate of 64
   resources required for 59
   rhythm of 64
   strength of 64–65
RAS. *see* reticulating activating system
real-life training 21
recording
   blood glucose 227–235
      anatomy and physiology in 227–228
      clinical findings in 234
      clinical rationale in 228–229, 228f, 229f
      clinical skill assessment process for 229
      hyperglycaemia in 234
      hypoglycaemia in 234
      normal values in 234
   12-lead electrocardiogram 78–87
      anatomy and physiology for 78–79
      breast interference in 86
      clinical findings for 86
      clinical rationale for 79
      clinical skill assessment process for 81
      ECG interpretation in 86
   tympanic temperature 217–225
      afebrile/normothermic temperature 223, 223t
      anatomy and physiology in 217
      assessment of 218–219, 218f, 219f
      axillary site of 218
      clinical findings in 223–224
      clinical rationale in 218–219
      clinical skill assessment process for 219
      febrile temperature 223
      hyperthermia 223
      hypothermia 223
      inaccurate readings of 223–224
      oral route of 218
      rectal temperature 218
      temporal evaluation in 218
rectal administration, medication delivery 374
rectum, absorption, oral medication 374
rectus femoris 424, 425f
reduction, anterior shoulder dislocation 561–571, 563f
   anatomy and physiology of 562, 562f
   clinical findings of 569–570
      attempt limitations 569
   clinical rationale of 562–565, 564f
      contraindications 564